A

▼ **Patient Teaching**

Of primary importance is th⸱⸱⸱ ⸱⸱⸱identify the offending allergen; sometimes this is done through skin testing. In the case of food allergies, an elimination diet is recommended. If an allergic reaction occurs, all food eaten should be eliminated and gradually reintroduced one at a time until the offending food is detected.

- Many allergic reactions, especially asthma and urticaria, may be aggravated by fatigue and emotional stress. The nurse can be instrumental in initiating a stress management program with patients.
- Control of allergic symptoms may require environmental control, including changing occupations, moving to a different climate, or giving up a pet. In the case of airborne allergens, sleeping in an air-conditioned room, damp dusting daily, and wearing a mask outdoors may be helpful.
- If the allergen is a drug, the patient should be instructed to avoid the drug. The patient also has the responsibility to make drug allergies well known to all health care providers. The patient should wear a medical-alert bracelet listing the particular drug allergy and have the drug listed on all medical and dental records.
- For patients allergic to insect stings, commercial bee-sting kits containing preinjectable epinephrine and a tourniquet are available. The nurse has the responsibility to instruct the patient about applying the tourniquet and self-injecting SC epinephrine. These patients also should wear medical-alert bracelets and carry bee-sting kits with them whenever they go outdoors.

ALZHEIMER'S DISEASE

Definition/Description

Alzheimer's disease (AD) is a type of dementia characterized by progressive deterioration in memory and other aspects of cognition. AD is increasingly recognized as a major health problem in the United States, particularly for persons over 65 years of age. It accounts for more than 50% of the cases of dementia (about 4 million cases).

Pathophysiology

The etiology of AD is still unclear, although age is the most important risk factor for developing AD.

- Pathologic changes associated with AD include neurofibrillary tangles and β-amyloid plaques in the cerebral cortex and hippocampus. There is also an excessive loss of cholinergic neurons, particularly in regions essential for memory and cognition.

- At least four chromosomes (1, 14, 19, 21) are involved in some forms of familial AD. Inheritance of the apo E-4 genotype (a gene responsible for making apolipoprotein) is a major genetic risk factor for developing AD.
- There are also data to suggest that estrogen protects against the development of AD. Estrogen may also slow the progression of AD in those who already have it.

Clinical Manifestations

- An initial sign is subtle deterioration in memory. Inevitably this progresses to more profound memory loss that interferes with the patient's ability to function. Recent events and new information cannot be recalled. Personal hygiene deteriorates as does the ability to maintain attention.
- Later in the disease, long-term memories cannot be recalled, and patients lose the ability to recognize family members. Eventually the ability to communicate and perform activities of daily living (ADLs) is lost.
- Progression of deterioration, which eventually leads to death, varies but can last as long as 20 years.
- AD must be distinguished from depression, a clinically similar condition, because depression is potentially reversible and often responds to appropriate treatment. A careful assessment can distinguish the two clinical conditions (Table 3).

Diagnostic Studies

The diagnosis of AD is a diagnosis of exclusion. When all other possible conditions that can cause mental impairment have been ruled out and manifestations of dementia persist, the diagnosis of AD can be made.

- A CT scan or MRI may show brain atrophy and enlarged ventricles in the later stages of the disease, although this finding occurs in other diseases and with aging in normal persons.
- Neuropsychologic testing can help document the degree of cognitive dysfunction in early stages.
- Definitive diagnosis of AD can be made only at autopsy when the presence of neurofibrillary tangles is observed.

Collaborative Care

Management of AD is aimed at improving or controlling the decline in cognition and undesirable symptoms that the patient may exhibit. Table 56-23, Lewis and others, *Medical-Surgical Nursing,* edition 5,

| | | **A** |

| Table 3 | **Differentiation of Depression and Dementia of Alzheimer's Disease** | |

Characteristic	Depression	Dementia
Onset	Abrupt (weeks)	Insidious
Psychiatric history	Previous depression common	Usually no history
Mental status	Pervasive dysphoria	Flattening of affect
	Normal or impaired cognition	Impaired cognition
	Variable performance	Stable performance
	Variable memory disturbance	Serious effects on memory
Sleep disturbance	Initial and early-morning insomnia	Frequent awakenings
Somatic complaints	Often multiple	Often none
Self-image	Poor	Normal
Suicidal ideation	Present	Present early in disease, then absent
Treatment	High effectiveness of antidepressants	Very limited usefulness of antidepressants
Weight loss	Yes, with appetite disturbance	Not until late in disease

p. 1704 details manifestations, drug therapy, and possible side effects of the prescribed drugs. It is important to be aware that these drugs do not significantly alter the disease course.

Recently drugs that inhibit the breakdown of acetylcholine in the brain and thereby enhance cognitive function have become available. Tacrine (Cognex), an acetylcholinesterase inhibitor, slows the decline in cognitive function. However, because of liver toxicity, frequent laboratory monitoring of liver function is required. Donepezil (Aricept) is another acetylcholinesterase inhibitor. It does not require laboratory monitoring, can be given once a day, and has been shown to either mildly improve or stabilize cognitive decline in some people with AD. Both drugs are used in the early and mid-stages of AD.

Nursing Management

Goals

The patient with AD will maintain functional ability for as long as possible, be maintained in a safe environment with a minimum of injuries, and have personal care needs met.

See NCP 56-5 for the patient with AD, Lewis and others, *Medical-Surgical Nursing,* edition 5, p. 1705.

Nursing Diagnoses

- Impaired physical mobility *related to* rigidity, bradykinesia, and akinesia.
- Altered thought processes *related to* effects of dementia
- Self-care deficits *related to* memory deficit and neuromuscular impairment
- Risk for injury *related to* impaired judgment, possible gait instability, muscle weakness, and sensory or perceptual alteration
- Ineffective management of therapeutic regimen *related to* decreasing level of cognitive functioning and memory
- Risk for violence: directed at others *related to* neurologic changes, sensory overload, lack of appropriate coping mechanisms, and unfamiliar environment

Nursing Interventions

Although there is no current treatment for reversing AD, there is a need for ongoing monitoring of both the patient and the patient's caregiver. An important nursing responsibility is to work collaboratively with the patient's physician to manage symptoms effectively as they change over time.

- The nurse is often responsible for teaching the caregiver to perform essential tasks for the patient. To aid in identifying caregiver problems, a nursing care plan for the caregiver of a person with AD is presented in NCP 56-5, Lewis and others, *Medical-Surgical Nursing,* edition 5, p. 1705.
- Adult day care is one of the options available to the person with AD. Common goals of all day-care programs are to provide respite for the family and a protective environment for the patient.
- The nursing care needs of the patient change as the disease progresses, emphasizing the need for regular assessment, monitoring, and support. Regardless of the setting, the severity of symptoms and amount of care required intensify over time.
- Patients with AD are subject to acute and other chronic illnesses. Their inability to communicate health symptoms and problems places responsibility for assessment and diagnosis

A

on caregivers and health professionals. Hospitalization of the patient can be a traumatic event for both patient and caregiver and can precipitate a worsening of the disease.
- Support groups for caregivers and family members have been formed throughout the United States by the Alzheimer's Association to provide an atmosphere of understanding and to give current information about the disease itself and related topics such as safety, legal, ethical, and financial issues.

AMYOTROPHIC LATERAL SCLEROSIS

Amyotrophic lateral sclerosis (ALS) is a rare, progressive neurologic disease characterized by a loss of motor neurons. This disease became known as Lou Gehrig's disease when the famous baseball player was stricken with it in the early 1940s. The onset is between the ages of 40 and 70 years, and twice as many men as women are affected. ALS usually leads to death in 2 to 6 years following diagnosis.
- For unknown reasons, motor neurons in the brainstem and spinal cord gradually degenerate in ALS. Consequently, messages originating in the brain never reach the muscles to activate them.
- Primary symptoms are weakness of the upper extremities, dysarthria, and dysphagia. Muscle wasting and fasciculations result from denervation of the muscles and lack of stimulation and use.
- Death usually results from respiratory infection secondary to compromised respiratory function.
- There is no cure for ALS. This illness is devastating because the patient remains cognitively intact while wasting away.
- Riluzole (Rilutek) was recently approved to slow the progression of ALS. This drug works to decrease the amount of glutamate (an excitatory neurotransmitter) in the brain. It was shown to delay the need for tracheostomy and to delay death by a few months in clinical trials.

The challenge of nursing care is to support the patient's cognitive and emotional functions by facilitating communication, providing diversional activities such as reading and human companionship, and helping the person and family with anticipatory grieving related to loss of motor function and ultimate death.

ANEMIA

Definition/Description
Anemia is a reduction in the number of red blood cells (RBCs) or erythrocytes, the quantity of hemoglobin (Hb), and the volume of packed red cells (hematocrit). Anemia can be caused by rapid blood loss, impaired production of erythrocytes, or increased destruction of erythrocytes.

- Because erythrocytes transport oxygen (O_2), erythrocyte disorders can lead to tissue hypoxia. This hypoxia accounts for many of the clinical manifestations of anemia.
- Anemia is not a specific disease; it is a manifestation of a pathologic process.
- Anemia is identified and classified by laboratory evaluation.
- Anemia can result from primary hematologic problems or can develop as a secondary consequence of defects in other body systems.

The different types of anemia can be classified according to either etiology or morphology.

- Etiologic classification is related to clinical conditions causing anemia, such as decreased erythrocyte production, blood loss, or increased erythrocyte destruction (Table 4).
- Morphologic classification is based on descriptive, objective laboratory information about erythrocyte size and color.

Although the morphologic system is the most accurate means of classifying anemia, it is easier to discuss patient care by focusing on the etiologic problem. Table 5 relates morphologic classifications to various etiologies.

Clinical Manifestations
Manifestations of anemia are primarily caused by the body's response to tissue hypoxia. The intensity of the manifestations varies depending on the severity of anemia and the presence of coexisting diseases. The severity of anemia may be determined by Hb levels.

- *Mild* states of anemia (Hb 10 to 14 g/dl [100 to 140 g/L]) may exist without causing symptoms. If symptoms develop, they are usually caused by the underlying disease or a compensatory response to heavy exercise. These symptoms include palpitations, dyspnea, and diaphoresis.
- In cases of *moderate* anemia (Hb 6 to 10 g/dl [60 to 100 g/L]), cardiopulmonary symptoms (e.g., increased heart rate) may be present with rest as well as activity.

Table 4	Etiologic Classification of Anemia

Decreased Erythrocyte Production
- Decreased Hb synthesis
  Iron deficiency
  Thalassemias (decreased globin synthesis)
  Sideroblastic anemia (decreased porphyrin)
- Defective DNA synthesis
  Cobalamin deficiency
  Folic acid deficiency
- Decreased number of erythrocyte precursors
  Aplastic anemia
  Anemia of leukemia and myelodysplasia
  Chronic diseases or disorders

Blood Loss
- Acute
  Trauma
  Blood vessel rupture
- Chronic
  Gastritis
  Menstrual flow
  Hemorrhoids

Increased Erythrocyte Destruction*
- Intrinsic
  Abnormal hemoglobin (HbS—sickle cell anemia)
  Enzyme deficiency (G6PD)
  Membrane abnormalities (paroxysmal nocturnal
    hemoglobinuria)
- Extrinsic
  Physical trauma (prosthetic heart valves, extracorporeal
    circulation)
  Antibodies (isoimmune and autoimmune)
  Infectious agents and toxins (malaria)

DNA, Deoxyribonucleic acid; *G6PD*, glucose-6-phosphate dehydrogenase;
Hb, hemoglobin; *HbS*, hemoglobin S.
*Hemolytic anemias.

Table 5	Relationship of Morphologic Classification and Etiologies of Anemia

Morphology	Etiology
Normocytic, normochromic	Acute blood loss, hemolysis, chronic renal disease, chronic disease, cancers, sideroblastic anemia, refractory anemia, diseases of endocrine dysfunction, aplastic anemia, pregnancy
Macrocytic, normochromic	Cobalamin (vitamin B_{12}) deficiency, folic acid deficiency, liver disease (including effects of alcohol abuse), postsplenectomy
Microcytic, hypochromic	Iron-deficiency anemia, thalassemia, lead poisoning

- Patients with *severe* anemia (Hb <6 g/dl [<60 g/L]) display many clinical manifestations that involve multiple body systems (Table 6).

Nursing Management

Goals
The patient with anemia will be able to assume normal activities of daily living (ADLs), maintain adequate nutrition, and develop no complications related to anemia.

See NCP 29-1, p. 740, for the patient with anemia; NCP 29-2, p. 759, for the patient with thrombocytopenia, and NCP 29-3, p. 769, for the patient with neutropenia, Lewis and others, *Medical-Surgical Nursing,* edition 5.

Nursing Diagnoses
- Activity intolerance *related to* weakness and malaise
- Altered nutrition: less than body requirements *related to* anorexia and treatment
- Ineffective management of therapeutic regimen *related to* lack of knowledge about lifestyle adjustments, appropriate nutrition, and drug therapy
- Self-care deficits *related to* weakness and fatigue

Nursing Interventions
The numerous causes of anemia necessitate different nursing interventions specific to patient needs. General components of care for all patients with anemia may include:
- Correction of the etiology of the anemia as the ultimate goal of therapy.

A

Table 6   Clinical Manifestations of Anemia

	Severity of anemia		
Body System	**Mild** (Hb 10-14 g/dl [100-140 g/L])	**Moderate** (Hb 6-10 g/dl [60-100 g/L])	**Severe** (Hb <6 g/dl [<60 g/L])
Integument	None	None	Pallor, jaundice,* pruritus*
Eyes	None	None	Icteric conjunctiva and sclera,* retinal hemorrhage, blurred vision
Mouth	None	None	Glossitis, smooth tongue
Cardiovascular	Palpitations	Increased palpitations	Tachycardia, increased pulse pressure, systolic murmurs, intermittent claudication, angina, CHF, MI
Pulmonary	Exertional dyspnea	Dyspnea	Tachypnea, orthopnea, dyspnea at rest
Neurologic	None	None	Headache, vertigo, irritability, depression, impaired thought processes
Gastrointestinal	None	None	Anorexia, hepatomegaly, splenomegaly, difficulty swallowing, sore mouth
Musculoskeletal	None	None	Bone pain
General	None	Fatigue	Sensitivity to cold, weight loss, lethargy

CHF, Congestive heart failure; Hb, hemoglobin; MI, myocardial infarction.
*Caused by hemolysis.

- Dietary and lifestyle changes that may reverse some anemias and return patients to their former state of health.
- Acute interventions such as blood transfusions, drug therapy (e.g., erythropoietin, vitamin replacements), and O_2 therapy.
- Chronic management that may require long-term transfusion therapy or erythropoietin injections.

Specific types of anemia are listed under separate headings.

ANEMIA, APLASTIC

Definition/Description

One of the most severe forms of anemia related to reduced red blood cell (RBC) or erythrocyte production is a group of disorders termed *aplastic, pancytopenic,* or *hypoplastic* anemias. These anemias are life-threatening stem cell disorders characterized by hypoplastic, fatty bone marrow that result in pancytopenia. Aplastic anemia is somewhat of a misnomer because in most cases all marrow elements—erythrocytes, leukocytes, and platelets—are quantitatively decreased, although qualitatively normal.

Pathophysiology

There are various etiologic classifications for aplastic anemia, but they can be divided into two major groups: congenital (idiopathic) or acquired.

- Congenital aplastic anemia is caused by chromosomal alterations.
- Acquired aplastic anemia is a result of exposure to ionizing radiation, chemical agents (e.g., benzene, insecticides, alcohol), viral and bacterial infections (e.g., hepatitis, miliary tuberculosis), and prescribed medications (e.g., alkylating agents, antiseizure medications, antimicrobials).

Clinical Manifestations

Aplastic anemia usually develops insidiously. Clinically the patient may have symptoms caused by suppression of any or all bone marrow elements.

- General manifestations of anemia such as fatigue and dyspnea, as well as cardiovascular and cerebral signs, may be seen (see Table 6, p. 25).
- The patient with granulocytopenia is susceptible to infection and generally has a fever.
- Thrombocytopenia is manifested by a predisposition to bleed (e.g., petechiae, ecchymoses, epistaxis).

Diagnostic Studies

Diagnosis is confirmed by laboratory studies.

- All marrow elements are affected: hemoglobin (Hb), white blood cell (WBC), and platelet values are often decreased (Table 7).
- Reticulocyte count is low and bleeding time is prolonged.
- Serum iron and total iron-binding capacity (TIBC) are elevated as initial signs of erythroid suppression.
- Bone marrow examination may be done for any anemic state. Findings are especially important in aplastic anemia because the marrow is hypocellular with increased yellow marrow (fat content), a finding called *dry tap*.

Nursing and Collaborative Management

Management of aplastic anemia is based on identifying and removing the causative agent (when possible) and providing supportive care until pancytopenia reverses.

Nursing interventions appropriate for the patient with pancytopenia from aplastic anemia are presented in the nursing care plans for patients with anemia, thrombocytopenia, and neutropenia (see NCPs 29-1, p. 740, 29-2, p. 759, and 29-3, p. 769, Lewis and others, *Medical-Surgical Nursing,* edition 5). Nursing actions are directed at preventing complications from infection and hemorrhage.

- Prognosis of untreated aplastic anemia is poor (approximately 75% fatal). However, advances in medical management, including bone marrow transplantation and immunosuppressive therapy with antithymocyte globulin (ATG) and cyclosporine have improved survival significantly. ATG is a horse serum containing polyclonal antibodies against human T cells. Rationale for this therapy is that aplastic anemia is an immune-mediated disease.
- Treatment of choice for adults less than 45 years of age who have a human leukocyte antigen (HLA)–matched sibling donor is allogeneic bone marrow transplantation. Best results occur in a younger patient who has not had previous blood transfusions. Prior transfusions increase the risk of graft rejection.
- For the older adult or the patient without HLA-matched siblings, the treatment of choice is immunosuppression with ATG or cyclosporine. Response to this therapy may only be partial, but usually transfusions can be avoided.

Table 7 Laboratory Study Findings in Anemias

	Iron deficiency	Thalassemia major	Cobalamin (vitamin B₁₂) deficiency	Folic acid deficiency	Aplastic anemia	Sickle cell anemia
Hb/Hct	↓	↓	↓	↓	↓	↓
MCV	↓	N	↑	↑	N	N
MCH	↓	N	N or slight ↓	N or slight ↓	N	N
MCHC	↓	N	↑	↑	N	N
Reticulocytes	N or ↓	↑	↓	N	↓	↑
Serum iron	↓	↑	N	N	± N	N to ↑
TIBC	↑	↑	N	N	± N	N to ↓
Bilirubin	N to ↓	↑	N	N	N	↑
Platelets	N or ↑	—	↓	—	↓	↑
Other findings	—	—	↓ cobalamin, positive Schilling test, achlorhydria	↓ folate	↓ WBC	See Table 29-11*

Hb, Hemoglobin; *Hct*, hematocrit; *MCH*, mean corpuscular hemoglobin; *MCHC*, mean corpuscular hemoglobin concentration; *MCV*, mean corpuscular volume; *N*, normal; *TIBC*, total iron-binding capacity; *WBC*, white blood cell.
*Lewis and others, *Medical-Surgical Nursing*, edition 5, p. 751.

ANEMIA, COBALAMIN DEFICIENCY

Definition/Description

There are many conditions in which cobalamin (vitamin B_{12}) deficiency anemia can occur. Normally a protein known as *intrinsic factor* (IF) is secreted by parietal cells of the gastric mucosa. IF is required for cobalamin (extrinsic factor) absorption in the distal ileum. Therefore if IF is not secreted, cobalamin cannot be absorbed.

- In *pernicious anemia,* which is one cause of cobalamin deficiency, the gastric mucosa is not secreting IF.

Pathophysiology

Cobalamin deficiency can occur in a patient who has a total gastrectomy, a small bowel resection involving the ileum, or Crohn's disease. Cobalamin deficiency results from the loss of IF-secreting gastric mucosal surface or impaired absorption of cobalamin in the distal ileum.

Pernicious anemia is an autoimmune disease of insidious onset that generally begins in middle age or later (usually after age 40). In this condition, IF secretion fails because of gastric mucosal atrophy, which probably results from destruction of parietal cells. Pernicious anemia occurs frequently in persons of Northern European ancestry (particularly Scandinavians) and African-Americans. In African-Americans, the disease tends to begin early (with a high frequency in women) and is often severe.

Clinical Manifestations

Manifestations of anemia related to cobalamin deficiency develop because of tissue hypoxia and neurologic changes (see Table 6, p. 25).

- GI manifestations include a sore tongue, anorexia, nausea, vomiting, and abdominal pain.
- Neuromuscular manifestations include weakness, paresthesias of feet and hands, reduced vibratory and position senses, ataxia, muscle weakness, and impaired thought processes ranging from confusion to dementia.
- Because cobalamin deficiency anemia has an insidious onset, it may take several months for these manifestations to develop.

Diagnostic Studies

Laboratory data reflective of cobalamin deficiency anemia are presented in Table 7.

- Erythrocytes appear large (macrocytic) and have abnormal shapes. This structure contributes to erythrocyte destruction because the cell membrane is very fragile.

- Serum cobalamin levels will be reduced.
- Gastric analysis may determine the cause of cobalamin deficiency.
- A Schilling test is diagnostic of pernicious anemia and assesses parietal cell function and absorption of cobalamin when IF is given parenterally.

Collaborative Care

Regardless of how much cobalamin is ingested, the patient is not able to absorb it if IF is lacking or if there is impaired ileum absorption, so dietary management is not used for cobalamin replacement.

- Parenteral administration of cobalamin (cyanocobalamin or hydroxocobalamin) is the treatment of choice. A typical treatment schedule consists of 1000 μg cobalamin intramuscular (IM) daily for 2 weeks, then weekly until hematocrit is normal, and then monthly for life. Hematologic manifestations can be completely reversed with supplemental cobalamin. However, most long-standing neuromuscular complications will not be reversed by this therapy.

Nursing Management

- Patients who have a positive family history of pernicious anemia should be evaluated for symptoms. Although disease development cannot be prevented, early detection and treatment can lead to reversal of symptoms.
- Nursing interventions for the patient with anemia are appropriate for the patient with cobalamin deficiency (see Anemia, p. 22). In addition to these measures, the patient should be protected from burns and trauma because of diminished sensation to heat and pain and peripheral neuropathy.
- Ongoing care is primarily related to ensuring patient compliance in receiving cobalamin supplementation. There must be careful follow-up to assess for neurologic difficulties that were not corrected by cobalamin replacement therapy. Because the potential for gastric carcinoma is increased in pernicious anemia, the patient should have frequent and careful evaluation for this problem.

ANEMIA, FOLIC ACID DEFICIENCY

Folic acid is required for deoxyribonucleic acid (DNA) synthesis leading to red blood cell (RBC) (erythrocyte) formation and maturation. Four common causes of folic acid deficiency are: (1) poor nutrition, especially a lack of leafy green vegetables, liver, citrus fruits, yeast, dried beans, nuts, and grains; (2) malabsorption syndromes, particularly small bowel disorders; (3) drugs that impede absorption and use of folic acid (e.g., methotrexate, oral contraceptives) and antiseizure medications (e.g., phenobarbital, phenytoin [Dilantin]); and (4) alcohol abuse and anorexia.

Clinical manifestations of folic acid deficiency are similar to those of cobalamin deficiency. The disease develops insidiously, and the patient's symptoms may be attributed to other coexisting problems such as cirrhosis or esophageal varices.

- GI disturbances include dyspepsia and a smooth, beefy red tongue.
- Absence of neurologic problems is an important diagnostic finding; this lack of neurologic involvement differentiates folic acid deficiency from cobalamin deficiency.
- Diagnostic findings for folic acid deficiency are presented in Table 7, p. 28. In addition, serum folate level is low, serum cobalamin level is normal, and gastric analysis is positive for hydrochloric acid.

Treatment for folic acid deficiency is by replacement therapy with the usual dose of 1 mg/day by mouth. In malabsorption states, up to 5 mg/day may be required. Duration of treatment depends on the reason for the deficiency. The patient should be encouraged to eat foods containing large amounts of folic acid.

ANEMIA, IRON DEFICIENCY

Definition/Description

Iron deficiency anemia, one of the most common chronic hematologic disorders, is found in 30% of the world's population. In the United States, iron deficiency anemia is most common in infants and children, those on poor diets, premenopausal and pregnant women, older adults, and individuals experiencing blood loss.

Pathophysiology

Iron deficiency may develop from inadequate dietary intake, malabsorption, blood loss, or hemolysis. Iron is obtained from dietary intake in which only 5% to 10% of all ingested iron is absorbed in the duodenum. This amount of dietary iron is adequate to meet needs of men and older women, but it may be inadequate for those individuals who have higher iron needs (e.g., children, pregnant women).

Malabsorption of iron may occur after certain types of GI surgery and in malabsorption syndromes. Surgical procedures for peptic ulcer disease may involve removal of or bypass of the duodenum.

Malabsorption syndromes may involve disease of the duodenum, where iron is normally absorbed.

Blood loss is a major cause of iron deficiency in adults. Major sources of chronic blood loss are from the GI and genitourinary (GU) systems.

- GI bleeding is often not apparent and therefore may exist for a considerable time before the problem is identified. Loss of 50 to 75 ml of blood from the upper GI tract is required to cause stools to appear black *(melena)*. This color results from iron in the red blood cells (RBCs).
- Common causes of adult GI blood loss are peptic ulcers, esophagitis, diverticuli, hemorrhoids, neoplasia, and gastritis. GU blood loss occurs primarily from menstrual bleeding. The average monthly menstrual blood loss is about 45 ml, which causes a loss of about 22 mg of iron.
- Pregnancy contributes to iron deficiency because of iron diversion to the fetus for erythropoiesis. Blood loss at delivery and lactation may also contribute to anemia.

Clinical Manifestations

In the early course of iron deficiency anemia, the patient may be free of symptoms. As the disease becomes chronic, any of the general manifestations of anemia may develop (see Table 6, p. 25). In addition, specific clinical symptoms may occur related to iron deficiency anemia.

- Pallor is the most common finding and *glossitis* (inflammation of tongue) is the second most common; another finding is *cheilitis* (inflammation of lips).
- In addition, the patient may report headache, paresthesias, and a burning sensation of the tongue, all of which are caused by lack of iron in the tissues.

Diagnostic Studies

Laboratory abnormalities characteristic of iron deficiency anemia are presented in Table 7, p. 28. Other diagnostic studies are done to determine the cause of iron deficiency. For example, endoscopy and colonoscopy may be used to detect GI bleeding.

Collaborative Care

The main goal in iron deficiency anemia is to treat the underlying cause of reduced intake (e.g., malnutrition, alcoholism) or malabsorption of iron. Efforts are directed toward replacing iron, which may be done through increasing iron intake.

- The patient should be taught which foods are good sources of iron. If nutrition is adequate, increasing iron intake by dietary

A

means may not be reasonable because it is difficult for nutritional intake to exceed 7 mg of iron per 1000 kcal without dietary supplement use. Consequently, oral parenteral iron supplements are used.

- If iron deficiency is from significant acute blood loss, transfusion of packed RBCs may be required (see Blood Transfusion Therapy, p. 629).

Nursing Management

It is important to recognize groups of individuals who are at increased risk for development of iron deficiency anemia, including infants, teenage girls, premenopausal and pregnant women, persons from low socioeconomic backgrounds, older adults, and individuals experiencing blood loss. Dietary teaching, with an emphasis on foods high in iron, is important for these groups. Supplemental iron is especially important for pregnant women.

Appropriate nursing measures are presented in NCP 29-1, Lewis and others, *Medical-Surgical Nursing,* edition 5, p. 740.

▼ **Patient Teaching**
- If anemia is present, it is important to discuss with the patient the need for diagnostic studies to identify the cause. The hemoglobin (Hb) level and RBC count should be reassessed to evaluate the response to therapy.
- Compliance with dietary and drug therapy needs to be emphasized. To replenish the body's iron stores, the patient should take iron therapy for 2 to 3 months after the Hb level returns to normal. An older adult patient may require lifelong iron supplementation.

ANEMIA, SICKLE CELL

Definition/Description

Sickle cell anemia is a genetic disorder characterized by production of abnormal hemoglobin (Hb), anemia, and acute and chronic tissue damage from vascular blockage by abnormal red blood cells (RBCs). In sickle cell anemia, abnormal Hb (hemoglobin S [HbS]), instead of normal hemoglobin A (HbA), is produced. The disease affects more than 50,000 Americans and is predominant in African-Americans, occurring in an estimated prevalence of 1 in 375 live births. It can also affect persons of Mediterranean, Caribbean, South and Central American, Arabian, or East Indian ancestry. It is an incurable type of anemia that is often fatal by middle age.

Pathophysiology

The mutation that causes HbS to develop involves one amino acid. One valine amino acid is substituted for a glutamic acid; this substitution leads to an abnormal linking reaction that causes development of deformed crescent-shaped cells when oxygen (O_2) tension is lowered.

- Sickle cell anemia is an autosomal recessive genetic disorder in which the person is homozygous for HbS.
- Some persons may have *sickle cell trait,* a mild condition that may be asymptomatic. A person with sickle cell trait is heterozygous, with approximately one fourth of the Hb in the abnormal S form and three fourths in the normal A form.

When hypoxia occurs in a patient with sickle cell disease, HbS assumes various crescent or sickle shapes. These sickled cells may clog the small capillaries. Erythrostasis causes further O_2 deprivation, which promotes more sickling. As blood vessels occlude, thrombosis occurs, which ultimately leads to ischemia and tissue infarction. All body systems are gradually involved with repeated infarction, especially the spleen, lungs, brain, and kidneys. The abnormal Hb shape is recognized by the body, and the cell is hemolyzed.

- Initially the sickling is reversible on reoxygenation but eventually becomes irreversible, with cells being hemolyzed. Acute episodes or *sickle cell crises* (exacerbations of sickling) develop if patients become extremely hypoxic.
- The frequency of sickle cell crises varies; crises may occur frequently and then may not recur for months or years. Each attack may last for 4 to 6 days.

Precipitating factors include conditions that cause hypoxia or deoxygenation of RBCs, including viral or bacterial infections (the most common cause), high altitudes, emotional or physical stress, surgery, and blood loss.

- Crises can also occur with elevated blood viscosity resulting from dehydration due to vomiting, diarrhea, or diaphoresis.

Clinical Manifestations

Infants do not manifest symptoms until 10 to 12 weeks of age, at which time most of the fetal hemoglobin (HbF) has been replaced by HbS.

- Children manifest a general impairment of growth and development and a failure to thrive. Puberty is delayed, but considerable growth occurs in late adolescence.
- Patients manifest signs of chronic anemia with pallor of the mucous membranes, fatigue, and decreased tolerance for exercise.
- The skin may have a grayish cast. Due to RBC hemolysis, jaundice is common and patients are prone to gallstones.

Sickle cell episodes may appear suddenly and affect various parts of the body, especially the chest, abdomen, bones, and joints. Organs that have a high need for O_2 are most immediately affected and form the basis for many of the complications of sickle cell disease, including an enlarged heart leading to congestive heart failure, retinal detachment and blindness, and thrombotic stroke. Additional chronic manifestations include hepatomegaly, osteoporosis, joint aching, and chronic leg ulcers.

- Severe pain with an acute episode usually begins in the extremities and lasts 4 to 6 days. Aplastic crises occur when a stressor significantly decreases erythropoiesis.
- The patient with sickle cell disease is prone to infections due to impairment of the spleen to phagocytize foreign substances. Pneumonia is the most common infection and needs to be treated vigorously with antibiotics.

Diagnostic Studies

- Hb level usually ranges from 5 to 11 g/dl (50 to 110 g/L) with a mean RBC survival time of 15 days.
- Findings of hemolysis (jaundice, elevated serum bilirubin levels) are noted with abnormal laboratory test results (see Table 7, p. 28).
- Skeletal x-rays will demonstrate bone and joint deformities and flattening.
- MRI of the brain may reveal cerebral ischemic damage due to blocked cerebral vessels from sickled cells.

Collaborative Care

Care is essentially supportive because there is no specific treatment.

- Therapy is directed toward alleviating symptoms from complications of the disease. For example, chronic leg ulcers may be treated with bed rest, antibiotics, warm saline soaks, debridement, and dressings.
- Sickle cell crises may require hospitalization. O_2 may be administered to treat hypoxia and control sickling. Rest is instituted to reduce metabolic requirements, and fluids and electrolytes are given to reduce blood viscosity and maintain renal function.
- Large, continuous doses of narcotic analgesics are used to treat pain during acute episodes.
- Blood transfusions may be indicated when an aplastic crisis occurs.
- Because these patients have an increased need for folic acid, it is important they obtain daily supplements. Iron therapy is generally not indicated.
- Hydroxyurea (Hydrea) is beneficial in decreasing the sickling process and incidence of crisis.

- Gene therapy and bone marrow transplantation may lead to a future cure.

Nursing Management

Because of the hereditary nature of sickle cell disease, genetic counseling is the only form of prevention. For genetic counseling to be effective, screening must be done to detect persons who have sickle cell trait.

- Basic care for patients with sickle cell anemia is discussed in NCP 29-1, Lewis and others, *Medical-Surgical Nursing,* edition 5, p. 740. Long-term care for the patient is based mostly on patient education. The patient and family must understand the basis of the disease and the reasons for supportive care.
- The patient must be taught ways to avoid crises, which include taking steps to reduce the chance of developing hypoxia, such as avoiding high altitudes, maintaining adequate fluid intake, and treating infections promptly.
- Education on pain control is also needed since the pain during a crisis may be severe and often requires considerable analgesia.

ANEURYSM

Definition/Description

An aneurysm is an outpouching or dilation of the arterial wall, commonly involving the aorta. Most aneurysms are found in the abdominal aorta below the level of the renal arteries. The aortic wall weakens and dilates with turbulent blood flow. The growth rate of an aneurysm is unpredictable, but the larger the aneurysm, the greater the risk of rupture.

Pathophysiology

Although the cause is unknown, there are several risk factors associated with development of aneurysms, including hypertension, smoking, and atherosclerosis.

- A common cause of aortic aneurysm is atherosclerosis with plaques composed of lipids, cholesterol, fibrin, and other debris deposited beneath the intima or lining of the artery. This plaque formation causes degenerative changes in the media (middle layer of arterial wall), leading to loss of elasticity, weakening, and eventual dilation of the aorta.
- A strong genetic component may exist in the development of abdominal aortic aneurysms.

- Other less common causes of aneurysm formation include trauma, acute or chronic infections (e.g., tuberculosis, syphilis), and anastomotic disruptions

Aneurysms are generally divided into two basic classifications, *true* and *false.*

- A *true aneurysm* is one in which the wall of the artery forms the aneurysm, with at least one vessel layer still intact. True aneurysms can be further subdivided into fusiform and saccular dilations. A fusiform aneurysm is circumferential and relatively uniform in shape; a saccular aneurysm is pouchlike with a narrow neck connecting the bulge to one side of the arterial wall.
- A *false aneurysm,* or *pseudoaneurysm,* is not an aneurysm but a disruption of all layers of the arterial wall resulting in bleeding that is contained or tamponaded by surrounding structures. False aneurysms may result from trauma, infection, or disruption of an arterial suture line after surgery.

Clinical Manifestations

Thoracic aneurysms are usually asymptomatic. When manifestations are present, they are varied, with deep, diffuse chest pain the most common sign.

Aneurysms in the ascending aorta and aortic arch can produce hoarseness due to pressure on the recurrent laryngeal nerve. Pressure on the esophagus can cause dysphagia. If the aneurysm presses on the superior vena cava, it can cause distended neck veins and head and arm edema. Pressure on pulmonary structures can lead to coughing, dyspnea, and airway obstruction.

Abdominal aneurysms are often asymptomatic and detected on routine physical examination or coincidentally when the patient is being examined for an unrelated problem (e.g., abdominal x-ray). On examination a pulsatile mass in the periumbilical area slightly to the left of midline may be detected. *Bruits* (murmurlike sounds resulting from turbulent blood flow) may be audible with a stethoscope placed over the aneurysm.

- Symptoms of an abdominal aortic aneurysm may mimic pain associated with any abdominal or back disorder. Symptoms may result from compression of nearby anatomic structures (e.g., back pain caused by lumbar nerve compression).
- Occasionally aneurysms, even small ones, spontaneously embolize plaque and thrombi. This can cause "blue toe syndrome" in which patchy mottling of the feet and toes occurs in the presence of pedal pulses.

Complications

Complications can be catastrophic, with the most common being rupture. If rupture occurs posteriorly into the retroperitoneal space,

bleeding may be tamponaded by surrounding structures, preventing exsanguination. In this case the patient has severe back pain and may or may not have back and/or flank ecchymosis (Turner's sign).
  - If rupture occurs anteriorly into the abdominal cavity, death from massive hemorrhage is likely. If the patient does reach the hospital, presenting signs are manifestations of shock such as tachycardia, hypotension, pale clammy skin, decreased urine output, and altered sensorium.

Diagnostic Studies
  - Chest x-ray demonstrates mediastinal silhouette and abnormal widening of the thoracic aorta.
  - Echocardiography may show aortic insufficiency related to ascending aortic dilation.
  - An ECG is done to rule out a myocardial infarction (MI).
  - CT scan determines anterior-posterior and cross-sectional diameter of the aneurysm.
  - MRI is used to diagnose and assess severity of the aneurysm.

Collaborative Care
The management goal is to prevent rupture of the aneurysm; therefore early detection and prompt treatment of the patient are imperative. Once an aneurysm is suspected, studies are performed to determine its exact size and location.

Generally, if coexisting problems are not severe, surgery is the treatment of choice, with the type of surgery depending on the location of the aneurysm.
  - The only effective treatment of an aortic aneurysm is surgery. Surgery is needed for aneurysms of any size that are expanding rapidly and causing the patient to be symptomatic. Before surgery, every effort is made to bring the patient into the best possible state of hydration and electrolyte balance.
  - If the aneurysm has ruptured, the treatment of choice is immediate surgical intervention. Even with prompt care, the mortality rate is high (about 50%) after rupture and increases with the patient's age.

Nursing Management
Goals
The patient with an aneurysm will have normal tissue perfusion, intact motor and neurologic function, and no complications related to surgical repair.
Nursing Diagnoses/Collaborative Problems
  - Risk for infection *related to* presence of a prosthetic vascular graft and invasive lines

- Altered peripheral tissue perfusion *related to* bypass graft occlusion
- Potential complication: hypovolemia *related to* hemorrhage, extravascular fluid redistribution, and prolonged diuresis
- Potential complication: altered renal perfusion *related to* renal artery embolism, prolonged hypotension, and prolonged aortic cross-clamping intraoperatively
- Potential complication: cardiac arrhythmias *related to* hypothermia, electrolyte imbalance, and coexisting coronary artery disease
- Potential complication: paralytic ileus *related to* bowel manipulation, pain medication, and immobility

Nursing Interventions

Special attention should be given to patients with a strong familial history of aneurysm or any evidence of other cardiovascular disease. Trauma victims with abdominal or back pain should be urged to seek medical attention even in the absence of symptoms.

- The patient should be encouraged to reduce risk factors known to be associated with atherosclerosis. This includes controlling hypertension, stopping smoking, and following a diet low in fat and cholesterol. These measures are also done to ensure continued graft patency following surgical repair.
- The nursing role during the preoperative period should include patient teaching, providing support to the patient and family, and carefully assessing all body systems. It is imperative that problems be identified early and proper intervention instituted.
- In the postoperative period adequate respiratory function, fluid and electrolyte balance, and pain control need to be maintained. The nurse needs to monitor graft patency and renal perfusion. The nurse can also assist in preventing ventricular arrhythmias, infections, and neurologic complications. Care of the patient with an aneurysm repair is described in NCP 36-1, Lewis and others, *Medical-Surgical Nursing,* edition 5, p. 984.

▼ Patient Teaching

The patient may be apprehensive about returning home after major surgery involving the aorta.

- Encourage the patient to express any concerns and reassure the patient that normal activities can be gradually resumed.
- Fatigue, poor appetite, and irregular bowel habits are to be expected.
- Heavy lifting is to be avoided for at least 4 to 6 weeks following surgery.
- Observation of incisions for signs and symptoms of infection should be encouraged. Any redness, increased pain, fever >100° F (>37.8° C), or drainage from incisions should be reported to the physician.

- Sexual dysfunction in male patients is not uncommon after aneurysm repair surgery. This may occur because the internal hypogastric artery is disrupted, leading to altered blood flow to the penis.
- The patient should be taught to observe for changes in extremity color or warmth and how to palpate peripheral pulses and assess for changes in their quality.
- The patient who has received a synthetic graft should be aware that prophylactic antibiotics may be required before future invasive procedures.
- Patients who do not undergo surgical repair should be urged to receive regular routine physical examinations and reminded that any symptom, no matter how minor, must be investigated if it persists.

ANGINA PECTORIS

Definition/Description

Angina pectoris is literally translated as pain *(angina)* in the chest *(pectoris).* Myocardial ischemia is expressed symptomatically as angina. More specifically, angina pectoris is transient chest pain due to myocardial ischemia. It usually lasts for only a few minutes (3 to 5) and commonly subsides when the precipitating factor (usually exertion) is relieved. Typical exertional angina should not persist longer than 20 minutes after rest or administration of nitroglycerin.

Pathophysiology

Myocardial ischemia develops when the demand for myocardial oxygen (O_2) exceeds the ability of the coronary arteries to supply it. The primary reason for insufficient flow is narrowing of coronary arteries by atherosclerosis. If myocardial O_2 needs are not met, coronary blood flow is increased through vasodilation and increased rate of flow.

- In the person with coronary artery disease (CAD), the coronary arteries are unable to dilate to meet increased metabolic needs because they are already chronically dilated beyond the obstructed area. In addition, the diseased heart has difficulty increasing the rate of blood flow, creating an O_2 deficit.
- Up to 90% of ischemia is asymptomatic, referred to as *silent ischemia.* Ischemia with pain (angina) or without pain has the same prognosis. Diabetes mellitus and hypertension are associated with an increased prevalence of silent ischemia.

- The myocardium becomes cyanotic within the first 10 seconds of coronary occlusion, and ECG changes appear. With total occlusion of the coronary arteries, contractility ceases after several minutes, depriving myocardial cells of glucose for aerobic metabolism. Myocardial nerve fibers are irritated by the increased lactic acid and transmit a pain message to cardiac nerves and upper thoracic posterior roots (the reason for referred cardiac pain to the left shoulder and arm).
- Under ischemic conditions, cardiac cells are viable for about 20 minutes. With restoration of blood flow, aerobic metabolism resumes and contractility is restored. Cellular repair begins.
- Extracardiac factors may precipitate myocardial ischemia and anginal pain, including physical exertion, strong emotions, consumption of a heavy meal (especially if exertion occurs afterward), hot or cold temperature extremes, cigarette smoking, sexual activity, stimulants (e.g., cocaine), and circadian rhythm patterns (CAD manifestations are more frequent in early morning on awakening).

Types of Angina

Stable angina (classic) refers to chest pain occurring intermittently over a long time with the same pattern of onset, duration, and intensity of symptoms. Stable angina is usually exercise induced. Pain at rest is unusual.

- An ECG usually reveals ST-segment depression, indicating subendocardial ischemia. Discomfort may be mild or severe and disabling, but it is usually infrequent.
- Stable angina can be controlled with medications on an outpatient basis. Because stable angina is often predictable, medications can be timed to provide peak effects during the time of day when angina is likely to occur.

Unstable angina (progressive, crescendo, or preinfarction angina) is different from stable angina in that it is unpredictable. Patients with stable angina may develop unstable angina, which can be the first clinical manifestation of CAD (see Coronary Artery Disease, p. 170).

- Unstable angina is associated with deterioration of a once stable atherosclerotic plaque. This unstable lesion is at increased risk of complete thrombosis of the lumen with progression to myocardial infarction (MI). These patients require immediate hospitalization with ECG monitoring and bed rest.
- Aspirin and systemic anticoagulation are the treatments of choice for unstable angina. If the patient is not already on antianginal agents, nitrates or β-blockers are the first line of treatment. Calcium channel blockers can be added if the patient is

already on adequate doses of nitrates or β-blockers, or if the patient cannot tolerate the other two drugs or has variant angina.

Prinzmetal's angina (variant angina) often occurs at rest, usually in response to spasm of a major coronary artery. It is a rare form of angina and may occur in the absence of CAD.

- Factors that may precipitate coronary artery spasm include increased myocardial O_2 demand and increased levels of a variety of vasoactive substances such as histamine, angiotensin, epinephrine, norepinephrine, and prostaglandins.
- When spasm occurs, the patient experiences pain and marked, transient ST-segment elevation. The pain may occur during rapid eye movement (REM) sleep when myocardial O_2 consumption increases. It may be relieved by some form of exercise, or it may disappear spontaneously.

Nocturnal angina occurs only at night but not necessarily when the person is in a recumbent position or sleeping. *Angina decubitus* is chest pain that occurs only while the person is lying down and is usually relieved by standing or sitting.

Clinical Manifestations

The most common initial symptom of angina is chest pain or discomfort. The exact cause of pain is unknown, but neurogenic pain at the site of ischemia is most likely.

- On direct questioning, some patients may deny feeling pain but will refer to a vague sensation, pressure, or ache in chest. It is an unpleasant feeling, often described as a constrictive, squeezing, heavy, choking, or suffocating sensation.
- Many persons complain of severe indigestion or burning. Although discomfort is usually felt substernally, the sensation may occur in the neck or radiate to various locations including the jaw, shoulders, and down the arms.
- Associated symptoms may include shortness of breath, cold sweat, weakness, or paresthesias of the arm(s). Relief of classic angina pectoris is usually obtained with rest or cessation of activity. Prinzmetal's angina differs from stable or unstable angina in that it is longer in duration and may wake people from sleep. See Table 32-9, Lewis and others, *Medical-Surgical Nursing,* edition 5, p. 854 for a comparison of the pain of angina pectoris and MI.

Diagnostic Studies

- Chest x-ray to detect cardiac enlargement, cardiac calcifications, and pulmonary congestion
- ECG to compare to earlier tracing when possible
- Serum enzyme levels to rule out MI

■ Serum lipid levels to screen for positive risk factors
■ Ambulatory 24- to 48-hour ECG monitoring to identify silent ischemia
■ Nuclear imaging studies to determine myocardial perfusion
■ Positron emission tomography (PET) to identify and quantify ischemia and infarction
■ Angiography studies for visualization of coronary arteries to determine extent of disease
■ Echocardiography with exercise to diagnose coronary artery stenosis

Collaborative Care

The most common initial therapy for angina is the use of nitrate therapy to enhance coronary blood flow. Emergency care of the patient with chest pain is presented in Table 32-11, Lewis and others, *Medical-Surgical Nursing,* edition 5, p. 857. Treatment of CAD may include *percutaneous transluminal coronary angioplasty* (PTCA), *stent placement, atherectomy, coronary artery bypass surgery,* and *laser angioplasty.*

Percutaneous transluminal coronary angioplasty. In a catheterization laboratory a catheter equipped with a balloon tip is inserted into the appropriate coronary artery. When the lesion is located, the catheter is passed through and just past the lesion, the balloon is inflated, and the atherosclerotic plaque is compressed, resulting in vessel dilation.

■ Advantages of PTCA are that (1) it provides an alternative to surgical intervention, (2) it is performed with local anesthesia, (3) it eliminates recovery from thoracotomy required for bypass surgery and its complications, (4) patient is ambulatory 24 hours after the procedure; (5) length of hospital stay is approximately 1 to 3 days compared with the 5- to 7-day stay of someone having open heart surgery with a coronary artery bypass graft (CABG), thus reducing hospital costs, and (6) there is rapid return to work (approximately 1 week after PTCA) instead of a 1- to 8-week convalescence after CABG.
■ PTCA is more frequently performed than CABG. Reduction of lesion size by >50% occurs in 90% of patients.
■ The most serious complication of PTCA is dissection of the dilated artery where the intimal lesion is pushed farther up or down the intimal lining instead of being compressed. If damage is extensive, the coronary artery could rupture, causing cardiac tamponade, a fall in cardiac output (CO), and possible death.
■ Risk of restenosis after PTCA is about 30% in the first 3 to 6 months. Restenosis occurs more commonly in smokers, diabetics, and patients with hypercholesteremia.

Stent placement. Stents are used to treat abrupt or threatened abrupt closure following PTCA. Stents are expandable meshlike structures designed to maintain vessel patency by compressing arterial walls and resisting vasoconstriction. Because stents are thrombogenic, patients are usually treated with antiplatelet agents such as aspirin.

- Primary complications from stent placement are hemorrhage and vascular injury. Additional complications are stent thrombosis, acute MI, need for emergency CABG, stent embolization, and coronary spasm. The possibility of arrhythmias is always present.

Atherectomy. The plaque is shaved off using a type of rotational blade. Atherectomy decreases the incidence of abrupt closure as compared to PTCA. It is superior to PTCA for lesions located in branches or attachment sites of a bypass graft, but carries the same risk for thrombosis and restenosis rate as conventional PTCA.

Laser angioplasty. A catheter is introduced through a peripheral artery into the diseased coronary artery. A small laser on the tip of the catheter vaporizes the plaqued areas of artery, thereby facilitating blood flow. A disadvantage of this procedure is that the technique needs refinement so that the proper laser strength for a given thickness of atherosclerotic plaque will be known.

Coronary artery bypass graft. Generally, CABG is recommended if the patient has (1) significant left main coronary artery obstruction, (2) triple vessel disease, or (3) two vessel disease unresponsive to medical therapy. Bypass surgery is usually recommended for the person with unstable angina who demonstrates a poor response to therapy, requiring repeat angioplasty. See Lewis and others, *Medical-Surgical Nursing,* edition 5, p. 908 for a discussion of CABG surgery.

Drug Therapy

- Antiplatelet aggregation therapy is the first line of drug therapy in the treatment of angina.
- Aspirin is the drug of choice to reduce the progression of unstable angina to MI.
- Nitrates, which are commonly classified as vasodilators, are the next step in the treatment of angina. Nitrates produce their principal effects by dilating peripheral blood vessels, coronary arteries, and collateral vessels. Nitroglycerin can be used prophylactically before undertaking an activity that the patient knows may precipitate an anginal attack.
- β-Blocking agents available for the prophylaxis of angina include propranolol (Inderal) and metoprolol (Lopressor). These drugs produce a direct decrease in myocardial contractility, heart rate, systemic vascular resistance, and BP, all of which reduce myocardial O_2 demand.
- Calcium-blocking agents such as nifedipine (Procardia), verapamil (Calan, Isoptin), and diltiazem (Cardizem) are the next

step in the management of angina. The primary effects of calcium channel blockers are systemic vasodilation with decreased systemic vascular resistance, decreased myocardial contractility, and coronary vasodilation.

Nursing Management

Goals
The patient with angina will experience pain relief, have reduced anxiety, have adequate knowledge of the problem and prescribed treatment, and modify risk factors.

Nursing Diagnoses
- Pain *related to* ischemic myocardium
- Anxiety *related to* diagnosis, pain and limited activity tolerance, and uncertainties about future, diagnostic tests, and pending surgery
- Decreased cardiac output *related to* myocardial ischemia affecting contractility
- Activity intolerance *related to* myocardial ischemia

Nursing Interventions
The main nursing objectives for the patient with angina are pain assessment, evaluation of treatment, and reinforcement of appropriate therapy. Because chest pain can be caused by many factors other than ischemia (e.g., pericarditis, valvular disease, MI), it is important to have a clear understanding of the patient's chest pain.

- The nurse needs to elicit a history of anginal pain. The nurse should determine whether breathing in or out or changing positions makes the patient's chest pain better or worse. Anginal pain does not vary with body position or respirations. In contrast, the pain of pericarditis does.
- It should be ascertained whether the pain is deep or superficial, mild or intense, diffuse or localized. Cardiac pain is usually described as deep and intense, but occasionally it may be characterized as a dull ache.
- The nurse should instruct the patient to quantify each pain experience by rating the pain on a scale from 1 to 10, with 10 being excruciating pain and 1 being barely noticeable. By doing this, the nurse can assess the effectiveness of treatment during a pain experience as well as discriminate between subsequent pain experiences.
- If a nurse is present during an anginal attack, the following measures should be instituted: (1) administration of O_2, (2) determination of vital signs, (3) 12-lead ECG, (4) prompt pain relief with a nitrate followed by a narcotic analgesic if needed, (5) physical assessment of the chest, and (6) comfortable positioning of the patient.

- Supportive and realistic assurance as well as a calm, soothing manner help to reduce patient anxiety.

▼ **Patient Teaching**

The patient needs to be reassured that a long, productive life is possible, even with angina.

- Patient teaching can be handled in a variety of ways. One-to-one contact between the nurse and patient is often the most effective. Time spent in providing daily care is often an ideal teaching period. Teaching tools, such as pamphlets, films at the bedside, a heart model, and especially written information, are important components of patient and family education.
- Prevention of angina is preferable to treatment.
- The patient needs to be educated regarding CAD and angina, precipitating factors, risk factors, and medications, including the proper use of sublingual nitroglycerin.
- The patient needs to be assisted in identifying factors that precipitate angina and given instruction on how to avoid or control these factors.
- The patient needs to be assisted in identifying personal risk factors for CAD. Once these risk factors are known, various methods of decreasing them should be discussed.
- Educating the patient and family about diets that are low in sodium and saturated fat may be appropriate. Maintaining ideal body weight is most important in controlling angina, since weight above this level increases myocardial workload and may cause pain. Eating large meals also contributes to angina, and patients may need to eat several small meals in place of three moderate to large meals each day.
- Adhering to a regular, individualized exercise program that conditions the heart rather than overstressing it is important. The nurse should consult with a physician or a physical therapist in instructing the patient regarding an exercise program.
- Counseling should be provided to assess psychologic adjustment of the patient and family to the diagnosis of CAD and resulting angina pectoris. Many patients feel a threat to their identity and self-esteem.

ANKYLOSING SPONDYLITIS

Definition/Description

Ankylosing spondylitis (AS) is a chronic inflammatory disease that primarily affects the sacroiliac joints, apophyseal and costovertebral joints of the spine, and adjacent soft tissues. Approximately

90% of Caucasian patients with AS are positive for HLA-B27. There appears to be a familial tendency, and the disease is unusual in African-Americans. The disease typically appears in adolescence or young adulthood.

Pathophysiology
The cause of AS is unknown. Genetic predisposition appears to play an important role in disease pathogenesis, but the precise mechanisms are unknown. Environmental factors and infectious agents are also suspected. Inflammation in joints and adjacent tissue causes the formation of granulation tissue and erodes vertebral margins, resulting in spondylitis. Calcification tends to follow the inflammation process, leading to bony ankylosis.

Clinical Manifestations
- The patient typically has lower back pain, stiffness, and limitation of motion that is worse during the night and in the morning but improves with mild activity.
- General constitutional features such as fever, fatigue, anorexia, and weight loss are rarely present.
- Other symptoms depend on the stage of disease and may include peripheral arthritis of the shoulders, hips, and knees and occasional ocular inflammation (iritis).
- Advancing kyphosis leads to a bent-over posture, and compensating hip-flexion contractures may occur. There is pronounced impairment of neck motion in all directions.
- Extraskeletal involvement may include iritis, aortic valvular regurgitation, and apical pulmonary fibrosis.

Diagnostic Studies
When abnormalities are present, they include sacroiliac joints that show pseudowidening of joint space and later obliteration with ankylosis.
- New bone formation (syndesmophytes) may be spotty or generalized (classic "bamboo spine").
- Erythrocyte sedimentation rate (ESR), alkaline phosphatase, and creatine kinase levels are usually elevated.
- Tissue typing is positive for HLA-B27 in the majority of patients.

Collaborative Care
Prevention of AS is not possible; however, families with diagnosed HLA-B27–positive rheumatic diseases should be alert to signs of lower back pain and arthritis symptoms so early therapy can be initiated.

Care of the patient is aimed at maintaining maximal skeletal mobility. Proper posture is important in all activities. Although drugs do not halt disease progression, nonsteroidal antiinflammatory drugs

(NSAIDs) such as diclofenac (Voltaren) and indomethacin (Indocin) can reduce inflammation, which makes proper posturing easier. Disease-modifying agents such as methotrexate can be used to delay disease progression. Surgery to correct extreme flexion deformities may be performed in certain cases. A total hip replacement is done for patients with crippling hip ankylosis.

Nursing Management

Nursing responsibilities include education about the nature of the disease and principles of therapy. A home management program consists of local heat and exercise and proper use of medications.

- Pain should be managed by appropriate medication, heat, massage, and gentle exercise. Application of moist heat should be followed by range-of-motion (ROM) exercises and daily chest expansion and deep-breathing exercises.
- Excessive physical exertion during periods of active inflammation should be discouraged.
- Proper positioning at rest is essential. The mattress should be firm, and pillows must be avoided. The patient should sleep on his or her back and avoid positions that encourage flexion deformity.
- Postural training emphasizes avoiding forward flexion (e.g., leaning over a desk), heavy lifting, and prolonged walking, standing, or sitting. Sports that facilitate natural stretching, such as swimming and racquet games, should be encouraged.
- Family counseling and vocational rehabilitation are important.

ANORECTAL ABSCESS

Anorectal abscesses are undrained collections of perianal pus that are due to perirectal infections in patients who have compromised local circulation or active inflammatory disease.

- The most common causative organisms are *Escherichia coli,* staphylococci, and streptococci. Manifestations include local pain and swelling, foul-smelling drainage, tenderness, and elevated temperature. Sepsis can occur as a complication.
- Surgical treatment consists of abscess drainage. If packing is used, it should be impregnated with petroleum jelly and the area should be allowed to heal by granulation. The packing is changed every day, and moist, hot compresses are applied to the area. Care must be taken to avoid soiling the dressing during urination or defecation. A low-residue diet is given. The patient may leave the hospital with the area open.

- Discharge teaching should include wound care, the importance of sitz baths, thorough cleaning after bowel movements, and follow-up visits to the physician.

ANOREXIA NERVOSA

Definition/Description
Anorexia nervosa is a specific psychiatric disorder characterized by a refusal to maintain body weight to >85% of that expected for age and height.

- Two subgroups of anorexia nervosa are the bulimic type and the restrictive type, depending on whether there are cycles of binging and purging.
- This condition is found predominantly in adolescent girls.
- Once anorexia nervosa has developed, the person will go to almost any extreme to hide eating behavior from parents or peers. Eating habits are severely disturbed. If purging is present, it is often accomplished by self-induced vomiting, use of cathartics, or enemas.
- If the eating pattern is permitted to continue for a prolonged time, body wasting and signs of severe malnutrition become evident. Restricted intake occurs even in the presence of hunger.

Clinical Manifestations
- Common signs and symptoms include amenorrhea, bradycardia, orthostatic hypotension, cold intolerance, breast atrophy, lanugo (soft, downlike hair normally associated with a fetus), dry skin, hair loss, severe constipation, and edema with altered fluid balance.
- Chronic anorexia nervosa places the patient at risk for serious complications affecting multiple organ systems such as the cardiovascular, musculoskeletal, GI, and endocrine systems.
- Life-threatening cardiac complications include hypotension, bradycardia, and malignant arrhythmias.
- Diagnostic studies often show iron deficiency anemia and an elevated blood urea nitrogen (BUN) level.

Collaborative Care
Multidisciplinary treatment must involve a combination of nutritional support and psychiatric care. Hospitalization may be necessary if there are severe physical complications that cannot be managed in an outpatient therapy program.

- Nutritional replenishment must be closely supervised, not merely for the few pounds the person can rapidly gain but for consistent and ongoing weight gains. The use of tube or parenteral feedings may be necessary. Improved nutrition, however, is not a cure for anorexia nervosa.
- The underlying psychologic problem must be addressed by identification of the disturbed patterns of individual and family interactions, followed by individual and family counseling.

AORTIC DISSECTION

Definition/Description
An aortic dissection is a longitudinal splitting of the medial layer of the artery by a column of blood, occurring most commonly in the thoracic aorta.

Pathophysiology
Aortic dissection results from a small tear in the intimal lining of the artery, allowing blood to "track" between the intima and media and creating a false lumen of blood flow.

- As the heart contracts, each systolic pulsation causes increased pressure, which further increases dissection. As it extends proximally or distally, it may occlude major branches of the aorta, cutting off blood supply to the brain, abdominal organs, spinal cord, and extremities.
- The exact cause is uncertain. Cystic medial necrosis (destruction of medial layer elastic fibers) may be the leading cause. Most people with dissection problems have hypertension. Persons with Marfan syndrome (a connective tissue disease) have a high incidence of dissection. Pregnancy also promotes vascular stress as a result of increased blood volume. Areas prone to dissection are the ascending aorta, aortic arch, and descending aorta beyond the origin of the left subclavian artery.

Clinical Manifestations and Complications
The patient with aortic dissection usually has sudden, severe pain in the back, chest, or abdomen. The pain is described as "tearing" or "ripping" and may mimic that of a myocardial infarction (MI). As the dissection progresses, pain may be located both above and below the diaphragm. Dyspnea may also be present.

- If the arch of the aorta is involved, the patient may exhibit neurologic deficiencies, including altered level of consciousness, dizziness, and weakened or absent carotid and temporal pulses.

- An ascending aortic dissection usually produces some degree of aortic valvular insufficiency and a murmur audible on auscultation.
- When either subclavian artery is involved, pulse quality and BP readings may vary between the left and right arms.
- As dissection progresses down the aorta, the abdominal organs and lower extremities may demonstrate evidence of altered tissue perfusion and ischemia.
- A severe complication of dissection of the ascending aortic arch is *cardiac tamponade,* which occurs when blood escapes from the dissection into the pericardial sac. Clinical manifestations include narrowed pulse pressure, distended neck veins, muffled heart sounds, and pulsus paradoxus.
- Because the aorta is weakened by medial dissection, it may rupture. Hemorrhage may occur into the mediastinal, pleural, or abdominal cavities.
- Dissection can lead to occlusion of the arterial supply to many vital organs, including the spinal cord, kidneys, and abdominal structures. Ischemia of the spinal cord produces symptoms varying from weakness to paralysis in lower extremities and decreased pain sensation. Renal ischemia is manifested by low urinary output. Signs of abdominal ischemia include abdominal pain, decreased bowel sounds, and altered bowel elimination.

Diagnostic Studies
- ECG to rule out MI
- Chest x-ray to determine widening of mediastinal silhouette and pleural effusion
- CT scan or MRI to assess presence and severity of dissection
- Echocardiogram to assess for left ventricular hypertrophy
- Aortography to determine extent of dissection

Collaborative Care
The goal of therapy for aortic dissection without complications is to lower BP and myocardial contractility to decrease the pulsatile forces within the aorta. The use of trimethaphan (Arfonad) and nitroprusside (Nitropress) IV rapidly reduces BP. IV β-blockers may also be used, such as propranolol (Inderal), or α-blockers and β-blockers, such as labetalol (Normodyne). Propranolol is used to decrease the force of myocardial contractility.

- The patient without complications can be conservatively treated for a long time. Supportive treatment is directed toward pain relief, blood transfusion (if required), and management of heart failure (if indicated).
- If dissection involves the ascending aorta, surgery is indicated. Surgery is also indicated when drug therapy is ineffective or

when complications of aortic dissection (e.g., heart failure, leaking dissection, occlusion of artery) are present. Surgery is delayed for as long as possible to allow time for edema in the area of dissection to resolve, to permit clotting of blood in the false lumen, and to allow the healing process to begin.

- Surgery for aortic dissection involves resection of the aortic segment containing the intimal tear and replacement with synthetic graft material.

Nursing Management

Interventions related to an aortic dissection include keeping the patient in bed in a semi-Fowler's position and maintaining a quiet environment. These measures assist in keeping systolic BP at the lowest possible level. Narcotics and tranquilizers should be administered as ordered. Pain and anxiety must be managed because they increase BP.

- Continuous IV administration of antihypertensive agents requires close nursing supervision. An ECG device is used and an intraarterial pressure line is usually inserted. The nurse should monitor for changes in the quality of peripheral pulses and for signs of increasing pain, restlessness, and anxiety. A widening pulse pressure may indicate increasing aortic valvular insufficiency. If blood vessels branching off the aortic arch are involved, decreased cerebral blood flow may alter sensorium and level of consciousness.
- Postoperative care after surgery to correct the dissection is similar to that after aortic aneurysm repair (see NCP 36-1, Lewis and others, *Medical-Surgical Nursing,* edition 5, p. 984.

▼ Patient Teaching
- The therapeutic regimen includes antihypertensive drugs, which are usually taken orally. The patient needs to understand that these drugs must be taken to control BP. Propranolol can be taken orally to continue to decrease myocardial contractility.
- Instruct the patient to seek help at the nearest health care facility if pain returns or other symptoms progress.

APPENDICITIS

Definition/Description

Appendicitis is an inflammation of the appendix, a narrow blind tube that extends from the inferior part of the cecum. Appendicitis occurs in 6% of the general population. Peak incidence is between 11 and 30 years of age.

Pathophysiology

The most common causes of appendicitis are obstruction of the lumen by a fecalith (accumulated feces), foreign bodies, intramural thickening due to lymphoid hyperplasia, or tumor of the cecum or appendix. Obstruction results in distention, venous engorgement, and the accumulation of mucus and bacteria, which can lead to gangrene and perforation.

Clinical Manifestations

Appendicitis typically begins with periumbilical pain, followed by anorexia, nausea, and vomiting. The pain is persistent and continuous, eventually shifting to the right lower quadrant and localizing at McBurney's point (located halfway between the umbilicus and right iliac crest).

- Further assessment reveals localized and rebound tenderness with muscle guarding. The patient usually prefers to lie still, often with right leg flexed. Low-grade fever may or may not be present. Coughing aggravates the pain. Rovsing's sign may be elicited by palpation of the left lower quadrant, causing pain to be felt in the right lower quadrant.

Complications of acute appendicitis are perforation, peritonitis, and abscesses.

Diagnostic Studies

- Palpation of the abdomen usually reveals tenderness and muscle guarding.
- White blood cell (WBC) count indicates leukocytosis.
- Urinalysis may be done to rule out genitourinary (GU) conditions that mimic manifestations of appendicitis.

Collaborative Care

Treatment is immediate surgical removal *(appendectomy)* if the inflammation is localized. If the appendix has ruptured and there is evidence of peritonitis or an abscess, conservative treatment, consisting of antibiotic therapy and parenteral fluids, may be used to prevent sepsis and dehydration for 6 to 8 hours before an appendectomy is performed.

Nursing Management

The patient with abdominal pain is encouraged to see a physician and to avoid self-treatment, particularly the use of laxatives and enemas. Increased peristalsis from these procedures may cause perforation.

- Until the patient is seen by the physician, nothing should be taken by mouth (NPO) to ensure that the stomach will be empty if surgery is needed.

- An ice bag may be applied to the right lower quadrant to decrease the flow of blood to the area and impede the inflammatory process. Heat is *never* used because it may cause the appendix to rupture.
- Surgery is usually performed as soon as a diagnosis is made.

Postoperative nursing management is similar to postoperative care of a patient after laparotomy (see Abdominal Pain, Acute, p. 3). In addition, the patient should be observed for evidence of peritonitis. Ambulation begins the day of surgery or the first postoperative day. Diet is advanced as tolerated.

- The patient is usually discharged on the first or second postoperative day, and normal activities are resumed 2 to 3 weeks after surgery.

ARRHYTHMIAS

Definition/Description

Arrhythmias are abnormal cardiac rhythms. Prompt assessment of an abnormal cardiac rhythm and the patient's response to the rhythm is critical. Disorders of impulse formation can initiate arrhythmias. A pacemaker from another site may be discharged in two ways. If the sinoatrial (SA) node discharges more slowly than a secondary pacemaker, electrical discharges from the secondary pacemaker may passively escape and discharge automatically at their intrinsic rates. Another way for secondary pacemakers to originate is when they discharge more rapidly than the normal pacemaker of the sinus node.

- Arrhythmias occur as the result of various abnormalities and disease states. The cause of arrhythmia influences the treatment of the patient. Common causes of arrhythmias are presented in Table 8.

Types of Arrhythmias

When assessing a cardiac rhythm, the recommended approach is to note rate, rhythm, P wave, QRS complex, relationship of P wave to QRS complex, PR interval, QRS interval, and QT interval. Examples of ECG tracings of the common arrhythmias are presented in Figs. 34-11 through 34-20, Lewis and others, *Medical-Surgical Nursing,* edition 5, pp. 925-934. Descriptive characteristics of common arrhythmias are discussed in Table 34-6, *Medical-Surgical Nursing,* p. 925.

Sinus bradycardia. This condition occurs when the sinus node discharges at a rate of <60 beats per minute (bpm); the rhythm is regular. It occurs in response to carotid sinus massage, Valsalva maneuver, hypothermia, increased vagal tone, and the administration

Table 8	**Common Causes of Arrhythmias**
Drug effects or toxicity	Cellular hypoxia
Myocardial cell degeneration	Edema
Hypertrophy of cardiac muscle	Acid-base imbalances
Emotional crisis	Myocardial ischemia
Connective tissue disorders	Degeneration of the
Alcohol	conduction system
Coffee, tea, tobacco	Metabolic conditions
Electrolyte imbalances	(e.g., thyroid dysfunction)

of parasympathomimetic drugs. Disease states associated with sinus bradycardia are hypothyroidism, increased intracranial pressure, and inferior wall myocardial infarction (MI).

- Clinical significance depends on how the patient tolerates bradycardia hemodynamically. Hypotension with decreased cardiac output (CO) may occur in some circumstances.
- Treatment consists of administration of atropine for patients with symptoms. Pacemaker therapy may be required.

Sinus tachycardia. This arrhythmia involves an increased discharge rate from the sinus node as a result of vagal inhibition or sympathetic stimulation. The sinus rate is >100 bpm; the rhythm is regular. Sinus tachycardia is associated with physiologic stressors such as exercise, fever, pain, hypovolemia, anemia, hypoxia, hypoglycemia, and congestive heart failure (CHF). It can also be an effect of drugs such as epinephrine, caffeine, theophylline, or nifedipine (Procardia).

- Clinical significance depends on the patient's tolerance of the increased heart rate (HR). Patient may have symptoms of dizziness, and hypotension may occur.
- Treatment is determined by underlying causes. In certain settings, β-blocker therapy (e.g., propranolol [Inderal]) is used to reduce HR and decrease myocardial oxygen (O_2) consumption.

Premature atrial contraction (PAC). PAC occurs as a result of contractions originating from an ectopic focus in the atrium in a location other than the sinus node. It originates in the left or right atrium and travels across the atria by an abnormal pathway, creating a distorted P wave. At the atrioventricular (AV) node it is stopped (nonconducted PAC), delayed (lengthened PR interval), or conducted normally. It moves through the AV node and in most cases is conducted normally through the ventricles. In a normal heart, a PAC can result from emotional stress or caffeine, tobacco, or alcohol use. A PAC can also result from disease states such as infection, thyrotoxicosis, chronic obstructive pulmonary disease (COPD), and heart disease (including atherosclerotic heart disease and valvular heart disease).

- HR varies with underlying rate and frequency of PAC and *rhythm* is irregular.
- Treatment depends on patient symptoms. Withdrawal of sources of stimulation such as caffeine may be warranted. Drugs such as digoxin, quinidine, procainamide (Pronestyl), flecainide (Tambocor), and β-blockers can be used.

Paroxysmal supraventricular tachycardia (PSVT). PSVT is an arrhythmia originating in an ectopic focus anywhere above the bifurcation of the bundle of His. *Paroxysmal* refers to an abrupt onset and termination. Some degree of AV block may be present. In the normal heart PSVT is associated with overexertion, emotional stress, deep inspiration, and stimulants such as caffeine and tobacco. In disease states PSVT is associated with rheumatic heart disease, Wolff-Parkinson-White (WPW) syndrome (conduction via accessory pathways), digitalis intoxication, coronary artery disease (CAD), or cor pulmonale.

- *HR* is 100 to 300 bpm and *rhythm* is regular.
- Clinical significance depends on symptoms and HR. A prolonged episode and HR >180 bpm may precipitate a decreased CO with hypotension and myocardial ischemia.
- Treatment includes vagal stimulation induced by carotid massage or Valsalva maneuver. Drug of choice is adenosine (Adenocard), a drug with a very short half-life (10 seconds) that successfully converts PSVT to sinus rhythm in a high percentage of patients. Verapamil (Calan), digitalis, and propranolol (Inderal) can also be used.

Atrial flutter. This condition is an atrial tachyarrhythmia identified by recurring, regular, sawtooth-shaped flutter waves. It is usually associated with a slower ventricular response. Because of the refractoriness of the AV node, there is usually some AV block in a fixed ratio of flutter waves to QRS responses (e.g., 2:1, 3:1). Atrial flutter is a relatively rare arrhythmia and rarely occurs in a normal heart. In disease states, it is associated with CAD, hypertension, mitral valve disorders, pulmonary embolus, cor pulmonale, and with the use of drugs such as digitalis, quinidine, and epinephrine.

- *Atrial rate* is 250 to 350 bpm. *Ventricular rate* varies according to conduction ratio. In 2:1 conduction, ventricular rate is typically about 150 bpm. *Atrial* and *ventricular rhythms* are usually regular.
- High ventricular rates can decrease CO and cause serious consequences such as heart failure.
- Primary goal in treatment is to slow ventricular response by increasing AV block. Electrical cardioversion may be used to

convert atrial flutter to sinus rhythm in an emergency situation. Drugs used include verapamil, digoxin, quinidine, procainamide, and β-blockers. A new drug, ibutilide (Covert), effectively terminates atrial flutter in closely monitored situations. Radiofrequency catheter ablation is increasingly being used to cure atrial flutter.

Atrial fibrillation. This condition involves a total disorganization of atrial electrical activity without effective atrial contraction. ECG demonstrates baseline fibrillatory waves or undulations of variable contour at a rate of 300 to 600 per minute. Ventricular response is irregular, and if the patient is untreated, ventricular rate will be 100 to 160 bpm. The arrhythmia may be chronic or intermittent and usually occurs in the patient with underlying heart disease. It is also associated with alcoholism, infection, and stress.

- *Atrial rate* may be as high as 350 to 600 bpm. *Ventricular rate* can vary from 50 to 180 bpm. *Atrial rhythm* is chaotic and *ventricular rhythm* is usually irregular.
- Atrial fibrillation can often result in a decrease in CO because of ineffective atrial contractions and rapid ventricular response. Thrombi may form in atria as a result of ineffective atrial contraction. Warfarin is used to prevent a stroke from an embolized clot.
- The goal of treatment is a decrease in ventricular response. In emergency situations, cardioversion may be used to convert atrial fibrillation to normal sinus rhythm. Medications used for pharmaceutical cardioversion or a decrease in ventricular response include digoxin, verapamil, diltiazem (Cardizem), quinidine, flecainide (Tambocor), propafenone (Rythmol), sotalol (Betapace), and β-blockers. IV ibutilide is also used in acute care settings.

First-degree AV block. In this type of AV block every impulse is conducted to the ventricles, but the duration of AV conduction is prolonged. This is manifested by a PR interval >0.2 second. After the impulse moves through the AV node, it is usually conducted normally through the ventricles. A first-degree AV block is associated with MI, chronic ischemic heart disease, rheumatic fever, hyperthyroidism, and drugs such as digitalis, flecainide, β-blockers, and IV verapamil.

- *HR* is normal and *rhythm* is regular.
- First-degree AV block may be a precursor of higher degrees of AV block.
- There is no treatment for first-degree AV block.

Second-degree AV block, type I (Mobitz I, Wenckebach phenomenon). This condition includes gradual lengthening of the PR interval, which occurs because of AV conduction time that is prolonged until an atrial impulse is nonconducted and a QRS complex is dropped. Once a ventricular beat is dropped, the cycle repeats itself with progressive lengthening of PR intervals until another QRS complex is dropped. The rhythm appears on the ECG in a pattern of grouped beats. Duration of the QRS complex is normal or prolonged. Type I AV block most commonly occurs in the AV node and may result from use of drugs such as digoxin or β-blockers. It may also be associated with ischemic cardiac disease and other diseases that can slow AV conduction.

- *Atrial rate* is normal, but *ventricular rate* may be slower as a result of dropped QRS complexes. *Ventricular rhythm* is irregular.
- Type I AV block is usually a result of inferior MI. It is almost always transient and well tolerated. However, it may be a warning signal of impending, significant AV conduction disturbance.
- If the patient is symptomatic, atropine is used to increase HR, or a temporary pacemaker may be needed, especially if the patient has an acute MI.

Second-degree heart block, type II (Mobitz II). In this type of heart block, the P wave is not conducted without progressive antecedent PR lengthening; this occurs when a bundle branch block is present. On conducted beats, the PR interval is constant. In a second-degree heart block a certain number of impulses from the sinus node are not conducted to the ventricles. This occurs in ratios of 2:1, 3:1, and so on when there are two P waves to one QRS complex, three P waves to one QRS complex, and so on. It may occur with varying ratios. Type II AV block almost always occurs in the His-Purkinje system and is associated with rheumatic and atherosclerotic heart disease, acute anterior MI, and digitalis toxicity.

- *Atrial rate* is usually normal. *Ventricular rate* depends on intrinsic rate and degree of AV block. *Sinus rhythm* is regular, but *ventricular rhythm* may be irregular.
- Type II AV block often progresses to third-degree AV block and is associated with a poor prognosis.
- Reduced HR may result in decreased CO with subsequent hypotension and myocardial ischemia.
- Type II AV block is an indication for therapy with a permanent pacemaker.
- Treatment before insertion of a permanent pacemaker involves the use of a temporary pacemaker (see Pacemakers, p. 677). Drugs such as atropine, epinephrine, or dopamine can be tried as temporary measures to increase HR until pacemaker therapy is available.

Third-degree AV heart block (complete heart block). This condition constitutes one form of AV dissociation in which no impulses from the atria are conducted to the ventricles. The atria are stimulated and contract independently of the ventricles. Ventricular rhythm is an escape rhythm, and focus may be above or below the bifurcation of the bundle of His. This rhythm is associated with fibrosis or calcification of the cardiac conduction system, CAD, myocarditis, cardiomyopathy, and open heart surgery.

- *Atrial rate* is usually a sinus rate of 60 to 100 bpm. *Ventricular rate* depends on the site of the block. If it is in the AV node, the rate is 40 to 60 bpm, and if it is in the Purkinje system, it is 20 to 40 bpm. *Atrial* and *ventricular rhythms* are regular but asynchronous.
- Third-degree AV block almost always results in reduced CO with subsequent ischemia and heart failure.
- A temporary pacemaker may be inserted or an external pacemaker may be applied on an emergency basis in the patient with acute MI. Use of drugs such as atropine, epinephrine, and dopamine are temporary treatments to increase HR and support BP before pacemaker insertion (see Pacemakers, p. 677).

Premature ventricular contractions (PVCs). These contractions originate in an ectopic focus in the ventricles. PVCs are a premature occurrence of the QRS complex, which is wide and distorted in shape. PVCs that are initiated from different foci appear different in contour from each other and are termed *multifocal PVCs.* When every other beat is a PVC, it is called *ventricular bigeminy.* When every third beat is a PVC, it is called *ventricular trigeminy.* Two consecutive PVCs are called *couplets.* Three consecutive PVCs are called *triplets. Ventricular tachycardia* occurs when there are three or more consecutive PVCs. When a PVC falls on the T wave of a preceding beat, the *R on T phenomenon* occurs and is considered to be quite dangerous because it may precipitate ventricular tachycardia or ventricular fibrillation. PVCs are associated with stimulants such as caffeine, alcohol, epinephrine, and digoxin. They are also associated with hypokalemia, fever, and emotional stress. Disease states associated with PVCs include MI, mitral valve prolapse, CHF, and CAD.

- *HR* varies according to the intrinsic rate and the number of PVCs. *Rhythm* is irregular because of premature beats.
- PVCs are usually a benign finding in a patient with a normal heart. In heart disease, PVCs may reduce CO and precipitate angina and heart failure. PVCs in ischemic heart disease or acute MI represent ventricular irritability.
- Indications for treatment in an appropriate clinical setting include (1) six or more PVCs occurring per minute, (2) ventricular couplets and triplets, (3) multifocal PVCs, and (4) R on T phenomenon. If treatment is not initiated, ventricular tachycardia or ventricular fibrillation may occur. For treating PVCs, lidocaine is the drug of choice. Procainamide is the second drug of choice if lidocaine is ineffective.

Ventricular tachycardia. This arrhythmia is a run of three or more PVCs that occurs when ectopic focus or foci fire repetitively and the ventricle takes control as the pacemaker. The ventricular rate is 110 to 250 bpm. Atria may also be depolarized by the ventricles in a retrograde fashion.

The appearance of ventricular tachycardia is an ominous sign because it usually indicates the presence of cardiac disease. It is considered to be a life-threatening arrhythmia because of decreased CO and the possibility of deterioration of ventricular tachycardia to ventricular fibrillation, which is a lethal arrhythmia. Ventricular tachycardia is associated with acute MI, CAD, significant electrolyte imbalances (e.g., potassium), cardiomyopathy, and coronary reperfusion after thrombolytic therapy. The arrhythmia has also been observed in patients who have no evidence of cardiac disease.

- If the patient is hemodynamically stable, treatment consists of administration of a lidocaine bolus with subsequent boluses as necessary. If this abolishes tachycardia, a continuous lidocaine infusion should be started. If lidocaine is ineffective, IV procainamide may be tried. If this treatment is successful, a continuous procainamide infusion should be started. A third drug of choice is IV bretylium.
- If a patient is unconscious or hemodynamically unstable, immediate cardioversion is recommended. A defibrillator is used in synchronized mode for cardioversion.

Ventricular fibrillation. This condition is a severe derangement of the heart rhythm characterized on the ECG by irregular undulations of varying contour and amplitude. This represents the firing of multiple ectopic foci in the ventricle. Mechanically, the ventricle is simply "quivering," and no effective contraction or CO occurs. This type of fibrillation occurs in acute MI and myocardial ischemia and in chronic diseases such as CAD and cardiomyopathy. It may occur during cardiac pacing or cardiac catheterization procedures due to catheter stimulation of the ventricle. Other clinical associations are accidental electrical shock, hyperkalemia, and hypoxemia.

- *HR* is not measurable. *Rhythm* is irregular and chaotic.
- Ventricular fibrillation results in unconsciousness, absence of pulse, apnea, and seizures. If left untreated, the patient will die.
- Treatment consists of immediate initiation of CPR and initiation of advanced cardiac life support (ACLS) measures with the use of defibrillation and definitive drug therapy.

See NCP 34-1 for the patient with arrhythmias, Lewis and others, *Medical-Surgical Nursing,* edition 5, p. 926.

ARTERIAL OCCLUSIVE DISEASE (CHRONIC PERIPHERAL)

A

Definition/Description

Chronic peripheral arterial occlusive disease involves the progressive narrowing, degeneration, and eventual obstruction of the arteries to the extremities, and it occurs predominately in the legs. It may affect the aortoiliac, femoral, popliteal, or tibial arteries; the peroneal vessels; or any combination of these arteries. Chronic arterial occlusion is a slowly progressive, insidious disease primarily attributed to the atherosclerotic process; hence the term *arteriosclerosis obliterans* is often used.

- It usually occurs in the sixth through eighth decades of life, primarily affects men, and has a familial tendency. It occurs at an earlier age in patients with diabetes mellitus.
- Although the process may be slowed or arrested through risk factor modification, there is no cure. All treatment is palliative.

Pathophysiology

The leading cause of chronic arterial occlusion is atherosclerosis, a gradual thickening of the intima and media, which leads to vessel lumen narrowing. Atherosclerosis primarily affects larger arteries. The involvement is generally segmental with normal segments interspersed between involved ones.

By the time symptoms occur, the vessel is about 75% narrowed. In advanced stages, multiple levels of occlusions are seen.

- The most significant risk factors are cigarette smoking, hyperlipidemia, and hypertension. Others are diabetes mellitus, a positive family history, obesity, and a sedentary lifestyle.

Clinical Manifestations

Severity of the manifestations depends on the site, extent of obstruction, and the extent and amount of collateral circulation.

- The classic symptom is *intermittent claudication,* which is ischemic muscle ache or pain that is precipitated by exercise and relieved by resting.
- Disease involving the femoral or popliteal arteries may cause claudication in the calf. Disease of the aortoiliac arteries may produce claudication in the buttocks and upper part of the thighs. If disease extends into the internal iliac (hypogastric) arteries, impotence may result.
- Pain at rest occurs as the disease worsens. Without revascularization, the limb may progress to ulceration, and gangrenous changes may occur.

- Paresthesia, manifested as numbness or tingling in the toes or feet, may result from nerve tissue ischemia. Gradually diminishing perfusion to neurons produces loss of both sensation and deep pain.
- Pallor or blanching on elevation indicates significant arterial ischemia. Hyperemia (redness) and a bluish or dusky appearance are observed when the limb is allowed to hang in a dependent position (dependent rubor). The skin becomes shiny and taut and there is hair loss on the lower legs. Diminished or absent pedal, popliteal, or femoral pulses may also be noted.

Common complications are ischemic ulcers and gangrene, which may result in lower extremity amputation. If atherosclerosis has been present for an extended period, collateral circulation may prevent the development of gangrene.

Diagnostic Studies

- Doppler ultrasound can determine blood flow
- Segmental BP readings of leg show low pressures
- Angiography or MRI delineates location and extent of disease

Collaborative Care

Conservative therapy goals include protecting the extremity from trauma, slowing progression of atherosclerosis, decreasing vasospasm, preventing and controlling infection, and improving collateral circulation.

- Patient risk factors should be assessed, and proper intervention should begin regarding cessation of smoking, weight reduction (if indicated), and control of lipid disorders. Hypertension also needs to be properly managed.
- Interventional radiologic procedures (e.g., percutaneous transluminal angioplasty) or surgery is indicated when (1) the symptoms of intermittent claudication become incapacitating, (2) the limb is so ischemic that the patient experiences pain at rest, or (3) ulceration or gangrene is severe enough to threaten limb viability.

Nursing Management

Goals

The patient with chronic arterial occlusive disease will have adequate tissue perfusion, relief of pain, increased exercise tolerance, and intact, healthy skin on extremities.

See NCP 36-2 for the patient with chronic arterial occlusive disease, Lewis and others, *Medical-Surgical Nursing,* edition 5, p. 993.

Nursing Diagnoses

- Altered peripheral tissue perfusion *related to* decreased arterial blood flow

- Impaired skin integrity *related to* decreased peripheral circulation, altered sensation, and increased susceptibility to infection
- Pain *related to* ischemia and exercise
- Activity intolerance *related to* imbalance between oxygen supply and demand
- Ineffective management of therapeutic regimen *related to* lack of knowledge of disease and self-care measures

Nursing Interventions

After surgical therapy, the operative extremity should be checked every 15 minutes initially and then every hour for color, temperature, capillary refill, and the presence of peripheral pulses distal to the operative site. Loss of palpable pulses necessitates immediate intervention.

After transfer from the recovery room, nursing care should focus on continued circulatory assessment and monitoring for the development of potential complications. These include bleeding, hematoma, thrombosis, embolization, and compartment syndrome. Severe ischemic pain, loss of palpable pulse or pulses, decreasing ankle-brachial indices, numbness or tingling, or cold temperature may indicate occlusion of the bypass graft and should be reported to the surgeon immediately.

- The patient's heels should be kept free of pressure. Knee-flexed positions should be avoided except for exercise.
- Sitting for long periods of time is discouraged because leg dependency may cause edema, resulting in discomfort and stress to suture lines and increased risk of deep vein thrombosis. If significant swelling develops, a reclining position is preferred, with the edematous leg elevated above heart level. Walking even short distances is desirable.

▼ **Patient Teaching**
- The patient should be consistently encouraged to abstain from smoking. Instruction regarding diet modification to reduce the intake of animal fat and refined sugars, proper foot care, and avoidance of injury to the extremities are also important.
- Promotion of a progressive exercise program often increases the patient's tolerance for exercise, enhances venous return, and improves the development of collateral circulation.
- Encourage rest when pain occurs so that tissue ischemia and pain are relieved or reduced and explain rationale to patient to increase cooperation. Teach relaxation techniques to decrease stress.
- Instruct the patient that footwear should be soft, roomy, and protective. Patients should learn to inspect their legs and feet daily for skin color changes, mottling, alterations in skin texture and subcutaneous fat, and reduction or absence of hair growth. Any ulceration or inflammation must be reported to the health care provider. Skin temperature should be noted with capillary refill of fingers and toes.

ASTHMA

Definition/Description

Asthma is a chronic inflammatory disease of the airways in which inflammation causes airway obstruction. This inflammation causes recurrent episodes of wheezing, breathlessness, chest tightness, and cough, particularly at night and in the early morning. The airway obstruction may reverse spontaneously or with treatment. The hyperresponsiveness of the airways is variable, producing spontaneous fluctuations in the severity of obstructions. The clinical course of asthma is unpredictable, ranging from paroxysms of dyspnea and wheezing to unremitting symptoms such as in status asthmaticus.

- Asthma affects an estimated 1 in 20 Americans with 14 to 15 million people affected. The incidence of asthma has increased 60% since the 1980s. It is not really known why the incidence has increased.

Pathophysiology

The hallmarks of asthma are airway inflammation and nonspecific hyperirritability or hyperresponsiveness of the tracheobronchial tree. The airway hyperresponsiveness seen in asthma is caused by bronchoconstriction in response to physical, chemical, or pharmacologic agents. Triggers of acute asthma attacks are listed in Table 9.

The prominent features of asthma are a reduction in airway diameter and an increase in airway resistance related to mucosal inflammation, constriction of bronchial smooth muscles, and excess production of mucus.

- The *early-phase response* in asthma is characterized by bronchospasm, which induces the inflammatory sequelae of the late-phase response. The early-phase response is triggered when an allergen or irritant cross-links with immunoglobulin E (IgE) receptors on mast cells found in the bronchial wall. The mast cells become activated with subsequent release of granules. Substances such as histamine, bradykinin, and prostaglandins are then released. These substances cause bronchial smooth muscle constriction, increased vasodilation, and epithelial damage. Signs include wheezing, chest tightness, dyspnea, and cough.
- The *late-phase response* peaks 5 to 6 hours after exposure to an allergen and may last for several hours or days. This response heightens airway reactivity, which may worsen the symptoms of future asthma attacks. Increased airway resistance leads to air being trapped in the alveoli and lung hyperinflation.

Table 9	Triggers of Acute Asthma Attacks

- Allergen inhalation
- Air pollutants
- Viral upper respiratory infection
- Sinusitis
- Exercise and cold, dry air
- Drugs
- Occupational exposure
- Food additives
  Sulfites (bisulfites and
    metabisulfites)
  Tartrazine
- Hormones/menses
- Gastroesophageal reflux

Clinical Manifestations

- Asthma attacks may have an abrupt or gradual onset, may last a few minutes to several hours, and a person may be asymptomatic with normal pulmonary function between attacks.
- Characteristic manifestations are wheezing, cough, dyspnea, a feeling of suffocation, and chest tightness. Expiration may be prolonged.
- Additional signs of hypoxemia include restlessness, increased anxiety, increased pulse and BP, and increased respiratory rate with the use of accessory muscles immediately after a meal.
- Percussion reveals hyperresonance of the lungs. Auscultation indicates inspiratory or expiratory wheezing.
- Severely diminished breath sounds are an ominous sign, indicating severe obstruction and impending respiratory failure.
  Table 10 presents a correlation between arterial blood gases (ABGs) and clinical manifestations during an acute asthma attack.

Complications

Status asthmaticus is a severe, life-threatening complication of asthma that may be refractory to usual treatment. It places the patient at risk for respiratory failure.

- Causes of status asthmaticus include viral illnesses, ingestion of aspirin or nonsteroidal antiinflammatory drugs (NSAIDs), emotional stress, an increase in allergen exposure, abrupt discontinuation of drug therapy (especially corticosteroids and theophylline), and abuse of aerosol medication. The patient usually reports a history of poorly controlled asthma progressing over days or weeks.
- Clinical manifestations are similar to those of asthma, but they are more severe and prolonged.
- Hypertension, sinus tachycardia, and ventricular arrhythmias may also occur.

Table 10   Arterial Blood Gas Results Correlated with Clinical Manifestations During an Acute Asthmatic Attack

Time frame	pH	$PaCO_2$	PaO_2	Physiologic event	Clinical manifestations
Early in attack	↑	↓	↓	Alveolar hyperventilation → hypocarbia Hypoxemia secondary to ventilation-perfusion mismatch	Use of all accessory muscles of ventilation to overcome increased airway resistance Increased heart rate, diaphoresis, chest tightness, cough, wheezing
Progressive attack	N	N	↓	Adequate alveolar ventilation CO_2 not being eliminated as well Decrease in effective alveolar ventilation	Tiring of patient and difficulty with increased work of breathing
Prolonged attack, status asthmaticus	↓	↓	↓	Hypercapnia indicating that ventilation is no longer adequate Alveolar hypoventilation → respiratory acidosis Worsening hypoxemia as result of hypoventilation and ventilation-perfusion mismatch	Exhaustion, diminished breath sounds, intubation and mechanical ventilation necessary

CO_2, Carbon dioxide; N, normal; $PaCO_2$, partial pressure of carbon dioxide in arterial blood; PaO_2, partial pressure of oxygen in arterial blood

- Complications include pneumothorax, pneumomediastinum, acute cor pulmonale, and respiratory muscle fatigue leading to respiratory arrest.
- Death from status asthmaticus is usually the result of respiratory arrest or cardiac failure.

Management focuses on correcting hypoxemia and improving ventilation, measures similar to those for acute asthma.

Diagnostic Studies

- Pulmonary function tests, including bronchodilator therapy response, are used to diagnose asthma and give an objective measurement of airflow obstruction.
- Sputum specimen (Gram stain and culture), if indicated, is used to rule out bacterial infection.
- Serum IgE levels and eosinophil count are measured.
- Chest x-ray during an attack shows hyperinflation.
- ABGs with mild attack show respiratory alkalosis and normal partial pressure of oxygen in arterial blood (PaO_2). Hypercapnia and respiratory acidosis indicate severe disease.
- Pulse oximetry is used to determine oxygenation status in mild asthma.
- Allergy testing may indicate the specific allergen causing the attack.

Collaborative Care

- Prevention management includes teaching the patient who has persistent airflow obstruction and frequent attacks of asthma to avoid triggers of acute attacks and to premedicate before exercising.
- The patient with mild to moderate asthma should use inhaled β-adrenergic agents or cromolyn (Intal) before exercising or when anticipating exposure to allergens.
- For moderate to severe asthma, inhaled corticosteroids, cromolyn, nedocromil (Tilade), inhaled or oral β-agonists, and theophylline can be used to prevent or alleviate symptoms.
- Some persons require continuous oral corticosteroids, which should be maintained at as low a dosage as possible and administered on alternate days (if possible) to reduce systemic side effects.

For a list of drugs used in the treatment of asthma and chronic obstructive pulmonary disease (COPD), see Table 27-6, Lewis and others, *Medical-Surgical Nursing,* edition 5, p. 669. Therapy should be continued until the patient is breathing comfortably, wheezing has disappeared, and pulmonary function study results are near baseline values.

Nursing Management

Goals

The patient with asthma will have normal or near normal pulmonary function, normal activity level, no recurrent exacerbations of asthma or a decreased incidence of attacks, and adequate knowledge to participate in and carry out a treatment plan.

See NCP 27-1 for the patient with asthma, Lewis and others, *Medical-Surgical Nursing,* edition 5, p. 677.

Nursing Diagnoses

- Ineffective breathing pattern *related to* increased airway resistance, bronchospasm, mucosal edema, and mucus production
- Anxiety *related to* difficulty breathing, perceived or actual loss of control, and fear of suffocation
- Risk for infection *related to* decreased pulmonary function and ineffective airway clearance
- Ineffective management of therapeutic regimen *related to* lack of knowledge about asthma and its treatment

Nursing Interventions

During an acute attack of asthma, it is important to monitor the patient's respiratory and cardiovascular systems. This includes auscultating lung sounds; taking pulse rate, respiratory rate, and BP; and monitoring ABGs, pulse oximetry, and peak expiratory flow rates.

- The patient's work of breathing (i.e., use of accessory muscles, degree of fatigue) and response to therapy should be evaluated. If the patient's condition deteriorates, the physician needs to be notified immediately to initiate prompt medical intervention.
- Nursing interventions include administering oxygen (O_2), bronchodilators, chest physical therapy, and medications.
- A calm, quiet, reassuring attitude may help the patient relax. The patient should be positioned comfortably (usually sitting) to maximize chest expansion. Staying with the patient and being available provide additional comfort. Encouraging slow breathing through pursed lips can be helpful.

▼ Patient Teaching

The nursing role in preventing asthma attacks or decreasing their severity focuses on teaching the patient and family.

- The patient should be taught to avoid known personal triggers for asthma (e.g., cigarette smoke, pet dander) and irritants (e.g., cold air, aspirin, foods, cats). If cold air cannot be avoided, dressing properly with a scarf or mask helps reduce the risk of an asthma attack. Aspirin and NSAIDs (e.g., indomethacin [Indocin]) should be avoided if they are known to precipitate an attack. Many over-the-counter (OTC) drugs contain aspirin, and the patient should be instructed to read labels carefully.

- β-Adrenergic blocking agents (e.g., propranolol [Inderal]) should not be used because they inhibit bronchodilation.

- The patient with asthma needs to learn about medications that may be recommended and to develop self-management strategies. Some patients may benefit from keeping a diary to record medication use, presence of wheezing or coughing, drug side effects, and activity level. This information will be valuable in helping the health care provider adjust the medication.

- The patient needs to be instructed to recognize triggers of acute exacerbation so that it will be possible to medicate early, continue medication according to individually predetermined protocols until symptoms improve, or seek emergency care at a predetermined place.

- It is most helpful for the physician or nurse to write a detailed individual protocol about what to do with medications once early warning signs of an acute exacerbation occur.

- Relaxation therapies (e.g., yoga, meditation, and breathing techniques) may be of value in helping the patient relax respiratory muscles and decrease respiratory rate.

- The patient should be taught to maintain a fluid intake of 2 to 3 L/day. Good nutrition and avoidance of overeating are other important measures. Physical exercise (e.g., swimming, walking, stationary cycling) within the patient's limit of tolerance is also beneficial.

- A plan should be developed with the patient and family that defines what can be done to help the patient during an asthmatic attack. Family members need to know where the patient's inhalers, oral medication, and emergency phone numbers are located. Family members can also be instructed on how to decrease patient anxiety if an asthma attack occurs.

- Counseling may be indicated to help the patient and family resolve personal, family, social, and occupational problems that have resulted from asthma.

BELL'S PALSY

Definition/Description

Bell's palsy (peripheral facial paralysis, acute benign cranial polyneuritis) is a disorder characterized by a disruption of motor branches of the facial nerve (CN VII) on one side of the face in the absence of any other disease such as a stroke.

- The exact etiology is not known, but current theories suggest that the herpes simplex virus (HSV) may be involved in the majority of cases.
- The onset of Bell's palsy is often accompanied by an outbreak of herpes vesicles in or around the ear.
- Bell's palsy is considered benign with full recovery after 6 months in about 85% of patients, especially if treatment is instituted immediately.

Clinical Manifestations

Paralysis of the motor branches of the facial nerve typically results in a flaccidity of the affected side of the face, with drooping of the mouth accompanied by drooling. An inability to close the bottom eyelid, with an upward movement of the eyeball when closure is attempted, is also evident.

- A widened palpebral fissure (opening between the eyelids), flattening of nasolabial fold, unilateral loss of taste, and inability to smile, frown, or whistle are also common.
- Fever, tinnitus, and a hearing deficit may occur.
- Decreased muscle movement may alter chewing ability, and some patients may experience a loss of tearing or excessive tearing.
- Pain may be present behind the ear on the affected side, especially before the onset of paralysis.

Complications can include psychologic withdrawal because of changes in appearance, malnutrition and dehydration, mucous membrane trauma, corneal abrasions, and facial spasms and contractures.

The diagnosis of Bell's palsy is one of exclusion. Diagnosis is indicated by observation of the typical pattern of onset and the testing of percutaneous nerve excitability by electromyogram (EMG).

Collaborative Care

- Corticosteroids, especially prednisone, are started immediately and the best results are obtained if corticosteroids are initiated before paralysis is complete. When the patient improves to the point that corticosteroids are no longer necessary, they should be tapered off over a 2-week period. Usually corticosteroid treatment decreases the edema and pain, but mild analgesics can be used if necessary.

- Because HSV is implicated in approximately 70% of cases of Bell's palsy, treatment with acyclovir (Zovirax) alone or in conjunction with prednisone is used. Newer drugs include valacyclovir (Valtrex) and famciclovir (Famvir).
- Other methods of treatment include moist heat, gentle massage, and electrical stimulation of the nerve. Stimulation may maintain muscle tone and prevent atrophy. Care is primarily focused on relief of symptoms and prevention of complications.

Nursing Management

Goals

The patient with Bell's palsy will be pain free or have pain controlled, maintain adequate nutritional status, not experience injury to the eye, return to normal or previous perception of body image, and be optimistic about disease outcome.

Nursing Diagnoses

- Pain *related to* the inflammation of CN VII
- Altered nutrition: less than body requirements *related to* inability to chew secondary to muscle weakness
- Risk for injury to the eye (corneal abrasion) *related to* inability to blink
- Body image disturbance *related to* change in facial appearance secondary to facial muscle weakness

Nursing Interventions

- Mild analgesics can relieve pain. Hot wet packs can reduce discomfort of herpetic lesions and relieve pain.
- The face should be protected from cold and drafts because trigeminal hyperesthesia may accompany the syndrome.
- Maintenance of good nutrition is important. The patient should be taught to chew on the unaffected side of the mouth to avoid trapping food and to improve taste. Thorough oral hygiene must be carried out after each meal to prevent development of parotitis, caries, and periodontal disease from accumulated residual food.
- Dark glasses may be worn for protective and cosmetic reasons. Artificial tears (methylcellulose) should be instilled frequently during the day to prevent corneal drying. Ointment and an impermeable eye shield can be used at night to retain moisture. In some patients taping the lids closed at night may be effective.
- A facial sling may be helpful to support affected muscles, improve lip alignment, and facilitate eating. Vigorous facial massage can break down tissues, but gentle upward massage has psychologic benefits. When function begins to return, active facial exercises are performed several times a day.

- The change in physical appearance can be devastating; the patient needs to be reassured that a stroke did not occur and that chances for a full recovery are good. The patient's need for privacy should be respected, especially during meals. Enlisting support from family and friends is important.

BENIGN PROSTATIC HYPERPLASIA

Definition/Description

Benign prostatic hyperplasia (BPH) refers to an increase in the amount of epithelial and especially stromal tissue within the prostate gland. It is the most common problem of the adult male genitourinary (GU) system.

- This problem occurs in about 50% of men over the age of 50 and 75% of men over the age of 70. BPH is most likely to develop in the innermost part of the prostate, whereas cancer is most likely to develop in the outer part of the prostate gland.
- Prostatic hyperplasia does not predispose a patient to the development of prostate cancer.

Pathophysiology

BPH begins with enlargement of the glandular tissue. Although the cause is not completely understood, it is thought that the increased number of cells results from endocrine changes associated with aging.

- Excessive accumulation of dihydroxytestosterone (the principal intraprostatic androgen), estrogen stimulation, and local growth hormone action are proposed causes.

Clinical Manifestations

The patient seeks assistance for relief of symptoms related to urinary obstruction. Symptoms are usually gradual in onset and may not be noticed until prostatic enlargement has been present for some time.

- With increasing blockage, obstructive symptoms of BPH develop, including a decrease in the caliber and force of the urinary stream, hesitancy in initiating voiding, dribbling at the end of urination, and a feeling of incomplete bladder emptying because of urinary retention.
- Irritative symptoms, including nocturia, dysuria, and urgency, can develop from inflammatory, infectious, or neoplastic causes.
- The patient is at increased risk for urinary tract infection because of the failure of the bladder to empty completely.

- Residual urine provides a favorable environment for bacterial growth, and calculi may develop due to alkalinization of residual urine.
- Breakage of tiny overstretched blood vessels in the bladder may produce hematuria.

Complications resulting from urinary retention are abnormally distended ureters (hydroureters), destruction of kidney parenchyma from back pressure of the urine (hydronephrosis), and pyelonephritis. These complications can lead to renal failure.

Diagnostic Studies

- Physical examination including digital rectal examination (DRE) for prostate enlargement and consistency
- Urinalysis with culture to indicate infection or inflammation
- Serum creatinine and blood urea nitrogen (BUN) levels to assess renal involvement with long-standing BPH
- Prostate specific antigen (PSA) examined as an indicator of prostate cancer
- Urodynamic flow studies and transrectal ultrasound scan of prostate
- Cystourethroscopy to evaluate bladder neck obstruction for surgical candidates

Collaborative Care

The primary treatment for BPH is referred to as "watchful waiting." If the patient begins to have signs or symptoms that indicate an increase in urethral obstruction, then further treatment is indicated. There are numerous treatment options for BPH.

Drug therapy. Hormonal manipulation can be used to cause regression of hyperplastic tissue through the suppression of androgens. Finasteride (Proscar) blocks the testosterone metabolite dihydroxytestosterone, the principal intraprostatic androgen. This results in a decrease in prostate size and increased urine flow.

- α-Adrenergic receptor blockers cause smooth muscle relaxation in prostate tissue, which ultimately facilitates urinary flow. Selective α-adrenergic blockers such as prazosin (Minipress), doxazosin (Cardura), and terazosin (Hytrin) are currently being used.

Nonsurgical invasive procedures. If BPH becomes symptomatic, nonsurgical invasive options may be tried before surgery. These outpatient options include microwave therapy, prostatic balloon dilation, laser ablation, and stents or coils.

- *Microwave therapy* involves the use of heat to reduce prostatic tissue. There are two types of microwave treatment. One is called hyperthermia and involves either a transurethral or transrectal (rarely used today) heated probe. A second type is transurethral microwave therapy (transurethral microwave antenna [TUMA]). In this treatment, a microwave urethral probe or catheter heats prostatic tissue to a temperature >113° F (>45° C) to produce tissue necrosis.

- A *prostatic balloon device* dilates the urethra by stretching, fracturing, or compressing the gland to enlarge the passage and allow for the free flow of urine. If the procedure is successful, an indwelling catheter is left in place for the first 24 hours to monitor urinary output and hematuria.

- *Stents* (stainless steel) or *coils* (titanium) placed in the prostatic urethra hold back the walls of the prostate to allow the unobstructed flow of urine. In the majority of cases the stents become completely covered by epithelium, reducing the risk of encrustation and infection. The procedure is used mostly for men who have contraindications to surgery, because only local anesthesia is required for this procedure.

Advantages and disadvantages of the various nonsurgical invasive treatment options are compared in Table 52-3, Lewis and others, *Medical-Surgical Nursing,* edition 5, p. 1556.

Surgical therapy. Surgery is indicated when there is a decrease in urine flow sufficient to cause discomfort, persistent residual urine, acute urinary retention because of obstruction with no reversible precipitating cause, or hydronephrosis.

- Treatment of symptomatic BPH primarily involves resection of the prostate. The selection of a surgical approach depends on size and position of the prostatic enlargement.

- Major postoperative complications of surgery are hemorrhage, infection, bladder spasm, and erectile problems.

Laser ablation using a transurethral ultrasound-guided laser-induced prostatectomy (TULIP) is another treatment that shrinks prostatic tissue.

The *transurethral resection* (TUR or TURP) approach is the most common route for partial removal of the prostate. A large three-way indwelling catheter with a 30 ml balloon containing sterile water is usually inserted into the bladder after the procedure to provide hemostasis and facilitate urinary drainage. The bladder is irrigated, either continuously or intermittently, for at least 24 hours to prevent obstruction from mucous threads and blood clots.

- TUR is the surgery of choice for the debilitated patient or for the patient with moderate prostatic enlargement. Advantages of TUR are that it does not involve an external incision and is less likely to result in erectile dysfunction or long-term incontinence. A disadvantage is that it does not completely remove all prostatic tissue, leaving the potential for recurrence of hyperplasia.

A *transurethral incision of the prostate* (TUIP) can be done in at-risk patients, those with mild obstruction, or in younger patients.

Transurethral slits or incisions are made into the prostatic tissue to relieve bladder neck obstruction. This method is usually used to treat intravesical obstruction related to BPH.

- The patient is discharged with an indwelling catheter for the first 24 hours to monitor urinary output and hematuria. Table 52-3, Lewis and others, *Medical-Surgical Nursing,* edition 5, p. 1556 lists the advantages and disadvantages of this procedure.

B

Nursing Management

Because the nurse is most directly involved with the care of patients having prostatic surgery, the focus of nursing management will be on preoperative and postoperative care.

Goals

Overall preoperative goals for the patient having prostatic surgery are to have restoration of urinary drainage, treatment of any urinary tract infection, and understanding of the upcoming surgery. Overall postoperative goals are that the patient will have no complications, complete bladder emptying, restoration of urinary control, and satisfying sexual expression.

See NCP 52-1 for the patient undergoing transurethral resection, Lewis and others, *Medical-Surgical Nursing,* edition 5, p. 1560.

Nursing Diagnoses/Collaborative Problems

Preoperative

- Pain *related to* bladder distention
- Fear *related to* actual or potential sexual dysfunction, possible diagnosis of cancer, and lack of knowledge regarding surgical procedure and postoperative care
- Risk for infection *related to* indwelling catheter, environmental pathogens, and urinary stasis

Postoperative

- Pain *related to* bladder spasms, presence of catheter, and surgical procedure
- Urge incontinence *related to* poor sphincter control
- Potential complication: hemorrhage *related to* surgical procedure

Nursing Interventions

Because the cause of BPH is poorly understood, the focus of health promotion is on early detection and treatment. The American Cancer Society recommends a yearly medical history and digital rectal exam for men over age 40 for early detection of prostate problems. After age 50 and when symptoms of prostatic hyperplasia become evident, further diagnostic screening may be necessary.

- Some men find that ingestion of alcohol and caffeine tends to increase prostatic symptoms because of the diuretic effect that increases bladder distention. Compounds found in common cough and cold remedies such as pseudoephedrine (in Sudafed) and phenylephrine (in Allerest or Coricidin preparations) often worsen BPH symptoms.

- Patients with obstructive symptoms should be advised to urinate every 2 to 3 hours or when they first feel the urge in order to minimize urinary stasis and acute urinary retention.

Preoperative care. Urinary drainage must be restored before surgery; a urethral catheter such as a Coudé (curved-tip) catheter may be needed.

- Any infection of the urinary tract must be treated before surgery. Restoring drainage and encouraging a high fluid intake are helpful.
- The patient is usually concerned about the impact of impending surgery on sexual function. The nurse should provide an opportunity for the patient to express his concerns.

Postoperative care. The plan of care should be adjusted to the type of surgery, reasons for surgery, and patient response to surgery.

- After prostatectomy the bladder may be continuously irrigated with sterile normal saline solution to remove clotted blood from the bladder and ensure drainage of urine. Some form of irrigation (continuous or intermittent) may be used for 24 hours or until no clots are noted draining from the bladder.
- Blood clots are normal for the first 24 to 36 hours. However, large amounts of bright red blood in the urine can indicate hemorrhage.
- Activities that increase abdominal pressure, such as sitting or walking for prolonged periods and straining to have a bowel movement, should be avoided.
- Bladder spasms occur as a result of irritation of the bladder mucosa from insertion of a resectoscope, the presence of a catheter, or clots leading to obstruction of the catheter. The patient should be instructed not to attempt to urinate around the catheter because this increases the likelihood of spasm. If bladder spasms develop, the catheter should be checked for clots. If present, the clots should be removed by irrigation so urine can flow freely. Belladonna and opium suppositories, along with relaxation techniques, are used to relieve pain and decrease spasm.
- Sphincter tone may be poor after catheter removal, resulting in incontinence or dribbling. Sphincter tone can be strengthened by having the patient practice Kegel exercises (pelvic floor muscle technique). Continence can improve for up to 12 months. If continence has not been achieved by that time, the patient may be referred to a continence clinic; a variety of methods, including biofeedback, have been used to achieve positive results. The patient can also use a penile clamp, condom catheter, or incontinent briefs to avoid embarrassment from dribbling.

- The patient should be observed for signs of postoperative infection. If an external wound is present, the area should be observed for redness, heat, swelling, and purulent drainage. Rectal procedures, such as rectal temperatures and enemas (except insertion of well-lubricated belladonna and opium suppositories), should be avoided.
- The catheter should be connected to a closed drainage system and not disconnected unless it is being removed, changed, or irrigated. Secretions that accumulate around the meatus can be cleansed daily with soap and water.
- Dietary intervention and stool softeners are important to prevent the patient from straining while having bowel movements. Straining increases intraabdominal pressure, which can lead to bleeding at the operative site. A diet high in fiber facilitates the passage of stool.

▼ **Patient Teaching**

Discharge planning and home care issues are important aspects of postprostatectomy care.

- Instructions include (1) caring for an indwelling catheter, if one is in place; (2) managing urinary incontinence; (3) maintaining oral fluids between 2000 and 3000 ml per day; (4) observing for signs and symptoms of urinary tract and wound infection; (5) preventing constipation; (6) avoiding heavy lifting (>10 pounds; >4.5 kg); and (7) refraining from driving or having intercourse for 6 weeks after surgery or as directed by the surgeon.
- Sexual counseling and treatment options may be necessary if erectile dysfunction becomes a chronic or permanent problem. Patients may also require counseling regarding treatment options, which include drug therapy, vacuum or constriction devices, implants, and surgery.
- Many men experience retrograde ejaculation after prostatectomy because of trauma to the internal sphincter. Semen is discharged into the bladder at orgasm and may produce cloudy urine when the patient urinates after orgasm. The nurse should discuss these changes with the patient and his partner and allow them to ask questions and express their concerns.
- The bladder may take up to 2 months to return to its normal capacity. The patient should be instructed to drink at least 1 to 2 L of fluid per day and to urinate every 2 to 3 hours. Bladder irritants such as caffeine products, citrus juices, and alcohol should be avoided or limited to small amounts.
- The patient must be advised that he should continue to have yearly DREs if he has had any procedure other than complete removal of the prostate. Hyperplasia or cancer can occur in the remaining prostatic tissue.

BLADDER CANCER

Definition/Description

Bladder cancer accounts for nearly one in every 20 cancers diagnosed in the United States. The most frequent malignant tumor of the urinary tract is transitional cell carcinoma of the bladder. Cancer of the bladder is most common between the ages of 60 and 70 years and is at least three times as common in men as in women.

Risk factors for bladder cancer include cigarette smoking, exposure to dyes used in the rubber and cable industries, and chronic abuse of phenacetin-containing analgesics. Individuals with chronic, recurrent stones and chronic lower urinary tract infections also have an increased risk of squamous cell bladder cancer.

Clinical Manifestations

- Gross, painless hematuria is the most common clinical finding in 85% to 90% of patients. Bladder irritability with dysuria, frequent urination, and intermittent bleeding may also occur.
- When cancer is suspected, urine specimens for cytology can be obtained to determine the presence of neoplastic or atypical cells.

Diagnostic Studies

Bladder cancer can be detected by intravenous pyelogram (IVP), ultrasound, CT, or MRI. Bladder cancer is confirmed by cytoscopy and biopsy. Clinical staging is determined by the depth of invasion of the bladder wall and surrounding tissue. Bladder tumors are staged using the Jewett-Strong-Marshall system or the TNM system (Table 11).

- The Jewett-Strong-Marshall system broadly classifies bladder cancer as a superficial, invasive, or metastatic disease.
- Pathologic grading systems are also used to classify the malignant potential of tumor cells, indicating a scale ranging from well differentiated to anaplastic categories.
- Low-stage, low-grade bladder cancers are most responsive to treatment and more easily cured.

Nursing and Collaborative Management

Surgical therapy may involve a variety of procedures including the following.

- *Transurethral resection and fulguration* (electrocautery) is used for diagnosis and treatment of superficial lesions with a low recurrence rate. This procedure is also used to control bleeding in patients who are poor operative risks or who have advanced tumors.

Table 11	TNM Classification System

Primary Tumor (T)
T_0 No evidence of primary tumor
T_{is} Carcinoma in situ
T_{1-4} Ascending degrees of increase in tumor size and
         involvement

Regional Lymph Nodes (N)
N_0 No evidence of disease in lymph nodes
N_{1-4} Ascending degrees of nodal involvement
N_x Regional lymph nodes unable to be assessed clinically

Distant Metastases (M)
M_0 No evidence of distant metastases
M_{1-4} Ascending degrees of metastatic involvement of the host,
         including distant nodes

- *Laser photocoagulation* can be repeated a number of times for superficial bladder cancer and recurrence. The advantages of this procedure include bloodless destruction of lesions, minimal risk of perforation, and the lack of a need for a urinary catheter.
- *Open loop resection* (snaring of polyp-type lesions) *and fulguration* is used to control bleeding for large superficial tumors and multiple lesions. Treatment of large lesions entails a segmental resection of the bladder.

Postoperative management of the patient who has had one of these surgical procedures includes instructions to drink large amounts of fluid each day, measurement of intake and output, avoidance of alcoholic beverages, use of analgesics and stool softeners (if necessary), and sitz baths to promote muscle relaxation and reduce urinary retention.

- The nurse should also help the patient and family cope with fears about cancer, surgery, and sexuality and should emphasize the importance of regular follow-up care. Frequent routine cystoscopies are required.

When the tumor is invasive or involves the trigone (area where ureters insert into the bladder) and the patient otherwise has a good life expectancy and no demonstrated metastases beyond the pelvic area, a *radical cystectomy* with urinary diversion is the treatment of choice.

- Radiation therapy is used with cystectomy or as the primary therapy when the cancer is inoperable or when surgery is refused (see Radiation Therapy, p. 681).

- Chemotherapy with local instillation of chemotherapeutic or immune-stimulating agents can be delivered into the bladder by a urethral catheter. Intravesical chemotherapeutic agents include bacille Calmette-Guérin (BCG), the drug of choice, and thiotepa if BCG fails and the cancer returns. These agents are instilled directly into the patient's bladder and retained for about 2 hours; position of the patient may be changed every 15 minutes for maximum contact in all areas of the bladder.

It is important for the nurse to encourage the patient to increase daily fluid intake and to quit smoking, assess the patient for secondary urinary infection, and stress the need for routine urology follow-up. The patient may have fears or concerns about sexual activity or bladder function that will also need to be addressed.

BONE CANCER

Definition/Description

Primary malignant bone neoplasms are rare in adults and account for <1% of all deaths attributed to cancer. They are characterized by their rapid metastasis and bone destruction. Primary neoplasms occur most frequently during childhood through young adulthood.

Types of bone cancers include osteogenic sarcoma, osteoclastoma, Ewing's sarcoma, and multiple myeloma (see Multiple Myeloma, p. 388).

Osteogenic Sarcoma (Osteosarcoma)

Osteogenic sarcoma is a primary neoplasm of bone that is extremely malignant and is characterized by rapid growth and metastasis. It usually occurs in the metaphyseal region of long bones of the extremities, particularly in regions of the distal femur, proximal tibia, and proximal humerus, as well as the pelvis. Osteogenic sarcoma has its highest incidence in 10- to 25-year-old males.

Clinical manifestations are usually associated with a past history of minor injury and gradual onset of pain and swelling, especially around the knee. The injury does not cause the neoplasm but rather serves to bring the preexisting condition to medical attention.

- The neoplasm grows rapidly and produces a noticeable increase in size of the general region, which can restrict joint motion.

Diagnosis is confirmed from biopsied tissue specimens, elevation of serum alkaline phosphatase and calcium levels, and x-ray findings.

Major advances are being made in treatment. Preoperative chemotherapy is used to decrease tumor size. As a result, limb-salvage surgical procedures are being used more frequently. Amputation (see p. 623) may be necessary. Adjunct chemotherapy following surgery has increased the survival rate.

Osteoclastoma

True osteoclastoma (giant cell tumor) is a malignant, destructive neoplasm that arises in the cancellous ends of long bones in young adults. Giant cell tumors most commonly occur between the ages of 20 and 35. These tumors are mostly (98%) benign.

Common sites are the distal ends of the femur, proximal tibia, and distal radius. The giant cell tumor is a locally destructive lesion, the growth of which extends from a few months to several years.

Clinical manifestations are swelling, local pain, and some disturbances in joint function. X-ray evidence of giant cell tumor is variable but usually reveals local areas of bone destruction and eventual expansion of bone ends.

Treatment initially includes a biopsy to establish the diagnosis followed by surgical curettage of the lesion with bone grafting. After treatment there is a >50% chance of recurrence. Recurrent giant cell tumors may subsequently make amputation necessary.

Ewing's Sarcoma

Ewing's sarcoma is the fourth most common primary malignant neoplasm of the bone, occurring most frequently in male patients under the age of 30. This neoplasm is characterized by rapid growth within the medullary cavities of long bones, especially the femur, pelvis, tibia, and ribs.

- The most frequent site of early metastasis is the lungs. The use of radiation, surgical excision, and chemotherapy has increased the 5-year survival rate to 70%.

Clinical manifestations are progressive local pain, palpable soft-tissue mass, noticeable increase in the size of the affected part, fever, and leukocytosis. Initially, x-rays show periosteal bone destruction.

Treatment usually involves radiation therapy and wide surgical resection of the tumor or amputation. Chemotherapeutic agents commonly used are cyclophosphamide (Cytoxan), vincristine (Oncovin), and doxorubicin (Adriamycin), actinomycin D, and ifosfamide (Ifex). Surgical resection of the tumor has helped decrease the rate of recurrence.

Nursing Management

Goals

The patient with bone cancer will have satisfactory pain relief; maintain preferred activities as long as possible; demonstrate acceptance of body image changes resulting from chemotherapy, radiation, and surgery; be free from injury; and verbalize a realistic idea of disease progression and prognosis.

Nursing Diagnoses

- Pain *related to* disease process, inadequate pain medication, and inadequate comfort measures
- Impaired physical mobility *related to* disease process, pain, weakness, and debility
- Body image disturbance *related to* possible amputation, deformity, swelling, and effects of chemotherapy
- Anticipatory grieving *related to* poor prognosis of disease
- Risk for injury (pathologic fracture) *related to* disease process and inadequate handling or positioning of affected body part

Nursing Interventions

Nursing care of the patient with a malignant bone neoplasm does not differ significantly from care given to the patient with a malignant disease of any other body system. However, special attention is required to reduce complications associated with prolonged bed rest and to prevent pathologic fractures. The patient is often reluctant to participate in therapeutic activities due to weakness and fear of pain. Regular rest periods should be provided between activities. Careful handling of the affected extremity is important to prevent pathologic fractures.

The nurse must be able to assist the patient in accepting the guarded prognosis associated with bone cancer. Inability to accomplish age-specific developmental tasks can increase the frustrations with this condition. General nursing principles related to cancer are applicable (see Cancer, p. 97). Special attention is necessary for problems of pain and dysfunction, chemotherapy, and specific surgery such as spinal cord decompression or amputation.

BREAST CANCER

Definition/Description

Breast cancer is the most common malignancy in North American women and is second only to lung cancer as the leading cause of death from cancer in women. This disease develops in one of every eight American women.

Although the vast majority of breast problems occur in women, men can have breast problems. One out of every 100 cases of breast cancer occurs in men.

Pathophysiology

Although the etiology is not completely understood, a number of factors are thought to be related to the development of breast cancer.

- Factors considered as contributory include long-term oral contraceptive use, young age at menarche and menopause, obesity, and alcohol intake. Environmental factors such as chemical and pesticide exposure and radiation may also play a role.
- Increasing age increases the risk of developing breast cancer. The incidence of breast cancer in women under 25 years of age is very low and increases gradually until age 60. After the age of 60 the incidence increases dramatically.
- A positive family history is an important risk factor, especially if the involved member with breast cancer was premenopausal, had bilateral disease, and was a first-degree relative (i.e., mother, sister, daughter). As many as 5% to 10% of all breast cancer patients may have inherited a specific genetic abnormality in the BRCA-1 and BRCA-2 genes that contributes to the development of breast cancer.

The various types of breast cancer are identified in Table 12. These types are based on histologic characteristics and tumor growth pattern. The natural history of breast cancer varies considerably from patient to patient. Cancer growth can range from slow to rapid.

- Factors that affect growth are axillary node involvement (the more nodes involved, the worse the prognosis), tumor differentiation (morphology of malignant cells), tumor size, estrogen and progesterone receptor status, and abnormal deoxyribonucleic acid (DNA) content.

Clinical Manifestations

Breast cancer is usually first detected as a single lump or as a mammographic breast abnormality. It occurs most often in the upper outer quadrant of the breast because most of the glandular tissue is there.

Table 12   Types of Breast Cancer

Type	Frequency of occurrence
Infiltrating ductal carcinoma (not otherwise specified)	80%
Medullary	5-8%
Colloid (mucinous)	2-4%
Tubular	1-2%
Papillary	1-2%
Infiltrating lobular carcinoma	10-15%
Noninvasive	4-6%
Ductal carcinoma in situ	2-3%
Lobular carcinoma in situ	2-3%

- If palpable, breast cancer is characteristically hard, irregularly shaped, poorly delineated, nonmobile, and nontender. Malignant lesions are characteristically painless and nontender.
- A small percentage of breast cancers present as nipple discharge. The discharge is usually unilateral and may be clear or bloody. Nipple retraction may occur.
- Plugging of the dermal lymphatics can cause skin thickening and exaggeration of the usual skin markings, giving skin the appearance of an orange peel *(peau d'orange)*.
- In large cancers, infiltration, induration, and dimpling (pulling in) of the overlying skin may occur.

Recurrence may be local or regional (skin or soft tissue near mastectomy site, axillary lymph nodes) or distant (most commonly bone, lung, brain, and liver).

Diagnostic Studies
- Physical examination of breast and lymphatics
- Mammography and ultrasound
- Biopsy
- Estrogen and progesterone receptor assays

Collaborative Care
Many prognostic factors are considered when treatment decisions are being made, including lymph node status, tumor size, and histologic classification. All of these factors enter into the *staging* of breast cancer. The most widely accepted staging method is the TNM system (see Table 11, p. 79).

- Breast conservation surgery (lumpectomy) with radiation therapy and modified radical mastectomy with or without reconstruction are currently the most common options for resectable breast cancer. Ten-year overall survival with lumpectomy and radiation is about the same as that with modified radical mastectomy.

Axillary node dissection is often performed regardless of the treatment option selected. Axillary lymph node involvement is one of the most important prognostic factors in breast cancer. The more nodes involved, the greater the risk of recurrence.

Lymphedema (accumulation of lymph in soft tissue) can occur as a result of excision or radiation of the lymph nodes. The patient may experience heaviness, pain, impaired motor function in the arm, and numbness and paresthesia of the fingers. Cellulitis and progressive fibrosis can also result.

- Frequent and sustained elevation of the arm, regular use of a custom-fitted pressure sleeve, and treatment with an inflatable sleeve (pneumomassage) are all helpful in preventing or reducing lymphedema.

Breast conservation surgery (lumpectomy) involves removal of the entire tumor along with a margin of normal tissue. A lymph node dissection is usually done along with a lumpectomy. Radiation therapy is delivered to the entire breast, ending with a boost to the tumor bed. If there is evidence of systemic disease, chemotherapy may be given before radiation therapy.

- One of the main advantages of breast conservation surgery and radiation is that it preserves the breast, including the nipple. The goal of combined surgery and radiation is to maximize the benefits of both cancer treatment and cosmetic outcome while minimizing the risks.

See Table 49-7, Lewis and others, *Medical-Surgical Nursing*, edition 5, p. 1484 for treatment options, side effects, complications, and patient issues related to common surgical procedures to treat breast cancer.

The *modified radical mastectomy* includes removal of the breast and axillary lymph nodes but preserves the pectoralis major muscle. This surgery is selected over breast conservation therapy if the tumor is too large to excise with good margins and attain a reasonable cosmetic result. Some patients may select this procedure over lumpectomy when presented with the choice of either procedure.

Follow-up care. After surgery, the woman must be followed up for the rest of her life at regular intervals. Most women have professional examinations every 3 months for the first 2 years, every 6 months for the next 3 years, and then annually thereafter.

- In addition, the woman must continue to practice monthly breast self-examinations (BSEs) on both breasts or the remaining breast and mastectomy site. The woman should also have yearly mammography of the remaining breast or breast tissue.
- The most common sites of cancer recurrence are at the surgical site and in the opposite breast.

Adjuvant therapy. The decision to recommend adjuvant (additional) therapy after surgery depends on the number of involved nodes, menstrual status, age, cell type, size and extent of the cancer, presence or absence of estrogen receptors, and other preexisting health problems that can complicate treatment.

Adjuvant therapies include radiation therapy and systemic therapies such as chemotherapy, hormonal manipulation, and biologic therapy.

Radiation therapy. The three situations in which radiation therapy may be used for breast cancer are (1) as primary treatment to destroy the tumor or as a companion to surgery to prevent local recurrence, (2) to shrink a large tumor to operable size, and (3) as palliative treatment for pain caused by local recurrence and metastases. Lumpectomy is almost always followed by radiation (see Radiation Therapy, p. 681).

Chemotherapy. Cytotoxic drugs are used to destroy cancer cells. The greatest benefits from chemotherapy have been achieved among premenopausal women with node findings that are positive for malignancy (see Chemotherapy, p. 643).

Hormonal therapy. Estrogen can promote growth of breast cancer cells if cells are estrogen-receptor positive. If the source of estrogen is removed, tumor regression may occur. The source of estrogen (especially estradiol) can be markedly reduced by surgical ablation (e.g., oophorectomy, adrenalectomy, and hypophysectomy) or with additive hormonal therapy.

- Tamoxifen citrate (an antiestrogen drug) is often the first treatment choice in postmenopausal, estrogen receptor–positive women with or without nodal involvement.
- Hormonal therapy is widely used to treat recurrent or metastatic cancer but may occasionally be used as an adjuvant to primary treatment.

Biologic therapy. The use of biologic therapy represents an attempt to stimulate the body's natural defenses to recognize and attack cancer cells. The use of high-dose chemotherapy and autologous or stem cell transplantation bone marrow are other potential treatments for patients with advanced disease. The use of these therapies is discussed in Chapter 14, Lewis and others, *Medical-Surgical Nursing,* edition 5. For further information on adjuvant therapy for breast cancer, see *Medical-Surgical Nursing,* p. 1483.

Nursing Management
Goals
The patient with breast cancer will actively participate in the decision-making process related to treatment options, fully comply with the therapeutic plan, manage side effects of adjuvant therapy, and be satisfied with support provided by significant others and health care providers.

See NCP 49-1 for the patient after a modified radical mastectomy, Lewis and others, *Medical-Surgical Nursing,* edition 5, p. 1487.

Nursing Diagnoses/Collaborative Problems
After a diagnosis of breast cancer and before a treatment plan has been selected, the following diagnoses would apply:

- Decisional conflict *related to* lack of knowledge about treatment options and their effects
- Fear *related to* diagnosis of breast cancer
- Body image disturbance *related to* anticipated physical and emotional effects of treatment modalities

If a modified radical mastectomy is planned, nursing diagnoses and collaborative problems may include:

- Pain *related to* surgical incision and manipulation of tissue
- Fear *related to* diagnosis of cancer

- Impaired physical mobility *related to* decreased arm and shoulder mobility
- Self-esteem disturbance *related to* altered body image and loss of body part
- Potential complication: lymphedema *related to* edema on operative side and lack of knowledge of preventive measures

Nursing Interventions

The time between the diagnosis of breast cancer and the selection of a treatment plan is a difficult period for the woman and her family. Although the primary care provider discusses treatment options, the woman often relies on the nurse to clarify and expand on these options.

- Appropriate nursing interventions during this period include exploring the woman's usual decision-making patterns, helping the woman accurately evaluate the advantages and disadvantages of the options, providing information relevant to the decision, and supporting the patient once a decision is made.
- Regardless of the surgery planned, the patient needs to be provided with sufficient information to ensure informed consent. Teaching in the preoperative phase includes instruction in turning and deep breathing, a review of postoperative exercises, and an explanation of the recovery period from the time of surgery until discharge.

The woman who has breast conservation surgery usually has an uneventful postoperative course with only a moderate amount of pain. The woman who has had a modified radical mastectomy needs nursing interventions specific to this surgery.

- Restoring arm function on the affected side after mastectomy and axillary lymph node dissection is an important goal.
- The woman should be placed in a semi-Fowler's position with the arm on the affected side elevated on a pillow. Flexing and extending the fingers should begin in the recovery room, with progressive increases in activity.

Postoperative discomfort can be minimized by administering analgesics about 30 minutes before initiating exercises. When showering is appropriate, warm water running over the involved shoulder often has a soothing effect and reduces joint stiffness. Whenever possible, the same nurse should work with the woman so that progress can be monitored.

Measures to prevent or reduce lymphedema must be taught. The patient must understand that she is at risk of developing lymphedema for the rest of her life.

- The affected arm should never be dependent, even while the person is sleeping.
- BP readings, venipunctures, and injections should not be done on the affected arm.

- The woman must be instructed to protect the arm on the operative side from even minor trauma such as a pinprick or sunburn.
- If trauma to the arm occurs, the area should be washed thoroughly with soap and water, and a topical antibiotic ointment and bandage should be applied.

Throughout interactions the nurse must keep in mind the extensive psychologic impact of the disease. All aspects of care must include sensitivity to the woman's efforts to cope with a life-threatening disease. The nurse can help meet the woman's psychologic needs by doing the following:

- Assisting her to develop a positive but realistic attitude.
- Helping identify sources of support and strength to her, such as her partner, family, and spiritual practices.
- Encouraging her to verbalize anger and fears about her diagnosis.
- Promoting open communication of thoughts and feelings between the patient and her family.
- Providing accurate and complete answers to questions about the disease, treatment options, and reproductive or lactation issues (if appropriate).
- Offering information about community resources, such as Reach to Recovery, Can Surmount, and local support organizations and groups.

▼ **Patient Teaching**

- The nurse should emphasize the importance of beginning and continuing BSE and annual mammography. Symptoms that should be reported to the clinician include new back pain, weakness, constipation, shortness of breath, and confusion.
- The nurse should stress the importance of wearing a well-fitting prosthesis designed for women who have had a mastectomy.
- A preoperative sexual assessment provides baseline data that the nurse can use to plan postoperative interventions. Often, the husband, sexual partner, or family members may need assistance in dealing with their emotional reactions to the diagnosis and surgery so that they can act as effective means of support for the patient.
- Depression may occur with the continued stress of a cancer diagnosis. Special nursing interventions are necessary for both psychologic support and self-care teaching if a recurrence is found.

Breast reconstruction is discussed in Chapter 49, Lewis and others, *Medical-Surgical Nursing,* edition 5.

BULIMIA

B

Definition/Description
Bulimia is a chronic eating disorder characterized by compulsive binge eating and purging through self-induced vomiting, laxative and exercise abuse, and diuretics. Food becomes an obsession and an addiction, an escape from the pressures of life. Unlike the person with anorexia, the patient caught up in the syndrome of bulimia usually maintains a normal or near-normal body weight.

- Bulimia is increasing in incidence and may be even more prevalent than anorexia nervosa. Female students of college age are the most susceptible to this disorder.

Pathophysiology
The cause of bulimia remains unclear but is thought to be similar to that of anorexia nervosa (see Anorexia Nervosa, p. 49).

Clinical Manifestations
- Unlike anorexia nervosa, the primary symptom is gorging rather than starvation.
- Characteristic skin lesions on the back of the hand, which are often over the metacarpophalangeal joint and are called Russell's sign, can result from repeated trauma to the skin from self-induced vomiting.
- Dental problems may develop from repeated vomiting.
- Swollen glands or salivary gland hypertrophy, sore throat, facial puffiness, chronic indigestion, irregular menstrual periods, electrolyte imbalances, and dehydration can also occur.
- Sudden death from cardiac arrest or fatal arrhythmia is not uncommon.
- Most bulimics have few, if any, noticeable signs of the illness.

Collaborative Care
Treatment is similar to that described for anorexia nervosa. The multidisciplinary approach consists of strategies that include individual psychotherapy, nutritional counseling (including discussion of the dangers involved in binge eating and purging), cognitive behavior therapy, and drug therapy.

- Antidepressants (e.g., fluoxetine [Prozac], amitriptyline [Elavil]) are useful for the depression associated with both anorexia nervosa and bulimia.
- Vitamin, mineral, and iron supplements may be prescribed. However, iron supplementation is not generally required if amenorrhea is present.

The return to normal eating habits may take several months to years to accomplish because relapses are frequent. Recovery is difficult. The abnormal eating behavior is hard to change because binge eating and purging provide the person with a feeling of satisfaction and of control over the body.

Nursing Management

For a discussion of the management of bulimia, see Malnutrition, p. 379.

BURNS

Definition/Description

Burns are a tissue injury resulting from exposure to or direct contact with hot objects, chemicals, electrical current, or smoke.

Pathophysiology

Burn wounds occur when there is contact between tissue and an energy source, such as heat, chemicals, electrical current, or radiation. The resulting effects are influenced by energy intensity, duration of exposure, and type of tissue injured. Immediately after the injury occurs, there is an increase in blood flow to the area surrounding the wound. This is followed by the release of various vasoactive substances from burned tissue, which results in increased capillary permeability. Fluid then shifts from the intravascular compartment to the interstitial space, producing edema and hypovolemia.

Types of Burn Injury

Various types of burn may be seen alone or in combination with other burns.

- Thermal injury is the most common type of burn and can be caused by flame, flash, scald, or contact with hot objects.
- Chemical injury is the result of tissue injury and destruction from necrotizing substances such as acids and alkali substances. Chemicals can cause respiratory, skin, eye, and systemic symptoms for up to 72 hours after the injury.
- Smoke and inhalation injury can cause damage to the respiratory tract. These injuries include carbon monoxide poisoning, thermal burn above the glottis, or chemical burn below the glottis.
- Electrical injury results from coagulation necrosis caused by intense heat from an electric current.

Classification of Burn Injury

The treatment of burns is related to injury severity. A variety of methods exist for determining burn severity.

1. The *depth of burn* is described according to the depth of skin destruction (epidermis, dermis, or subcutaneous tissue) (Table 13).
   - Partial-thickness burn
     Superficial (first degree) with erythema, pain, mild swelling, no vesicles or blisters
     Deep (second degree) with fluid-filled vesicles, severe pain, mild to moderate edema
   - Full-thickness burn (third and fourth degree) with dry, waxy, leathery, or hard skin; pain insensitivity; possible bone, muscle, and tendon involvement
2. The *extent of burn* is calculated as the percent of total body surface area (TBSA) that has been burned. Burn extent is determined by one of two methods:
   - Lund-Browder chart, which takes into account the patient's age and relative body area
   - Rule of Nines chart, which is easy to remember and adequate for initial assessment (Fig. 1)
3. *Burn location* has a direct relationship to the severity of the injury. For example, face and neck burns may inhibit respiratory function; hands, feet, joint, and eye burns may limit self-care and functioning.
4. *Age of patient* influences burn severity because infants (immature immune system) and older patients (decreased defense mechanisms) are less able to cope.
5. *Preexisting disorders* such as cardiovascular, pulmonary, or renal disease reduce the patient's ability to recover from the tremendous demands of burn injury.

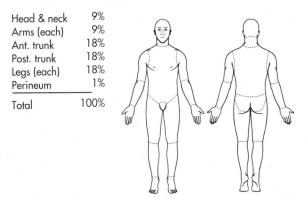

Head & neck	9%
Arms (each)	9%
Ant. trunk	18%
Post. trunk	18%
Legs (each)	18%
Perineum	1%
Total	100%

Fig. 1 Rule of Nines chart.

Table 13   Classification of Burn Injury Depth

Classification	Clinical appearance	Cause	Structure
Partial-thickness skin destruction			
■ Superficial (First-degree)	Erythema, blanching on pressure, pain and mild swelling, no vesicles or blisters (although after 24 hr skin may blister and peel)	Superficial sunburn Quick heat flash	Only superficial devitalization with hyperemia is present. Tactile and pain sensation intact.
■ Deep (Second-degree)	Fluid-filled vesicles that are red, shiny, wet (if vesicles have ruptured); severe pain caused by nerve injury; mild-to-moderate edema	Flame Flash Scald Contact burns Chemical tar	Epidermis and dermis involved to varying depth. Some skin elements, from which epithelial regeneration can occur, remain viable.
Full-thickness skin destruction			
■ (Third- and fourth-degree)	Dry, waxy white, leathery, or hard skin; visible thrombosed vessels; insensitivity to pain and pressure because of nerve destruction; possible involvement of muscle, tendons, and bones	Flame Scald Chemical Tar Electrical current	All skin elements and nerve endings destroyed. Coagulation necrosis present.

Table 14 American Burn Association Adult Burn Classification

Magnitude of burn injury	Partial thickness* (second-degree)	Full thickness* (third-degree)	Other factors
Minor	<15%	<2%	Does not involve special care areas (eyes, ears, face, hands, feet, perineum); excludes electrical injury, inhalation injury, complicated injury (fractures), all poor-risk patients (extremes of age, concomitant disease)
Moderate uncomplicated	15-25%	2-10%	Excludes electrical injury, inhalation injury, complicated injury, all poor-risk patients; does not involve special care areas
Major	>25%	>10%	Includes all burns involving hands, face, eyes, ears, feet, or perineum; includes inhalation injury, electrical injury, complicated burn injury, and all poor-risk patients; patient should be transferred to a burn unit

*Figures indicate percentage of total body surface area involved.

A major adult burn is classified as >25% TBSA for a partial-thickness (second-degree) burn or >10% for a full-thickness (third-degree) burn (Table 14).

Diagnostic Studies
- Routine laboratory tests
- Serum electrolytes, especially sodium (Na^+) and potassium (K^+)
- Chest x-ray, arterial blood gases (ABGs), and sputum for inhalation injury
- Urine output and specific gravity to assess renal function
- White blood cell (WBC) count and wound cultures if infection is suspected

Collaborative Care
Burn management can be classified into three phases: *emergent* (resuscitative), *acute,* and *rehabilitative.*

Emergent (resuscitative) *phase* is the period of time required to resolve immediate problems resulting from burn injury. This phase may last from burn onset to 5 or more days, but it usually lasts 24 to 48 hours. This phase begins with fluid loss and edema and continues until fluid mobilization and diuresis begin.
- From the onset of the burn event until the patient is stabilized, therapy predominantly consists of airway management, fluid therapy, and wound care.
- Drug therapy includes analgesics and narcotics for comfort and pain control and topical antibacterial agents.

Acute phase begins with mobilization of extracellular fluid and subsequent diuresis. The acute phase is concluded when the burned area is completely covered or when the wounds are healed. This may take weeks or many months.
- Predominant management in the acute phase is fluid replacement, physical therapy, wound care, and early excision and grafting.
- Pain management includes the use of multiple drugs and alternate methods of pain relief such as guided imagery.
- Nutritional management is to minimize energy demands and provide adequate calories (often 5000 kcal/day) to promote healing.

Rehabilitation phase begins when the burn wound is covered with skin or healed and the patient is capable of assuming some self-care activity. This can occur as early as 2 weeks to as long as 2 or 3 months after the injury.
- Rehabilitation goals are to assist the patient in resuming a functional role in society and to accomplish functional and cosmetic reconstruction.

Clinical Manifestations

- *Emergent phase:* Characterized by possible shock from pain and hypovolemia, intense thirst, minimal urine output, shivering as a result of heat loss or anxiety, and possible disorientation. Complications may include arrhythmias, airway obstruction, and acute tubular necrosis and renal failure.

- *Acute phase:* Wounds may or may not have intact blisters and are painful to touch. Complications may include infection progressing to bacteremia, acute delirium at night, contractures, Curling's ulcer, occult blood in stool, and stress diabetes.

- *Rehabilitative phase:* Contractures may occur if range of motion (ROM) is not adequate, and the healing site, which is extremely sensitive to trauma, may itch. Complications are skin and joint contractures and hypertrophic scarring.

Nursing Management

Goals

The patient with a burn injury will have self-care activities resumed, an absence of contractures, weight loss not >10% of body weight, rapid control if wound becomes infected, no pain or a tolerable level of pain, and verbalization of realistic goals.

See NCP 23-1 for the burn patient, Lewis and others, *Medical-Surgical Nursing,* edition 5, p. 534.

Nursing Diagnoses

- Risk for fluid volume deficit *related to* evaporative loss, plasma loss, and fluid shift
- Pain *related to* burn injury and treatments
- Anticipatory grieving *related to* change in body image
- Self-care deficits *related to* pain, immobility, and perceived helplessness
- Risk for infection *related to* impaired skin integrity
- Impaired physical mobility *related to* contractures secondary to pain and immobility
- Altered nutrition: less than body requirements *related to* increased caloric demands

Nursing Interventions

- *Emergent phase:* Assess adequacy of airway management and fluid therapy, provide pain medication and wound care, and offer support to patient and family.

- *Acute phase:* Wound care, fluid therapy, comfort, hygiene measures, and ROM exercises continue. A critical function is pain assessment and management.

- *Rehabilitative phase:* Responsibility is shared among the health care team to return the patient to optimal functioning.

▼ Patient Teaching

- Describe to the patient and family the burn injury process and the expected signs and symptoms related to phases of burn management.
- Explain therapeutic interventions, precautionary measures, gowning and handwashing, and institution visiting policy to elicit cooperation and decrease anxiety.
- Teach the patient to watch for injuries to new skin.
- Instruct the patient and family about the signs and symptoms of infection so early treatment can be initiated.
- Teach the family how to perform dressing changes to ensure proper technique and increase their sense of control.
- Emphasize the importance of exercise and appropriate physical therapy to the patient and family. Plan a daily program with the patient and offer appropriate resources to provide a continuing activity program as needed.
- Assist the patient and family in setting realistic future expectations because anticipatory guidance decreases anxiety and inaccurate perceptions. The patient and family will need anticipatory guidance to know what to expect physiologically as well as psychologically during recovery.
- Provide avenues for the patient and family to maintain contact with hospital personnel after discharge to promote continuity of care and minimize anxiety.

CANCER

Definition/Description

Cancer is a group of more than 200 diseases characterized by un-regulated growth of cells. Cancer is currently the second leading cause of death in the United States. There are differences in the incidence of certain cancers in men and women (Table 15). The death rate from cancer is leveling off or decreasing except for an increasing rate of deaths from lung cancer in women (Table 16).

Table 15 — Cancer Incidence by Site and Sex in 1998*

Male		Female	
Type	**Percentage**	**Type**	**Percentage**
Prostate	29	Breast	30
Lung	15	Lung	13
Colon/rectum	10	Colon/rectum	11
Urinary tract	9	Uterus	8
Leukemia/ lymphoma	8	Leukemia/ lymphoma	7

From *Cancer Statistics 1998,* American Cancer Society, 1998.
*Excluding basal and squamous cell skin cancers and carcinoma in situ.

Table 16 — Estimates of Cancer Deaths by Site and Sex in 1998

Male		Female	
Type	**Percentage**	**Type**	**Percentage**
Lung	32	Lung	25
Prostate	13	Breast	16
Colon/rectum	9	Colon/rectum	11
Leukemia/ lymphoma	9	Leukemia/ lymphoma	8

From *Cancer Statistics 1998,* American Cancer Society, 1998.

Pathophysiology

Two major dysfunctions present in the process of cancer are *defective cellular proliferation* (growth) and *defective cellular differentiation*. The cause and development of each type of cancer is likely to be multifactorial. Tumors may have a chemical, environmental, genetic, immunologic, or viral origin.

Cancer is theorized to develop through the following stages:

- *Initiation* is the irreversible alteration in cellular genetic structure by a chemical, physical, or biologic agent.
- *Promotion* is the reversible proliferation of altered, initiated cells. Promoting factors include dietary fat, obesity, and cigarette smoking. Additional factors that promote cancer development are listed in Table 14-6, Lewis and others, *Medical-Surgical Nursing*, edition 5, p. 274.
- *Progression* involves increased tumor growth, invasiveness, and metastasis. *Metastasis* refers to tumor spread to distant organ sites via the vascular and lymph systems and by implantation (cancer cells embedded along body serosal surfaces).

Tumors can be classified according to:

- Anatomic site (e.g., leukemia originates from hematopoietic tissue)
- Histologic analysis (grading of tumor cells from well differentiated to anaplasia)
- Extent of disease (staging of cancer from 0 to IV)
- The TNM classification system (see Table 11, p. 79), which is used to describe the extent of the disease process according to tumor size (T), degree of regional spread to lymph nodes (N), and absence of metastasis (M).

Clinical Manifestations

Clinical manifestations are dependent on the type of cancer and may include:

- Change in respiratory status with increased frequency of infections and change in cough
- Occult bleeding, diarrhea, constipation, pain, and black tarry stools
- Dysuria and hematuria
- Abnormal uterine bleeding, pain, and change in menstrual pattern
- A sore that does not heal or a change in a wart or mole
- Lump, thickening discharge from the nipple, and breast pain

Table 17 lists the seven warning signs of cancer.

Complications resulting from cancer can include infection, paraneoplastic syndrome, hypercalcemia, superior vena cava syndrome, third space syndrome, and spinal cord compression.

Table 17	Seven Warning Signs of Cancer

C hange in bowel or bladder habits
A sore that does not heal
U nusual bleeding or discharge from any body orifice
T hickening or a lump in the breast or elsewhere
I ndigestion or difficulty in swallowing
O bvious change in a wart or mole
N agging cough or hoarseness

Diagnostic Studies

Various diagnostic studies may be done depending on the suspected primary or metastatic site(s) of the cancer and may include:

- Cytology studies (e.g., Pap smear)
- Chest x-ray
- Oncofetal antigens such as carcinoembryonic (CEA) and α-fetoprotein (AFP) antigens
- Bone marrow examination for hematolymphoid malignancy
- MRI and CT scan
- Proctoscopic examination
- Radioisotope scans (liver, brain, bone, and lung)
- Radiographic studies (e.g., mammogram)
- Biopsy (needle, incisional, and excisional), which can definitively diagnose cancer

Collaborative Care

The goal of cancer treatment is cure, control, or palliation. Factors that determine treatment modality are (1) cell type of the cancer, (2) location and size of the tumor, and (3) extent of the disease. The physiologic and psychologic status and the expressed needs of the patient also play an important part in determining the treatment plan, modalities chosen, and length of treatment administration.

Cancer treatment modalities include:

- Surgery can be used for cure and control (e.g., lumpectomy), supportive care (e.g., colostomy for rectal abscess), and palliation of symptoms (e.g., cordotomy for pain relief).
- Radiation therapy can be given externally or internally (a procedure in which radioactive materials are placed in or near the tumor). Goals of therapy are cure, control, or palliation (see Radiation Therapy, p. 681)
- Chemotherapy, the systemic use of chemicals (drugs), is used to reduce the size of the primary tumor and kill metastatic cancer cells (see Chemotherapy, p. 643)

- Biologic therapy alters the host's biologic response to tumor cells. Two examples are α-interferon and interleukin-2.

Nursing Management

Goals

The patient with cancer will maintain body weight, have adequate energy, demonstrate adequate self-care knowledge, experience adequate relief from pain, have no oral mucosal infections, and effectively communicate with significant others.

See NCP 14-1 for the patient with cancer, Lewis and others, *Medical-Surgical Nursing,* edition 5, p. 307.

Nursing Diagnoses/Collaborative Problems

- Pain *related to* effects of the disease or its treatment
- Altered nutrition: less than body requirements *related to* anorexia, nausea, and vomiting
- Altered family processes *related to* cancer diagnosis of family member
- Fatigue *related to* effects of cancer and treatment
- Ineffective individual coping *related to* depression
- Body image disturbance *related to* hair loss, surgery, and weight loss
- Risk for infection *related to* leukopenia
- Potential complication: bleeding *related to* thrombocytopenia

Nursing Interventions

- Actively listen to the patient's concerns while awaiting diagnostic study results.
- Assess and intervene for adequate relief of pain.
- Manage the commonly experienced side effects associated with radiation therapy, chemotherapy, and biologic therapy.
- Assist with nutritional intake to minimize protein and calorie malnutrition.
- Monitor for signs of complications resulting from cancer.
- Facilitate development of a hopeful attitude.
- Encourage the use of relaxation techniques to reduce anxiety.

▼ Patient Teaching

A predominant role of the nurse is the prevention and early detection of cancer to increase survival rate. The nurse should instruct the patient to:

- Reduce or avoid exposure to known or suspected carcinogens.
- Eat a balanced diet that includes vegetables, fresh fruits, whole grains, and low levels of fats and preservatives.
- Participate in regular exercise and obtain adequate, consistent periods of rest (at least 6 to 8 hours/night).
- Have a health examination on a consistent basis that includes health history, physical examination, and specific diagnostic tests for common cancers.

- Educate the public about the recommended screening guidelines for specific cancer sites (see Cancer Screening Guidelines, p. 712).
- Eliminate, reduce, or change perception of stressors.
- Learn and practice breast and testicular self-examination, and know the seven warning signs of cancer.
- Seek immediate medical care if cancer is suspected.

Education is an extremely important nursing role related to chemotherapy and radiation therapy. Fear and anxiety can be associated with both treatment modalities. The patient must be told what to expect during a course of treatment. The patient also needs to know the possible side effects of chemotherapy and radiation therapy. The nurse needs to provide guidance to the patient and family in setting realistic expectations.

Specific types of cancer are listed under separate headings.

CARDIOMYOPATHY

Definition/Description

Cardiomyopathy (CMP) is a term used to describe a group of heart muscle diseases of unknown etiology that primarily affect the structural and functional abilities of the myocardium. A diagnosis of CMP is based on the patient's clinical manifestations and on noninvasive and invasive cardiac procedures to rule out other causes of dysfunction.

CMP can be classified as primary or secondary:

- *Primary CMP* includes those conditions in which the etiology of the heart disease is unknown. The heart muscle in this instance is the only portion of the heart involved, and other cardiac structures are unaffected.
- In *secondary CMP* the myocardial disease is known and is secondary to another disease process. Common causes of secondary CMP are ischemia, viral infections, illicit drug abuse, and pregnancy.

The World Health Organization has classified CMP conditions into three general types: *dilated (congestive), hypertrophic,* and *restrictive*. Each of these types has its own pathogenesis, clinical presentation, and therapeutic management. All types of CMP can lead to cardiomegaly and congestive heart failure (CHF) (Table 18).

Dilated Cardiomyopathy

Pathophysiology. *Dilated (congestive) cardiomyopathy* is the most common type of CMP, accounting for >90% of all cases, and is characterized by cardiomegaly with ventricular dilation, impairment of

Table 18   Characteristics of Cardiomyopathies

	Dilated	Hypertrophic	Restrictive
Etiology:	Idiopathic condition, alcoholism, pregnancy, myocarditis, nutritional deficiency (vitamin B_1), exposure to toxins and drugs, genetic disease	Inherited disorder (autosomal dominant), possible chronic hypertension	Amyloidosis, postradiation, post-open heart surgery, diabetes mellitus
Major manifestations:	Fatigue, weakness, palpitations, dyspnea, dry cough	Exertional dyspnea, fatigue, angina, syncope, palpitations	Dyspnea, fatigue, palpitations
Cardiomegaly:	Moderate to marked	Mild	Mild to moderate
Contractility:	Decreased	Increased or decreased	Normal or decreased
Valvular incompetence:	Atrioventricular valves, particularly mitral	Mitral valve	Mitral valve
Arrhythmias:	Sinoatrial tachycardia, atrial and ventricular arrhythmias	Tachyarrhythmias	Atrial and ventricular arrhythmias
Cardiac output:	Decreased	Decreased	Normal or decreased
Stroke volume:	Decreased	Normal or increased	Decreased
Ejection fraction:	Decreased	Increased	Normal or decreased
Outflow tract obstruction:	None	Increased	None

systolic function, atrial enlargement, and stasis of blood in the left ventricle (LV). Deterioration is rapid after the development of symptoms.

- No specific cause has been identified, although dilated CMP often follows an infectious myocarditis. Thyrotoxicosis, diabetes mellitus, toxins (especially alcohol and cocaine), and drugs causing a hypersensitivity reaction have all been associated with the development of dilated CMP.

Clinical manifestations. The patient may have signs and symptoms of CHF, including fatigue, dyspnea, orthopnea, palpitations, and anorexia. Signs can include S_3, S_4, tachycardia, pulmonary crackles, edema, pallor, hepatomegaly, and jugular venous distention. The patient may also present with arrhythmias or systemic embolism.

Diagnostic studies. A diagnosis is made on the basis of patient history and ruling out other conditions that cause CHF.

- Chest x-ray shows cardiomegaly.
- ECG may reveal tachycardia and arrhythmias.
- Echocardiography is useful in distinguishing dilated CMP from other structural abnormalities, including ventricular chamber size and heart muscle thickness.
- Cardiac catheterization and coronary angiography are used to evaluate manifestations of dilated CMP.
- Left ventriculogram may reveal abnormal wall motion caused by the dilation within a thinned wall and dilated ventricles.

Nursing and collaborative management. Interventions focus on controlling CHF by enhancing myocardial contractility and decreasing afterload (similar to treatment for chronic CHF).

- Digitalis is used in the presence of atrial fibrillation, diuretics are used to decrease preload, and diuretics and vasodilators such as angiotensin converting enzyme (ACE) inhibitors are used to reduce afterload.
- Drug therapy, nutritional therapy, and cardiac rehabilitation may help to alleviate the symptoms of CHF and improve cardiac output (CO).
- A patient with secondary dilated CMP must be treated for the underlying disease process. For example, the patient with alcohol-induced dilated CMP must abstain from all alcohol intake.
- The patient with terminal end-stage CMP may require cardiac transplantation. This patient is in great need of emotional support.
- Patients with dilated CMP are very ill people with a grave prognosis who need expert nursing care. The patient's family must learn CPR and how to access emergency care in their neighborhood.
- Nursing care should focus on observing the patient's response to medications, monitoring for arrhythmias, and preventing or rapidly detecting emboli.

- The nurse should also educate the patient about the disease process and how to space daily activities to allow for rest periods.

Hypertrophic Cardiomyopathy

Pathophysiology. Hypertrophic cardiomyopathy (HCM), also called idiopathic hypertrophic subaortic stenosis (IHSS), produces asymmetric myocardial hypertrophy without ventricular dilation. HCM occurs less commonly than dilated CMP and is more common in men than in women. HCM seems to have an autosomal dominant genetic basis. It is usually diagnosed in young adulthood and is often seen in active, athletic individuals.

- The primary defect of HCM is diastolic dysfunction. Impaired ventricular relaxation inhibits adequate filling of ventricles during diastole. Decreased ventricular filling and obstruction to outflow can result in decreased CO, especially during exertion when increased CO is needed.

Clinical manifestations. Manifestations of HCM include exertional dyspnea, fatigue, angina, and syncope. The most common symptom is dyspnea, which is caused by an elevated left ventricular diastolic pressure.

- Palpitations are common and are most often due to arrhythmias. Common arrhythmias include atrial fibrillation, ventricular tachycardia, and ventricular fibrillation. Any of these arrhythmias may lead to loss of consciousness or sudden cardiac death, which is the most common cause of death.

Diagnostic studies. Chest x-ray is usually normal except in patients with severe disease causing an increased cardiac silhouette.

- Increased voltage and duration of the QRS complex are the most common abnormalities on the ECG; these findings usually indicate ventricular hypertrophy. Ventricular arrhythmias are also frequently seen, with ventricular tachycardia the most common.
- Echocardiogram is the primary diagnostic tool revealing the classic feature of HCM, which is LV hypertrophy; the echocardiogram may also demonstrate wall motion abnormalities and diastolic dysfunction.
- Cardiac catheterization will document a pressure gradient and depressed diastolic left ventricular compliance if HCM is present.

Nursing and collaborative management. The goal of therapy is to improve ventricular filling by reducing ventricular contractility and relieving LV outflow obstruction. This can be accomplished with the use of β-blockers or calcium channel blockers.

- Antiarrhythmics are used to control arrhythmias; however, their use has not proven to prevent sudden death in this group. An alternative treatment for ventricular arrhythmias may be an implantable defibrillator.
- Some patients may be candidates for surgical treatment (ventriculomyotomy and myectomy) of their hypertrophied septum.

Indications for surgery include severe symptoms refractory to therapy with marked obstruction to aortic outflow.

- Most patients have good symptomatic improvement after surgery and improved exercise tolerance.

Nursing interventions focus on relieving symptoms, observing for and preventing complications, and providing emotional and psychologic support.

- Education should focus on teaching the patient to adjust his or her lifestyle to avoid strenuous activity and dehydration. Any activity or procedure that causes an increase in systemic vascular resistance (thus increasing obstruction to forward blood flow) is dangerous for this patient and should be avoided. The patient should be taught to space activities and allow for rest periods.

Restrictive Cardiomyopathy

Pathophysiology. Restrictive cardiomyopathy is the least common of cardiomyopathic conditions. It is a disease of the heart muscle that impairs diastolic volume and stretch.

- Although a specific etiology of restrictive CMP is unknown, a number of pathologic processes may be involved. These include myocardial fibrosis, hypertrophy, and infiltration, which produce stiffness of the ventricular wall.
- The principal characteristic of restrictive CMP is cardiac muscle stiffness characterized by the loss of ventricular compliance. The ventricles are resistant to filling and therefore demand high diastolic filling pressures to maintain CO.

Clinical manifestations

- Angina, syncope, fatigue, exercise intolerance, and dyspnea on exertion are common signs.
- Additional signs and symptoms are similar to CHF. The patient may have signs of both left-sided and right-sided heart failure, including peripheral edema, ascites, and hepatic dysfunction.
- Kussmaul's sign (bulging of internal jugular neck veins on inspiration) may also be present.

Diagnostic studies

- Chest x-ray may be normal or show cardiomegaly.
- ECG may reveal tachycardia at rest. The most common arrhythmias are atrial fibrillation and complex ventricular arrhythmias.
- Echocardiogram may reveal the thickened ventricular wall of restrictive CMP, small ventricular cavities, and dilated atria.
- Endomyocardial biopsy, CT scan, and nuclear imaging may be helpful in a definitive diagnosis.

Nursing and collaborative management. Currently, no specific treatment for restrictive CMP exists. Interventions are aimed at improving diastolic filling and the underlying disease process. Treatment includes conventional therapy for CHF and arrhythmias. Heart transplant may also be a consideration.

Nursing care is similar to the care of a patient with CHF. As in the treatment of patients with HCM, patients should be taught to avoid situations that impair ventricular filling, such as strenuous activity, dehydration, and increases in systemic vascular resistance (SVR).

CARPAL TUNNEL SYNDROME

Definition/Description

Carpal tunnel syndrome is a condition caused by compression of the median nerve beneath the transverse carpal ligament. This occurs within the narrow confines of the carpal tunnel located at the wrist. This condition is frequently due to pressure from trauma or edema caused by inflammation of a tendon (tenosynovitis), neoplasm, rheumatoid synovial disease, or soft tissue masses such as ganglia.

- Carpal tunnel syndrome occurs most frequently in middle-aged or postmenopausal females and persons who are employed in occupations that require continuous wrist movement (e.g., butchers, secretaries, carpenters, computer operators).

Clinical Manifestations

Manifestations include weakness (especially of the thumb), pain and numbness, impaired sensation in the distribution of the median nerve, and clumsiness in performing fine hand movements. Numbness and tingling may be present and may awaken the patient at night.

- Holding the wrist in acute flexion for 60 seconds will produce tingling and numbness over the distribution of the median nerve, palmar surface of the thumb, index finger, middle finger, and part of the ring finger. This is known as a positive *Phalen's sign.*
- In late stages there is atrophy of thenar muscles. This syndrome can result in recurrent pain and eventual dysfunction of the hand.

Nursing and Collaborative Management

Therapy is directed toward relieving the underlying cause of the nerve compression. Early symptoms can usually be relieved by placing the hand and wrist at rest by immobilizing them in a hand splint. If the cause is inflammation, injection of hydrocortisone directly into the carpal tunnel may provide relief.

- If the problem continues, the median nerve may have to be surgically decompressed by longitudinal division of the transverse carpal ligament under regional anesthesia. Endoscopic carpal tunnel release is a new procedure in which decompression is done through a small puncture site.

Prevention of carpal tunnel syndrome involves educating employees and employers to identify risk factors.

- Adaptive devices such as wrist splints may be worn to relieve pressure on the median nerve. Special keyboard pads are available for computer operators to help prevent carpal tunnel syndrome or a worsening of symptoms if present.

Comfort should be maintained through the use of medication and splints to relieve pain and protect the area. Sensation may be impaired; therefore the patient should be instructed to avoid hazards such as extreme heat because of the risk of thermal injury.

Nursing care usually occurs in the office or outpatient setting. The patient may be required to consider occupational changes because of discomfort and sensory and functional changes.

- If the surgery is performed, the neurovascular status of the hand should be evaluated regularly. The patient should be instructed in assessments to perform at home since surgery is done on an outpatient basis.

CATARACTS

Definition/Description

A cataract is an opacity within the crystalline lens of one or both eyes, causing a gradual decline in vision. Approximately 50% of Americans between the ages of 65 and 74 have some degree of cataract formation. Cataract removal is a common surgical procedure for Americans older than 65

Pathophysiology

Although most cataracts are age related (senile cataracts), they can be associated with other factors, including blunt or penetrating trauma, congenital factors (e.g., maternal rubella), radiation or ultraviolet (UV) light exposure, certain drugs such as systemic corticosteroids or long-term topical corticosteroids, and ocular inflammation. The patient with diabetes mellitus tends to develop cataracts at a younger age than does a patient in the nondiabetic population.

- In senile cataract formation, altered metabolic processes within the lens cause water accumulation and alterations in the fiber structure of the lens.

Clinical Manifestations
- The patient may complain of decreased vision, abnormal color perception, and glare that worsens at night.
- Visual decline is gradual, but the rate of cataract development varies from patient to patient.
- Secondary glaucoma may also occur if the enlarging lens causes increased intraocular pressure.

Diagnostic Studies
- Opacity directly observable by ophthalmoscopic or slit-lamp microscopic examination
- Visual acuity measurement
- Glare testing
- Keratometry and A-scan ultrasound if surgery is planned

Collaborative Care
The presence of a cataract does not necessarily indicate a need for surgery. For many patients the diagnosis is made long before they actually decide to have surgery. Other therapy may postpone or even negate the need for surgery.
- Helpful palliative measures include a change in eyeglass prescription, strong reading glasses or magnifiers, an increased amount of light for reading, and avoidance of night-time driving.
- Surgery may be performed when the patient's decreasing vision interferes with normal activities such as driving, reading, and watching television. The goal of surgery is to remove the source of visual impairment and restore vision. Surgical treatment can involve lens removal (e.g., phacoemulsification) and correction (e.g., intraocular lens implantation and contact lenses).

Nursing Management
Goals
Until surgery is necessary, the patient will wear sunglasses and avoid unnecessary radiation. Preoperatively, the patient will make informed decisions and experience minimal anxiety. Postoperatively, the patient will understand and comply with therapy. Comfort will be maintained and the patient will remain free of infection.
Nursing Diagnoses
- Decisional conflict *related to* lack of knowledge about condition and treatment options
- Self-care deficits *related to* visual deficit
- Anxiety *related to* lack of knowledge about the surgical and postoperative experience

Nursing Interventions

For the patient who chooses not to have surgery, suggest vision enhancement techniques and modification of activities and lifestyle to accommodate visual deficits.

For the patient who elects surgery, provide information, support, and reassurance about the surgical and postoperative experience to reduce or alleviate patient anxiety. Inform all patients that they will not have depth perception until their patch is removed (usually within 24 hours).

- Postoperatively, offer mild analgesics for slight scratchiness or mild eye pain. The physician needs to be notified for severe pain, increased or purulent drainage, increased redness, or decreased visual acuity.
- Assess the patient's ability to follow the postoperative regimen (see NCP 20-1 for the patient following eye surgery, Lewis and others, *Medical-Surgical Nursing,* edition 5, p. 457).

▼ **Patient Teaching**

- Written and verbal discharge teaching should include postoperative eye care, activity restrictions, medications, follow-up visit schedule, and signs of possible complications. (For more on patient teaching following eye surgery, see Table 20-7, Lewis and others, *Medical-Surgical Nursing,* edition 5, p. 456).
- The patient's family should be included in the instruction since some patients may have difficulty with self-care activities, especially if vision in the unoperated eye is poor. Provide an opportunity for the patient and family to present return demonstrations of any necessary self-care activities.
- Suggest ways for the patient and family to modify activities and environment to maintain a level of safe functioning. Suggestions may include getting assistance with steps, removing area rugs and other potential obstacles, preparing meals for freezing before surgery, and obtaining audio books for diversion until visual acuity improves.

CEREBROVASCULAR ACCIDENT (STROKE)

Definition/Description

A cerebrovascular accident (CVA) or stroke is a broad term that includes a variety of disorders that influence blood flow to the brain. CVAs result when there is an inadequate blood supply to the brain (cerebral ischemia) or cerebral hemorrhage within the brain. Regardless of the cause, the damaged brain no longer performs cognitive, sensory, motor, or emotional functions. The effects of a CVA may vary from minor to severe disability.

- Stroke is the third most common cause of death and is the leading cause of serious, long-term disability in the United States and Canada. Strokes are considered a major public health problem in terms of mortality and morbidity as 500,000 to 600,000 persons experience CVAs annually.
- About 31% of people who have an initial stroke die within a year. This percentage is higher among people age 65 and older.
- Although one third of individuals having a stroke die within a month of occurrence, 2 to 3 million people live with disability as a direct result of strokes. Rehabilitation is a realistic option for 90% of older adults who have had a stroke.

Risk factors associated with stroke can be divided into nonmodifiable and potentially modifiable.

- Nonmodifiable risk factors include gender, age, race, and heredity. The incidence of stroke is higher for men than for women, with the risk of stroke increasing with age until age 75. African-Americans experience a higher incidence of stroke, which is associated with an increased incidence of hypertension. Persons with a family history of stroke or transient ischemic attacks (TIAs) are also at higher risk for stroke.
- Potentially modifiable risk factors are hypertension, cardiac disease, diabetes mellitus, sickle cell anemia, and certain lifestyle habits such as cigarette smoking, a diet high in fat content, and drug abuse. Control of hypertension is the most significant contributor to the prevention of stroke.

Types of Strokes

CVAs are classified as *ischemic* or *hemorrhagic* strokes on the basis of their underlying pathophysiology (Table 19).

- *Ischemic strokes* result from a decreased blood flow to the brain secondary to partial or complete occlusion of an artery. They occur much more frequently than hemorrhagic strokes. The most common types of ischemic stroke are thrombotic and embolic (see below).
- *Hemorrhagic strokes* are generally the result of spontaneous bleeding into the brain tissue itself (intracerebral or intraparenchymal hemorrhage) or into the subarachnoid space or ventricles (subarachnoid hemorrhage).

Pathophysiology

Thrombotic stroke. Thrombosis results from the formation of a blood clot that causes narrowing of the lumen of a blood vessel with eventual occlusion. It is the most common cause of cerebral infarction.

Table 19   Types of Stroke

Type	Gender/age	Warning	Time of onset	Course/prognosis
Ischemic				
Thrombotic	Men more than women, oldest median age	TIA (30-50% of cases)	During or after sleep	Stepwise progression, signs and symptoms develop slowly, usually some improvement, recurrence in 20-25% of survivors
Embolic	Men more than women	TIA (uncommon)	Lack of relationship to activity, sudden onset	Single event, signs and symptoms develop quickly, usually some improvement, recurrence common without aggressive treatment of underlying disease
Hemorrhagic				
Intracerebral	Slightly higher in women	Headache (25% of cases)	Activity (often)	Progression over 24 hr; poor prognosis, fatality more likely with presence of coma
Subarachnoid	Slightly higher in women, youngest median age	Headache (common)	Activity (often), sudden onset Most commonly related to head trauma	Single sudden event usually, fatality more likely with presence of coma

C

- Two thirds of strokes caused by thrombosis are associated with hypertension or diabetes mellitus, both of which are conditions that accelerate the atherosclerotic process.
- Thrombosis may be preceded by prodromal episodes, such as paralysis, paresis (decreased strength and motion of an extremity), mental confusion, and aphasia (disturbance of language function). The prodromal symptoms are considered *transient ischemic attacks* (TIAs) and usually last 5 to 30 minutes.

Thrombotic stroke is characterized by a pattern of (1) a single attack where symptoms occur over several hours, (2) intermittent progression toward a stroke occurring over hours to days, (3) partial stroke with permanent neurologic deficits, or (4) a series of TIAs followed by a stroke with permanent neurologic deficits.

- The extent of the stroke depends on rapidity of onset, size of the lesion, and presence of collateral circulation.

Embolic stroke. Cerebral embolism is the occlusion of a cerebral artery by an embolus, resulting in necrosis and edema of the area supplied by the involved blood vessel. Embolism is the second most common cause of stroke.

The majority of emboli originate from the heart with plaques or tissue breaking off from the endocardium and entering the circulation. The emboli travel to smaller vessels and become a source of obstruction. Emboli are associated with heart conditions such as atrial fibrillation and myocardial infarction (MI).

- Onset of an embolic stroke is usually sudden and may or may not be related to activity. The patient usually maintains consciousness, although a headache may develop on the side where the embolus is lodged.
- Recurrence is common unless the underlying cause is aggressively treated.

Temporal Development of Cerebrovascular Accidents

The temporal development of CVAs includes TIAs, reversible ischemic neurologic deficit, stroke-in-evolution or progressing stroke, and completed stroke (stable stroke). Knowledge of this classification is useful in planning nursing care.

TIAs are brief episodes of neurologic deficit that occur but leave no residual effects. The deficits usually clear completely in less than 24 hours.

- It is thought that TIAs are caused by microemboli breaking off from atherosclerotic plaques found in extracranial arteries.
- A TIA is considered a warning signal of progressive cerebrovascular disease.
- Signs and symptoms vary according to the part of the brain affected. If the carotid system is involved, the patient may report a temporary loss of vision in one eye, transient hemiparesis, or a sudden inability to speak.

- Symptoms related to vertebrobasilar insufficiency are tinnitus, vertigo, darkened or blurred vision, diplopia, dysphagia, and unilateral or bilateral numbness or weakness.

Reversible ischemic neurologic deficit is a neurologic deficit that remains after 24 hours but leaves no residual signs or symptoms after days to weeks. It is considered by some to be a completed stroke with minimal to no residual deficit.

Stroke-in-evolution or a *progressing stroke* develops over a period of hours or days. A stepwise or intermittent progression of deteriorating neurologic findings is common.

Completed stroke (stable stroke) occurs when the neurologic deficit remains unchanged over a 2-day period. An embolic stroke may demonstrate this characteristic from the onset. With the exception of stroke secondary to a ruptured aneurysm, a completed stroke signals readiness for more aggressive rehabilitative treatment.

Clinical Manifestations

Table 55-2, Lewis and others, *Medical-Surgical Nursing,* edition 5, p. 1650 lists manifestations seen with specific cerebral artery involvement. Figure 2 illustrates manifestations of right-sided and left-sided stroke.

Neuromotor function. Motor deficits are the most obvious effect of stroke and are caused by destruction of motor neurons in the pyramidal pathway. This destruction can result in the loss of skilled voluntary movements *(akinesia),* impairment of integration of movements, and alterations in muscle tone and reflex activity.

- Hyporeflexia that initially occurs with stroke progresses to hyperreflexia for most patients.

Communication. The left hemisphere is dominant for language skills in all right-handed persons and in the majority of left-handed persons.

- Language disorders involve the expression and comprehension of written or spoken words. The patient may experience *aphasia* (total loss of comprehension and use of language) when a stroke damages the dominant hemisphere of the brain.
- When the stroke involves Wernicke's area of the brain, the patient experiences *receptive aphasia;* neither the sounds of speech nor its meaning can be understood, and comprehension of both written and spoken language is impaired.
- The stroke causing *expressive aphasia* affects Broca's area, the motor area for speech. This patient has difficulty in speaking and writing.
- Most stroke patients also experience *dysarthria,* a disturbance in the muscular control of speech.

Affect. Patients with a stroke may demonstrate loss of control of their emotions; emotional responses may be exaggerated or unpredictable.

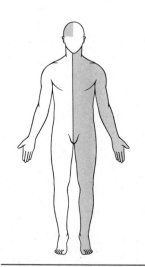 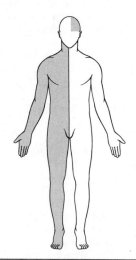

Right brain damage	**Left brain damage**
• Paralyzed left side	• Paralyzed right side
• Spatial-perceptual deficits	• Speech-language deficits (if left brain dominant)
• Behavioral style: quick, impulsive	• Behavioral style: slow, cautious
• Memory deficits: performance	• Memory deficits: language
• Indifference to the disability	• Distress and depression in relation to the disability

Fig. 2 Manifestations of right-sided and left-sided stroke.

Additional manifestations include impairment of memory and judgment, deficits in spatial-perceptual orientation, and transient problems with bowel and bladder function.

Diagnostic Studies
Various tests are carried out to determine the cause and location of the stroke and to guide decisions about therapy.

- CT scan, the primary diagnostic test, can indicate lesion size and location and differentiate between hemorrhage and infarction.
- MRI is the best imaging technique to differentiate types of infarcts.

- Positron emmission tomography (PET) shows brain chemical activity and extent of tissue damage.
- Electroencephalogram (EEG) may show low-voltage, slow waves with ischemic infarction and high-voltage slow waves with hemorrhage.
- Arteriography can demonstrate cerebral and cerebrovascular occlusion, arteriosclerotic plaques, and vessel malformation.

Collaborative Care

Prevention. The goals of stroke prevention include management of modifiable risk factors, prevention of stroke for those with a history of TIA, and prevention of additional strokes for those who have had a CVA.

- Patients with known risk factors, such as diabetes mellitus, hypertension, or cardiac dysfunction, should be followed closely. Measures designed to prevent the development of a thrombus or embolus are used; low-dose aspirin or dipyridamole (Persantine) can reduce the risk of stroke. The platelet-aggregation inhibitor called ticlopidine hydrochloride (Ticlid) has been shown to be as effective as aspirin in reducing the incidence of stroke.
- Surgical therapy for the patient with TIAs includes carotid endarterectomy, transluminal angioplasty, and extracranial-intracranial (EC-IC) bypass. Following these procedures, patients are at risk for stroke and require close, long-term assessment and management.

Acute care. The focuses of acute care are preservation of life, prevention of additional brain damage, and the lessening of disability. Treatment differs according to the type of stroke.

- The first goal is to maintain a patent airway, which may be compromised due to decreased consciousness. Oxygen administration, an artificial airway, intubation, and mechanical ventilation may be indicated.
- The patient is monitored closely for signs of increasing neurologic deficit. Table 55-5, Lewis and others, *Medical-Surgical Nursing,* edition 5, p. 1654 outlines emergency management of the patient with a CVA.
- Patients with ischemic strokes may be treated with hypervolemic hemodilution and volume expansion with crystalloids or colloids. The goal of treatment is to decrease blood viscosity, which promotes blood flow to the area of the stroke.
- Fluid and electrolyte balance must be controlled carefully. While the goal is to maintain perfusion to the brain, overhydration may further compromise perfusion by increasing cerebral edema. Adequate fluid intake during acute care via oral, IV administration, or tube feedings should be 2000 to 3000 ml/day. Patients are monitored for urine output.

- Management of increased intracranial pressure (ICP) includes practices that enhance venous drainage, including elevation of the head of the bed as ordered, maintenance in alignment of the patient's head and neck, and the avoidance of hip flexion.
- Additional measures include the treatment of pain, avoidance of hypervolemia, and management of constipation. Diuretic medications, such as mannitol (Osmitrol) and furosemide (Lasix), may be used to decrease cerebral edema.

Surgical therapy for stroke includes an immediate evacuation of blood occurring with strokes due to aneurysm-induced hematomas or cerebellar hematomas larger than 3 cm.

Drug Therapy

Thrombolytic therapy. Recombinant tissue plasminogen activator (tPA) is used to reestablish blood flow and prevent cell death for patients with ischemic strokes. Thrombolytic drugs such as tPA act to produce localized fibrinolysis by binding to the fibrin in the thrombi

The major side effect of tPA is cerebral hemorrhage. During infusion of the drug the patient's vital signs are monitored to assess for improvement or deterioration related to intracerebral hemorrhage. Control of BP is critical during treatment and for 24 hours following treatment.

Platelet inhibition/anticoagulant therapy. Patients with stroke caused by thrombi and emboli (ischemic strokes) may also be treated with platelet inhibitors and anticoagulants (after the first 24 hours if treated with tPA) to prevent the formation of more clots. Common anticoagulants include heparin and warfarin (Coumadin). IV heparin or low molecular weight heparin may be given in the situation of rapidly evolving strokes or strokes due to emboli traveling from the heart.

Other drug therapies. Aspirin or acetaminophen (Tylenol) is given to treat hyperthermia. Cooling blankets may be used cautiously to lower core temperatures. The nurse needs to closely monitor the patient's body temperature. Antiseizure medication, such as phenytoin (Dilantin), may be administered if seizure activity is present.

Nutritional Therapy

The stress of illness contributes to a catabolic state that can interfere with recovery.

- The patient may initially be receiving IV fluids. The first oral feeding should be approached with caution because the gag reflex may be impaired. Before initiation of feeding, the gag reflex may be assessed by gently stimulating the back of the throat with a tongue blade. The patient should remain in a high Fowler's position, preferably in a chair with the head flexed forward for the feeding and for 30 minutes following feeding.

After the acute phase, the dietitian can assist in determining the appropriate daily caloric intake based on the patient's size, weight, and activity level. If the patient is unable to take in an adequate oral diet, enteral feedings via a nasogastric tube may be used.

Rehabilitation care. After the stroke has stabilized for 12 to 24 hours, care shifts from the preservation of life to the lessening of disability and the attainment of optimal function. Depending on the patient's status, the patient's rehabilitation potential, and the available resources, the patient may be transferred to a rehabilitation facility or unit. Other approaches for rehabilitation include outpatient therapy or home care–based rehabilitation.

C

Nursing Management

Goals

The patient who has experienced a stroke will maintain a stable or improved level of consciousness, attain maximum physical functioning, maintain stable body functions (e.g., bladder control), maximize communication abilities, attain maximum self-care abilities and skills, maintain adequate nutrition, avoid complications of stroke, and maintain effective personal and family coping.

See NCP 55-1 for the patient with a stroke, Lewis and others, *Medical-Surgical Nursing,* edition 5, p. 1659.

Nursing Diagnoses

- Altered tissue perfusion (cerebral) *related to* decreased cerebral blood flow secondary to thrombus, embolus, hemorrhage, edema, or vasospasm
- Impaired physical mobility *related to* generalized weakness, muscle atrophy, or paralyzed extremities
- Self-care deficits *related to* motor weakness, paralysis, and loss of ability to effectively perform activities of daily living (ADLs)
- Impaired swallowing *related to* weakness or paralysis of affected muscles
- Altered urinary elimination *related to* impaired impulse to void or inability to reach toilet or manage tasks of voiding
- Risk for ineffective airway clearance *related to* inability to raise secretions
- Unilateral neglect *related to* visual field cut and sensory loss on one side of body
- Self-esteem disturbance *related to* actual or perceived loss of function

Nursing Interventions

Respiratory system. During the acute phase of a stroke the nursing priority is management of respiratory function.

- An oropharyngeal airway may be used in comatose patients to hold the tongue in place, prevent airway obstruction, and make suctioning accessible. Interventions include frequent assessment of airway patency and function, suctioning, patient mobility, positioning of the patient to prevent aspiration, and encouragement of deep breathing.

Neurologic system. The patient's neurologic status needs to be monitored closely to detect stroke in evolution or increased ICP.

- The Glasgow Coma Scale (GCS) is used for neurologic assessment and contains the essential factors of level of consciousness, mental status, pupillary responses, and movement and strength of extremities. (The GCS is shown on p. 720-721.)
- A decreasing level of consciousness is the earliest and most sensitive sign of increasing brain ischemia. Vital signs are closely monitored and documented.

Cardiovascular system. Nursing goals for the cardiovascular system are aimed at maintaining homeostasis.

- Fluid retention plus overhydration can result in fluid overload; it can also increase cerebral edema. The nurse should closely monitor intake and output. IV therapy is also carefully regulated.
- After a stroke the patient is at risk for thrombophlebitis and deep vein thrombosis in the weak or paralyzed lower extremity. The most effective prevention is to keep the patient moving. Active range-of-motion (ROM) exercises should be taught if the patient has voluntary movement in the affected extremity. For the patient with hemiplegia, passive ROM exercises should be done several times a day.
- Additional measures often used to prevent thrombophlebitis include positioning to minimize the effects of dependent edema and the use of elastic compression gradient stockings.

Musculoskeletal system. The goal for the musculoskeletal system is to maintain optimal function, which is accomplished by prevention of joint contractures and muscular atrophy

- In the acute phase, ROM exercises and positioning are important interventions. Passive ROM exercise is begun on the first day of hospitalization. Muscle atrophy secondary to lack of innervation and to inactivity can develop within a month following stroke.
- The paralyzed or weak side needs special attention when the patient is positioned. Each joint should be positioned higher than the joint proximal to it. Specific deformities on the affected side of the patient with stroke are shoulder adduction; flexion contractures of the hand, wrist, and elbow; external rotation of the hip; and plantar flexion of the foot.

Integumentary system. The patient's skin is particularly susceptible to breakdown because of the loss of sensation, diminished circulation, and immobility.

- The patient should not be left in any position longer than 2 hours. Time spent lying on the paralyzed or weak side should be limited to 30 minutes at a time.

Gastrointestinal system
- The most common bowel problem is constipation. The patient should be checked every 2 days for impaction.
- Depending on the patient's fluid balance status and swallowing ability, fluid intake should include 1800 to 2000 ml/day and fiber intake up to 25 g/day. Physical activity also promotes bowel function.

Urinary system. In the acute stage of stroke, the primary urinary problem is poor bladder control, resulting in incontinence.
- Efforts should be made to promote normal bladder function and avoid the use of an indwelling catheter.
- Long-term use of an indwelling catheter is associated with urinary tract infections and delayed bladder retraining. An intermittent catheterization program may be used for patients with urinary retention.

Communication. During the acute stage the nurse's role in meeting the psychologic needs of the patient is primarily supportive.
- An alert patient is usually anxious due to a lack of understanding of what has happened and the inability to communicate. If the patient cannot understand words, gestures may be used to support verbal cues. It may help to speak slowly and to calmly use relatively simple words.

Sensory-perceptual alterations. *Homonymous hemianopsia* (blindness in the same half of each visual field) is a common problem after a stroke.
- Initially the nurse helps the patient to compensate by arranging the environment within the patient's perceptual field, such as arranging the food tray so that all food is on the right side or the left side to accommodate for field of vision.
- Later, the patient is instructed to consciously attend to the neglected side. The weak or paralyzed extremities are carefully noted for adequacy of dressing, hygiene, and trauma.
- Visual problems may include diplopia, loss of the corneal reflex, and ptosis, particularly if the stroke is in the vertebrobasilar distribution. Diplopia is often treated with the use of an eye patch. If the corneal reflex is absent, the patient is at risk for a corneal abrasion and should be observed closely and protected against eye injuries.

Coping. A stroke is usually a sudden, extremely stressful event for the patient, close family members, and significant others.
- Reactions vary considerably but may involve fear, apprehension, denial of severity of the stroke, depression, and anger.
- During the acute phase of caring for the patient and family, nursing interventions designed to facilitate coping involve providing information and emotional support.

- Explanations to the patient about what has happened and about diagnostic and therapeutic procedures should be clear and understandable. It will be particularly challenging to keep the aphasic patient adequately informed.
- Because family members usually have not had time to prepare for the illness, they may need assistance in arranging care for family members or pets and in arranging transportation and finances.

Home care and rehabilitation. Nurses have an excellent opportunity to prepare the patient and family for hospital discharge through education, demonstration and return demonstration, practice, and evaluation of self-care skills prior to discharge. Total care is considered in discharge planning in relation to medications, nutrition, mobility, exercises, hygiene, and toileting.

- Follow-up care is carefully planned to permit continuing nursing, physical, occupational, and speech therapy, as well as medical care. Community resources should also be identified.

The goals of rehabilitation are to prevent deformity and to maintain and improve function.

- These goals are mutually set by the patient, family, nurse, and other members of the rehabilitation team. The goals typically include (1) learning techniques to self-monitor and maintain physical wellness, (2) demonstrating self-care skills, (3) exhibiting problem-solving skills with self-care, (4) avoiding complications associated with stroke, (5) establishing and maintaining a useful communication system, (6) maintaining nutritional and hydration status, (7) listing community resources for equipment, supplies, and support, and (8) establishing flexible role behaviors to promote family cohesiveness.

Rehabilitation and long-term management of the stroke patient are further described in chapter 55 of Lewis and others, *Medical-Surgical Nursing.*

▼ **Family and Patient Teaching**

- The care provider needs instruction and practice in necessary areas of home care while the patient is hospitalized. This allows for support and encouragement as well as opportunities for feedback. Adjustments in the home environment, such as the removal of a door to accommodate a wheelchair, can be made before discharge.
- Specific areas for instruction related to home care include exercise and ambulation techniques; dietary requirements; recognition of signs indicating the possibility of another stroke (e.g., headache, vertigo, numbness, visual disturbances); understanding of emotional lability and the possibility of depression; medication routine; and time, place, and frequency of follow-up activities, such as occupational therapy and physical therapy.

- To assist the caregiver to stay healthy after the patient is discharged, it is important to plan for respite or time away from caregiving activities on a regular basis.

CERVICAL CANCER

C

Definition/Description

The number of deaths from cervical cancer has fallen steadily over the past 40 years. This is attributable to earlier and better diagnosis with widespread use of the Pap test. In addition to cancer, the Pap test detects precancerous changes called cervical intraepithelial neoplasia (CIN) or dysplasia. By treating dysplasia, progression to cervical cancer can be prevented.

- African-American, Hispanic, and Native-American women have a higher incidence of cervical cancer than Caucasians.
- An increased risk of cervical cancer is associated with low economic status, early sexual activity (before 17 years of age), multiple sexual partners, infection with human papillomavirus (HPV), and smoking.

Precancerous changes are asymptomatic, which highlights the importance of routine screening. CIN occurs mainly in young women. The peak incidence of CIN is in women in their early 30s. The average age for women with invasive cervical cancer is 50.

Pathophysiology

The progression from normal cervical cells to dysplasia and on to cervical cancer appears to be related to repeated injuries to the cervix. The progression occurs slowly over years rather than months. There is a relationship between certain subtypes of HPV and cervical cancer. Women who smoke have a 50% higher risk for developing cervical cancer than nonsmokers.

Clinical Manifestations

Early cervical cancer is generally asymptomatic, but leukorrhea and intermenstrual bleeding eventually occur.

- A vaginal discharge that is usually thin and watery becomes dark and foul smelling as the disease advances.
- Vaginal bleeding is initially only spotting, but as the tumor enlarges, it becomes heavier and more frequent.
- Pain is a late symptom and is followed by weight loss, anemia, and cachexia.

Diagnostic Studies

- Pap test, Schiller iodine test, colposcopy, and biopsy are performed for diagnostic purposes.
- The Bethesda System is used for classifying the stage of cervical cancer (see Table 51-13, Lewis and others, *Medical-Surgical Nursing,* edition 5, p. 1542).
- Type and extent of the biopsy may vary with abnormality seen. A punch biopsy may be done on an outpatient basis with special punch biopsy forceps.
- Excision of a cone-shaped section of the cervix may be used for both diagnosis and treatment. Conization is accomplished using one of several techniques. The choice of procedure is determined by the provider's experience and the availability of equipment.
- *Cryotherapy* (freezing) and laser cone vaporization destroy the tissue. Laser cone excision and *loop electrosurgery excision procedure* (LEEP) remove the identified tissue and allow for histologic examination.

Collaborative Care

Treatment is guided by the tumor stage, the patient's age, and the patient's general health state.

- Conization may be the only therapy needed for CIN if analysis of removed tissue indicates that a wide area of normal tissue surrounds the excised malignancy.
- Laser treatments, in which a directed infrared beam causes boiling and vaporization of intracellular water, are effective in destruction of dysplastic tissue.
- Cautery and cryosurgery may also be used.

Invasive cancer of the cervix is treated with surgery, radiation, or a combination of the two to remove or destroy the involved areas and lymphatic drainage.

- Surgical procedures commonly carried out include hysterectomy, radical hysterectomy, and, rarely, pelvic exenteration (Table 20). Radiation may be external (e.g., cobalt) or internal (e.g., cesium or radium). Standard radiation treatment is 5 to 6 weeks of external radiation followed by one or two internal implants (see Radiation Therapy, p. 681).

Nursing Management: Cancers of the Female Reproductive System

Malignant tumors of the female reproductive system can be found in the cervix, endometrium, ovaries, vagina, and vulva. The patient with any of these malignant tumors may experience a variety of clinical manifestations, including leukorrhea (white discharge from the vagina), bowel and bladder dysfunction, and vulvar itching and

C

Table 20 Surgical Procedures on the Female Reproductive Tract

Type of surgery	Description
Subtotal hysterectomy	Removal of uterus without cervix (rarely done today)
Total hysterectomy	Removal of uterus and cervix
Panhysterectomy (TAH-BSO)	Removal of uterus, cervix, fallopian tubes, and ovaries
Simple vulvectomy	Excision of vulva and wide margin of skin
Radical vulvectomy	Excision of tissue from anus to few cm above symphysis pubis (skin, labia majora and minora, and clitoris) with superficial and deep lymph node dissection

TAH-BSO, total abdominal hysterectomy and bilateral salpingo-oophorectomy.

Continued

Table 20   Surgical Procedures on the Female Reproductive Tract—cont'd

Type of surgery	Description
Vaginectomy	Removal of vagina
Radical hysterectomy (Wertheim)	Panhysterectomy, partial vaginectomy, and dissection of lymph nodes in pelvis
Pelvic exenteration	Radical hysterectomy, total vaginectomy, removal of bladder with diversion of urinary system and resection of bowel with colostomy
Anterior pelvic exenteration	Above operation without bowel resection
Posterior pelvic exenteration	Above operation without bladder removal

burning. Assessment for these signs and symptoms is an important nursing responsibility.

Goals

The patient with a malignant tumor of the female reproductive system will actively participate in treatment decisions, achieve satisfactory pain and symptom management, recognize and report problems promptly, maintain preferred lifestyle as long as possible, and continue to practice cancer detection strategies.

Nursing Diagnoses

- Anxiety *related to* threat of a malignancy and lack of knowledge about the disease process and prognosis
- Pain *related to* pressure secondary to enlarging tumor
- Body image disturbance *related to* loss of body part and loss of good health
- Altered sexuality patterns *related to* physiologic limitations and fatigue

Nursing Interventions

Through their contact with women in a variety of settings, nurses can teach women the importance of routine screening for cancers of the reproductive system. Cancer can be prevented from occurring when screening reveals precancerous conditions of the vulva, cervix, or endometrium. Also, routine screening increases the chance that a cancer will be identified in its early stage. Nurses can assist women in viewing routine cancer screening as an important self-care activity.

- Educating women about risk factors for cancers of the reproductive system is also very important. Limiting sexual activity during adolescence, using condoms, having fewer sexual partners, and not smoking reduce the risk of cervical cancer.

Hysterectomy. Preoperatively, the patient is prepared for surgery with the standard perineal or abdominal preparation. A vaginal douche and enemas may be given according to surgeon preference. The bladder should be emptied before the patient is sent to the operating room. An indwelling catheter is often inserted.

- After surgery the patient who has had a hysterectomy will have an abdominal dressing (abdominal hysterectomy) or a sterile perineal pad (vaginal hysterectomy) (see NCP 51-2 for care of a patient after a total abdominal hysterectomy, Lewis and others, *Medical-Surgical Nursing,* edition 5, p. 1538). The dressing should be observed frequently for any sign of bleeding during the first 8 hours after surgery. A moderate amount of serosanguineous drainage on the perineal pad is expected following a vaginal hysterectomy.

Food and fluids may be restricted if the patient is nauseated. A rectal tube may be prescribed to relieve abdominal flatus. Ambulation is encouraged. A Fleet enema or suppository may be given on the third postoperative day.

Special care must be taken to prevent the development of thrombophlebitis in the pelvic or leg veins. Frequent position changes and avoidance of the high Fowler's position will minimize blood flow stasis and pooling. Leg exercises to promote circulation and the use of compression stockings or elastic bandages are also helpful.

The loss of the uterus may bring about grief responses similar to any great personal loss. The ability to bear children is central to society's image of being a female. Eliciting the woman's feelings and concerns about her surgery will provide needed information to give understanding care.

When surgery removes the ovaries as well, women experience surgical menopause. Estrogen is no longer available from the ovaries, so symptoms of estrogen deficiency (e.g., hot flashes) will arise. To counter this, hormone replacement therapy may be initiated in the early postoperative period.

The patient should be prepared for what to expect following surgery (e.g., she will not menstruate). Teaching should include specific activity restrictions. Intercourse should be avoided until the wound is healed (about 4 to 6 weeks). If a vaginal hysterectomy is performed, the woman needs to know that there may be a temporary loss of vaginal sensation.

- Physical restrictions are limited for a short time. Heavy lifting should be avoided for 2 months. Activities that may increase pelvic congestion, such as dancing and brisk walking, should be avoided for several months, whereas activities such as swimming may be both physically and mentally helpful.
- Wearing a girdle is allowed and may provide comfort. Once the patient has been assured that healing is complete, all previous activities can be resumed.

Salpingectomy and oophorectomy. Postoperative care of the woman who has undergone removal of a fallopian tube *(salpingectomy)* or an ovary *(oophorectomy)* is similar to that for any patient having abdominal surgery. When both ovaries are removed (bilateral oophorectomy), surgical menopause results. Symptoms are similar to those of regular menopause but may be more severe because of the sudden withdrawal of hormones. Replacement therapy with estrogen is given to most patients to avoid symptoms of menopause and osteoporosis.

Pelvic exenteration. When other forms of therapy are ineffective in stopping cancer spread and no metastases have been found outside of the pelvis, pelvic exenteration may be performed. Although different types are done, this radical surgery usually involves removal of the uterus, ovaries, fallopian tubes, vagina, bladder, urethra, and pelvic lymph nodes. In some situations, the descending colon, rectum, and anal canal may also be removed. Postoperative care involves that of a patient who has had a radical hysterectomy, an abdominal perineal resection, and an ileostomy or colostomy. Physical, emotional, and social adjustments to life on the part of the woman and her family are great. There are urinary or fecal diversions in the abdominal wall, a reconstructed vagina, and the onset of menopausal symptoms.

- The patient's rehabilitative process should keep pace with her acceptance of the situation. Much understanding and support is needed from the nursing staff during a long hospital stay.
- The patient should be encouraged to regain her independence. She needs to verbalize her feelings about her altered body to an interested and concerned listener.
- Inclusion of the family in the plan of care is very important.

CHLAMYDIAL INFECTION

Definition/Description
Chlamydia trachomatis, a gram-negative bacteria, is recognized as a genital pathogen responsible for a variety of illnesses.

- There are numerous strains of *C. trachomatis.* Some cause urogenital infection (e.g., nongonococcal urethritis [NGU] in men and cervicitis in women), some cause ocular trachoma, and others cause lymphogranuloma venereum.
- Chlamydia is now a reportable disease in almost all states. *C. trachomatis* infections are the most prevalent bacterial sexually transmitted diseases (STDs) in the United States.

Risk factors include an age of less than 25 years, multiple sex partners, history of STDs, use of nonbarrier contraception, and bleeding inducible by swabbing of cervical mucosa.

- Because of the high prevalence of asymptomatic infections in both men and women, screening of high-risk populations is needed to identify those infected.

Clinical Manifestations
As with gonorrhea, chlamydial infections result in a superficial mucosal infection that can become more invasive.

- Signs and symptoms in men include urethritis (dysuria, urethral discharge), epididymitis (unilateral scrotal pain, swelling, fever), and proctitis (rectal discharge and pain during defecation).
- Signs and symptoms in women include cervicitis (mucopurulent discharge and hypertrophic ectopy [area that is edematous and bleeds easily]), urethritis (dysuria and frequent urination), bartholinitis (purulent exudate), and pelvic inflammatory disease (abdominal pain, vomiting, fever, abnormal vaginal bleeding,

and menstrual abnormalities). A large number of women with chlamydial cervicitis have been found to have a male partner with NGU.

Complications often develop from poorly managed, inaccurately diagnosed, or undiagnosed chlamydial infections.

- Infection in men may result in epididymitis with possible infertility and Reiter's disease.
- Women may develop pelvic inflammatory disease (PID) and ectopic pregnancy.
- A chlamydial infection may be transmitted from a mother to a newborn, causing inclusion conjunctivitis or pneumonia.

Diagnostic Studies

In men a diagnosis of chlamydial infection is made by excluding gonorrhea; specifically, if no gram-negative intracellular diplococci are found on a Gram-stained smear of male urethral discharge or sediment of a first-catch urine specimen, a culture is done. If both these tests are negative and signs of inflammation are present (e.g., polymorphonuclear leukocytes [PMNs] on the Gram-stained smear), a diagnosis of NGU-*Chlamydia* infection can be made.

Screening in both men and women is now more effective due to the availability of nonculture tests, including direct fluorescent antibody (DFA) tests, enzyme immunoassay (EIA), and DNA hybridization tests. These tests do not require special handling of specimens, are less expensive, and are easier to perform than cell cultures. Culturing for chlamydial organisms should be done if laboratory facilities are available.

Collaborative Care

Chlamydial infections respond to treatment with doxycycline or azithromycin (Zithromax). Erythromycin or amoxicillin are the drugs of choice for use in pregnant patients.

- Follow-up care should include advising the patient to return if symptoms persist or recur, the treatment of sex partners, and encouraging the use of condoms during all sexual contacts.

Nursing Management: Sexually Transmitted Diseases

Goals

The patient with a STD will demonstrate an understanding of the mode of transmission of STDs and the risk posed by them, complete treatment and return for appropriate follow-up, notify or assist in notification of contacts about their need for testing and treatment, abstain from intercourse until infection is resolved, and demonstrate knowledge of safe sex practices.

Nursing Diagnoses

- Risk for infection *related to* lack of knowledge about mode of transmission, inadequate personal and genital hygiene, and failure to practice precautionary measures
- Altered health maintenance *related to* knowledge about disease process, appropriate follow-up measures, and possibility of reinfection
- Anxiety *related to* impact of condition on relationships, disease outcome, and lack of knowledge of disease

Nursing Interventions

The diagnosis of chlamydia or any other STD may be met with a variety of emotions, such as shame, guilt, anger, or a desire for vengeance. The nurse should try to help the patient verbalize feelings. A referral for professional counseling to explore the ramifications of a STD may be indicated.

All patients should return to the treatment center for a repeat culture from infected sites or for serologic testing at designated times to determine effectiveness of treatment.

- Informing the patient that cures are not always obtained on first treatment can reinforce the need for a follow-up visit.
- The patient should also be advised to inform sexual partners of the need for treatment, regardless of whether they are free of symptoms or experiencing symptoms.

The patient with a STD should have certain hygiene measures emphasized.

- An important measure is frequent handwashing and bathing; this results in the destruction of many of the causative organisms of STDs.
- Bathing and cleaning of involved areas can provide local comfort and prevent secondary infection.
- Douching may spread infection and is therefore contraindicated.
- Sexual abstinence is indicated during the communicable phase of the disease. If sexual activity occurs before treatment of the patient has been completed, the use of condoms may prevent the spread of infection and reinfection.

▼ **Patient Teaching**

- Nurses should be prepared to discuss safe sex practices with all patients, not only those who are perceived to be at risk. These practices include abstinence, monogamy with an uninfected partner, avoidance of certain high-risk sexual practices, and the use of condoms and other barriers to limit contact with potentially infectious body fluids or lesions. A patient teaching guide related to the patient with an STD is presented in Table 50-10, Lewis and others, *Medical-Surgical Nursing,* edition 5, p. 1507.

- All sexually active women should be screened for cervical cancer. Women with a history of STDs are at greater risk for cervical cancer than those women without this history.
- The nurse can initiate an interview to establish the patient's risk for contracting a STD. Questions to ask include number of partners, type of birth control used, use of condoms, and use of IV drugs. Patient education can be planned based on responses to these questions.
- Teach the patient to inspect the sexual partner's genitals before coitus is initiated. The presence of discharge, sores, blisters, or rash should be viewed with concern.
- Men should be told that some protection is provided if they void immediately following intercourse and wash their genitalia and adjacent areas with soap and water.
- Women may also benefit from postcoital voiding and washing. Spermicidal jellies and creams have a mild detergent effect that may reduce the risk of contracting STDs.
- Proper use of a latex condom provides a highly effective mechanical barrier to infection. The condom should be undamaged and correctly in place throughout all phases of sexual activity. The use of a spermicide such as nonoxynol-9, which inactivates most STD organisms, in the vagina and concurrent use of a condom can further reduce the risk of disease.
- Sexual contact with persons known or suspected to have HIV infection should be avoided. Sexually active individuals can reduce their risk by minimizing the number of sexual contacts. Unprotected anal intercourse should be eliminated, and condoms should be used if sexual contact continues.
- Nurses can actively encourage their communities to provide better education related to STDs for their citizens. Teenagers, who are known to have a high incidence of infection, should be a prime target for such educational programs.

CHOLELITHIASIS/CHOLECYSTITIS

Definition/Description

The most common disorder of the biliary system is *cholelithiasis* (stones in the gallbladder). *Cholecystitis* (inflammation of the gallbladder) is usually associated with cholelithiasis. The stones may be lodged in the neck of the gallbladder or in the cystic duct. Cholecystitis may be acute or chronic, with these conditions also occurring together.

- The incidence of cholelithiasis is higher in women, especially multiparous women, and persons over 40 years of age.

- Other predisposing factors for gallbladder disease are sedentary lifestyle, familiar tendency, and obesity.

Pathophysiology

The actual cause of gallstones is unknown. Cholelithiasis develops when the balance that keeps cholesterol, bile salts, and calcium in solution is altered so that precipitation of these substances occurs. Conditions that upset this balance include infection and disturbances in the metabolism of cholesterol.

- The stones may remain in the gallbladder or migrate to the cystic duct or common bile duct. They cause pain as they pass through the ducts and may lodge in the ducts and produce an obstruction.

Cholecystitis is most commonly associated with stones. When it occurs in the absence of stones, it is thought to be caused by bacteria reaching the gallbladder via the vascular or lymphatic route or chemical irritants in the bile.

- *Escherichia coli,* streptococci, and salmonellae are the most common causative bacteria.
- Other etiologic factors include adhesions, neoplasms, bile stasis, extensive fasting, frequent weight fluctuations, anesthesia, and some narcotics.
- During an acute attack of cholecystitis the gallbladder is edematous and hyperemic. It may be distended with bile or pus. The cystic duct is also involved and may become occluded.
- The wall of the gallbladder becomes scarred after an acute attack. Decreased functioning occurs if large amounts of tissue are fibrosed.

Clinical Manifestations

Cholelithiasis may produce severe symptoms or none at all. Many patients have silent cholelithiasis. The severity of symptoms depends on whether the stones are stationary or mobile and whether obstruction is present

- When a stone is lodged in the ducts or when stones are moving through the ducts, spasms may result. This sometimes produces very severe pain, which is termed *biliary colic.* The pain can be accompanied by tachycardia, diaphoresis, and prostration. The severe pain may last up to an hour, and when it subsides there is residual tenderness in the right upper quadrant.
- Attacks of pain frequently occur 3 to 6 hours after a high fat meal or when the patient assumes a recumbent position.
- When total obstruction occurs, symptoms related to bile blockage are manifested; these include steatorrhea, bleeding tendencies, and jaundice.

Manifestations of cholecystitis vary from indigestion to moderate to severe pain, leukocytosis, fever, and jaundice.

- Initial symptoms include indigestion and pain and tenderness in the right upper quadrant, which may be referred to the right shoulder and scapula.
- Pain may be acute and is accompanied by restlessness, diaphoresis, and nausea and vomiting.
- Symptoms of chronic cholecystitis include a history of fat intolerance, dyspepsia, heartburn, and flatulence.

Complications

Complications of cholecystitis include subphrenic abscess, pancreatitis, cholangitis (inflammation of biliary ducts), fistulas, and rupture of gallbladder, which can produce bile peritonitis. Many of the same complications can occur from cholelithiasis; these include cholangitis, carcinoma, and peritonitis.

Diagnostic Studies

- Ultrasonography diagnoses gallstones.
- Oral cholecystogram detects radiopaque stones.
- IV cholangiogram outlines the gallbladder and ducts.
- Percutaneous transhepatic cholangiography diagnoses obstructive jaundice and locates stones within the bile ducts.
- Laboratory studies may demonstrate liver function test abnormalities, elevated serum enzymes and pancreatic enzymes, increased white blood cell (WBC) count, elevated direct and indirect bilirubin levels, and urinary bilirubin.

Collaborative Care

During an acute episode of cholecystitis the focus is on control of pain, control of possible infection with antibiotics, and maintenance of fluid and electrolyte balance. Treatment is mainly supportive and symptomatic.

- If nausea and vomiting are severe, gastric decompression may be used to prevent further gallbladder stimulation. Anticholinergics to decrease secretions (which prevents biliary contraction) and counteract smooth muscle spasms may be administered. Analgesics are given to decrease pain.

There are currently several options for management of cholelithiasis. These include cholesterol solvents such as methyl tertiary terbutyl ether (MTBE), oral drugs that dissolve stones, endoscopic sphincterotomy, extracorporeal shock-wave lithotripsy (ESWL), and surgery. Supportive treatment, similar to that given for cholecystitis, may also be necessary.

- If stones cause an obstruction, additional treatment consists of replacement of fat-soluble vitamins, administration of bile salts to facilitate digestion and vitamin absorption, and a low-fat diet.

Surgical intervention for cholelithiasis is frequently indicated and may consist of one of several procedures.

- Cholecystectomy is considered by many surgeons to be the preferred surgical procedure. Currently 90% of all cholecystectomies are performed laparoscopically. In a laparoscopic procedure the gallbladder is removed through one of four small punctures in the abdomen. Most patients experience minimal postoperative pain and are discharged the day of surgery or the day after. In most cases they are able to resume normal activities and return to work after 2 or 3 days.

- Advantages of a laparoscopic cholecystectomy include decreased postoperative pain, a shorter hospital stay, and an earlier return to work and full activity. The main complication is injury to the common bile duct.

Drug therapy for gallbladder disease includes analgesics, anticholinergics (antispasmodics, such as atropine), fat-soluble vitamins, and bile salts. Meperidine (Demerol) is used if a narcotic analgesic is required. This drug causes less spasm in the ducts than opiates such as morphine sulfate.

Nutritional therapy with cholelithiasis and cholecystitis is a low-fat diet, which decreases stimulation of the gallbladder. If obesity is a problem, a reduced-calorie diet is indicated.

Nursing Management
Goals
The patient with gallbladder disease will have relief of pain and discomfort, no complications postoperatively, and no recurrent attacks of cholecystitis or cholelithiasis.
Nursing Diagnoses
- Pain *related to* surgical incision and presence of drains and bulky dressing
- Ineffective management of therapeutic regimen *related to* lack of knowledge of diet and postoperative management
Nursing Interventions
Nursing objectives for the patient undergoing conservative therapy include relieving pain, relieving nausea and vomiting, providing comfort and emotional support, maintaining fluid and electrolyte balance and nutrition, making accurate assessments for effectiveness of treatment, and observing for complications.

The patient with cholecystitis or cholelithiasis is frequently experiencing severe pain; medications ordered to relieve pain should be given as required before the pain becomes more severe.

- The nurse should assess what medications relieve pain and how much medication is required. Observations for side effects of medications must be part of the continued assessment.

- Nursing comfort measures, such as a clean bed, comfortable positioning, and oral care, are appropriate.

Postoperative nursing care following a laparoscopic cholecystectomy includes:

- Monitoring for complications such as bleeding, making the patient comfortable, and preparing the patient for discharge.
- Relieving pain with narcotic analgesics such as oxycodone and acetaminophen with codeine (Percodan, Percocet).
- Assisting the patient with clear liquids and ambulation to the bathroom.

▼ **Patient Teaching**

- When the patient is on conservative therapy, dietary teaching is usually necessary. The diet is usually low in fat, and sometimes a weight-reduction diet is also recommended. The patient may need to take fat-soluble vitamin supplements.
- Instructions should be provided regarding observations the patient should make indicating obstruction (stool and urine changes, jaundice, and pruritus).

The patient who undergoes a laparoscopic cholecystectomy is discharged soon after surgery, so teaching is essential.

- The patient should be instructed to remove bandages on the puncture sites the day after surgery and bathe or shower.
- The patient should be instructed to report signs and symptoms of complications, such as redness, swelling, or bile-colored drainage or pus from any incision; severe abdominal pain; nausea and vomiting; and fever and chills.
- The patient can gradually return to normal activity and may return to work within a week after surgery.

CHRONIC FATIGUE SYNDROME

Definition/Description

Chronic fatigue syndrome (CFS) is a disorder characterized by debilitating fatigue and a variety of associated complaints, including joint and muscle pain, lymph node tenderness, headaches, unrefreshing sleep, sore throat, self-reported impairment in short-term memory, and postexertional malaise greater than 24 hours.

- Patients with CFS are three times more likely to be women as men and are generally 25 to 45 years of age. Prevalence of this syndrome is difficult to determine.
- CFS is poorly understood. Although some health care providers doubt the existence of this disorder, it does exist and can have a devastating impact on the patient's life.

Pathophysiology

Despite numerous attempts to determine the etiology and pathology of CFS, its precise mechanisms remain unknown. An unremarkable flulike illness or other acute stress is often identified as a triggering event.

- A dysfunction may exist in the hypothalamus-pituitary-adrenal axis.
- There may be a reduced production of corticotropin-releasing hormone in the hypothalamus. Serum cortisol levels are low and adrenocorticotropic hormone (ACTH) levels are correspondingly high. These changes could cause decreased energy and altered mood states.
- Several viruses may precipitate the syndrome, including herpesviruses (e.g., Epstein-Barr virus, cytomegalovirus), enteroviruses, and retroviruses, as antibody titers to many infectious agents are elevated in patients with CFS.
- Immune alterations that have been shown to occur with CFS include decreased immunoglobulin production, altered natural killer cell activity, decreased lymphocyte proliferation, and increased CD4/CD8 ratio. These alterations do not occur in all patients and have not been shown to correlate with CFS severity.
- Because mild to moderate depression occurs in about 70% of the patients, it has been proposed that CFS is a psychiatric disorder. However, it is difficult to determine if depression is a cause or an effect of debilitating chronic fatigue.

Clinical Manifestations

In about one half of the cases, CFS develops insidiously, or the patient may have intermittent episodes that gradually become chronic. In other situations, CFS arises suddenly in a previously active, healthy individual.

- Incapacitating fatigue is the most common symptom that causes the patient to seek health care. Associated symptoms (described earlier) may fluctuate in intensity over time.
- The patient may become angry and frustrated with the inability of the physician to treat the problem. The disorder may have a major impact on work and family responsibilities. Some individuals may even need help with activities of daily living (ADLs).

Diagnostic Studies

Physical examination and diagnostic studies can be used to rule out other possible causes of the patient's symptoms. No laboratory test can diagnose CFS or measure its severity. In general, it remains a diagnosis of exclusion.

Nursing and Collaborative Management

Because there is no definitive therapy for CFS, supportive management is essential. The patient should be informed about what is known about the disease and all complaints should be taken seriously.

- Nonsteroidal antiinflammatory drugs (NSAIDs) can be used to treat headaches, muscle and joint aches, and fever. Antihistamines and decongestants can be used to treat allergic symptoms. Antidepressants (e.g., fluoxetine [Prozac], paroxetine [Paxil]) can improve mood and sleep disorders.
- Total rest is not advised as it can potentiate the self-image of being an invalid. On the other hand, strenuous exertion can exacerbate the exhaustion. Therefore it is important to plan a carefully graduated exercise program.
- Behavioral therapy may be used to promote a positive outlook as well as improve overall disability, fatigue, and other symptoms.

Chronic fatigue syndrome does not appear to progress. Although most patients recover or at least improve over time, they suffer from substantial occupational and psychosocial impairments and loss, including the social pressure and isolation from being characterized as lazy or crazy.

CHRONIC OBSTRUCTIVE PULMONARY DISEASE: EMPHYSEMA AND CHRONIC BRONCHITIS

Definition/Description

Chronic obstructive pulmonary disease (COPD) is defined as a disease state characterized by the presence of airway obstruction due to chronic bronchitis or emphysema. The airway obstruction is generally progressive, may be partially reversible, and is often accompanied by airway hyperreactivity.

- More than 15 million persons in the United States suffer from emphysema and chronic bronchitis. COPD is the fourth leading cause of death in the United States.

Etiology

Cigarette smoking is the major risk factor for developing COPD. Cigarette smoke has several direct effects on the respiratory tract.

- The irritating effect of smoke causes hyperplasia of cells, which subsequently results in increased mucus production. Hyperplasia reduces airway diameter and increases the difficulty in clearing secretions. Smoking also reduces ciliary activity and produces abnormal dilation of the distal air space with destruction of alveolar walls.

- Recurring respiratory tract infections are another major contributing factor to the aggravation and progression of COPD. Recurring infections impair normal defense mechanisms, making the bronchioles and alveoli more susceptible to injury. The most common causative organisms are *Haemophilus influenzae, Streptococcus pneumoniae,* and *Moraxella catarrhalis.* Retained secretions provide a medium for their proliferation.

- Inhaled irritants cause a nonspecific inflammatory response. The incidence of COPD is higher in urban than in rural areas due to inhaled irritants. This difference may be partially explained by air pollution and occupational irritants (e.g., coal dust, potash) to which persons are exposed.

A form of heredity primary emphysema is related to a deficiency of alpha$_1$-antitrypsin (AAT) that normally has an inhibitory effect on proteolytic enzymes. Emphysema results when lysis of lung tissues by proteolytic enzymes from neutrophils and macrophages occurs because of AAT deficiency. Smoking greatly exacerbates the disease process in these patients.

Some degree of emphysema is common in the lungs of older persons, even nonsmokers. Aging results in changes in the lung structure, thoracic cage, and respiratory muscles. Clinically significant emphysema is usually not caused by aging alone.

Pathophysiology

It is clinically common to find a combination of emphysema and chronic bronchitis in the same person, often with one condition predominating.

Emphysema is a lung condition characterized by abnormal, permanent enlargement of air spaces distal to the terminal bronchioles, accompanied by destruction of their walls and without obvious fibrosis. Structural changes include (1) hyperinflation of alveoli, (2) destruction of alveolar walls, (3) destruction of alveolar capillary walls, (4) narrowed, tortuous, small airways, and 5) loss of lung elasticity.

Chronic bronchitis is excessive production of mucus in the bronchi accompanied by a recurrent cough that persists for at least 3 months of the year during at least 2 successive years.

- Pathologic changes in the lung consist of (1) hyperplasia of mucus-secreting glands in the trachea and bronchi, (2) increase in goblet cells, (3) disappearance of cilia, (4) chronic inflammatory changes and narrowing of small airways, and (5) altered function of alveolar macrophages leading to increased bronchial infections.

- Frequently the airways are colonized with organisms; infections can occur when organisms increase in number. Eventually scarring of bronchial walls may occur.
- In contrast to emphysema, alveolar structure and capillaries are normal.

Clinical Manifestations

Manifestations of COPD vary from those of pure emphysema to those of pure chronic bronchitis. Most patients with COPD have features of both (Table 21).

- An early symptom of emphysema is dyspnea, which becomes progressively more severe. The person is characteristically thin and underweight; the exact cause for this is not well understood.
- Later in the course of emphysema, secondary chronic bronchitis may develop. In advanced stages, finger clubbing may be present in both emphysema and chronic bronchitis.
- The earliest symptom in chronic bronchitis is usually a frequent, productive cough during most winter months. Frequent respiratory infections are another common manifestation. Somewhat later, dyspnea on exertion may develop.
- Bluish-red color of the skin with chronic bronchitis results from polycythemia and cyanosis. Polycythemia develops as a result of increased production of red blood cells (RBCs) secondary to the body's attempt to compensate for chronic hypoxemia.
- A person with chronic bronchitis is usually of normal weight or heavyset, with a robust appearance.

Complications

Cor pulmonale is hypertrophy of the right side of the heart, with or without heart failure, resulting from pulmonary hypertension. In COPD, pulmonary hypertension is caused primarily by constriction of pulmonary vessels in response to alveolar hypoxia, with acidosis further potentiating vasoconstriction. Overt manifestations of cor pulmonale may include jugular venous distention, hepatomegaly with right upper quadrant tenderness, ascites, epigastric distress, peripheral edema, and weight gain.

- Management of cor pulmonale is continuous low-flow oxygen (O_2). Long-term O_2 therapy can reverse the progression of pulmonary hypertension in COPD. Although the use of digitalis is not indicated for cor pulmonale, it is used when congestive heart failure (CHF) is present. Dietary salt restriction is sometimes recommended, especially if overt CHF is present. Although diuretics are generally used, they are prescribed with caution because of their tendency to deplete potassium and chloride and reduce intravascular volume and cardiac output (CO).

Table 21   Comparison of Emphysema and Chronic Bronchitis*

Clinical Features	Emphysema	Chronic bronchitis
Age	30-40 yr (onset)	20-30 yr (onset)
	60-70 yr (disabling)	40-50 yr (disabling)
Body build	Thin	Tendency toward obesity
Health history	Generally healthy, occasional insidious dyspnea, smoking	Recurrent respiratory tract infections, smoking
Weight loss	Often marked	Absent or slight
Dyspnea	Slowly progressive and eventually disabling	Variable, relatively late
Sputum	Scanty, mucoid	Copious, mucopurulent
Cough	Negligible	Considerable
Chest examination	Marked increase in AP diameter, quiet or diminished breath sounds, limited diaphragmatic excursion	Slight to marked increase in AP diameter, scattered crackles, rhonchi, wheezing
Cor pulmonale	Rare except terminally	Frequent with many episodes

AP, Anteroposterior.
*Most persons with COPD have features of both pulmonary emphysema and chronic bronchitis.

Continued

Table 21   Comparison of Emphysema and Chronic Bronchitis—cont'd

	Emphysema	Chronic bronchitis
Diagnostic Study Results		
ABGs	Near normal, mild ↓ PaO_2, normal or ↓ $PaCO_2$	↓ PaO_2, ↑ $PaCO_2$
Chest x-ray	Hyperinflation, flat diaphragm, attenuated peripheral vessels, small or normal heart, widened intercostal margins	Cardiac enlargement, normal or flattened diaphragm, evidence of chronic inflammation, congested lung fields
Lung volumes		
Total lung capacity	Increased	Normal or slightly increased
Residual volume	Increased	Increased
Vital capacity	Decreased	Decreased
Hematocrit and hemoglobin	Normal until late in disease	Increased

ABGs, Arterial blood gases; *$PaCO_2$,* partial pressure of carbon dioxide in arterial blood; *PaO_2,* partial pressure of oxygen in arterial blood.

The most common event leading to acute respiratory failure in COPD is acute respiratory tract infection (usually viral) or acute bronchitis.

The incidence of peptic ulcer disease is increased with COPD. The reason for this occurrence is not known; it may be related to side effects from long-term use of bronchodilator or corticosteroid drugs or to the stressful nature of the disease (see Peptic Ulcer Disease, p. 454).

Gastroesophageal reflux, which may or may not be associated with hiatal hernia, occurs frequently with COPD and may aggravate respiratory symptoms (see Hiatal Hernia, p. 305 and Gastroesophageal Reflux Disease, p. 249).

Pneumonia is a frequent complication of COPD with the most common causative agents being *S. pneumoniae, H. influenzae,* and viruses. The most common manifestation is purulent sputum. Systemic manifestations of pneumonia such as fever, chills, and leukocytosis may not be present (see Pneumonia, p. 466).

Diagnostic Studies

See the diagnostic study results in Table 21.

Collaborative Care

The primary goals of care for the patient with COPD are to (1) improve ventilation, (2) promote secretion removal, (3) prevent complications and progression of symptoms, (4) promote patient comfort and participation in care, and (5) improve quality of life as much as possible.

- Cessation of cigarette smoking in the early stages is probably the most significant factor in slowing the progression of the disease. The health care provider has a responsibility to inform each patient who smokes about the effects of smoking, offer suggestions and guidelines on how to quit, and refer them to a smoking cessation program. The use of nicotine replacement therapy and non-nicotine medication (bupropion [Zyban]) may be helpful in minimizing the effects of nicotine withdrawal. These adjunctive therapies should be combined with other modalities such as support groups, educational materials, and behavior modification programs.
- Bronchodilator drug therapy is often helpful in relieving symptoms. Although patients with COPD do not respond as dramatically as those with asthma to bronchodilator therapy, a reduction in dyspnea and an increase in FEV_1 are usually achieved.
- O_2 therapy is used to supply the patient with adequate O_2 to maximize the O_2-carrying ability of the blood. O_2 may be prescribed for continuous use, only at night, or with exercise (see Oxygen Therapy, p. 676).

- Respiratory care is a collaborative effort involving respiratory therapists and nurses. Respiratory care includes breathing retraining, effective cough techniques, chest physiotherapy, and aerosol-nebulization therapy. (See Lewis and others, *Medical-Surgical Nursing,* edition 5, pp. 669 to 702 for further information on respiratory care.)

The patient with COPD should try to keep his or her body weight for height in the standard range. Weight loss and malnutrition are commonly seen in patients with severe emphysema.

- To decrease dyspnea and conserve energy, the patient should rest at least 30 minutes before eating and should select foods that can be prepared in advance. The patient should eat 5 to 6 small, frequent meals to avoid feelings of bloating and early satiety when eating.
- The patient who is overweight, a condition more commonly seen in chronic bronchitis, needs to be placed on a low-fat diet to assist in weight reduction.

Nursing Management
Goals
The patient with COPD will have a return of baseline respiratory function, the ability to perform activities of daily living (ADLs), relief from dyspnea, no complications related to COPD, knowledge and ability to implement a long-term treatment regimen, and overall improved quality of life.

See NCP 27-2 for the patient with chronic obstructive pulmonary disease, Lewis and others, *Medical-Surgical Nursing,* edition 5, p. 704.

Nursing Diagnoses
- Ineffective airway clearance *related to* expiratory airflow obstruction, ineffective cough, and infection in airways
- Impaired gas exchange: hypercapnia *related to* alveolar hypoventilation
- Impaired gas exchange: hypoxemia *related to* alveolar hypoventilation
- Sleep pattern disturbance *related to* anxiety, depression, and shortness of breath
- Self-care deficits *related to* lowered energy level, hypoxemia, and depression
- Altered nutrition: less than body requirements *related to* poor appetite, lowered energy level, shortness of breath, gastric distention, and sputum production
- Risk for infection *related to* decreased pulmonary function, possible corticosteroid therapy, ineffective airway clearance, and lack of knowledge regarding signs and symptoms of infection and preventive measures

Table 22	Patient and Family Teaching Guide: Chronic Obstructive Pulmonary Disease

Goal: To assist patient and family in improving quality of life through education and promotion of lifestyle practices that support successful living with COPD.

Teaching topic	Resources
What is COPD?	
▪ Basic anantomy and physiology of lung	Help Yourself to Better Breathing (American Lung Association)
▪ Basic pathophysiology of lung with COPD	Videos (American Lung Association)
▪ Signs and symptoms of COPD, respiratory infection, heart failure	
Breathing Retraining	
▪ Pursed-lip breathing	Demonstration and return demonstration
▪ Abdominal (diaphragm) breathing	
Energy Conservation Techniques	
▪ Pacing and pursing (pacing activity and using pursed-lip breathing with activities)	Around the Clock with COPD: Helpful Hints for Respiratory Patients (American Lung Association)
Medications	
▪ Types (include mechanism of action) Methylxanthines β-Adrenergic agonists Corticosteroids Anticholinergics Antibiotics	Understanding Lung Medications: How They Work—How to Use Them (American Lung Association) Write out medication list and schedule
▪ Establishing medication schedule	
Correct Use of Metered-Dose Inhaler/Spacer and Nebulizer	
	Figure 27-5, Lewis and others, *Medical-Surgical Nursing*, edition 5, p. 674

COPD, Chronic obstructive pulmonary disease.

| Table 22 | Patient and Family Teaching Guide: Chronic Obstructive Pulmonary Disease—cont'd |

Teaching topic	Resources
Home Oxygen ■ Explanation of rationale for use ■ Guide for home O_2 use	About Oxygen Therapy at Home (American Lung Association) Table 27-19, Lewis and others, *Medical-Surgical Nursing*, edition 5, p. 698
Psychosocial Emotional Issues ■ Concerns about inter-personal relationships Dependency Intimacy ■ Problems with emotions Depression Anxiety Panic Effects of medications ■ Support and rehabilitation groups	Intimacy and Lung Disease (American Lung Association) Open discussion (sharing with patient, significant other, and family)
COPD Management Plan ■ Focus on self-management ■ Knowing usual signs/symptoms ■ Need to report changes ■ Cause of flare-ups ■ Recognition of signs and symptoms of respiratory infection, heart failure ■ Yearly follow-up	Nurse and patient develop and write up COPD manage-ment plan that meets indi-vidual needs
Healthy Nutrition ■ Strategies to lose weight (if overweight) ■ Strategies to gain weight (if underweight)	Consultation with dietitian

COPD, Chronic obstructive pulmonary disease; O_2, oxygen.

Nursing Interventions

Nurses need to participate actively in developing policies establishing smoke-free working environments for themselves and others, controlling smoking in public places, requiring self-extinguishing cigarettes to prevent fire deaths and injuries, prohibiting advertising and tobacco promotions, and mandating health warning labels on cigarette packages.

- Early diagnosis and treatment of respiratory tract infections is another way to decrease COPD incidence. Avoiding exposure to large crowds in peak periods for influenza may be necessary, especially for the older adult and the person with a history of respiratory problems. Influenza and pneumococcal pneumonia vaccines are recommended for the patient with COPD.

The patient with COPD will require acute intervention for complications such as pneumonia, cor pulmonale, and acute respiratory failure. Once the crisis in these situations has been resolved, the nurse can assess the degree and severity of the underlying respiratory problem. The information obtained will help to plan nursing care.

▼ **Patient Teaching**

The most important aspect in long-term care of the patient with COPD is education.

- Help the patient understand that it is possible to plan treatment aimed at preserving lung function and slowing the progression of the disease. Patient and family participation in the treatment plan is essential. Respiratory care, as well as other related approaches, will need to be ongoing.
- A sample teaching plan on the signs of respiratory infection may include when to notify the physician, increasing fluid intake, increasing nebulizer treatments (e.g., from twice a day to four times a day) with physician's order, beginning taking prescribed antibiotics, monitoring symptoms, and notifying the physician regarding effects of these interventions.
- Further components of a teaching plan are discussed in Table 22.

CIRRHOSIS

Definition/Description

Cirrhosis is a chronic progressive disease of the liver characterized by extensive degeneration and destruction of liver parenchymal cells. Excessive alcohol ingestion is the single most common cause of cirrhosis. The four types of cirrhosis, in order of incidence, are as follows:

1. *Alcoholic* (previously *Laennec's) cirrhosis,* also called portal or nutritional cirrhosis, is usually associated with alcohol abuse. The first change in the liver from excessive alcohol intake is an accumulation of fat in the liver cells. Uncomplicated fatty changes in the liver are potentially reversible if the person stops drinking alcohol.
2. *Postnecrotic cirrhosis* is a complication of viral, toxic, or idiopathic hepatitis. Broad bands of scar tissue form within the liver.
3. *Biliary cirrhosis* is associated with chronic biliary obstruction and infection. There is diffuse fibrosis of the liver.
4. *Cardiac cirrhosis* results from long-standing severe right-sided heart failure in patients with cor pulmonale, constrictive pericarditis, and tricuspid insufficiency.

Pathophysiology
In cirrhosis, cell necrosis occurs and the destroyed liver cells are replaced by scar tissue. Eventually, irregular, disorganized regeneration, poor cellular nutrition, and hypoxia caused by inadequate blood flow and scar tissue result in decreased liver function.

Clinical Manifestations
The onset of cirrhosis is usually insidious. Occasionally there is an abrupt onset of manifestations.

- Early manifestations include anorexia, dyspepsia, flatulence, nausea and vomiting, and change in bowel habits (diarrhea or constipation). Other early manifestations are fever, lassitude, abdominal pain, slight weight loss, and enlargement of the liver and spleen.
- Later manifestations may be severe and result from liver failure and portal hypertension. Jaundice, peripheral edema, and ascites develop gradually. Other late symptoms include skin lesions, hematologic disorders, endocrine disturbances, and peripheral neuropathies. In advanced stages the liver becomes small and nodular. (See Fig. 41-5, Lewis and others, *Medical-Surgical Nursing,* edition 5, p. 1204 for the systemic manifestations of cirrhosis.)

Complications
Major complications are portal hypertension with resultant esophageal varices; peripheral edema and ascites; hepatic encephalopathy (coma); and hepatorenal syndrome.

Portal hypertension and *esophageal varices* result because of structural liver changes from cirrhosis; there is compression and destruction of the portal and hepatic veins and sinusoids. Pathophysiologic changes resulting from portal hypertension include the development of collateral circulation in an attempt to reduce high portal pressure and also to reduce increased plasma volume and lymphatic flow.

- Common areas where collateral channels form are the lower esophagus (anastomosis of the left gastric vein and azygos veins), anterior abdominal wall, parietal peritoneum, and rectum.
- Varicosities may develop in areas where collateral and systemic circulations communicate, resulting in esophageal and gastric varices, caput medusae (ring of varices around the umbilicus), and hemorrhoids.

Esophageal varices are a common complication, occurring in two thirds to three fourths of all patients with cirrhosis. These collateral vessels contain little elastic tissue and are quite fragile. They tolerate high pressure poorly, and the result is distended, tortuous veins that bleed easily.

- Bleeding esophageal varices are the most life-threatening complication of cirrhosis.
- Varices rupture and bleed in response to ulceration and irritation. Factors producing ulceration and irritation include alcohol ingestion; swallowing of poorly masticated food; ingestion of coarse food; acid regurgitation from the stomach; and increased intraabdominal pressure caused by nausea, vomiting, straining at stool, coughing, sneezing, or lifting heavy objects.
- Patients may have melena or hematemesis. There may be slow oozing or massive hemorrhage, which is a medical emergency.

Peripheral edema results from decreased colloidal osmotic pressure from impaired liver synthesis of albumin and increased portocaval pressure from portal hypertension. Peripheral edema occurs as ankle and presacral edema.

Ascites is an accumulation of serous fluid in the peritoneal or abdominal cavity. When BP is elevated in the liver, as occurs in portal cirrhosis, proteins move from the blood vessels via larger pores of the sinusoids (capillaries) into the lymph space. When the lymphatic system is unable to carry off excess proteins and water, proteins leak through the liver capsule into the peritoneal cavity. A second mechanism of ascites formation is hypoalbuminemia resulting from the inability of the liver to synthesize albumin. A third mechanism of ascites, hyperaldosteronism, results when aldosterone is not metabolized by damaged hepatocytes, which causes increased renal reabsorption of sodium.

- Ascites is manifested by abdominal distention with weight gain. If ascites is severe, the umbilicus may be everted. Abdominal striae with distended abdominal wall veins may also be present.
- The patient has signs of dehydration (e.g., dry tongue and skin, sunken eyeballs, muscle weakness), with a decrease in urinary output.

- Hypokalemia is common and is due to an excessive loss of potassium from the effects of aldosterone and the use of diuretic therapy to treat ascites.

Hepatic encephalopathy, or coma, is a frequent terminal complication in liver disease. Encephalopathy can occur in any condition in which liver damage causes ammonia to enter the systemic circulation without liver detoxification.

- The main pathogenic agents appear to be nitrogenous ammonia and aromatic amino acids. When blood is shunted past the liver via collateral anastamoses or the liver is unable to convert ammonia to urea, large quantities of ammonia remain in the systemic circulation. Ammonia crosses the blood-brain barrier and produces neurologic toxic manifestations.
- A number of factors may precipitate hepatic encephalopathy because they increase the amount of circulating ammonia, including GI hemorrhage, constipation, infection, hypokalemia, hypovolemia, dehydration, and metabolic alkalosis.

Hepatorenal syndrome is a serious complication of cirrhosis. It is characterized by functional renal failure with advancing azotemia, oliguria, and intractable ascites.

- There is no structural abnormality of the kidneys and the exact cause of decreased renal function is unknown. It is thought to be related to a redistribution of blood flow from the kidneys to the peripheral and splanchnic circulation or to hypovolemia secondary to ascites.
- This syndrome frequently follows diuretic therapy, GI hemorrhage, or paracentesis. It is also associated with a deterioration in renal function.
- Treatment measures, which are usually unsuccessful, include salt-poor albumin, salt and water restrictions, and diuretic therapy.

Diagnostic Studies
- Liver function studies demonstrate an elevation in alkaline phosphatase, aspartate aminotransferase (AST), alanine aminotransferase (ALT), and gamma-glutamyltransferase (GGT).
- Liver biopsy (percutaneous needle) and scan.
- Esophagogastroduodenoscopy.
- Angiography (percutaneous transhepatic portography).
- Prothrombin time is prolonged.
- Serum albumin and protein levels are decreased.
- Complete blood count (CBC) and stool for occult blood.

Collaborative Care
Although there is no specific therapy for cirrhosis, certain measures can be taken to promote liver cell regeneration and prevent or treat complications.

- Rest is significant in reducing the metabolic demands of the liver and allowing for recovery of liver cells. At various times during the progress of cirrhosis, rest may have to take the form of complete bed rest.

Management of ascites is focused on sodium restriction (250 to 500 mg/day), diuretic therapy (e.g., spironolactone [Aldactone]), and fluid removal (paracentesis). Peritoneovenous shunt insertion provides for the continuous reinfusion of ascitic fluid into the venous system.

The main therapeutic goal related to esophageal varices is avoidance of bleeding and hemorrhage. The patient who has esophageal varices should avoid ingesting alcohol, aspirin, and irritating foods. Upper respiratory infections should be treated promptly and coughing should be controlled.

- Management related to bleeding esophageal varices includes the use of vasopressin (VP) and nitroglycerin (NTG), β-adrenergic blockers, balloon tamponade, sclerotherapy, ligation of varices, and shunt therapy.
- Supportive measures during an acute variceal bleed include administration of fresh frozen plasma and packed red blood cells (RBCs), vitamin K (Aquamephyton), and histamine blockers such as cimetidine (Tagamet). Neomycin administration may be started to prevent the occurrence of hepatic encephalopathy from the breakdown of blood and the release of ammonia in the intestine.

The goal of management in hepatic encephalopathy is the reduction of ammonia formation. This consists mainly of protein restriction and reduction of ammonia formation in the intestines. Lactulose (Cephulac) discourages bacterial growth, traps ammonia in the gut, and expels ammonia from the colon. Constipation should be prevented with cathartics and enemas to decrease bacterial action.

- Treatment of hepatic encephalopathy also involves controlling GI hemorrhage and removing blood from the GI tract to decrease protein in the intestine. Electrolyte and acid-base imbalances and infections should also be treated.

Additional Management

There is no specific drug therapy for cirrhosis. A number of medications may be used to treat symptoms and complications of advanced liver disease. Specific nutritional therapy varies with the degree of liver damage and the danger of encephalopathy; generally, protein and sodium are restricted.

Liver transplantation should be considered in patients with recurring hepatic encephalopathy and end-stage liver disease. Transplantation depends on a number of factors, including the cause of the cirrhosis and other systemic medical problems.

Nursing Management

Goals

The patient with cirrhosis will have relief of discomfort, will have minimal to no complications (ascites, esophageal varices, hepatic encephalopathy), and will return to as normal a lifestyle as possible.

See NCP 41-2 for the patient with cirrhosis, Lewis and others, *Medical-Surgical Nursing,* edition 5, p. 1214.

Nursing Diagnoses/Collaborative Problems

- Ineffective breathing pattern *related to* pressure on diaphragm and reduced lung volume secondary to ascites
- Ineffective airway clearance *related to* inability to remove and swallow secretions and bleeding from esophageal varices.
- Risk for infection *related to* leukopenia and increased susceptibility to environmental pathogens
- Activity intolerance *related to* fatigue, anemia, ascites, dyspnea, treatment schedule, and cardiac deconditioning
- Altered nutrition: less than body requirements *related to* anorexia, impaired utilization and storage of nutrients, and nausea
- Risk for injury *related to* diminished sensory perception secondary to peripheral neuropathy
- Impaired skin integrity *related to* edema, ascites, and pruritus
- Potential complication: hemorrhage *related to* bleeding tendency secondary to altered clotting factors
- Potential complication: hepatic encephalopathy *related to* increased formation of ammonia and aromatic amino acids

Nursing Interventions

Prevention and early treatment of cirrhosis must focus on the primary etiology.

- Alcoholism must be treated; adequate nutrition, especially for the alcoholic and other individuals at risk for cirrhosis, is essential to promote liver regeneration.
- Hepatitis must be identified and treated early so that it does not progress to chronic hepatitis.
- Biliary disease must be treated so that stones do not cause obstruction and infection.
- The underlying cause (e.g., chronic lung disease) of right-sided heart failure must be treated so that the heart failure does not lead to cirrhosis.

The focus of acute nursing interventions is on conserving the patient's strength. Rest enables the liver to restore itself. Complete bed rest may not always be necessary.

- Anorexia, nausea and vomiting, pressure from ascites, and poor eating habits all create problems in the maintenance of an adequate intake of nutrients. Nursing measures relating to nutrition for patients with hepatitis also apply here, including oral hygiene and between-meal nourishment.

- A semi-Fowler's or Fowler's position allows for maximal respiratory efficiency when dyspnea is a problem. Pillows can be used to support arms and chest and may increase patient comfort and ability to breathe.

- Meticulous skin care is essential because edematous tissues are subject to breakdown. An alternating-air pressure mattress or other special mattress should be used. A turning schedule (minimum of every 2 hours) must be adhered to rigidly. The abdomen may be supported with pillows.

- Accurate recordings of intake and output, daily weights, and measurements of extremities and abdominal girth help in the ongoing assessment of edema.

- When a paracentesis is done, have the patient void immediately before the procedure to prevent puncture of the bladder. After the procedure, monitor for hypovolemia and electrolyte imbalances, and check the dressing for bleeding and leakage.

- If the patient has esophageal varices, monitor for signs of bleeding from varices, such as hematemesis and melena. If hematemesis occurs, assess patient for hemorrhage.

- The focus of care with hepatic encephalopathy is on sustaining life and assisting with measures to reduce the formation of ammonia. Factors that are known to precipitate coma should be controlled as much as possible.

▼ **Patient Teaching**

The patient and family need to understand the importance of continuous health care and medical supervision. They should be taught symptoms of complications and when to seek medical attention.

- Measures to achieve and maintain remission should be encouraged, including proper diet, rest, avoidance of potentially hepatotoxic over-the-counter drugs such as acetaminophen, and abstinence from alcohol.

- Provide information regarding community support programs such as Alcoholics Anonymous.

- Other health teaching should include instruction about adequate rest periods, how to detect early signs of complications, skin care, drug therapy precautions, observation for bleeding, and protection from infection.

- Counseling information regarding sexual problems may be needed.

- Referral to a community or home health nurse may be helpful to ensure adequate patient compliance with prescribed therapy.

COLD-RELATED INJURIES

Definition/Description

Cold injuries may be localized (frostbite) or systemic (hypothermia). Contributing factors include age, duration of exposure, environmental temperature, preexisting conditions (e.g., diabetes), medications that suppress shivering (narcotics, heroin, psychotropic agents, and antiemetics), and alcohol intoxication, which causes peripheral vasodilation and depresses shivering.

- Smokers have an increased risk of cold-related injury due to the vasoconstrictive effects of nicotine.

Frostbite occurs with peripheral vasoconstriction in response to cold exposure, which decreases blood flow. As cellular temperature decreases and ice crystals form in intracellular spaces, intracellular sodium and chloride increase and the cell membrane is destroyed. The depth of frostbite is the result of ambient temperature, length of exposure, type and condition (wet or dry) of clothing, and contact with metal surfaces. Other factors that affect severity include skin color (dark-skinned people are more prone to frostbite), exhaustion, and poor peripheral vascular status.

Superficial frostbite involves skin and subcutaneous tissue, usually the ears, nose, fingers, and toes. The skin is pale, waxy, and feels crunchy and frozen. The patient may complain of tingling, numbness, or a burning sensation. The damaged area should be handled carefully and never squeezed, massaged, or scrubbed.

- The affected area should be elevated and warm soaks (104° to 110° F [40° to 43° C]) applied. The patient often experiences a warm, stinging sensation as tissue thaws.
- Blisters form within a few hours. The blisters should be debrided and a sterile dressing applied.

Deep frostbite involves muscle, bone, and tendon. The skin is white, hard, and insensitive to touch. The area has the appearance of deep thermal injury with mottling gradually progressing to gangrene.

- The affected extremity is submersed in a circulating water bath (104° to 108° F [40° to 42° C]) until distal flush occurs. Significant edema may begin within 3 hours with blistering in 6 hours to days.
- Parenteral analgesia is required in severe frostbite due to the pain associated with tissue thawing.
- Amputation may be required if the injured area is untreated or treatment is unsuccessful.
- The patient is admitted to the hospital for observation for 24 to 48 hours, with bed rest, elevation of the injured part, and prophylactic antibiotics if the wound is at risk for infection.

Hypothermia, in which a person's core temperature is <95° F (<35° C), occurs when the individual is exposed to freezing temperatures, cold winds, and wet, damp terrain in the presence of physical exhaustion, inadequate clothing, and inexperience.

- Near drowning and water immersion are also associated with hypothermia. The elderly are more prone to hypothermia due to diminished energy reserves, decreased shivering response, decreased sensory perception, and medications that alter body defenses.
- Hypothermia mimics cerebral or metabolic disturbances causing ataxia, confusion, and withdrawal, so the patient may be misdiagnosed.
- Patients with *mild hypothermia* (90° to 95° F [33° to 35° C]) have shivering, lethargy, confusion, and minor heart rate (HR) changes. Shivering disappears at temperatures <92° F (<32° C).
- *Moderate hypothermia* (87° to 90° F [31° to 33° C]) causes rigidity, bradycardia, slowed respiratory rate, BP obtainable only by Doppler, metabolic and respiratory acidosis, and hypovolemia.
- *Profound hypothermia* (<87° F [<30.5° C]) makes the person appear dead. Metabolic rate, HR, and respirations are so slow they may be difficult to detect. Reflexes are absent and the pupils are fixed and dilated. The cause of death is usually refractory ventricular fibrillation. Every effort is made to warm the patient to >90° F (>32° C) before the person is pronounced dead.

Treatment focuses on rewarming the patient, correcting dehydration and acidosis, maintaining a patent airway, and treating cardiac arrhythmias.

- *Passive rewarming* is used for mild hypothermia. The patient is moved to a warm, dry place; damp clothing is removed; and warm blankets are applied.
- *Active external rewarming* with warm blankets, radiant heat lamps, hot water bottles, and hot water baths is used for moderate hypothermia. The patient should be closely monitored for marked vasodilation and hypotension. *Active core rewarming* refers to heat applied directly to the core. Techniques include heated, humidified oxygen (O_2) at 105° to 115° F (40.5° to 46.1° C) and installation of heated fluids via IV infusions, gastric lavage, hemodialysis and heart-lung bypass.

Ventricular arrhythmias do not respond to conventional therapy at low core temperatures, so only one defibrillation attempt is recommended. Core temperatures should be carefully monitored during rewarming procedures. Rewarming should be discontinued once the core temperature reaches 93° F (34° C). (See Table 64-11 for the emergency management of hypothermia, Lewis and others, *Medical-Surgical Nursing,* edition 5, p. 1968.)

- Discharge teaching focuses on educating the patient to avoid future problems. Essential information includes dressing in layers for cold weather, covering the head, carrying high-carbohydrate foods for extra calories, and developing a plan for survival should an accident occur. Homeless individuals should be sheltered until fully recovered.

COLORECTAL CANCER

Definition/Description
Colorectal cancer is the second most common cause of cancer death in the United States. Cancer of the colon and rectum may occur at any age but is most prevalent over the age of 50. The 5-year survival rate for early, localized colorectal cancers is 91%; the rate is 63% for cancer that has spread to adjacent organs and lymph nodes.

Pathophysiology
The causes of colorectal cancer remain unclear. Age is a risk factor in both men and women. Risk for development in the general population increases slightly after age 40 and then rises rapidly in the following decades.

- The high-caloric, high-fat Western diet is an important environmental factor that has been closely associated with the development of colon cancer.
- Individuals with ulcerative colitis and familial polyposis have an increased risk for colon cancer.

Adenocarcinoma is the most common type of colon cancer. Most colorectal cancers appear to arise from adenomatous polyps. All tumors tend to spread through the walls of the intestine and into the lymphatic system. Tumors commonly spread to the liver because venous blood flow is through the portal vein.

Clinical Manifestations
Manifestations are usually nonspecific or do not appear until the disease is advanced.

- Rectal bleeding is the most common symptom of colorectal cancer. Other common manifestations include alternating constipation and diarrhea, change in stool caliber (narrow, ribbon-like), and sensation of incomplete evacuation.
- Colorectal cancer may also be asymptomatic. Vague abdominal discomfort or crampy, colicky abdominal pain may be present.

Iron deficiency anemia and occult bleeding dictate further investigation. Weakness and fatigue result from anemia.

Diagnostic Studies

- Complete blood count (CBC) and stool testing for occult blood.
- Digital rectal examination.
- Air-contrast barium enema and sigmoidoscopy if colorectal cancer is suspected. Colonoscopy is the procedure of choice if a questionable lesion is found on sigmoidoscopy or barium enema.
- CT scan of abdomen and pelvis and endorectal ultrasonography to localize the lesion.
- Carcinoembryonic antigen (CEA) serum test to follow the progress of the patient after surgery.

Collaborative Care

Prognosis and treatment correlate with pathologic staging of colon cancer. Several methods of staging are currently being used. The most widely known is Dukes' classification. Surgical removal of the primary lesion is the treatment for Dukes' stages A, B, and C. Prognosis for Dukes' stage A (negative nodes, lesion limited to mucosa) is 90% to 100% 5-year survival, compared to <15% with Dukes' stage D (distant, unresectable metastases). Another classification system for colorectal cancer is the TNM system (see Table 11, p. 79).

Several noninvasive procedures may be performed through a colonoscope to treat certain types of colorectal cancer effectively.

- Endoscopic polypectomy is a highly effective and safe procedure. Adequate treatment is thought to be obtained if the resected margin of the polyp is free of cancer, the cancer is well differentiated, and there is no apparent lymphatic or blood vessel involvement.
- Laser therapy may be used to ablate nonresectable tumors. This is usually used only as palliative therapy in patients with obstructive symptoms.

Surgical Therapy

Surgery is the only curative treatment for colorectal cancer; the type of surgery performed is determined by the location and extent of the cancer. The success of the surgery depends on resection of the tumor with an adequate margin of healthy bowel and resection of regional lymph nodes.

- *Right hemicolectomy* is performed when the cancer is located in the cecum, ascending colon, hepatic flexure, or transverse colon to the right of the middle colic artery. *Left hemicolectomy* involves resection of the left transverse colon, splenic flexure, descending colon, sigmoid colon, and upper portion of the rectum. *Abdominal-perineal resection* is most often performed when the cancer is located within 5 cm of the anus.

- *Low anterior resection* may be indicated for tumors of the rectosigmoid and mid to upper rectum.
- *Sphincter-sparing procedures* are being performed on patients who are poor operative risks and for patients with early disease. In these procedures a local resection is performed and anal sphincters are left intact.

Radiation Therapy and Chemotherapy

Radiation may be used preoperatively or as a palliative measure for patients with advanced lesions. As a palliative measure, its primary objective is to reduce the tumor size and provide symptomatic relief (see Radiation Therapy, p. 681). Chemotherapy is recommended when the patient has positive lymph nodes at the time of surgery or has metastatic disease. No drug is available that can cure malignant colon or rectal tumors. The most commonly used drugs are 5-fluorouracil (5-FU) and methotrexate. Nitrosoureas, carmustine (BCNU), levamisole, and semustine (MeCCNU) are sometimes used in combination with 5-FU (see Chemotherapy, p. 643).

Nursing Management

Goals

The patient with cancer of the colon or rectum will have no metastasis or recurrence of cancer, normal bowel elimination patterns, quality of life appropriate to disease progression, relief of pain, and feelings of comfort and well-being.

Nursing Diagnoses

- Diarrhea or constipation *related to* altered bowel elimination patterns
- Pain *related to* difficulty in passing stools due to partial or complete obstruction from tumor
- Fear *related to* diagnosis of colon cancer, surgical or therapeutic interventions, and possible terminal illness
- Ineffective individual coping *related to* diagnosis of cancer and side effects of treatment

Nursing Interventions

Screening recommendations from the American Cancer Society for colorectal cancer in patients who are not at high risk include annual digital rectal examination and fecal testing for occult blood beginning at age 40. Starting at age 50, flexible sigmoidoscopy should be done every 3 to 5 years, after two negative examinations done 1 year apart. Positive findings should be followed with colonoscopy or air-contrast barium enema.

- For high-risk patients screening usually begins with colonoscopy and continues at more frequent intervals that vary according to risk factors.

Preoperative care. Acute nursing care for patients with colon resections is similar to the care of the patient having a laparotomy (see Abdominal Pain, Acute, p. 3). The patient should be taught side-to-side positioning and made to understand that short walks are better than sitting. The nurse should teach and assist the patient in proper positioning for taking a sitz bath.

Postoperative care. After an abdominal-perineal resection, there are two wounds, and a stoma has been surgically constructed in the left lower quadrant.

- Management of the perineal incision differs depending on the type of wound. Three techniques are used: (1) packing of the entire open wound, (2) partial closure with Penrose drains for open drainage, and (3) primary closure of the perineal wound with closed-suction drainage of pelvic cavity.

- A patient who has open and packed wounds requires meticulous care. During the immediate postoperative period the perineal dressing is reinforced and changed frequently because drainage can be profuse for several hours after surgery. All drainage is carefully assessed for the amount, color, and consistency; drainage is usually serosanguinous.

- The nurse should examine the wound regularly and record bleeding, excessive drainage, and unusual odor. The nurse should also observe for signs of edema, erythema, drainage around the suture line, fever, and elevated white blood cell (WBC) count.

- The patient may complain of pain and itching in and around the wound. Antipruritic agents and sitz baths are usually ordered. Use of a pressure-reducing chair cushion provides comfort when sitting. Sitting on a toilet for prolonged periods is discouraged until the perineal wound is well healed.

- The perineal wound may not be completely healed before discharge. After discharge the patient is usually seen by the physician, home health nurse, and enterostomal therapist in an outpatient clinic. The wound is usually irrigated and debrided; if necessary, the infected area may be cauterized with silver nitrate. The nurse should report drainage because it may also indicate the presence of a foreign body, fistula, osteomyelitis, or rectal tissue not removed during surgery. The patient and significant others are taught management of the wound and the procedure to take a sitz bath at home.

- Sexual dysfunction is a possible complication of an abdominal-perineal resection and should be included in the plan of care. The enterostomal therapy nurse can often provide correct and factual information concerning sexual dysfunction.

- Psychologic support for patient as well as for family is important. The recovery period is long and the possibility of recurrence of cancer is always present.

- The patient and family should be aware of all community services available for assistance.

CONGESTIVE HEART FAILURE

Definition/Description

Congestive heart failure (CHF) is a cardiovascular condition in which the heart is unable to pump an adequate amount of blood to meet the metabolic needs of body tissues. CHF is not a disease; it is a syndrome caused by a variety of pathophysiologic processes including coronary artery disease (CAD), rheumatic heart disease, cor pulmonale, arrhythmias, and anemia. CHF is characterized by left ventricular dysfunction, reduced exercise tolerance, diminished quality of life, and shortened life expectancy.

Risk factors for CHF include CAD, advancing age, hypertension, diabetes mellitus, cigarette smoking, obesity, and high cholesterol levels.

Pathophysiology

CHF may be caused by any interference with the normal mechanisms regulating cardiac output (CO). CO depends on (1) preload, (2) afterload, (3) myocardial contractility, (4) heart rate (HR), and (5) metabolic state of the individual. Any alteration in these factors can lead to decreased ventricular function and subsequent CHF.

- Major causes of CHF may be divided into two subgroups: (1) underlying cardiac diseases, such as CAD and cardiomyopathy, and (2) precipitating factors, such as anemia, infection, and nutritional deficiencies. (See the complete listing of causes in Tables 33-1 and 33-2, Lewis and others, *Medical-Surgical Nursing,* edition 5, pp. 888-889.) Precipitating factors are generally more amenable to treatment than cardiac diseases.

Ventricular failure can be described as (1) a defect in systolic function that results in impaired ventricular emptying or (2) a defect in diastolic function that causes an impairment in ventricular filling. Patients with heart failure comprise three distinct groups: (1) those with failure of systolic ejection, (2) those with abnormal resistance to diastolic filling, and (3) those presenting with mixed systolic and diastolic dysfunction.

Systolic failure, the most common cause of CHF, is a defect in the ability of the cardiac myofibrils to shorten, which decreases the muscles' ability to contract (pump). Systolic failure is caused by impaired contractile function (e.g., myocardial infarction), increased afterload (e.g., hypertension), or mechanical abnormalities (e.g., valvular heart disease).

Diastolic failure is characterized by high filling pressures and the resultant venous engorgement in both the pulmonary and systemic systems. The diagnosis of diastolic failure is based on the presence of pulmonary congestion and pulmonary hypertension in the setting of normal ejection fraction. Diastolic failure is commonly seen in older adults as a result of myocardial fibrosis and hypertension.

Mixed systolic and diastolic failure is seen in disease states such as dilated cardiomyopathy (DCM), in which poor systolic function (weakened muscle function) is further compromised by dilated left ventricular walls that are unable to relax.

The patient with ventricular failure of any type has low systemic arterial BP, low CO, and poor renal perfusion. When pulmonary congestion and edema are present, the diagnosis of CHF may be made. Whether a patient arrives at this point acutely (from a myocardial infarction [MI]) or chronically (from worsening cardiomyopathy or hypertension), the body's response to this low CO is to mobilize compensatory mechanisms to maintain CO and BP. The main compensatory mechanisms include (1) ventricular dilation, (2) ventricular hypertrophy, (3) increased sympathetic nervous system stimulation, and (4) hormonal response.

CHF is usually manifested by biventricular failure, although one ventricle may precede the other in dysfunction.

- The most common form of initial heart failure is left-sided failure. CHF occurs in a retrograde fashion, progressing from the left ventricle (LV) to the pulmonary system to the right ventricle (RV). LV failure will usually lead to and is the main cause of right-sided failure.
- Right-sided failure can occur without preceding LV failure as a result of right ventricular MI or cor pulmonale. CHF will eventually develop in the majority of persons with moderate to severe cardiac disease.

Acute Clinical Manifestations

Regardless of etiology, acute heart failure typically presents as pulmonary edema. The most common factor in the onset of pulmonary edema is LV failure due to CAD.

- Manifestations of pulmonary edema are unmistakable: the patient may be agitated, pale, and possibly cyanotic, with clammy and cold skin.
- The patient has severe dyspnea, as evidenced by obvious use of respiratory accessory muscles, respiratory rate >30 breaths per minute, and orthopnea. Wheezing and coughing with production of frothy, blood-tinged sputum may also occur.
- Auscultation of the lungs may reveal bubbling crackles, wheezes, and rhonchi. The patient's HR is rapid, and BP may be elevated or decreased depending on the severity of edema.

Chronic Clinical Manifestations

Manifestations of chronic CHF depend on the patient's age, underlying type and extent of heart disease, and which ventricle is failing to pump effectively. Table 23 lists manifestations of LV and RV failure. The patient with chronic CHF will probably have manifestations of biventricular failure.

- Fatigue is one of the earliest symptoms. The patient notices fatigue after activities that normally are not tiring.
- Dyspnea is a common sign. The shortness of breath makes the patient conscious of air hunger that prompts rapid, shallow respirations. Dyspnea can occur with mild exertion or at rest (orthopnea).
- Paroxysmal nocturnal dyspnea (PND) occurs when the patient is asleep. The patient awakens in a panic, has feelings of suffocation, and has a strong desire to seek respiratory relief by sitting up.
- Other common signs include tachycardia; edema in the legs, liver, abdominal cavity, and lungs; nocturia; cool and dusky skin; restlessness and confusion; angina-type chest pain; and weight changes.

Complications

Pleural effusion results from increasing pressure in the pleural capillaries. The pleural effusion usually develops in the right lower lobe initially.

Left ventricular thrombus may occur with acute or chronic CHF in which the enlarged LV and poor CO combine to increase the chance of thrombus formation in the LV. Many health care providers will administer anticoagulants to decrease the development of thrombus formation in patients with chronic CHF.

Hepatomegaly may result as liver lobules become congested with venous blood. Hepatic congestion leads to impaired liver function; eventually liver cells die, fibrosis occurs, and cirrhosis can develop.

Diagnostic Studies

- Serum chemistries, renal profile, and liver function tests.
- Chest x-ray to assess and monitor heart failure.
- ECG to confirm cardiac changes. Exercise-stress testing and nuclear imaging studies add additional information to ECG findings.
- Echocardiography measures ventricular and valvular function and measures size of cardiac chambers.
- Hemodynamic monitoring via a pulmonary artery catheter directly assesses cardiac function.
- Cardiac catheterization and angiocardiography help detect underlying heart disease.

Nursing and Collaborative Management: Acute Congestive Heart Failure and Pulmonary Edema

The goal of therapy is to improve left ventricular function by decreasing intravascular volume, decreasing venous return, decreasing

Table 23   Clinical Manifestations of Heart Failure

Right-sided heart failure	Left-sided heart failure
Signs RV heaves Murmurs Peripheral edema Weight gain Edema of dependent body parts (sacrum, anterior tibias, pedal edema) Ascites Anasarca (massive generalized body edema) Jugular venous distention Hepatomegaly (liver engorgement) Right-sided pleural effusion **Symptoms** Fatigue Dependent edema Right upper quadrant pain Anorexia and GI bloating Nausea	**Signs** LV heaves Cheyne-Stokes respirations Pulsus alternans (alternating pulses: strong, weak) Increased HR PMI displaced inferiorly and posteriorly (LV hypertrophy) ↓ PaO_2, slight ↑ $PaCO_2$ (poor oxygen exchange) Crackles (pulmonary edema) S_2 and S_4 heart sounds **Symptoms** Fatigue Dyspnea (shallow respirations up to 32-40/min) Orthopnea (paroxysmal nocturnal dyspnea) Dry, hacking cough Pulmonary edema Nocturia

GI, Gastrointestinal; *HR*, heart rate; *LV*, left ventricle; *PaCO$_2$*, partial pressure of carbon dioxide in arterial blood; *PaO$_2$*, partial pressure of oxygen in arterial blood; *PMI*, point of maximal impulse; *RV*, right ventricle.

C

afterload, improving gas exchange and oxygenation, increasing CO, and reducing anxiety. Major components of management include:

- Decreasing intravascular volume with the use of diuretics by reducing venous return to the failing LV. A loop diuretic (e.g., furosemide [Lasix], bumetanide [Bumex]) is the drug of choice for decreasing volume, since it may be administered quickly by IV push and acts rapidly within the kidney.
- The use of IV nitroglycerin (NTG), which reduces circulating volume by decreasing preload. NTG also increases coronary artery circulation by dilating coronary arteries.
- Decreasing venous return, which reduces amount of volume returned to the LV. This can be accomplished by placing the patient in a high Fowler's position with feet horizontal in bed or dangling at bedside.
- The use of IV nitroprusside (Nipride), which reduces preload and afterload. Because of its potent vasodilator effects, this is the drug of choice for the patient with pulmonary edema.
- Morphine also reduces preload and afterload. It dilates both the pulmonary and systemic blood vessels, thereby decreasing pulmonary pressures and improving gas exchange.
- Administration of oxygen (O_2), which helps to increase the percentage of O_2 in inspired air (see Oxygen Therapy, p. 676). In severe pulmonary edema the patient may need to be intubated and placed on a mechanical ventilator.
- Improvement of LV function through the use of digitalis increases contractility but also increases myocardial O_2 consumption. Newer inotropic drugs (e.g., dobutamine [Dobutrex], amrinone [Inocor]) increase myocardial contractility without increasing O_2 consumption.

Hemodynamic monitoring may become necessary if rapid resolution of symptoms does not occur with diuretics, morphine, and NTG or if the patient becomes hypotensive (see the section on hemodynamic monitoring, Lewis and others, *Medical-Surgical Nursing*, edition 5, p. 1917).

Nursing care focuses on continual physical assessment, hemodynamic monitoring, and monitoring patient response to treatment.

Collaborative Care: Chronic Congestive Heart Failure

One of the most important goals in the treatment of chronic CHF is to treat the underlying cause. If arrhythmias have precipitated the failure, they should be treated accordingly. If the underlying cause is hypertension, antihypertensives should be used in treatment. Valvular defects can be treated with surgery.

- If cardiac dysfunction is a result of ischemic heart disease, specific interventions such as thrombolytic therapy, percutaneous transluminal coronary angioplasty (PTCA), or coronary artery bypass surgery may be needed.

Additional management includes:

- Administration of O_2 to improve saturation and assist in meeting tissue oxygen needs, thereby decreasing dyspnea and fatigue.
- Physical and emotional rest so the patient may conserve energy and decrease the need for additional O_2. A patient with severe CHF needs to be on bed rest with limited activity. A patient with mild CHF can be ambulatory with a restriction on strenuous activity.

General objectives of drug therapy for CHF are (1) correction of sodium and water retention and volume overload, (2) reduction of cardiac workload, (3) improvement of myocardial contractility, and (4) control of precipitating and complicating factors. Because CHF is a complex syndrome, it is unlikely that any single drug therapy would be successful alone. A combination of drugs has been the most successful in treating patients with CHF.

- Positive inotropic agents (e.g., digitalis) are used to improve cardiac contractility.
- β-Adrenergic agonists (e.g., dopamine) are used in the short-term treatment of acute CHF. These agents increase cardiac contractility and urine output (decreasing preload).
- Diuretics mobilize edematous fluid, reduce pulmonary venous pressure, and reduce preload. Three potent loop diuretics are furosemide (Lasix), ethacrynic acid (Edecrin), and bumetanide (Bumex).
- LV volume overload (increased preload and afterload) exerts a major role in the development of LV dysfunction and has led to the addition of vasodilators (e.g., angiotensin converting enzyme [ACE] inhibitors) in the treatment plan.
- Carvedilol (Coreg), a β-adrenergic blocking agent, is used in chronic CHF and halts the negative effects of the sympathetic nervous system on the failing heart.

Nutritional Therapy

Diet education and weight management are critical to the control of chronic CHF.

- The patient should be taught what foods are low and high in sodium and ways to enhance food flavors without the use of salt (e.g., substituting lemon juice and various spices). A commonly prescribed diet for a patient with mild CHF is a 2 g sodium diet. (For sample menu plans for a 2 g sodium diet, see Table 33-10, Lewis and others, *Medical-Surgical Nursing*, edition 5, p. 898.) For more severe CHF, sodium intake is restricted to 500 to 1000 mg.

- Fluid restrictions are not commonly prescribed for mild to moderate CHF. Diuretic therapy and digitalis preparations act as effective diuretics to promote fluid excretion. However, in moderate to severe CHF, fluid restrictions are usually implemented.
- When weight reduction is indicated to decrease cardiac workload, the nurse and dietitian can assist the patient and family in menu planning. Patients should be instructed to weigh themselves at the same time each day, preferably before breakfast, while wearing the same type of clothing. This helps to identify early signs of fluid retention.

Nursing Management: Chronic Congestive Heart Failure

Goals

The patient with CHF will have decreased peripheral edema, decreased shortness of breath, increased exercise tolerance, compliance with prescribed medications, and no complications related to CHF

See NCP 33-1 for the patient with CHF, Lewis and others, *Medical-Surgical Nursing,* edition 5, p. 900.

Nursing Diagnoses

- Fluid volume excess *related to* pump failure
- Activity intolerance *related to* fatigue secondary to cardiac insufficiency, pulmonary congestion, and inadequate nutrition
- Impaired gas exchange *related to* increased preload, mechanical failure, or immobility
- Sleep pattern disturbance *related to* nocturnal dyspnea, inability to assume favored sleep position, and nocturia
- Anxiety *related to* dyspnea or perceived threat of death
- Risk for impaired skin integrity *related to* edema or immobility
- Ineffective management of therapeutic regimen *related to* lack of knowledge regarding signs and symptoms of CHF, proper diet, and medications

Nursing Interventions

An important measure used to prevent heart failure is the treatment or control of underlying heart disease. For example, in rheumatic valvular disease, valve replacement should be planned before lung congestion develops.

- Early and continued treatment of hypertension is important. Hyperlipidemic states in persons with CAD should be managed with diet, exercise, and medication.
- The use of antiarrhythmic agents or pacemakers is indicated for people with serious arrhythmias or conduction disturbances.
- When a patient is diagnosed with CHF, preventive care should focus on slowing the progression of the disease. Knowledge of the importance of following the medication, diet, and exercise regimen is paramount.

Many persons with CHF do not experience an acute episode. If they do, they are usually initially managed in a critical care unit and later transferred to a general unit when their condition has stabilized. Nursing management for the patient with CHF applies to the patient with stabilized acute or chronic CHF.

CHF is a chronic illness for most persons. Important nursing responsibilities are (1) educating the patient about physiologic changes that have occurred and (2) assisting the patient to adapt to both physiologic and psychologic changes. It must be emphasized to the patient that it is possible to live productively with this health problem.

- Home health care is a vital factor in preventing future hospitalization for this patient. Home nursing care will follow up with ongoing clinical assessments and monitoring of vital signs and response to therapies. (See Table 33-13, Lewis and others, *Medical-Surgical Nursing,* edition 5, p. 902.)
- It must be stressed that the disease is chronic and that medication must be continued to keep the heart failure under control. The patient must understand the importance of maintaining adequate drug levels, as well as the danger of omitting or making up missed doses.
- The patient should also be taught to recognize signs of digitalis toxicity, how to take pulse rate, the symptoms of hypokalemia, and energy-saving behaviors.
- Small achievable goals and possible lifestyle changes need to be discussed with the patient and family.

CONJUNCTIVITIS

Definition/Description

Conjuctivitis is an inflammation or infection of the conjunctiva and one of the most common inflammatory eye diseases. Conjunctivitis may be caused by bacterial, viral, or chlamydial microorganisms, with inflammation resulting from exposure to allergens or chemical irritants (including cigarette smoke). The *tarsal conjunctiva* (lining of the lid interior surface) may become inflamed as a result of a chronic foreign body in the eye, such as a contact lens or an ocular prosthesis.

Acute bacterial conjunctivitis (pinkeye) is a common infection. Although it occurs in every age group, epidemics commonly occur in children because of poor hygiene. In adults and children the most common causative microorganism is *Staphylococcus aureus.*

Clinical Manifestations

- Bacterial conjunctivitis: irritation, tearing, redness, and mucopurulent drainage. Although this typically occurs initially in one eye, it spreads rapidly to the unaffected eye.
- Viral conjunctivitis: tearing, foreign body sensation, redness, and mild photophobia. Unless other ocular structures become involved, this condition is usually mild and self-limiting.
- Allergic conjunctivitis: itching, burning, redness, tearing, and white or clear exudate. Allergic conjunctivitis is caused by exposure to certain allergens and can be mild, transitory, or severe enough to cause significant swelling, sometimes even ballooning the conjunctiva beyond the eyelids.

Collaborative Care

- Bacterial conjunctivitis is usually self-limiting, but treatment with antibiotic drops will shorten the course of the disorder. Careful handwashing and the use of individual or disposable towels will help prevent the spread of infection.
- Viral conjunctivitis treatment is usually palliative. If the patient is severely symptomatic, topical corticosteroids provide temporary relief but have no benefit in the final outcome. Antiviral drops are ineffective and therefore not indicated.
- Allergic conjunctivitis treatment includes artificial tears to dilute the allergen and wash it from the eye. Effective topical medications include antihistamines, cromolyn (Intal), and corticosteroids.

CONSTIPATION

Description/Definition

Constipation may be defined as a decrease in the frequency of bowel movements from what is "normal" for the individual—hard, difficult-to-pass stool; a decrease in stool volume; or retention of feces in the rectum. Normal bowel elimination may vary from three times a day to once every 3 days.

- Frequently, constipation may be due to insufficient dietary fiber, inadequate fluid intake, medication use, and lack of exercise. Constipation may also be due to ignoring the urge to defecate, chronic laxative abuse, and multiple organic causes. Changes in diet, mealtime, or daily routines are a few environmental factors that may cause constipation. Depression and stress can also result in constipation.

Clinical Manifestations

Constipation may vary from a chronic discomfort to an acute event mimicking an "acute abdomen." Clinical manifestations are presented in Table 24.

- Hemorrhoids are the most common complication of chronic constipation. They result from venous engorgement due to repeated Valsalva maneuvers (straining) and venous compression from hard impacted stool (see Hemorrhoids, p. 291).
- Diverticulosis is another potential complication of chronic constipation (see Diverticulitis/Diverticulosis, p. 209).
- In the presence of obstipation or fecal impaction secondary to constipation, colonic perforation may occur. Perforation, which is life-threatening, causes abdominal pain, nausea, vomiting, fever, and an elevated white blood cell (WBC) count.

Diagnostic Studies

A thorough history and physical examination should be performed so that the underlying cause of constipation can be identified.

- Abdominal x-rays, barium enema, colonoscopy, sigmoidoscopy, and anorectal manometry may be helpful in the diagnosis.
- In severe constipation, anorectal manometry, GI tract transit studies, and sigmoidoscopic rectal biopsies may be performed.

Collaborative Care

Most cases of constipation can be managed with diet therapy, including fiber and fluids, and an exercise program. Laxatives should always be used cautiously; with chronic overuse they may become a cause of constipation. Enemas are fast acting and beneficial in the immediate treatment of constipation but should be limited in their use for long-term treatment. Soapsuds enemas should be avoided because they may lead to inflammation of colon mucosa. Oil-retention enemas may be used to soften fecal impactions.

Table 24	Clinical Manifestations of Constipation
Hard, dry stool	Increased flatulence
Abdominal distention	Nausea
Abdominal pain	Anorexia
Decreased frequency of bowel movements	Headache
	Palpable mass
Straining	Stool with blood
Rectal pressure	Dizziness
Tenesmus	Urinary retention

- The patient with severe constipation related to a motility or mechanical disorder may require more intensive treatment. In a patient with unrelenting constipation, a subtotal colectomy with ileorectal anastomosis is the procedure of choice.

Many patients experience an improvement in their symptoms when they increase their intake of dietary fiber and fluids. The diet should include a fluid intake of at least 3000 ml/day, unless contraindicated by heart or renal disease. Increasing fiber intake without increasing fluids may predispose the patient to impaction or obstruction.

Nursing Management

Goals

The patient with constipation will increase dietary intake of fiber and fluids; have passage of soft, formed stools; and not have any complications, such as bleeding hemorrhoids.

Nursing Diagnoses

- Constipation *related to* inadequate dietary intake of fiber, inadequate fluid intake, and decreased physical activity

Nursing Interventions

Interventions should be based on the assessment and symptoms of the patient.

- Proper position is important when defecating. For a patient in bed, the head of the bed should be elevated as high as the patient can tolerate. For the person who can sit on a toilet, a footstool may be placed in front of toilet. Placing feet on a footstool promotes flexion of the thighs, which assists in defecation.
- The patient with poor muscle tone should be encouraged to exercise the abdominal muscles and can be taught to contract abdominal muscles several times a day. Sit-ups and straight leg raises can also be used to improve abdominal muscle tone.
- Some patients may have to be encouraged to increase their social activities as well as their physical activity; this is especially true of older adults who may become depressed and socially isolated.

▼ Patient Teaching

- Teach the patient the importance of dietary measures to prevent constipation. Emphasis should be placed on maintenance of a high-fiber diet, increased fluid intake, and a regular exercise program.
- The patient should be taught to establish a regular time to defecate and to not suppress the urge to defecate. In many persons the urge to defecate occurs after breakfast because of stimulation of the gastrocolic reflex.
- The patient should be discouraged from using laxatives and enemas to achieve fecal elimination.

COR PULMONALE

Cor pulmonale is enlargement of the right ventricle (RV) secondary to diseases of the lung, thorax, or pulmonary circulation. Pulmonary hypertension is usually a preexisting condition in the individual with cor pulmonale. Cor pulmonale may be present with or without overt cardiac failure.

- The most common cause of acute cor pulmonale is a massive pulmonary embolism. However, cor pulmonale is usually chronic, resulting from alveolar hypoxia in chronic obstructive pulmonary disease (COPD). Almost any disorder that affects the respiratory system can cause cor pulmonale.

Clinical Manifestations

Manifestations include dyspnea, chronic productive cough, wheezing respirations, retrosternal or substernal pain, and fatigue.

- If heart failure accompanies cor pulmonale, additional manifestations, such as peripheral edema, weight gain, distended neck veins, full, bounding pulse, and enlarged liver, will also be found.

Collaborative Care

Management is directed at treating the underlying pulmonary problem that precipitated the heart problem. Low-flow oxygen (O_2) therapy is used to correct hypoxemia and reduce vasoconstriction in chronic states of respiratory disorders. In acute states (e.g., those caused by pulmonary emboli), higher concentrations of O_2 may be required.

- If fluid and electrolyte and acid-base imbalances are present, they need to be corrected.
- Diuretics and a low-sodium diet will help to decrease the plasma volume and the load on the heart.
- Bronchodilator therapy is indicated if the underlying respiratory problem is due to an obstructive disorder.
- Antibiotic therapy is indicated if cor pulmonale was precipitated by an infection.
- Digitalis may be used if there is left-sided heart failure.
- Phlebotomies may be needed in the patient with hematocrits >60 g/dl (>600 g/L).

Chronic management of cor pulmonale resulting from COPD is similar to that described for COPD (see p. 136). Continuous low-flow O_2 during sleep, exercise, and small, frequent meals may allow the patient to feel better and be more active. Other treatments include those for pulmonary hypertension and include vasodilator therapy, calcium channel blockers, and anticoagulants. When medical treatment fails, lung transplantation may be an option.

CORONARY ARTERY DISEASE

Definition/Description

Coronary artery disease (CAD) is a type of blood vessel disorder that is included in the general category of atherosclerosis. *Atherosclerosis* is derived from two Greek words: *athere,* meaning "fatty mush," and *skleros,* meaning "hard." Atherosclerosis is often referred to as "hardening of the arteries." Although this condition can occur in any artery in the body, the atheromas (fatty deposits) have a preference for coronary arteries.

- Arteriosclerotic heart disease (ASHD), cardiovascular heart disease (CVHD), ischemic heart disease (IHD), coronary heart disease (CHD), and CAD are synonymous terms used to describe this disease process.
- Cardiovascular diseases are the major cause of death in the United States. Myocardial infarctions (MIs) are the leading cause of all cardiovascular disease deaths and deaths in general.

Pathophysiology

Atherosclerosis is the major cause of CAD. It is characterized by a focal deposit of cholesterol and lipids, primarily found within the arterial intimal wall. Plaque formation is the result of complex interactions between components of the blood and the elements forming the vascular wall. Table 32-1, Lewis and others, *Medical-Surgical Nursing,* edition 5, p. 843 summarizes the theories of atherogenesis, with endothelial injury being the leading theory.

- The endothelial lining can be altered as a result of chemical injuries, such as hyperlipidemia (nondenuding), or high-shear stress, such as hypertension (denuding). With either type of endothelial alteration, platelets are activated and release a growth factor that stimulates smooth muscle proliferation. Smooth muscle cell proliferation entraps lipids, which are calcified over time and form an endothelium irritant upon which platelets adhere and aggregate.
- CAD takes many years to develop. When it becomes symptomatic, the disease process is usually well advanced. Stages of development in atherosclerosis are (1) fatty streak, (2) raised fibrous plaque resulting from smooth muscle cell proliferation, and (3) complicated lesion.

The three most significant risk factors for atherosclerosis are elevated serum lipids, hypertension, and cigarette smoking. Risk factors can be categorized as unmodifiable and modifiable (Table 25). Unmodifiable risk factors are age, gender, race, and genetic inheritance. Modifiable risk factors include elevated serum lipids, hypertension,

Table 25	Risk Factors for Coronary Artery Disease

Unmodifiable	Modifiable
Age	Major
Gender (men > women until	Elevated serum lipids
60 yrs of age)	Hypertension
Race (African-Americans	Cigarette smoking
< Caucasians)	Obesity
Genetic predisposition and	Physical inactivity
family history of heart	Contributing
disease	Diabetes mellitus*
	Stressful lifestyle

*May be hereditary.

smoking, obesity, sedentary lifestyle, and stress in daily living. Although control of diabetes mellitus is recommended, it has not been proven to decrease the incidence of CAD.

Clinical Manifestations
The three major clinical manifestations of CAD include angina pectoris (see Angina Pectoris, p. 40), acute MI (see Myocardial Infarction, p. 398), and sudden cardiac death.

Collaborative Care
Treatment usually begins with dietary calorie restriction, decreased dietary fat content, lower cholesterol intake, and exercise instruction. Serum cholesterol levels are reassessed after 6 months of diet therapy. If they remain elevated, drug therapy may be started.
   Drug Therapy
   Various drugs are used to treat hyperlipidemia. Two bile acid sequestering agents, cholestyramine (Questran) and colestipol (Colestid), are commonly used. These resins primarily lower low-density lipoprotein (LDL) cholesterol and also cause an increase in high-density lipoprotein (HDL).
   Nicotinic acid (niacin, a B vitamin) is highly effective in lowering cholesterol and triglyceride levels by interfering with their synthesis. Clofibrate (Atromid) is effective primarily in lowering serum triglyceride levels and has some cholesterol-lowering activity as well. It appears to act by decreasing the synthesis of lipids. Gemfibrozil (Lopid) is primarily effective in lowering very low-density lipoprotein (VLDL) levels and triglycerides, and it also increases

HDL cholesterol. Lovastatin (Mevacor), pravastatin (Pravachol), simvastatin (Zocor), fluvastatin (Lescol), atorvastatin (Lipitor), and cerivistatin (Baycol) are all competitive inhibitors of the biosynthesis of cholesterol.

- Drug therapy for hyperlipidemia is likely to be prolonged, perhaps continuing for a lifetime. It is essential that diet modification be used to minimize the need for drug therapy. The patient must fully understand the rationale and goals of treatment as well as any medication side effects.

Nursing Management

In both the acute care setting and the community, the nurse needs to identify persons at high risk for CAD. Screening involves obtaining personal and family health histories. Environmental factors, such as eating habits, type of diet, and level of exercise, are also assessed. A psychosocial history is included to determine smoking habits, alcohol ingestion, recent life-stressing events, sleeping habits, and presence of anxiety or depression.

- The nurse needs to identify patient attitudes and beliefs about health and illness. This information can give some indication of how disease and lifestyle changes may affect the patient and can reveal possible misconceptions about heart disease.
- Knowledge of the patient's educational background is frequently helpful in deciding at what level to begin teaching.
- Once a high-risk person is identified, preventive measures can be taken. Risk factors such as age, gender, and genetic inheritance cannot be modified. However, the person with any of these unmodifiable risk factors can change his or her modifiable risk factors and thus alter the additive effects of both the modifiable and unmodifiable risk factors.
- Persons who have modifiable risk factors needs to be encouraged and motivated to make changes in their lifestyle to reduce their risk of heart disease. For highly motivated persons, knowing how to reduce this risk may be the only information needed to get them to make changes.

CROHN'S DISEASE

Definition/Description

Crohn's disease is a chronic, nonspecific inflammatory bowel disorder of unknown origin that can affect any part of the GI tract. Crohn's disease occurs most often between the ages of 15 and 30 years. Similar to ulcerative colitis, it occurs more often in Jewish and upper-middle-class urban populations.

- Crohn's disease is a chronic disorder with unpredictable periods of recurrence and remission. Attacks are intermittent, usually recurring over a period of several weeks to months, with diarrhea and abdominal pain subsiding spontaneously.
- Crohn's disease and ulcerative colitis are compared in Table 26.

Pathophysiology

Crohn's disease is characterized by inflammation of segments of the GI tract. It can affect any part of the GI tract but is most often seen in the terminal ileum, jejunum, and colon. Involvement of the esophagus, stomach, and duodenum is rare. The inflammation involves all layers of the bowel wall (i.e., transmural).

- Areas of involvement are usually discontinuous, with segments of normal bowel occurring between diseased portions. Typically, ulcerations are deep and longitudinal and penetrate between islands of inflamed edematous mucosa, causing the classic cobblestone appearance.
- Thickening of the bowel wall occurs, as well as narrowing of the lumen with stricture development. Abscesses or fistula tracts that communicate with other loops of bowel, skin, bladder, rectum, or vagina may develop.

Clinical Manifestations

Manifestations depend largely on the anatomic site of involvement, extent of the disease process, and presence or absence of complications. Onset is usually insidious, with nonspecific complaints such as nonbloody diarrhea, fatigue, abdominal pain, weight loss, and fever. Pain may be severe and intermittent or constant, depending on the cause.

- Extraintestinal manifestations, such as arthritis and finger clubbing, may precede the onset of bowel disease.
- As the disease progresses, there is weight loss, malnutrition, dehydration, electrolyte imbalances, anemia, increased peristalsis, and pain around the umbilicus and right lower quadrant.

Complications are common in Crohn's disease and may include:

- Strictures and obstruction as scar tissue from inflammation narrows the lumen of the intestine.
- Fistulas, which are a cardinal feature, may develop between segments of the bowel. Fistulas communicating with the urinary tract may cause urinary tract infections.
- Inflammation of all intestinal layers, which may result in perforation (peritonitis) and the formation of intraabdominal abscesses.
- Impaired absorption, causing various nutritional abnormalities as a result of damage to the intestinal mucosa. Fat malabsorption causes a deficiency in fat-soluble vitamins, and the patient

Table 26 Comparison of Ulcerative Colitis and Crohn's Disease

Characteristic	Ulcerative colitis	Crohn's disease
Clinical		
Age at onset	Young to middle age	Young (usually)
Diarrhea	Common	Common
Abdominal cramping pain	Possible	Common
Fever (intermittent)	During acute attacks	Common
Weight loss	Common	Severe
Rectal bleeding	Common	Infrequent
Tenesmus	Severe	Rare
Malabsorption and nutritional deficiencies	Minimal incidence	Common
Pathologic		
Location	Starts distally and spreads in a continuous pattern up the colon	Occurs anywhere along GI tract in characteristic skip lesions; most frequent site is terminal ileum
Distribution	Continuous	Segmental

Depth of involvement	Mucosa and submucosa	Entire thickness of bowel wall (transmural)
Granulomas	Absent	Common
Cobblestoning of mucosa	Rare	Common
Pseudopolyps	Common	Rare
Small bowel involvement	Minimal	Common
Complications		
Fistulas	Rare	Common
Strictures	Rare	Common
Anal abscesses	Rare	Common
Perforation	Common	Common
Toxic megacolon	Common	Rare
Carcinoma	Increased incidence after 10 yr of disease	Slightly > general population
Recurrence after surgery	Cure with colectomy	70% or more recurrence after segmental resections of small or large intestine

GI, Gastrointestinal.

may have an intolerance to gluten (a protein found in barley, rye, and wheat).

Systemic complications are similar to those of ulcerative colitis and include arthritis, liver disease, renal disorders, cholelithiasis (especially with ileal involvement), ankylosing spondylitis, erythema nodosum, and uveitis.

Diagnostic Studies
- Complete blood count (CBC) and stool for occult blood
- Barium enema of small and large intestine to determine disease location and extent
- Flexible sigmoidoscopy and colonoscopy with biopsy to detect early inflammatory mucosal changes and the presence of granulomas

Collaborative Care
The goal of management is to control the inflammatory process, relieve symptoms, correct metabolic and nutritional problems, and promote healing. Drug and nutritional therapy are the mainstays of treatment.

Drug Therapy
- Sulfasalazine (Azulfidine) is effective when the disease involves the large intestine but is less effective when only the small intestine is involved.
- Corticosteroid therapy is effective in reducing inflammation and suppressing disease; dosage and route of administration depend on the severity of illness and the area involved. Once clinical symptoms subside, the dosage should be tapered.
- Immunosuppressive agents (e.g., azathioprine [Imuran]) may be tried if repeated trials with corticosteroids fail.
- Metronidazole (Flagyl) is useful in treating Crohn's disease of the perianal area.
- Marked exacerbations have been reported when drug therapy is stopped.

Balloon dilation of strictures may be effective in relieving symptoms; this is usually performed through a colonoscope or under fluoroscopic guidance.

Nutritional Therapy
Elemental diets and total parenteral nutrition (TPN) (see Total Parenteral Nutrition, p. 684) may be used. The elemental diet provides a high-calorie, high-nitrogen, fat-free, no-residue substrate that is absorbed in the proximal small bowel. TPN may be given to patients with severe disease, small bowel fistulas, or short bowel syndrome. It is given before and after surgery to promote wound healing, reduce complications, and hasten recovery.
- Vitamin deficiencies may develop as a result of malabsorption. Cobalamin (vitamin B_{12}) injections every month may be needed

because of the inability of the terminal ileum (if affected) to absorb this vitamin.

Surgical Therapy

Surgery is used in patients with severe symptoms that are unresponsive to therapy and in patients with life-threatening complications. The majority of patients eventually require surgery at least once in the course of the disease. Unlike ulcerative colitis, which can be cured by total proctocolectomy, Crohn's disease is not cured by surgery; the recurrence rate after surgery is high. The surgical procedure depends on the affected area and the condition of the patient. Conservative intestinal resection with anastomosis of the healthy bowel is the procedure of choice.

Nursing Management

Acute care of the patient is very similar to that of the patient with ulcerative colitis (see Ulcerative Colitis, p. 590). As the patient's condition improves, the nurse should allow for more self-care, provide frequent rest periods, and advise the patient of the importance of rest and avoidance or control of emotional stress. Initially this may be difficult for the patient when told the nature of the disease and the limitations of treatment. Special skin care may be needed by patients who have perianal fistulas or abscesses. Postoperative care should be the same as for exploratory laparotomy (see Abdominal Pain, Acute, p. 3).

▼ **Patient Teaching**

- In the majority of patients the disease course is chronic and intermittent, regardless of the site of involvement. The patient and significant others may need help in setting realistic short-term and long-term goals.
- Specific teaching strategies should include (1) the importance of rest and diet management, (2) perianal care, (3) the action and side effects of medications, (4) the symptoms of recurrence of disease, (5) when to seek medical care, and (6) the use of diversional activities to reduce stress.

CUSHING'S SYNDROME

Definition/Description

Cushing's syndrome is composed of a spectrum of clinical abnormalities that are caused by excess corticosteroids, particularly glucocorticoids. Several conditions can cause Cushing's syndrome; the most common cause is iatrogenic administration of exogenous corticosteroids. *Cushing's disease* is specifically caused by an adrenocorticotropic hormone (ACTH)–secreting pituitary tumor.

- Other causes of Cushing's syndrome include adrenal tumors and ectopic ACTH production by tumors outside the hypothalamic-pituitary-adrenal axis (usually in the lung or pancreas).

Clinical Manifestations

Manifestations can be seen in most body systems and are related to excess levels of corticosteroids (see Table 47-13, Lewis and others, *Medical-Surgical Nursing*, edition 5, p. 1436). Although manifestations of glucocorticoid excess usually predominate, symptoms of mineralocorticoid and androgen excess may also be seen.

- *Glucocorticoid excess* causes pronounced changes in personal appearance. Weight gain, the most common feature, results from accumulation of adipose tissue in the trunk, face, and cervical neck area. Transient weight gain from sodium and water retention may be present because of the mineralocorticoid effects of cortisol. Glucose intolerance occurs because of cortisol-induced insulin resistance and increased gluconeogenesis by the liver.
- *Protein wasting* is caused by the catabolic effects of cortisol on peripheral tissue. Muscle wasting leads to muscle weakness, especially in the extremities. Loss of bone protein matrix leads to osteoporosis with pathologic fractures, vertebral compression fractures, and bone and back pain. Loss of collagen makes the skin weaker, thinner, and easier to bruise. The skin and mucous membranes may take on a bronze color because of the melanotropic activity of ACTH.
- *Mineralocorticoid excess* may cause hypertension and hypokalemia, whereas adrenal androgen excess may cause pronounced acne and masculinization in women.

Clinical presentation, as revealed by the history and physical examination, is the first indication of Cushing's syndrome. Of particular importance are a combination of centripedal obesity and protein wasting as indicated by slender extremities and thin, friable skin; "moon facies" (fullness of face); purplish-red striae on abdomen, breast, or buttocks; premenopausal osteoporosis; and unexplained hypokalemia.

Diagnostic Studies

- Plasma and urine cortisol levels may be elevated with loss of diurnal variation.
- Plasma ACTH levels may be low, normal, or elevated depending on the underlying problem.
- Dexamethasone suppression test.
- 24-hour urine collection for free cortisol levels.

- Complete blood count (CBC) findings of granulocytosis, lymphopenia, eosinopenia, and polycythemia.
- Serum potassium and glucose levels reveal hypokalemia and hyperglycemia.
- CT scan and MRI for tumor localization.

Collaborative Care

The treatment of choice is transsphenoidal surgical removal of a pituitary adenoma. Adrenalectomy is indicated for adrenal tumors or hyperplasia. Patients with ectopic ACTH-secreting tumors are managed with treatment of the neoplasm.

- In inoperable cases or cases in which residual disease remains, treatment with o,p'-DDD (mitotane) may be used. This drug suppresses cortisol production, alters peripheral metabolism of cortisol, and decreases plasma and urine steroid levels by actually destroying adrenocortical cells. The action of this drug results in a "medical adrenalectomy."
- Metyrapone and aminoglutethimide (Cytadren) may be used to inhibit cortisol synthesis. Occasionally, bilateral adrenalectomy is necessary. Ketoconazole (Nizoral), which inhibits synthesis of gonadal and adrenal steroids, may also be used.

If Cushing's syndrome has developed during the course of prolonged administration of glucocorticoids, one or more of the following alternatives may be tried: (1) gradual discontinuance of glucocorticoid therapy, (2) reduction of glucocorticoid dose, and (3) conversion to an alternate-day regimen.

Nursing Management

Goals

The patient with Cushing's syndrome will experience relief of symptoms with no serious complications, maintain a positive self-image, and actively participate in the therapeutic plan.

See NCP 47-4 for the patient with Cushing's syndrome, Lewis and others, *Medical-Surgical Nursing,* edition 5, p. 1438.

Nursing Diagnoses

- Risk for infection *related to* lowered resistance to stress and suppression of immune system
- Altered nutrition: more than body requirements *related to* increased appetite and inactivity
- Self-esteem disturbance *related to* altered body image, emotional lability, and diminished physical capabilities
- Risk for injury *related to* decreased muscle strength, fatigue, osteoporosis, and increased protein catabolism
- Impaired skin integrity *related to* excess steroids, immobility, and altered skin fragility

Nursing Interventions

Because the therapeutic interventions have many side effects, the focus of assessment is on the signs and symptoms of hormone and drug toxicity and on complicating conditions such as cardiovascular disease, diabetes mellitus, infection, nephrolithiasis, and pathologic fractures. Daily nursing assessment includes the following:

- Vital signs every 4 hours, particularly BP, glucose monitoring, and daily weights (gain possibly indicating volume excess)
- Signs and symptoms of infection, especially pain, loss of function, and purulent drainage, because other signs such as fever and redness may be minimal or absent
- Location, time, and duration of abdominal pain. Bone pain or limitations of range of motion, especially in the lower back
- Signs of abnormal thromboembolic phenomena, such as sudden chest pain, dyspnea, or tachypnea
- Changes in mental status, particularly depression

The patient needs a great deal of emotional support. Changes in appearance, such as centripedal obesity, multiple bruises, hirsutism in females, and gynecomastia in males, can be very distressing. The nurse can help by offering respect and unconditional acceptance. The patient can be reassured that the physical changes and much of the emotional lability are related to the side effects of drug therapy and will resolve when hormone levels return to normal.

If treatment involves surgical removal of a pituitary adenoma, an adrenal tumor, or one or both adrenal glands, nursing care will have an additional focus on preoperative and postoperative care. Surgery on glandular structures poses risks beyond those of other types of operations. Because glands are highly vascular, the risk of hemorrhage is increased. Manipulation of glandular tissue during surgery may release large amounts of hormone into the circulation, producing great fluctuations in metabolic processes affected by these hormones (e.g., hypertension, susceptibility to infection).

Preoperative care. Before surgery, hypertension and hyperglycemia need to be controlled, with hypokalemia corrected by diet and potassium supplements; a high-protein meal plan helps correct protein depletion.

- Information and instruction about exercises, coughing, and deep breathing are particularly important since patients are prone to thrombosis and infection.

Postoperative care. Because of hormone fluctuations, the patient's BP, fluid balance, and electrolyte levels tend to be unstable after surgery. High doses of glucocorticoid (cortisone) are administered IV during surgery and for several days afterward to ensure adequate responses to the stress of the procedure.

- Any rapid or significant changes in BP, respirations, or heart rate (HR) should be reported.
- Fluid intake and output should be monitored carefully and assessed for potential imbalance.
- If glucocorticoid dosage is tapered too rapidly after surgery, acute adrenal insufficiency may develop. Vomiting after the nasogastric tube is removed, increased weakness, dehydration, and hypotension may indicate hypocortisolism. In addition, the patient may complain of painful joints, pruritus, or peeling skin and may experience severe emotional disturbances.

The nurse must constantly be alert for signs of glucocorticoid imbalance. After surgery the patient is usually maintained on bed rest until the BP stabilizes. The nurse must also be alert for subtle signs of postoperative infections. Meticulous care must be used when changing the dressing and during any other procedures that necessitate access to body cavities, circulation, or areas under skin.

▼ **Patient Teaching**

Discharge instructions are based on the patient's lack of endogenous cortisol and resulting inability to react to stressors physiologically.

- Patients should wear medical-alert bracelets at all times and carry medical identification and instructions in a wallet or purse. Exposure to extremes of temperature, infections, and emotional disturbances should be avoided as much as possible.
- Stress may produce or precipitate acute adrenal insufficiency because the remaining adrenal tissue cannot meet an increased hormonal demand. Many patients can be taught to adjust their corticosteroid replacement therapy in accordance with stress levels.
- If the patient cannot adjust his or her own medication or if weakness, fainting, fever, or nausea and vomiting occur, the patient should notify the clinician for a possible adjustment in corticosteroid dosage.
- Lifetime replacement therapy is required by many patients, but it may take several months to satisfactorily adjust the hormone dose.

CYSTIC FIBROSIS

Definition/Description

Cystic fibrosis (CF) is an autosomal recessive, multisystem disease characterized by altered function of the exocrine glands involving primarily the lungs, pancreas, and sweat glands.

CF was once exclusively a pediatric disease. However, due to improvements in therapy, approximately 34% of patients reach adulthood and nearly 10% live past the age of 30. The average life span is 28 years. Each person has an individual spectrum of the disease and time course of deterioration.

Pathophysiology

The basic pathophysiologic mechanism is obstruction of the exocrine gland ducts with thick, viscous secretions that adhere to the lumen of the ducts. Thick secretions obstruct bronchioles and lead to air trapping and lung hyperinflation. Stasis of mucus provides an excellent growth medium for bacteria.

- Exocrine function of the pancreas is altered and may stop completely. Pancreatic enzymes such as trypsinogen and amylase do not reach the intestine to digest nutrients. There is malabsorption of fat, protein, and fat-soluble vitamins. Fat malabsorption results in steatorrhea, and protein malabsorption results in failure to grow and gain weight.
- Lung disorders can result, including pneumonia, bronchiolitis, bronchitis, bronchiectasis, atelectasis, and emphysema. There is progressive loss of lung tissue from inflammation and scarring, and chronic hypoxia leads to pulmonary hypertension and cor pulmonale. Death usually results from extensive respiratory infection.

Clinical Manifestations

Manifestations vary depending on the disease severity. Early childhood signs are failure to grow, clubbing, persistent cough with mucus production, tachypnea, and large, frequent bowel movements. A large, protuberant abdomen may develop with emaciated appearance of extremities.

- As the disease progresses, periods of clinical stability are interrupted by exacerbations characterized by increased cough, weight loss, and decreases in pulmonary function.
- Small amounts of blood in the sputum are common with lung infection. Massive hemoptysis is life threatening. Respiratory failure and cor pulmonale are late complications of CF.

Diagnostic Studies

- Sweat chloride test (pilocarpine iontophoresis method) to measure sweat production and sodium and chloride concentrations
- Chest x-ray, pulmonary function tests, fecal analysis for fat, and duodenoscopy for enzyme quantification

Collaborative Care

The objectives of therapy are to promote clearance of secretions, control infection in the lungs, and provide adequate nutrition.

Management of pulmonary problems is focused on relieving airway obstruction and controlling infection. Drainage of thick bronchial mucus is assisted by aerosol and nebulization treatments that liquefy mucus and facilitate coughing. Aerobic exercise also seems to be effective in clearing airways. Early intervention with antibiotics for lung infection is useful, with long courses of antibiotics generally prescribed.

Management of pancreatic insufficiency includes pancreatic enzyme replacement (e.g., lipase, pancrease, Cotazym-S, and Creon) administered before each meal and snack. A high-calorie, high-protein diet and multivitamins are recommended. Fat-soluble vitamins need to be supplemented. Added dietary salt is indicated whenever sweating is excessive, such as during hot weather, in the presence of fever, or from intense physical activity.

Lung transplantation has resulted in significant improvement of pulmonary function with no recurrence of lung disease.

Nursing Management

Goals

The patient with cystic fibrosis will have adequate airway clearance, a reduction of risk factors associated with respiratory infections, the ability to perform activities of daily living (ADLs), no complications related to CF, and active participation in the planning and implementing of a therapeutic regimen.

Nursing Diagnoses

- Ineffective airway clearance *related to* thick bronchial mucus, weakness, and fatigue
- Impaired gas exchange *related to* recurring lung infections
- Altered nutrition: less than body requirements *related to* altered enzyme production, dietary intolerances, and intestinal gas

Nursing Interventions

The nurse can assist young adults to gain independence by helping them assume responsibility for their care and for their vocational or school goals. Crises and life transitions that must be dealt with include building confidence and self-respect on the basis of achievements, persevering with employment goals, developing a motivation to achieve, learning to cope with the treatment program, and adjusting to the need for dependence if health fails. For a couple considering children, genetic counseling may be suggested.

▼ Patient Teaching

- For the young adult a major problem that needs to be discussed is sexuality. Delayed or irregular menstruation is not uncommon. There may also be delayed development of secondary sex characteristics, such as breasts in girls, or prolonged short stature in boys.

- Home management of CF includes an aggressive plan of postural drainage with percussion and vibration, aerosol-nebulization therapy, and breathing retraining.
- The patient is taught controlled coughing techniques, deep breathing exercises, and progressive exercise conditioning such as a bicycling program or arm ergometry.

CYSTITIS

Definition/Description
Cystitis is a type of urinary tract infection (UTI) in which there is an inflammation of the bladder. Although the majority of patients with cystitis are women, other groups with a high incidence are older men and young children (especially girls).

- The adult female urethra is short, and its proximity to the rectum and vagina predisposes females to the risk of bladder contamination. Bacterial contamination of the bladder can result from poor personal hygiene practices and sexual intercourse.
- In children and older men, UTIs are often associated with other preexisting problems. In children, vesicoureteral reflux is usually the preexisting abnormality. In older men, infection is usually related to obstruction caused by benign prostatic hyperplasia (BPH).

Pathophysiology
Not all bacterial invasions of the bladder result in cystitis or cause spread to the upper urinary tract *(pyelonephritis)*. Once cystitis has occurred, it may remain localized in the urinary bladder for years without ascension to the kidneys or may be completely resolved after initial treatment. The risk of recurrent symptomatic infection is increased when there are urinary tract abnormalities.

Clinical Manifestations
- Manifestations of cystitis are frequency and urgency of urination, suprapubic pain, dysuria, pyuria, and foul-smelling urine. In some persons, hematuria may be present.
- Presence of fever, nausea and vomiting, and flank tenderness usually indicates pyelonephritis.
- About one half of all persons with significant bacteriuria have no symptoms or may exhibit nonspecific signs such as increased fatigue, anorexia, or changes in cognitive ability.

Diagnostic Studies

- Urinalysis for the presence of white blood cells (WBCs), with urine culture or urine Gram stain to detect bacteriuria.
- Further evaluation of urinary tract may include intravenous pyelogram (IVP), voiding cystourethrogram, cystoscopy, and pelvic examination.

Collaborative Care

Once cystitis has been diagnosed, appropriate antimicrobial therapy is initiated. Sulfamethoxazole combined with trimethoprim (Bactrim, Septra) has proved to be effective in the treatment of UTIs. When these drugs are combined, resistance seems to develop less rapidly. Systemic antibiotics such as cephalexin (Keflex), norfloxacin (Chibroxin), nitrofurantoin (Furadantin), and ciprofloxacin (Cipro) can also be used.

- Phenazopyridine (Pyridium) may be used in cystitis to provide an analgesic effect on urinary mucosa; this drug should relieve the burning sensation. The azo dye in the drug stains urine reddish orange; it is important to tell the patient about the color change so that he or she does not think it is related to the infection.
- Antibiotic therapy is not usually recommended for asymptomatic bacteriuria unless symptoms develop or there is evidence of obstructive uropathy. Prophylactic antibiotics may be ordered when a patient with asymptomatic bacteriuria undergoes surgery or genitourinary instrumentation.
- High-dose single therapy is effective when the infection is localized to the bladder and the organism is sensitive to antibiotics. Fosfomycin (Monurol) is a single-dose medication indicated exclusively for the treatment of UTI.

Nursing Management

Goals

The patient with cystitis will have relief from dysuria, no upper urinary tract complications, and no recurrent episodes.

See NCP 43-1 for the patient with a UTI, Lewis and others, *Medical-Surgical Nursing*, edition 5, p. 1265.

Nursing Diagnoses

- Altered urinary elimination *related to* UTI
- Risk for reinfection *related to* lack of knowledge regarding measures to prevent recurrence
- Pain *related to* inflammation of mucosal tissue of urinary tract
- Hyperthermia *related to* infection

Nursing Interventions

Health promotion measures include recognizing groups with a higher than normal incidence of UTIs. Especially for these individuals, health promotion activities can help decrease the frequency of infections and promote early detection of infection. These activities include teaching preventive measures, such as emptying the bladder regularly and completely, wiping the perineal area from front to back after urination and defecation, and drinking an adequate amount of liquid each day. In addition, it is important to teach the patient to seek early treatment once symptoms are identified.

- The nurse can play a major role in prevention of nosocomial infections. Debilitated persons, older adults, patients with severe underlying disease (cancer, diabetes), and patients being treated with immunosuppressive drugs or radiation are at increased risk for UTIs. The patient undergoing instrumentation of the urinary tract is also at risk for developing nosocomial infections; aseptic techniques should always be followed for these procedures.

Acute intervention includes an adequate fluid intake if this is not contraindicated. Explain to the patient that fluids will increase frequency at first, but will also dilute the urine, making the bladder less irritable. Caffeine, alcohol, citrus juices, chocolate, and highly spiced foods should be avoided because they are potential bladder irritants. Treatment of cystitis does not usually require hospitalization.

If the patient has been compliant with drug therapy, relapse suggests possible renal involvement. For the individual who has more than three episodes in 1 year, prophylactic antibiotic therapy may be ordered.

▼ Patient Teaching

- The patient needs to be instructed about prescribed drug therapy. It is important for the patient to take the full course of antibiotics. Sometimes a second medication or a reduced dose of medication is ordered to suppress bacterial growth in certain patients susceptible to recurrent UTI.
- The patient should be instructed to watch for any changes in the color or consistency of urine and a decrease in or cessation of symptoms as a sign of therapy effectiveness.
- The patient must understand the need for follow-up care with urine culture to determine that the infection has been adequately treated. Relapse with bacteria of the same species usually occurs within 1 to 2 weeks after completion of therapy.

DIABETES INSIPIDUS

Definition/Description

Diabetes insipidus (DI) is a condition that occurs when any organic lesion of the hypothalamus, infundibular stem, or posterior pituitary interferes with antidiuretic hormone (ADH) synthesis, transport, or release. Causes of DI include brain tumors, pituitary or other cranial surgery, closed head trauma, central nervous system (CNS) infections, and vascular disorders.

D

Clinical Manifestations

The primary characteristic is excretion of large quantities of urine (5 to 20 L/day) with a very low specific gravity. In the milder form, urinary output may be lower (2 to 4 L/day).

- The patient compensates for fluid loss by drinking great amounts of water so that serum osmolality is normal or only moderately elevated.
- The patient is usually fatigued from nocturia. If oral fluid intake cannot keep up with urinary losses, severe fluid volume deficit results. This is manifested by weight loss, poor tissue turgor, hypotension, tachycardia, constipation, and shock.
- The patient also shows CNS manifestations ranging from irritability and mental dullness to coma. These symptoms are related to rising serum osmolality and hypernatremia.

Diagnostic Studies

Because DI may be pituitary, renal, or psychogenic in origin, identification of the cause of the DI is the initial step.

- A complete history and physical are done. An attempt is made to rule out psychogenic DI related to emotional disturbances. *Psychogenic DI* is associated with overhydration and hypervolemia rather than with dehydration and hypovolemia as seen in other forms of DI.
- *Neurogenic DI* that results from head trauma is usually self-limiting and improves with treatment of the underlying problem. DI following cranial surgery may be permanent.

Collaborative Care

The therapeutic goal is the maintenance of fluid and electrolyte balance. This may be accomplished by IV administration of fluid (saline and glucose) and by hormone replacement with ADH administered by subcutaneous (SC), intramuscular (IM), or IV methods.

- In acute DI, fluids should be administered at a rate that decreases serum sodium by about 1 mEq/L every 2 hours. Clofibrate

(Atromid), carbamazepine (Tegretol), and thiazide diuretics may
be prescribed.

- For long-term therapy, desmopressin (DDAVP), an analogue of
  ADH that is administered as a nasal or SC preparation and does
  not have the vasoconstrictive effect, is the preferred therapy.

Nursing Management

Care of the patient with DI is based on clinical symptoms.

- Fluids must be replaced orally or IV, depending on the patient's
  condition and ability to drink copious amounts of fluids. Adequate fluids should be kept at the bedside.
- If IV glucose is used, urine should be assessed for glucose. If
  positive, the physician should be notified because glycosuria
  increases fluid volume deficit.
- Accurate records of intake and output, urine specific gravity,
  and daily weights are mandatory in the assessment of fluid volume status. Fluid volume deficit manifested by hypotension,
  tachycardia, and rapid, shallow respirations can be detected
  early by frequent assessment.
- Polyuria and nocturia can cause disturbances in rest and sleep
  patterns. The patient is often listless, tired, and discouraged.
  Support and reassurance that the sleep disturbances are temporary can be helpful.
- Perineal care should be done at least twice daily in bedridden
  female patients to cleanse urine from the perineum.

When the patient affected by DI is hospitalized, often for emergency treatment of hypertonic encephalopathy, the therapeutic goal
is to restore fluid balance. DDAVP is administered as a nasal or SC
preparation. Adequacy of treatment is assessed by monitoring fluid
intake and output and urine specific gravity. Increased urine volume
with lower specific gravity is related to an inadequate pharmacologic effect, and the physician should be notified immediately.

▼ **Patient Teaching**

- The patient who requires long-term ADH replacement needs
  instruction in self-management.
- DDAVP acetate is usually taken intranasally twice daily. Nasal
  irritation, headache, and nausea may indicate overdosage,
  whereas failure to improve may indicate underdosage. The
  need for close follow-up should be stressed.

DIABETES MELLITUS

Definition/Description

Diabetes mellitus (DM) is a group of genetically and clinically heterogeneous disorders characterized by abnormalities in glucose homeostasis resulting in hyperglycemia. The hyperglycemia associated with diabetes is caused by a decrease in the secretion or activity of insulin. These insulin alterations result in the disordered metabolism of carbohydrate, fat, and protein. In time, structural abnormalities occur in a variety of organs, especially the heart, kidneys, and eyes.

D

The diagnosis of DM is made when the fasting plasma glucose level exceeds 126 mg/dl (7.0 mmol/L), when a plasma glucose measurement exceeds 200 mg/dl (11.1 mmol/L), or when plasma glucose 2 hours after a glucose challenge is >200 mg/dl (>11.1 mmol/L).

- *Type 1 diabetes* results from progressive destruction of β-cell function as a result of an autoimmune process in susceptible individuals. Islet cell antibodies and insulin autoantibodies cause a reduction in β cells of 80% to 90% of normal before hyperglycemia and symptoms occur.
- *Type 2 diabetes* is a combination of genetically determined defects in skeletal muscle, fat, and liver receptors for insulin and β-cell secretory exhaustion. Excessive hepatic glucose production eventually adds to the fasting and postprandial hyperglycemia.

A comparison of types 1 and 2 diabetes is presented in Table 27.

Pathophysiology

Type 1 Diabetes Mellitus

In type 1 diabetes, autoimmune β-cell destruction is attributed to a genetic predisposition coupled with one or more viral agents and possibly chemical agents. It is not known conclusively that these are the only factors involved.

- Onset and progression of hyperglycemic symptoms is usually more rapid and acute in type 1 diabetes as compared to type 2. Successful treatment depends on insulin replacement. If the disease process is allowed to progress without treatment, diabetic ketoacidosis (DKA) with nausea and vomiting, electrolyte imbalance, weight loss, and muscle wasting may develop.
- Without treatment (i.e., insulin) ketoacidosis can progress to coma and death. Once treatment is initiated, patients may go into a remission (often called honeymoon) phase. During this time, very little insulin is needed to control blood glucose. Eventually, blood glucose levels climb, more insulin is needed, and the honeymoon period ends.

Table 27 Characteristics of Type 1 and Type 2 Diabetes Mellitus

Factor	Type 1 diabetes mellitus	Type 2 diabetes mellitus
■ Age at onset	Usually in young person but possible at any age	Usually >35 yr but possible at any age
■ Type of onset	Signs and symptoms abrupt, but disease process may be present for several years	Insidious
■ Genetic susceptibility	HLA-DR3, -DR4, and others	Frequent genetic background, no relation to HLA
■ Environmental factors	Virus, toxins	Obesity, lack of exercise
■ Islet cell antibodies	Often present at onset	Absent
■ Endogenous insulin	Minimal or absent	Possibly excessive; adequate but delayed secretion or reduced but not absent secretion
■ Nutritional status	Thin, catabolic state	Obese or possibly normal
■ Symptoms	Thirst, polyuria, polyphagia, fatigue	Frequently none or mild
■ Ketosis	Prone at onset or during insulin deficiency	Resistant except during infection or stress
■ Dietary management	Essential	Essential, possibly sufficient for glycemic control
■ Insulin	Required for all	Required for 30-40%
■ Oral agents	Not beneficial	Usually beneficial
■ Vascular and neurologic complications	In majority of patients after ≥5 yr	Frequent

HLA, Human leukocyte antigens.

Type 2 Diabetes Mellitus

Approximately 90% of people with DM have type 2. Type 2 diabetes has a strong genetic influence (almost 100% concordance in monozygotic twins), but no correlation with human leukocyte antigens (HLA) type has been found.

Pathophysiologic factors that have been identified in type 2 diabetes include decreased tissue (e.g., fat, muscle) responsiveness to insulin as a result of receptor or postreceptor defects, eventual decreased secretion of insulin due to β-cell exhaustion, and abnormal hepatic glucose regulation. These events are often referred to as peripheral insulin resistance. Obesity appears to play a major role in type 2 diabetes.

Clinical Manifestations

Normally, insulin and its counterregulatory hormones maintain blood glucose within a range of 70 to 110 mg/dl (3.9 to 6.0 mmol/L). When an absolute insulin deficiency or decreased insulin activity occurs, glucose is not used properly. Glucose remains in the bloodstream and produces an osmotic effect on intracellular and interstitial fluid. This shift in fluid balance results in symptoms of frequent urination *(polyuria)* and thirst *(polydipsia)*. Without sufficient insulin the patient may experience hunger *(polyphagia)* as the body turns to other energy sources besides glucose—first fat and then protein.

- Varying degrees of polyuria, polydipsia, and polyphagia are the hallmark symptoms of DM.
- In type 2 DM the onset of hyperglycemic symptoms may occur over a long period. The person may "adjust" to persistent feelings of fatigue, thirst, polyuria, and blurred vision without realizing that the disease process is producing the symptoms.

Acute Complications

The acute problems of diabetic ketoacidosis (DKA) and hyperglycemic hyperosmolar nonketosis (HHNK) coma result from hyperglycemia and insufficient insulin. A problem that may arise from too much insulin or an excessive dose of an oral antidiabetes agent (OA) is *hypoglycemia* (also referred to as *insulin reaction* or *low blood glucose*), which occurs when the level of available blood glucose falls. It is important for the health care provider to be able to distinguish between hyperglycemia and hypoglycemia because hypoglycemia can constitute a serious threat and requires immediate attention.

Diabetic ketoacidosis. DKA, also referred to as diabetic acidosis and diabetic coma, may develop quickly or over several days or weeks. It can be caused by too little insulin accompanied by increased caloric intake, physical or emotional stress, or undiagnosed diabetes.

- DKA is most likely to occur in type 1 diabetes but may be seen in type 2 in conditions of severe illness or stress when the extra demand for insulin cannot be met by the pancreas.
- Manifestations include dehydration signs (such as dry and loose skin), soft and sunken eyeballs, hypotension with a weak and rapid pulse, vomiting, Kussmaul's respirations, and a sweet fruity odor of acetone on the breath. Eventually renal failure and coma occur. If not treated, death is inevitable.

Hyperglycemic hyperosmolar nonketosis. HHNK occurs in the patient with diabetes who is able to produce enough insulin to prevent DKA but not enough to prevent severe hyperglycemia, osmotic diuresis, and extracellular fluid depletion.

- This complication causes neurologic abnormalities such as somnolence, coma, seizures, hemiparesis, and aphasia.
- HHNK often occurs in the older adult patient with type 2 diabetes.
- There is usually a history of inadequate fluid intake, increasing mental depression, and polyuria.

Hypoglycemia. Hypoglycemia, or *low blood glucose,* occurs when proportionately too much insulin is in the blood for the available glucose. This causes the blood glucose level to drop to <50 mg/dl (<2.8 mmol/L).

- Manifestations include cold sweats, nervousness, pallor, irritability, and increased heart rate (HR). Other various signs may include confusion, fatigue, dizziness, and tremors.

Chronic Complications

Chronic complications are primarily those of end-organ disease from angiopathy and neuropathy. *Angiopathy,* or blood vessel disease, is estimated to account for the majority of deaths in patients with diabetes. Many factors are being investigated in the development of angiopathy. These chronic blood vessel problems are divided into two categories: macroangiopathy and microangiopathy.

Macroangiopathy, or disease of the large and medium-sized blood vessels, is essentially atherosclerosis and arteriosclerotic vascular disease characterized by a higher frequency and earlier onset than in the nondiabetic population. The degree of vascular damage appears to be related to the duration of the diabetes and not to its severity. Tight glucose control may help delay the atherosclerotic process. Complications resulting from macroangiopathy are cerebrovascular, cardiovascular, and peripheral vascular disease.

Microangiopathy, or disease of the small blood vessels, is different from macroangiopathy in that it is specific to diabetes. Although microangiopathy can be found throughout the body, the areas most noticeably affected are the eyes *(retinopathy),* kidneys *(nephropathy),* and skin *(dermopathy).*

Peripheral vascular disease (PVD) is a combination of microangiopathy and macroangiopathy. The legs and feet are most often affected in diabetes. The sequelae of PVD can lead to infection, gangrene, and amputation. Signs of PVD include intermittent claudication, pain at rest, cold feet, loss of hair, delayed capillary filling, and dependent rubor.

Diabetic retinopathy refers to the microangiopathic process of the retina seen in patients with diabetes. The primary problems are microvascular damage and occlusion of retinal capillaries. Patients may go blind without treatment.

Diabetic nephropathy is now the leading cause of end-stage renal disease (ESRD) in the United States. This occurs as a result of microvascular abnormalities associated with DM by processes not clearly understood.

Neuropathy. Neuropathy is probably one of the most common complications of diabetes in adults; its cause is unclear.

- Two major categories of diabetic neuropathy are (1) neuropathic conditions of the peripheral nervous system, including symmetric peripheral polyneuropathy, mononeuropathic disorders, and diabetic amyotrophy; and (2) autonomic neuropathic conditions, including cardiovascular abnormalities, GI abnormalities, urinary bladder abnormalities, and sexual dysfunction.
- Symmetric peripheral polyneuropathy affects all extremities, but it most often affects the legs. The patient has pain and paresthesias. Hand neuropathy causes atrophy of small muscles, limiting fine movement.

Diagnostic Tests

- Blood tests, including fasting blood glucose; postprandial blood glucose; glycosylated hemoglobin; lipid, cholesterol, and triglyceride levels; blood urea nitrogen (BUN); serum creatinine; and electrolytes
- Urine for complete urinalysis, microalbuminuria, culture and sensitivity, glucose, and acetone
- Neurologic and funduscopic examination
- BP and monitoring of weight
- Doppler scan to determine the presence and degree of peripheral vascular disease

Collaborative Care

Management of DM is primarily aimed at achieving a balance of diet, activity, and medications together with appropriate monitoring and patient and family education. Management of neuropathies is also important.

Drug Therapy

Two types of glucose-lowering agents used in the treatment of diabetes are insulin and OAs.

Insulin

Exogenous insulin is needed when a patient has inadequate insulin to meet specific metabolic needs and the combination of nutritional therapy, exercise, and OAs cannot maintain a satisfactory blood glucose level. Exogenous insulin is required in the management of type 1 diabetes. Exogenous insulin may be prescribed for patients with type 2 diabetes during periods of severe stress, such as illness or surgery, or when attempts at glycemic control by means of diet, exercise, or OAs fail.

Exogenous insulin had previously been obtained from the pancreases of pigs and cows. Today, biosynthetic human insulin is used almost exclusively. The advantages of these new insulins are a reduced allergic response and a more predictable insulin activity. In addition to origin and purity, insulins differ in regard to onset, peak action, and duration. The specific properties of each type of insulin are matched with the patient's diet and activity. (For information on administering an insulin injection, see Table 46-6, Lewis and others, *Medical-Surgical Nursing,* edition 5, p. 1376.)

Nursing care related to insulin therapy. Nursing responsibilities for the patient receiving insulin include proper administration, assessment of patient use of and response to insulin therapy, and education of the patient regarding administration, adjustment to, and side effects of insulin. The patient with newly diagnosed diabetes should be assessed for the ability to understand the purpose of insulin therapy; the interaction of insulin, diet, and activity; and the side effects.

- The patient or significant other also has to be able to prepare and inject the insulin. If the patient or family lacks the psychomotor skills to prepare insulin, the nurse may have to find additional resources to assist the patient.
- Follow-up of the patient who has been using insulin therapy includes inspection of insulin sites for allergic reactions, a review of the insulin preparation and injection technique, a history pertaining to the occurrence of hypoglycemic episodes, and the patient's method for handling hypoglycemic episodes.
- A review of the patient's record of urine and blood glucose tests is also important in assessing overall glycemic control.

Oral Antidiabetes Agents

There are currently five classes of drugs used in the treatment of type 2 diabetes. The first class of drugs includes sulfonylureas. The first generation of these drugs included tolbutamide (Orinase), tolazamide (Tolinase), and chlorpropamide (Diabinese). A second generation of sulfonylureas includes glipizide (Glucotrol), glyburide (Micronase), and glimepiride (Amaryl).

- Second-generation drugs have fewer adverse effects, are about 100 times more potent by weight, and have more predictable times of action and half-lives. The main disadvantage is their increased expense.

A second class of drugs includes metformin (Glucophage), which is a biguanide glucose-lowering agent that is widely used as a monotherapy and in combination with a sulfonylurea. The glucose-lowering effect occurs without stimulation of insulin secretion and results mainly by decreasing the rate of hepatic glucose production (gluconeogenesis).

A third class of drugs is the carbohydrate absorption inhibitors that work in the small intestines. α-Glucosidase inhibitors, such as acarbose (Precose) and miglitol (Glyset), slow the breakdown of disaccharides and polysaccharides. These drugs can be used as a monotherapy or in combination with other OAs or insulin.

The fourth class of drugs includes thiazolidinediones that improve insulin resistance in skeletal muscle without stimulating insulin secretion. Troglitazone (Rezulin), the first thiazolidinedione, was approved in 1997 and works by decreasing peripheral insulin resistance in muscles without stimulating insulin secretion. Side effects are minimal.

- Troglitazone requires 4 to 6 weeks for full efficacy to be reached. It can be used in combination with sulfonylureas or insulin.

The fifth class of drugs is meglitinides.

- Repaglinide (Prandin), an example of this class, stimulates a rapid and short-lived release of insulin from the pancreas.

Nursing care related to oral agents. OAs are not oral insulin or a substitute for insulin. The patient must have some functioning endogenous insulin for OAs to be effective. Nursing responsibilities for the patient taking OAs are similar to those for the patient taking insulin. Proper administration, assessment of patient's use of and response to OAs, and education of the patient and family are all part of the nurse's role.

- The nurse's assessment can be invaluable in determining the most appropriate OA for a patient. The assessment includes the patient's mental status, eating habits, home environment, attitude toward diabetes, and use of OAs.
- The patient needs to understand the importance of diet and not skipping meals.
- The patient also needs to know that hypoglycemic reactions may be severe and prolonged and that health care provider supervision may be necessary, particularly for older patients.
- The patient should also be instructed to contact a physician if periods of illness or extreme stress occur. During such a period, insulin therapy may be required to prevent or treat hyperglycemic symptoms and HHNK.

Nutritional Therapy

Nutritional therapy is the cornerstone of care. Today there is no one "diabetic" or "American Diabetes Association (ADA)" diet. The recommended diet can only be defined as a dietary prescription based on nutritional assessment and goals. Because of the complexity of nutrition issues, it is recommended that a registered dietitian with expertise in diabetes management be a member of the treatment team. Monitoring of glucose and glycohemoglobin, lipids, and renal status is essential to evaluate nutrition-related outcomes.

- *Type 1 diabetes.* Meal planning should be based on the individual's usual food intake with insulin therapy integrated into the usual eating and exercise patterns. It is recommended that individuals using insulin therapy eat meals at consistent times synchronized with the time-action of the insulin preparation used.

- *Type 2 diabetes.* The emphasis for nutritional therapy in type 2 diabetes should be placed on achieving glucose, lipid, and blood pressure goals. Weight loss and hypocaloric diets usually improve short-term glycemic levels and have the potential to increase long-term metabolic control. (See Table 46-4 for dietary strategies for type 1 and type 2 diabetes, Lewis and others, *Medical-Surgical Nursing,* edition 5, p. 1373.)

Diet principles that both the nurse and dietitian should teach and reinforce include:

- Eat according to the prescribed meal plan. A dietary prescription is individualized to reflect dietary needs related to a specific patient's body weight, occupation, age, activities, and type of diabetes. Individual responses to a dietary prescription should be monitored, and appropriate adjustments should be made as necessary.

- Never skip meals. This is particularly important for the patient taking insulin or OAs. The body requires food at regularly spaced intervals throughout the day; omission or delay of meals can result in hypoglycemia.

- Learn to recognize appropriate food portions; practice can result in accurate portion allotments.

Nursing Management

Goals

The patient with DM will be an active participant in the management of the diabetes regimen; experience minimal or no episodes of DKA, HHNK, or hypoglycemia; prevent or delay the occurrence of chronic complications of diabetes; and adjust lifestyle to accommodate the diabetes regimen with a minimum of stress.

See NCP 46-1 for the patient with diabetes, Lewis and others, *Medical-Surgical Nursing,* edition 5, p. 1386.

Nursing Diagnoses/Collaborative Problems

- Ineffective management of therapeutic regimen *related to* lack of knowledge of exercise program, diet and weight control, administration and potential side effects and complications of glucose-lowering agents (GLA), glucose monitoring, and care during acute minor illness
- Risk for infection *related to* depressed immune system, inadequate circulation, and environmental pathogens
- Self-esteem disturbance *related to* lifestyle changes imposed by diabetes and its treatment, and frustration at progression of disease
- Potential complication: hypoglycemia *related to* low blood glucose secondary to too much insulin
- Potential complication: DKA and HHNK *related to* inadequate insulin and excess blood glucose secondary to increased caloric intake, physical or emotional stress, or undiagnosed diabetes

Nursing Interventions

The nurse may be involved in any or all aspects of management, but the focus of nursing care has two aims: (1) to care for the patient during acute episodes and (2) to assist the patient in learning to live with diabetes. Both aims require the nurse to be thoroughly familiar with diabetes and its management and to educate the patient.

- The effect of the diagnosis of diabetes cannot be overestimated. An assessment of the patient's perception of what it means to have diabetes must be carefully made before education is designed and implemented.
- The nurse should foster a positive attitude about the prescribed regimen and assist the patient in developing an individualized management plan. Learning goals should be mutually determined by the patient and nurse on the basis of individual needs as well as therapeutic requirements.
- The nurse needs to assess patient feelings and facilitate acceptance of diabetes and its treatment over time.

Glucose monitoring. Glucose levels must be determined daily to monitor interactions and effect of diet, exercise, and medication on an individual's diabetic regimen. Detection of extreme or episodic hyperglycemia is necessary to avoid DKA and HHNK. Urine testing for ketonuria is a valuable aid in determining the advent of DKA and is recommended for all patients with type 1 diabetes when they are experiencing hyperglycemia or acute illness.

- Patient self-monitoring of blood glucose using capillary blood glucose monitoring (CBGM) is a reliable technique for measuring blood glucose. CBGM patient training should be emphasized not only at the initial session, but also at follow-up visits with the health care team. Patient technique should be reassessed after initial training.

Foot care. Proper care of the feet is crucial for the patient with diabetes; guidelines for foot care are listed in Table 46-25, Lewis and
others, *Medical-Surgical Nursing,* edition 5, p. 1399.

Exercise. Regular, consistent exercise is considered an essential part
of diabetic management. Exercise contributes to weight loss, reduces
triglycerides and cholesterol, increases muscle tone, and improves
circulation. Guidelines for exercise are listed in Table 46-11, Lewis
and others, *Medical-Surgical Nursing,* edition 5, p. 1382.

Effects of stress. Emotional and physical stress can increase blood
glucose levels and result in hyperglycemia. Common stress-evoking
situations include acute illness and the stress of surgery. The patient
with diabetes who has a minor illness such as a cold or the flu
should continue drug therapy and food intake.

- Blood glucose monitoring should be done every 1 to 2 hours
  by either the patient or a person who can assume responsibility
  for care during the illness. Urine output and the presence and
  degree of ketonuria should be monitored, particularly when
  fever is present. Fluid intake should be increased to prevent
  dehydration, with a minimum of 4 oz per hour for an adult.
- Surgery is controlled stress, and adjustments in the diabetes regimen can be planned to ensure glycemic control. The patient is
  given IV fluids and insulin immediately before, during, and after
  surgery when there is no oral intake. The type 2 DM patient receiving OAs usually has the OAs discontinued 48 hours before
  surgery and is treated with insulin during the surgical period.
- The nurse caring for an unconscious surgical patient receiving
  insulin must be alert for hypoglycemic signs such as sweating,
  tachycardia, and tremors. The nurse should be aware that blood
  glucose monitoring must also be done frequently.

DKA and HHNK. When a patient is hospitalized, the nurse is responsible for monitoring blood glucose and urine for output and
ketones, as well as using laboratory data to direct care.

- Areas that need monitoring are administration of IV fluids to
  correct dehydration, administration of insulin therapy to reduce
  blood glucose and serum acetone, administration of electrolytes to correct electrolyte imbalance, assessment of renal
  status, assessment of cardiopulmonary status related to hydration and electrolyte levels, and monitoring of the level of
  consciousness.
- The nurse must also monitor the signs of potassium (K^+) imbalance resulting from hypoinsulinemia and osmotic diuresis.
- Vital signs should be assessed often to determine the presence
  of fever, hypovolemic shock, tachycardia, and Kussmaul's
  respirations.

Hypoglycemia. The preferred treatment of hypoglycemia is prevention. If hypoglycemia does occur, the patient should be able to

reverse the situation before medical assistance is required. The patient's ability to do this depends on the state of alertness, ability to swallow, and availability of a quick-acting carbohydrate source.

- At the first sign of hypoglycemia the patient should ingest 5 to 20 g of a simple (fast-acting) carbohydrate, such as 120 to 180 ml of orange juice, 180 to 240 ml of regular soft drink, two packets of sugar, or five or six hard candies. Overtreatment with large quantities of quick-acting carbohydrates, such as a whole candy bar, should be avoided.
- If the symptoms are still present after 10 to 15 minutes, ingestion of 5 to 20 g of carbohydrate should be repeated. Once the symptoms have improved, the patient should eat a longer-lasting carbohydrate, such as bread or milk, to prevent symptoms from recurring.
- If there is little improvement in the patient's condition after two to three doses of 5 to 20 g of simple carbohydrate within 30 minutes or if the patient is not alert enough to swallow, 1 mg of glucagon may be administered with the same technique used for an insulin injection. The blood glucose level must be carefully monitored during the treatment.
- With effective treatment, hypoglycemia can be quickly reversed. Once acute hypoglycemia has been reversed, the nurse should explore with the patient the reasons why the situation developed. This assessment may indicate a need for additional education of the patient and family to avoid future episodes of hypoglycemia. The danger of hypoglycemic reactions must be stressed because memory and learning impairment can result from repeated episodes of severe hypoglycemia.

▼ **Patient Teaching**

- The patient should be instructed to carry identification at all times indicating diabetes. An identification card can supply valuable information, such as the name of the health care provider and the type and dose of insulin or OA. A medical-alert bracelet or necklace should be worn by all persons with diabetes.
- The major educational objective is a level of self-management appropriate to the individual patient. Ideally, the patient should be taught about the disease and encouraged to achieve self-management with guidance only from the health care provider.
- A knowledgeable patient should be able to make minor adjustments in insulin dosage and diet prescription to compensate for special circumstances, such as illness or increased exercise.
- Not all patients with diabetes are capable of self-management. If the patient is not able to manage the disease, a family member may be able to assume this role. If the patient or family cannot make decisions related to diabetes management, the

nurse may identify appropriate resources outside the family. These resources can assist the patient and family in outlining a feasible treatment program that meets their capabilities.

DIARRHEA

Definition/Description

Diarrhea is not a disease but a symptom. The term is commonly used to denote an increase in stool frequency or volume, as well as an increase in stool looseness.

- Causes can be divided into the general classifications of decreased fluid absorption, increased fluid secretion, motility disturbances, or a combination of these. Causes of acute infectious diarrhea are listed in Table 28.

Clinical Manifestations and Complications

Diarrhea may be acute or chronic. *Acute* diarrhea most commonly results from infection. Bacterial or viral infection of the intestine may result in explosive watery diarrhea, *tenesmus* (spasmodic contraction of the anal sphincter with pain and persistent desire to defecate), and abdominal cramping pain. Perianal skin irritation may also develop. Acute diarrhea is often self-limiting in the adult with symptoms continuing until the irritant or causative agent is excreted.

- Systemic manifestations may include fever, nausea, vomiting, and malaise. Leukocytes, blood, and mucus may be present in the stool, depending on the causative agent (see Table 28).

Diarrhea is considered *chronic* when it persists for at least 2 weeks or when it subsides and returns more than 2 to 4 weeks after the initial episode. Severe diarrhea may be debilitating and life-threatening.

- A patient may have severe dehydration (water and sodium loss) and electrolyte disturbances. Malabsorption and malnutrition are also sequelae of chronic diarrhea.

Diagnostic Studies

An accurate diagnosis requires a thorough history, physical examination, and when indicated, laboratory tests.

- A history of travel, medication use, diet, previous surgery, and interpersonal contacts, as well as family history, should be obtained.
- Blood tests may identify anemia, elevated white blood cell (WBC) count, iron and folate deficiencies, liver enzyme increases, and electrolyte disturbances.

Table 28   Causes of Acute Infectious Diarrhea

	Onset	Duration	Symptoms and signs
Viral			
Rotavirus, Norwalk	18-24 hr	24-48 hr	Explosive, watery diarrhea; nausea; vomiting; abdominal cramps
Bacterial			
Escherichia coli	4-24 hr	3-4 days	Four or five loose stools per day, nausea, malaise, low-grade fever
Enterohemorrhagic *E.coli* (0157:H7)	4-24 hr	4-9 days	Bloody diarrhea; difficile severe cramping; fever
Shigella	24 hr	7 days	Watery stools containing blood and mucus, tenesmus, urgency, severe cramping, fever
Salmonellae	6-48 hr	2-5 days	Watery diarrhea, nausea, vomiting, abdominal cramps, fever
Campylobacter species	24 hr	<7 days	Profuse, watery diarrhea; malaise, nausea, abdominal cramps, low-grade fever
Clostridium perfringens	8-12 hr	24 hr	Watery diarrhea, abdominal cramps, vomiting
Clostridium difficile	4-9 days after start of antibiotics	24 hr	Associated with antibiotic treatment; symptoms range from mild, watery diarrhea to severe abdominal pain, fever, leukocytosis, leukocytes in stool

Continued

D

Table 28 Causes of Acute Infectious Diarrhea—cont'd

	Onset	Duration	Symptoms and signs
Parasitic			
Giardia lamblia	1-3 wk	Few days to 3 months	Sudden onset; malodorous, explosive, watery diarrhea; flatulence, epigastric pain and cramping, nausea
Entamoeba histolytica	4 days	Weeks to months	Frequent soft stools with blood and mucus (in severe cases, watery stools), flatulence, distention, abdominal cramps, fever, leukocytes in stool
Cryptosporidium	2-10 days	1-6 months	Watery diarrhea, nausea, vomiting, abdominal cramps, weight loss in AIDS

AIDS, acquired immunodeficiency syndrome.

- Stools may be examined for blood, mucus, WBCs, and parasites. Stool cultures may help in identifying infectious organisms.
- In a patient with chronic diarrhea, measurement of stool electrolytes, pH, and osmolality may help to determine whether diarrhea is related to decreased fluid absorption or increased fluid secretion (secretory diarrhea).
- Measurement of stool fat and undigested muscle fibers may be indicative of fat and protein malabsorption conditions, including pancreatic insufficiency.
- Endoscopy may be used to examine mucosa and to obtain specimens for examination.
- Upper and lower barium studies may be helpful in detecting mucosal disease.

Collaborative Care

Treatment is based on the cause and is aimed at replacing fluids and electrolytes and decreasing the number, volume, and frequency of stools. Oral solutions containing glucose and electrolytes (e.g., Gatorade, Pedialyte) are often sufficient to replace losses due to mild diarrhea. In severe diarrhea, parenteral administration of fluids, electrolytes, vitamins, and (potentially) nutrition is warranted.

Once the cause has been determined, antidiarrheal agents may be given to coat and protect mucous membranes, inhibit GI motility, decrease intestinal secretions, and decrease central nervous system (CNS) input to the GI tract.

- Antiperistaltic agents are not given to a patient who has infectious diarrheal syndromes because of the potential for prolonging exposure to the infectious agent. Antidiarrheal medications should not be given over a prolonged time.
- Antibiotics are reserved for treating specific bacterial organisms. Antibiotics can cause diarrhea by altering normal bowel flora.

Nursing Management: Acute Infectious Diarrhea

Goals

The patient with diarrhea will not transmit the microorganism causing the infectious diarrhea, will cease having diarrhea and resume normal bowel patterns, will have normal fluid and electrolyte and acid-base balance, will have normal nutritional intake, and will have no perianal skin breakdown.

See NCP 40-1 for the patient with acute infectious diarrhea, Lewis and others, *Medical-Surgical Nursing,* edition 5, p. 1139.

Nursing Diagnoses

- Diarrhea *related to* acute infectious process
- Fluid volume deficit *related to* excessive fluid loss and decreased fluid intake secondary to diarrhea

■ Impaired skin integrity of perianal area *related to* contact with
   diarrheal stools and inadequate perianal hygiene

Nursing Interventions

Adherence to infection control precautions for infectious diseases
is important because some cases of acute diarrhea are infectious.
All cases of acute diarrhea should be considered infectious until the
cause is determined.

■ Handwashing is the most important measure in the prevention
   of the transfer of microorganisms. Hands should be washed before and after contact with each patient and when excretions
   of any kind are handled.

▼ **Patient Teaching**

■ The patient should be taught the principles of hygiene, infection control precautions, and potential dangers of an illness that
   is infectious to themselves and others.

■ Proper handling, cooking, and storage of food should be discussed with patients suspected of having infectious diarrhea.

■ Teach the patient to be alert for the recurrence of diarrhea,
   fever, and other symptoms and for evidence of the same symptoms in family members.

■ Assist the patient in identifying factors that precipitated diarrhea
   to avoid causing reinfection of self or transmission to others.

■ Explain the importance of seeking medical care when diarrhea
   and other symptoms begin so early treatment can be initiated.

DISLOCATION AND SUBLUXATION

Definition/Description

A *dislocation* is a severe injury of the ligamentous structures that
surround a joint. It results in the complete displacement or separation
of joint articular surfaces. A *subluxation* is a partial or incomplete
displacement of the joint surface. Manifestations of a subluxation
are similar to those of a dislocation but are less severe. Treatment of
a subluxation is similar to that of a dislocation, but subluxation requires less healing time.

Dislocations characteristically result from overwhelming forces
transmitted to the joint that cause a disruption of the soft tissues.
Joints most frequently dislocated in the upper extremity include the
thumb, elbow, and shoulder. In the lower extremity, the hip is vulnerable to dislocation occurring as a result of severe trauma, often
associated with motor vehicle accidents.

Clinical Manifestations

The most obvious manifestation of a dislocation is asymmetry of the musculoskeletal contour. For example, if a hip is dislocated, the limb is shorter on the affected side.

- Additional manifestations include local pain, tenderness, loss of function of the injured part, and swelling of the soft tissues in the region of the joint.

Complications of a dislocated joint are open joint injuries, avascular necrosis, intraarticular fractures, fracture dislocation, and damage to adjacent neurovascular tissue.

Diagnostic Studies

- X-ray studies determine the extent of shifting of the involved structures.
- Joint aspiration determines the presence of fat cells. If fat cells from the exposed marrow are found in the synovial fluid, an intraarticular fracture is present.

Collaborative Care

A dislocation requires prompt attention. The longer the joint remains unreduced, the greater the possibility of *avascular necrosis* (bone cell death as a result of inadequate blood supply). The hip joint is particularly susceptible to avascular necrosis.

The goal of management is to realign the dislocated portion of the joint in its original anatomic position. This can be accomplished by a closed reduction, which may be performed under local or general anesthesia. In some situations, open reduction may be necessary.

- After reduction, the extremity is usually immobilized by taping or using a sling to allow the torn ligaments and capsular tissue time to heal.
- Observation is indicated for the patient with a posterior sternoclavicular dislocation because delayed intrathoracic complications, such as pneumothorax or subclavian vessel injury, may occur.

Nursing Management

Nursing care is directed toward symptomatic relief of pain and support and protection of the injured joint. After the joint has been immobilized, motion is usually restricted.

- A carefully regulated rehabilitation program can prevent the formation of contractures. The patient should not stretch the joint beyond its limits because the torn capsule and ligament may heal in a shortened position with fibrous scar tissue that is not as strong as the original tissue.
- An exercise program slowly and methodically restores the joint to its original range of motion without causing another dislocation.

- Activity restrictions of the affected joint may be imposed to decrease the risk of dislocating the joint on a chronic basis.

DISSEMINATED INTRAVASCULAR COAGULATION

Definition/Description

Disseminated intravascular coagulation (DIC) is a serious bleeding disorder resulting from abnormally initiated and accelerated clotting. Decreases in clotting factors and platelets may lead to uncontrollable hemorrhage. The term *DIC* can be misleading because it suggests that blood is clotting. The paradox of this condition is that profuse bleeding results from depletion of platelets and clotting factors. DIC is always caused by an underlying disease; the underlying disease must be treated for DIC to resolve.

Pathophysiology

DIC is an abnormal response of the normal clotting cascade stimulated by a disease process or disorder. The diseases and disorders known to predispose patients to DIC include shock, septicemia, abruptio placentae, severe head injury, heat stroke, and pulmonary emboli.

- DIC can occur as an acute, catastrophic condition, or it may exist at a subacute or chronic level. Each condition may have one or multiple triggering mechanisms to start the cascade.

Initially in DIC, normal coagulation mechanisms are enhanced. Intravascular thrombin is produced and it catalyzes the conversion of fibrinogen to fibrin and enhances platelet aggregation. There is widespread fibrin and platelet deposition in capillaries and arterioles, resulting in thrombosis. Excessive clotting activates the fibrinolytic system, which in turn lyses newly formed clots, creating fibrin-split (fibrin-degradation) products (FSPs), which inhibit normal blood clotting. Ultimately the blood loses its ability to form a stable clot at injury sites, which predisposes the patient to hemorrhage.

- Chronic DIC is most commonly seen in patients with long-standing illnesses such as malignant disorders or autoimmune diseases.

Clinical Manifestations

There is no well-defined sequence of events in acute DIC. Bleeding in a person with no previous history or obvious cause should be questioned because it may be one of the first manifestations of acute DIC.

Other nonspecific manifestations include weakness, malaise, and fever. There are both bleeding and thrombotic manifestations in DIC.

- *Bleeding manifestations* of DIC are multifactorial and result from consumption and depletion of platelets and coagulation factors; manifestations include petechiae, oozing blood, tachypnea, hemoptysis, tachycardia, hypotension, bloody stools, hematuria, dizziness, headache, changes in mental status, and bone and joint pain.
- *Thrombotic manifestations* are a result of fibrin or platelet deposition in the microvasculature; manifestations include acute respiratory distress syndrome (ARDS), oliguria, ECG changes, venous distention, and paralytic ileus.

Diagnostic Studies

- Prolonged prothrombin time and partial thromboplastin time
- Prolonged activated partial thromboplastin time and thrombin time
- Reduced fibrinogen, antithrombin III (AT III), and platelets
- Elevated FSPs and elevated D-dimers (cross-linked fibrin fragments)
- Reduced levels of factors V, VII, VIII, X, and XIII

Collaborative Care

It is important to diagnose DIC quickly, institute therapy that will resolve the underlying causative disease or problem, and provide supportive care. Treatment of DIC remains controversial and under investigation as researchers determine how to suitably manage this dangerous syndrome. It is imperative that the nurse maintain an ongoing awareness of current modes of therapy. Regardless of etiology, treating the primary disease process is essential to the resolution of DIC. Depending on its severity, a variety of different methods are used to provide supportive and symptomatic management of DIC (Fig. 3).

- If chronic DIC is diagnosed in a patient who is not bleeding, no therapy for DIC is necessary. Treatment of the underlying disease may be sufficient to reverse DIC (e.g., antineoplastic therapy when DIC is due to malignancy).
- When the patient with DIC is bleeding, therapy is directed toward providing support with necessary blood products while treating the primary disorder. Blood products are administered on the basis of specific component deficiencies; platelets are given to correct thrombocytopenia, cryoprecipitate replaces factor VIII and fibrinogen, and fresh-frozen plasma (FFP) replaces all clotting factors except platelets and provides a source of antithrombin (see Blood Transfusion Therapy, p. 629).
- A patient with manifestations of thrombosis is often treated by anticoagulation with either unfractionated (low- or high-dose)

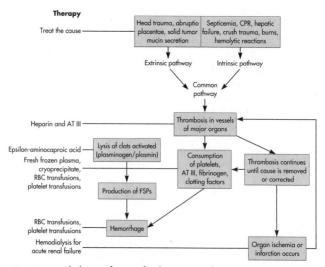

Fig. 3 Intended sites of action for therapies in disseminated intravascular coagulation. *AT III,* Antithrombin III; *CPR,* cardiopulmonary resuscitation; *FSP,* fibrin-split product; *RBC,* red blood cell. (Modified from Thelan LA and others: *Textbook of critical care nursing: diagnosis and management,* ed 2, St Louis, 1994, Mosby.)

or low molecular weight heparin. Use of heparin in the treatment of DIC remains controversial. AT III, a cofactor of heparin that becomes depleted during DIC, has been used alone or in conjunction with heparin when levels of this factor are low.

- Hirudin, a thrombin inhibitor and neutralizer, is being studied as a blocker of the abnormal coagulation process.
- Another treatment that has been used is epsilon aminocaproic acid (EACA [Amicar]) because of its ability to inhibit fibrinolysis. The use of EACA is controversial because it can enhance thrombosis.

Therapy will stabilize a patient, prevent exsanguination or massive thrombosis, and permit institution of definitive therapy to treat the underlying cause.

Nursing Diagnoses

- Altered cerebral, cardiopulmonary, renal, GI, and peripheral tissue perfusion *related to* bleeding and sluggish or diminished blood flow secondary to thrombosis
- Pain *related to* bleeding into tissues and diagnostic procedures
- Decreased cardiac output (CO) *related to* fluid volume deficit and hypotension

■ Anxiety *related to* fear of the unknown, disease process, diagnostic procedures, and therapy

Nursing Interventions

Nurses must be alert to the precipitating factors and possible development of DIC. The nurse must remember that because DIC is secondary to an underlying disease, appropriate care for managing the causative problem must be provided while providing supportive care related to the manifestations of DIC. Correcting the primary disease (when possible) will help resolve DIC.

■ Nursing care for the patient with thrombocytopenia is appropriate for the patient with DIC (see Thrombocytopenic Purpura, p. 570).

■ Early detection of bleeding, both occult and overt, must be a primary goal. The patient should be thoroughly assessed for signs of external bleeding (e.g. petechiae, oozing at IV or injection sites) and signs of internal bleeding (e.g., changes in mental status, increasing abdominal girth, pain).

■ Any sites of bleeding should be carefully monitored for progression or response to supportive therapies. Tissue damage should be minimized and the patient protected from additional foci of bleeding.

■ An additional nursing responsibility is to administer blood products properly when ordered. Infusing cryoprecipitate or FFP is similar to giving other blood products (see Blood Transfusion Therapy, p. 629).

DIVERTICULITIS/DIVERTICULOSIS

Definition/Description

A diverticulum is a saccular dilation or outpouching of the mucosa through the circular smooth muscle of the intestinal wall. Clinically, diverticular disease occurs in two forms, diverticulosis and diverticulitis. Multiple noninflamed diverticula are present with diverticulosis. The patient is most often free of symptoms but may have some abdominal discomfort. In diverticulitis, inflammation of the diverticula occurs. Diverticula may occur at any point within the GI tract but are most commonly found in the sigmoid colon.

Pathophysiology

There is no known cause of diverticular disease, but a deficiency in dietary fiber has been associated with it. The disease is more prevalent in Western populations that consume diets that are low in fiber and high in refined carbohydrates, and it is virtually unknown in areas of the world, such as rural Africa, where high-fiber diets are consumed.

■ When diverticula form, the smooth muscle of the colon wall becomes thickened. Lack of dietary fiber slows transit time and more water is absorbed from the stool, making it more difficult to pass through the lumen. Decreased bulk of stool, combined with a more narrowed lumen in the sigmoid colon, causes high intraluminal pressures. These factors are believed to contribute to the formation of diverticula.

The cause of diverticulitis is related to the retention of stool and bacteria in the diverticulum, which form a hardened mass called a *fecalith.* This causes inflammation of the diverticulum that spreads to the surrounding area in the colon, causing the tissue to become edematous. Abscesses may form, or complete perforation with peritonitis may occur.

Clinical Manifestations and Complications

The majority of patients with *diverticulosis* have no symptoms. Those with symptoms typically have crampy, abdominal pain located in the left lower quadrant that is usually relieved by the passage of flatus or a bowel movement. Alternating constipation and diarrhea may be present. Approximately 15% of patients with diverticulosis progress to acute diverticulitis.

In patients with *diverticulitis* abdominal pain is localized over the involved area of the colon. A tender, left lower quadrant mass may be felt on palpation of the abdomen. Fever, chills, nausea, anorexia, and leukocytosis may also be present. Elderly patients with diverticulitis are frequently afebrile with little to no abdominal tenderness.

Complications of diverticulitis include perforation with peritonitis, abscess and fistula formation, bowel obstruction, ureteral obstruction, and bleeding. Bleeding is a common complication of diverticulitis and is manifested by *hematochezia* (maroon stools). Bleeding usually stops spontaneously.

Diagnostic Studies

■ Complete blood count (CBC), urinalysis, and fecal occult blood test
■ Barium enema to diagnose diverticular disease
■ Sigmoidoscopy
■ Colonoscopy to rule out polyps or lesions

Collaborative Care

Uncomplicated diverticular disease is treated with a high-fiber diet and bulk laxatives, such as psyllium hydrophilic mucilloid (Metamucil). Anticholinergic drugs such as dicyclomine (Bentyl) and Donnatal may be used to relieve discomfort due to spasm of the bowel. In acute diverticulitis, broad-spectrum antibiotic therapy is required. The patient is kept on nothing by mouth (NPO) status and bed rest and is given parental fluids. The white blood cell (WBC) count is monitored. A nasogastric (NG) tube may be necessary.

- Approximately 30% of the patients with acute diverticulitis will require surgical intervention. Surgical intervention is necessary to drain abscesses or to resect an obstructing inflammatory mass. Usual surgical procedures involve resection of involved colon with a temporary diverting colostomy. The colostomy is reanastomosed after the colon is healed.

Nursing Management

Uncomplicated diverticular disease is primarily treated by a high-fiber diet. Fluids should be increased because fibers retain water, thus decreasing the amount absorbed by the body. If the patient is obese, a reduction in weight is needed.

- Increased intraabdominal pressure should be avoided because it may precipitate an attack. Factors that increase intraabdominal pressure are straining at stool, vomiting, bending, lifting, and tight, restrictive clothing.

In acute diverticulitis, the goal of treatment is to allow the colon to rest and inflammation to subside. The patient needs to be observed for signs of possible peritonitis.

- When the acute attack subsides, oral fluids progressing to a semisolid diet are allowed. Ambulation is also permitted. At this stage the patient needs to be observed for a recurrent attack.
- If the patient has a bowel resection or colostomy, nursing care is the same as for these procedures.
- The patient should be provided with a full explanation of the condition. The better the patient understands the disease process and adheres to the prescribed regimen, the less likely the exacerbation of the disease and the onset of complications.

DYSMENORRHEA

Definition/Description

Dysmenorrhea is cramping abdominal pain or discomfort associated with menstrual flow. The degree of pain and discomfort varies with the individual. Two types of dysmenorrhea exist: *primary,* when no pathology exists, and *secondary,* when a pelvic disease or condition is the underlying cause.

- Approximately 50% of all women experience dysmenorrhea, making it one of the most common gynecologic problems.

Pathophysiology

Primary dysmenorrhea is caused by either an excess of or an increased sensitivity to prostaglandin $F_{2\alpha}$ ($PGF_{2\alpha}$).

- Prostaglandins increase myometrial contractions and constriction of small endometrial blood vessels, with consequent tissue ischemia and increased sensitization of the pain receptors.
- Prostaglandins are also known to cause headaches, diarrhea, and vomiting, which are other manifestations of dysmenorrhea.

Secondary dysmenorrhea is usually acquired after adolescence, occurring most commonly in persons in their 30s and 40s. Secondary dysmenorrhea is due to pelvic diseases such as endometriosis, chronic pelvic inflammatory disease (PID), uterine leiomyomas (fibroids), and adenomyosis.

Clinical Manifestations

Primary dysmenorrhea starts 12 to 24 hours before the onset of menses. The pain is most severe the first day of menses and rarely lasts more than 2 days

- Characteristic manifestations include lower cramping abdominal pain that is colicky in nature, frequently radiating to the lower back and upper thighs. The abdominal pain is often accompanied by nausea, diarrhea or loose stools, fatigue, headache, and lightheadedness

Secondary dysmenorrhea usually occurs after the woman has experienced problem-free periods for some time. The pain, which may be unilateral, is generally more constant in nature and continues for a longer time than primary dysmenorrhea.

- Depending on the cause, symptoms such as dyspareunia (painful intercourse), painful defecation, or irregular bleeding may occur at times other than menstruation.

Collaborative Care

Evaluation begins with distinguishing primary from secondary dysmenorrhea. A complete health history with special attention to menstrual and gynecologic history should be obtained. A pelvic exam is also done.

- If the pelvic exam is normal and the history reveals an onset shortly after menarche with symptoms only associated with menses, the probable diagnosis is primary dysmenorrhea.
- If any cause or etiology for the pain is evident, the diagnosis is secondary dysmenorrhea. Further evaluation of the cause would then be indicated.

Non-drug treatment for primary dysmenorrhea includes heat applied to the lower abdomen or back and regular exercise. Regular exercise is thought to be beneficial because it may reduce endometrial hyperplasia and subsequently reduce prostaglandin production.

Drug therapy involves nonsteroidal antiinflammatory drugs (NSAIDs) such as ibuprofen. NSAIDs are started at the first sign of menses and continued every 4 to 8 hours for the duration of the usual discomfort.

- Birth control pills provide another choice for drug therapy. Birth control pills can decrease dysmenorrhea by reducing endometrial hyperplasia.

Nursing Management

- The nurse should instruct the woman that during acute pain, relief may be obtained by lying down for short periods, drinking hot beverages, applying heat to the abdomen, and taking an antiinflammatory drug for mild to moderate pain.
- The nurse can also suggest noninvasive pain-relieving practices such as distraction and guided imagery.
- Other health care measures that can decrease discomfort include regular exercise, maintenance of proper nutritional habits, avoidance of constipation, maintenance of good body mechanics, and avoidance of stress and overfatigue, particularly during the time preceding menstrual periods.
- Staying active and interested in activities may also help.
- Education and supportive therapy can provide women with a foundation for coping with this common occurrence and increase feelings of control and self-reliance.

ENCEPHALITIS

Encephalitis, an acute inflammation of the brain, is usually caused by a virus. Many different viruses have been implicated in encephalitis; some of them are associated with certain seasons of the year and endemic to certain geographic areas. *Epidemic encephalitis* is transmitted by ticks and mosquitoes, whereas *nonepidemic encephalitis* may occur as a complication of measles, chickenpox, or mumps.

- Encephalitis is a serious, sometimes fatal disease with mortality rates of 5% to 20%.
- Herpes simplex virus (HSV) encephalitis is the most common form of viral encephalitis. Cytomegalovirus encephalitis is one of the common complications in patients with AIDS.

The disease is characterized by diffuse damage to the nerve cells of the brain, perivascular cellular infiltration, proliferation of glial cells, and increasing cerebral edema. Sequelae of encephalitis include mental deterioration, amnesia, personality changes, and hemiparesis.

- Manifestations resemble those of meningitis, but they have a more gradual onset; these include headache, high fever, seizures, and a change in the level of consciousness.
- Diagnostic studies for encephalitis are described in Table 29.

Collaborative and nursing management is symptomatic and supportive. Cerebral edema is a major problem, with diuretics (mannitol) and corticosteroids (dexamethasone) used to control it. Vidarabine suspension (Vira-A) is used in the treatment of HSV encephalitis. Acyclovir (Zovirax) is also used for the treatment of HSV encephalitis. It has fewer side effects than vidarabine and is often the preferred treatment. For maximal benefit, antiviral agents must be started before the onset of coma.

See NCP 54-3 for the patient with an inflammatory condition of the brain, Lewis and others, *Medical-Surgical Nursing,* edition 5, p. 1640.

ENDOCARDITIS, INFECTIVE

Definition/Description
Infective endocarditis, previously known as bacterial endocarditis, is an infection of the endocardial surface with microorganisms present in the lesion. Inflammation from infective endocarditis frequently affects the cardiac valves. Although the most common cause of infective endocarditis is bacterial infection, it may be caused by

Table 29   Cerebral Inflammatory Conditions

	Bacterial meningitis*	Encephalitis	Brain abscess
Causative organisms	Bacteria (pneumococci, meningococci, streptococci)	Bacteria, fungi, parasites, herpes simplex virus (HSV), other viruses	Streptococci, staphylococci through bloodstream
CSF			
Pressure (normal, 60-150 mm H_2O)	Increased	Normal to slight increase with increased ICP	Increased
WBC count (normal, 0-8/μl)	>500/μl (mainly PMN)	<500/μl, PMN (early), lymphocytes (later)	25-300/μl (PMN)
Protein (normal, 15-45 mg/dl [0.15-0.45 g/L])	High	Slight increase	Normal
Glucose (normal, 45-75 mg/dl [2.5-4.2 mmol/L])	Low or absent	Normal	Low or absent
Appearance	Turbid, cloudy	Clear	Clear
Diagnostic studies	Gram stain, smear, culture	Viral studies, MRI HSV DNA	CT scan, EEG, skull x-ray
Treatment	Antibiotics with sensitivity tests, supportive care, prevention of symptoms of increased ICP	Supportive care, prevention of symptoms of increased ICP, acyclovir (Zovirax) for HSV	Antibiotics, incision and drainage Supportive care

CSF, Cerebrospinal fluid; CT, computed tomography; DNA, deoxyribonucleic acid; EEG, electroencephalogram; ICP, intracranial pressure; PMN, polymorphonuclear cells; WBC, white blood cell.
*Meningitis can also be caused by virus, yeast, and fungi.

E

a variety of microorganisms. Before the era of antibiotics, infective endocarditis was almost always fatal.

Classification

Two forms of infective endocarditis, *subacute* and *acute,* have been described.

- The *subacute form* has a longer clinical course of more insidious onset with less toxicity, and the causative organism is usually of low virulence (most often *Streptococcus viridans*).
- In contrast, the *acute form* has a shorter clinical course with a more rapid onset, increased toxicity, and a more pathogenic causative organism (usually *Staphylococcus aureus*).

Although this classification system has been historically used and may be conceptually useful, clinicians prefer to classify infective endocarditis based on etiologic agent.

Pathophysiology

The term *bacterial endocarditis* has been replaced by *infective endocarditis* because the causative organisms include fungi, chlamydiae, rickettsiae, and bacteria. Streptococci and staphylococci account for the majority of cases.

Infective endocarditis occurs when turbulence within the heart allows the causative organism to infect previously damaged valves or other endothelial surfaces. The damage may occur in individuals with underlying cardiac conditions such as rheumatic heart disease, prosthetic valves, and mitral valve prolapse with murmur. A variety of invasive procedures (e.g., surgical interventions, IV injection, and diagnostic procedures) can allow large numbers of organisms to enter the bloodstream and trigger the infectious process.

- *Vegetations,* the primary lesions of infective endocarditis, consist of fibrin, leukocytes, platelets, and microbes that adhere to the valve surface or endocardium.
- The loss of portions of this friable vegetation into the circulation results in embolization. Systemic embolization occurs from left-sided heart vegetation, progressing to organ (particularly kidney, spleen, and brain) and limb infarction. Right-sided heart lesions embolize to the lungs.
- The infection may spread locally to cause damage to valves or their supporting structures.
- The resulting valvular incompetence and eventual invasion of the myocardium in the infectious disease results in congestive heart failure (CHF), generalized myocardial dysfunction, and sepsis.

Clinical Manifestations

The clinical manifestations are nonspecific and can involve multiple organ systems. Fever occurs in more than 90% of patients with endocarditis.

- *Nonspecific manifestations* that may accompany fever include chills, weakness, malaise, fatigue, and anorexia. Arthralgias, myalgias, abdominal discomfort, back pain, weight loss, headache, and clubbing of fingers may occur in subacute forms of endocarditis.
- *Vascular manifestations* include *splinter hemorrhages* (black longitudinal streaks) that may occur in the nailbeds. Petechiae, as a result of fragmentation and microembolization of vegetative lesions, are common in the conjunctivae, lips, buccal mucosa, palate, and over the ankles, feet, antecubital, and popliteal areas. *Osler's nodes* (painful, tender, red or purple, pea-size lesions) may be found on the fingertips or toes. *Janeway lesions* (flat, painless, small, red spots) may be found on the palms and soles. Funduscopic examination may reveal hemorrhagic retinal lesions called *Roth's spots.*
- Onset of a new murmur is frequently noted, with the aortic and mitral valves most commonly affected.

Clinical manifestations secondary to embolization in various body organs may also be present: (1) embolization to the spleen may result in sharp, left upper quadrant pain and splenomegaly, local tenderness, and abdominal rigidity; (2) embolization to the kidneys may cause pain in the flank, hematuria, azotemia, and glomerulonephritis; (3) emboli may lodge in the small peripheral blood vessels of the arms and legs and cause gangrene; (4) embolization to the brain may cause an embolic stroke with hemiplegia, ataxia, aphasia, visual changes, and a change in the level of consciousness; and (5) pulmonary emboli may occur in right-sided endocarditis.

Diagnostic Studies

A recent health history should be obtained with inquiry made regarding any recent dental, urologic, surgical, or gynecologic procedures including normal or abnormal obstetric delivery. Previous history of heart disease, recent cardiac catheterization, and skin, respiratory, or urinary tract infections (UTIs) should also be documented.

- Blood culture and sensitivity may reveal positive cultures.
- White blood cell (WBC) count with differential may demonstrate mild leukocytosis.
- Proteinuria and rheumatoid factor are found in some patients.
- Chest x-ray is used to detect CHF.
- ECG may reveal changes.
- Echocardiography may identify vegetation and abscesses on valves.

- Cardiac catheterization is done when surgical intervention is considered.

Prophylactic Treatment

Cardiac lesions, prosthetic valves, acquired valvular disease, mitral valve prolapse, prior endocarditis, and noncardiac diseases are the principal risk factors for infective endocarditis. Procedure-associated risks include IV injection of recreational drugs and specific dental, medical, or surgical procedures.

- Antibiotic prophylaxis is recommended for patients with specific cardiac conditions before they undergo certain dental or surgical procedures.
- Antibiotic prophylaxis should also be instituted in high-risk patients who are to undergo removal or drainage of infected tissue, have indwelling cardiac pacemakers, undergo renal dialysis, and have ventriculoatrial shunts for management of hydrocephalus.

Collaborative Care

Accurate identification of the infecting organism is the key to successful treatment. The appropriate antibiotic (usually given IV) is chosen on the basis of sensitivity studies (see Table 35-6, Lewis and others, *Medical-Surgical Nursing,* edition 5, p. 951). Complete eradication of the organism generally takes weeks to achieve and relapses are common.

- The patient's antibiotic serum levels should be monitored periodically. Subsequent blood cultures may be done to evaluate the effectiveness of antibiotic therapy. Blood cultures that remain positive indicate inadequate or inappropriate antibiotic administration, aortic root or myocardial abscess, or the wrong diagnosis (e.g., an infection elsewhere).
- Fever may persist for several days after treatment has been started and is treated with aspirin, acetaminophen, fluids, and rest.
- Complete bed rest is usually not indicated unless the temperature remains elevated or there are signs of heart damage.

The results of drug therapy alone are generally poor in patients with fungal endocarditis and prosthetic valve endocarditis. Early valve replacement followed by prolonged drug therapy is recommended in these situations.

Nursing Management

Goals

The patient with infective endocarditis will have normal cardiac function, have no residual cardiac damage, be able to perform activities of daily living (ADLs) without fatigue, and understand the therapeutic regimen to prevent recurrence of endocarditis.

See NCP 35-1 for the patient with infective endocarditis, Lewis and others, *Medical-Surgical Nursing,* edition 5, p. 952.

Nursing Diagnoses

- Decreased cardiac output *related to* valvular insufficiency and fluid overload
- Activity intolerance *related to* generalized weakness and alteration in oxygen transport secondary to valvular dysfunction
- Anxiety *related to* critical illness and prolonged hospitalization
- Fever *related to* infection of cardiac tissue
- Altered health maintenance *related to* lack of knowledge about the disease and treatment process

Nursing Interventions

The incidence of infective endocarditis can be decreased by identifying individuals who are at risk for the development of endocarditis. Assessment of the patient's history and an understanding of the disease process are crucial for planning and implementing appropriate health maintenance strategies.

Infective endocarditis generally requires treatment with antibiotics for 4 to 6 weeks. The patient usually requires in-hospital stabilization, and then may be treated with outpatient parenteral antibiotic therapy.

- Fever, chronic or intermittent, is a common early sign of infective endocarditis. Frequent assessment of body temperature is important because persistent, prolonged temperature elevations may mean that the drug therapy is ineffective.
- The patient needs adequate periods of physical and emotional rest. Bed rest may be necessary when fever is present or there are complications (e.g., heart damage). Otherwise the patient may ambulate and perform moderate activity.
- Laboratory data should be monitored to determine the effectiveness of long-term, high-dose antibiotic therapy received by the patient.
- IV lines should be monitored for patency, and antibiotics should be given when scheduled. The patient should be monitored continuously for undesirable side effects of drugs.
- To prevent problems because of immobility, the patient should wear elastic compression gradient stockings, perform range-of-motion (ROM) exercises, and turn, cough, and deep breathe every 2 hours.
- The patient may experience anxiety and fear associated with the illness. The nurse must recognize this problem and implement strategies to help reduce the patient's fears and anxieties.

Patients who receive outpatient antibiotics will require vigilant home nursing care. Patients with active endocarditis are at risk for life-threatening complications such as cerebral emboli and pulmonary edema.

- Adequacy of the home environment in terms of in-home companions and hospital access must be determined for successful management.
- After therapy is completed in either the home or hospital setting, management will focus on educating the patient about the nature of the disease and on reducing the risk of reinfection.

▼ **Patient Teaching**

Education is crucial for the patient's understanding of and adherence to the planned treatment regimen.

- The patient should understand the need to avoid persons with infections, especially upper respiratory ones, and to report cold, flu, and cough symptoms.
- The importance of avoiding excessive fatigue and the need to plan rest periods before and after activities should be carefully explained to the patient.
- Good oral hygiene, including daily care and regular dental visits, is also important.
- The patient must inform all health care providers performing dental, medical, or surgical procedures of his or her history of heart disease.
- The patient should understand the significance of the prescribed prophylactic antibiotic therapy given before any invasive procedure.
- Once therapy has been completed, the patient should be instructed about symptoms that may indicate recurrent infection such as fever, fatigue, malaise, and chills. If any of these symptoms occur, the patient should be aware of the importance of notifying the physician.
- Explain to the patient the relationship of follow-up care, good nutrition, and early treatment of common infections (e.g., colds) to maintain good health.

ENDOMETRIAL CANCER

Definition/Description

Cancer of the endometrium has become the most common gynecologic malignancy, accounting for nearly 50% of female genital tract neoplasms. However, it has a relatively low mortality, with a survival rate of 94% if the cancer has not spread at the time of diagnosis. About 25% of endometrial cancer is diagnosed before menopause. The average age at the time of diagnosis is 61.

- The major risk factor for endometrial cancer is estrogen, in particular unopposed estrogen. Additional risk factors include increasing age, nulliparity, obesity, hypertension, and diabetes mellitus (DM). Pregnancy and birth control pills are protective factors.

Pathophysiology

This type of cancer arises from the endometrium lining. The precursor may be a hyperplastic state that progresses to invasive carcinoma. Direct extension develops into the cervix and through the uterine serosa. As invasion of the myometrium occurs, regional lymph nodes, including the paravaginal and paraaortic, become involved. Hematogenous metastases develop concurrently. The usual sites of metastases are the lung, bone, liver, and eventually the brain. Endometrial cancer grows slowly, metastasizes late, and is amenable to therapy if diagnosed early.

E

Clinical Manifestations

- The first symptom is abnormal uterine bleeding, usually in postmenopausal women.
- Because perimenopausal women have sporadic periods for a time, it is important that this sign not be ignored or automatically blamed on menopause.
- Pain occurs late in the disease process, and other symptoms that may arise are related to metastasis to other organs.

Diagnostic Studies

Endometrial biopsy has replaced dilation and curettage (D & C) as a diagnostic procedure for endometrial cancer.

- Endometrial biopsy can be done as an office procedure and involves obtaining endometrial tissue from the uterus. Occurrence of breakthrough bleeding in a postmenopausal woman mandates obtaining a tissue sample to exclude endometrial cancer.
- The Pap test is not a reliable diagnostic tool for endometrial cancer, but it can rule out cervical cancer.

Collaborative Care

Treatment is by total hysterectomy, which includes bilateral salpingooophorectomy and total hysterectomy with selective node biopsies. Surgery may be followed by radiation therapy, either to the pelvis or abdomen externally or intravaginally, to decrease local recurrence (see Radiation Therapy p. 681). Treatment of advanced or recurrent disease is difficult. Hormonal therapy (e.g., progesterone) is the treatment of choice when the progesterone receptor is positive and the tumor is well differentiated. Chemotherapy is considered when progesterone therapy is unsuccessful. The most common agents used are doxorubicin (Adriamycin) and cisplatin (Platinol).

Nursing Management: Cancers of the Female Reproductive Tract

See Cervical Cancer, p. 121.

ENDOMETRIOSIS

Definition/Description

Endometriosis is the presence of normal endometrial tissue in sites outside the endometrial cavity. The most frequent sites are in or near the ovaries, uterosacral ligaments, and uterovesical peritoneum. However, endometrial tissues can be in many other locations such as the stomach, lungs, and spleen.

- The endometrial tissue responds to hormones of the ovarian cycle and undergoes a mini-menstrual cycle similar to uterine endometrium.
- Endometriosis appears to cause infertility in 30% to 60% of cases.

Although many theories about the cause of endometriosis have been advanced, the etiology remains unknown. A widely held view is that retrograde menstrual flow passes through the fallopian tubes, carrying viable endometrial tissues into the pelvis and attaching to various sites.

Clinical Manifestations

A wide range of symptoms and severity exist. The magnitude of a woman's symptoms do not match the clinical extent of her endometriosis.

- The most common symptoms are secondary dysmenorrhea, infertility, pelvic pain, dyspareunia, and irregular bleeding.
- Less common symptoms include backache, painful bowel movements, and dysuria.
- Symptoms may or may not correspond to the woman's menstrual cycles. With menopause, estrogen is no longer produced in the ovaries, which may lead to the disappearance of symptoms.
- When a cyst ruptures, the pain may be acute and the resulting irritation promotes the formation of adhesions, which fix the affected area to another pelvic structure. The adhesions may become severe enough to cause a bowel obstruction or painful micturition. Adhesions involving the uterus, fallopian tubes, or ovaries may result in infertility.

Diagnostic Studies

Diagnosis is frequently confirmed by patient history and the palpation of firm nodular lumps in the adnexa on bimanual examination. Laparoscopic examination is necessary for a definitive diagnosis.

Collaborative Care

Treatment is influenced by a patient's age, desire to get pregnant, and symptom severity. When symptoms are not disruptive, a "watch and wait" approach is used.

Drug Therapy

Drug therapy is used to reduce symptoms. Hormonal therapy can control but not cure endometriosis.

- Continuous use (for 9 months) of combined progestin and estrogen causes regression of endometrial tissue. Ovulation is suppressed and pseudopregnancy (hyperhormonal amenorrhea) is produced.
- Another approach to hormonal treatment is danazol (Danocrine), a synthetic androgen that inhibits the anterior pituitary. The drug produces a pseudomenopause (ovarian suppression), with consequent atrophy of ectopic endometrial tissue. Subjective relief of symptoms is noted within 6 weeks of danazol use.
- Another drug therapy is an injectable gonadotropin-releasing hormone agonist (leuprolide acetate [Lupron]). It causes a hypoestrogenic state resulting in amenorrhea.

Surgical Therapy

The only cure for endometriosis is surgical removal of all the endometrial implants. Surgical therapy may be conservative or definitive. *Conservative surgery* is done to confirm the diagnosis or to remove implants. It involves removal or destruction of endometrial implants and the lysing or excision of adhesions by means of laparoscopic laser surgery and laparotomy.

- For women wishing to get pregnant, conservative surgical therapy is used to remove implants that may block the fallopian tube. Adhesions are also removed from the tubes, ovaries, and pelvic structures.

Definitive surgery involves the removal of the uterus, tubes, ovaries, and as many endometrial implants as possible. Each woman should be actively involved in making the decision about preserving part or all of her ovaries if surgically possible. Her feelings about maintaining her cyclical ovarian function need to be explored.

Nursing Management

- Dysmenorrhea after years of relatively pain-free menses and infertility after a period of trying to achieve pregnancy may serve as clues to the presence of this disease.
- Education of the patient and reassurance that a health-threatening situation does not exist may permit her to accept a conservative and progressive treatment. The nurse is often the person who counsels the patient in the use of the prescribed drugs.

- Psychologic support may be needed for the patient experiencing severe disabling pain, sexual difficulties secondary to dyspareunia, and infertility.
- If conservative surgery is the treatment selected, nursing care is similar to general preoperative and postoperative care of a patient undergoing laparotomy (see Abdominal Pain, Acute, p. 3).
- If definitive surgery is planned, nursing care is similar to the patient undergoing an abdominal hysterectomy. (See NCP 51-2 for the patient undergoing an abdominal hysterectomy, Lewis and others, *Medical-Surgical Nursing,* edition 5, p. 1538).

EPIDIDYMITIS

Epididymitis is an inflammatory process of the epididymis, usually secondary to an infectious process (sexually or nonsexually transmitted), trauma, or urinary reflux down the vas deferens. Swelling may progress to the point that the epididymis and testis are indistinguishable. The problem may be associated with prostatitis and is usually painful.
- In younger men less than 35 years of age, the most common cause is the sexual transmission of either gonorrhea or chlamydia.

Conservative treatment consists of bed rest with elevation of the scrotum, the use of ice packs, and analgesics. Ambulation places the scrotum in a dependent position and increases pain.
- The use of antibiotics is important for both partners if transmission is through sexual contact.
- Most tenderness subsides within 1 week, although swelling may last for weeks or months.

ERECTILE DYSFUNCTION

Definition/Description

Erectile dysfunction is the inability to attain or maintain an erect penis that allows for satisfactory sexual performance. Erectile dysfunction is increasing in all segments of the sexually active male population. In younger men the increase is attributed to an increase in substance abuse, such as the abuse of recreational drugs and alcohol. Middle-aged men are affected by disease and modern medical technology such as major organ transplants, bypass surgeries, and chemotherapeutic agents.

- Stress factors associated with modern lifestyles are affecting men of all ages and contribute greatly to the psychologic causes of erectile failure.
- The problem can occur at any age, although it is most common among males between the ages of 55 and 65 years.

Pathophysiology

Erection is a parasympathetic nervous system reflex initiated mainly by certain tactile, visual, and mental stimuli. It consists of dilation of the arteries and arterioles of the penis, which in turn fills and distends spaces in its erectile tissue and compresses its veins. Therefore more blood enters the penis through dilated arteries than leaves it through constricted veins. Hence the penis become larger and rigid; in other words, erection occurs. Problems occur when these spaces (corporeal bodies) fail to fill when desired or when they empty before orgasm.

- There are two classifications of erectile dysfunction: *primary dysfunction* occurs when patient has never been able to have an adequate erection with any type of sexual experience; *secondary dysfunction* occurs when patient has lost the ability to achieve erection or is able to have an erection only with assistance.

Causative factors may be physiologic, psychologic, or both. These include anatomic anomalies (e.g., congenital deformities and cardiorespiratory disorders [emphysema]), drug-induced problems (e.g., caffeine and diuretics), endocrine imbalances (e.g., diabetes mellitus [DM]), genitourinary disorders (e.g., prostatitis), psychogenic factors (e.g., depression and fatigue), and neurologic problems (e.g., spinal cord trauma). (See Table 52-9, Lewis and others, *Medical-Surgical Nursing,* edition 5, p. 1573.)

The major complication is that the man's inability to perform sexually can cause distress in his interpersonal relationships and may interfere with his concept of himself as a man. See Table 52-10, *Medical-Surgical Nursing,* p. 1573 for normal age-related changes in sexual performance.

Diagnostic Studies

- Detailed sexual history, including practices and techniques
- Psychosocial and neurologic evaluation
- Testosterone, prolactin, follicle-stimulating hormone (FSH), and luteinizing hormone (LH) levels
- Prostate specific antigen (PSA) levels
- Intracavernosal vasoactive and nocturnal penile tumescence testing to distinguish psychogenic from neurogenic or vascular causes
- Vascular flow studies (e.g., duplex Doppler, cavernosogram)
- Tests to exclude unrecognized systemic disease: complete blood count (CBC), serum chemistry profile, urinalysis, creatinine, lipid profile, fasting blood sugar, and thyroid function studies

Collaborative Care

Treatment is based on the cause. Whenever possible, collaboration should occur between the primary physician providing the medical care and the urologist treating the erectile dysfunction.

- Treatment of psychologic causes of erectile dysfunction should be carried out by a qualified therapist. The approach may be behavioral, psychologic, or, in some patients, may also involve interventions to temporarily restore self-confidence. The goal of therapy is to have the man and his partner develop a satisfactory sexual relationship that includes good communication skills.
- When the problem is physical, interventions are directed at correcting or eliminating the cause or restoring function through medical means. The results of these interventions are usually quite satisfactory when both partners are involved in the decision-making process and have realistic expectations of the treatment.

Drug Therapy

Elimination of or substitution for a medication that causes erectile dysfunction (e.g., methyldopa [Aldomet], propranolol [Inderal]) is sometimes all that is necessary to alleviate the problem.

- When there is an established diagnosis of testicular failure (hypogonadism), androgen replacement therapy may sometimes be effective in improving erectile dysfunction. It should be given as an intramuscular (IM) injection of testosterone enanthate or testosterone orcypionate. The effectiveness of testosterone supplementation for older men experiencing a normal, gradual decline is doubtful.
- Penile vasoactive drug therapy enhances blood flow in the penile arteries. These medications are available in pill, gel, patch, pellet, and injection form. Current vasoactive medications include papaverine, alprostadil (Caverject, Prostin), phentolamine (Regitine), and, in combination with other vasoactive medications, vasoactive intestinal peptide (VIP) and sildenafil (Viagra).

Aids or Devices

Suction devices applied to the flaccid penis produce an erection by pulling blood up into the corporeal bodies. A penile ring or other device placed around the base of the penis causes vasoconstriction and prevents detumescence (subsidence of swelling).

- Special care must be taken in using these devices to prevent tissue damage. Suction devices are sometimes used in conjunction with intracorporeal injection therapy in those patients with moderate-to-severe venous leaks of the penile veins.

Alternative Methods

Patients experiencing temporary loss of erection or who are awaiting surgical interventions may use a variety of methods to achieve sexual satisfaction. Sexual counselors or therapists acting as consultants can provide support and suggest alternative forms of sexual expression.

Surgical Therapy

Penile implants are used to treat erectile dysfunction; these paired devices can be semirigid, malleable, or inflatable. They are implanted into the corporeal bodies to provide an erection firm enough for penetration.

- All implants provide a usable erection and should be chosen carefully based on the man's mental and physical capabilities, surgical risk factors, personal lifestyle, insurance, and financial resources.
- The main problems associated with penile prostheses are mechanical failure, infection, and erosions.
- For essentially healthy men the surgical procedure may be done on an outpatient basis, with patients being periodically monitored. Complete recovery time varies from 4 to 6 weeks.
- Sexual counseling is often recommended before and after surgery.

Nursing Management

The patient experiencing erectile dysfunction requires a great deal of emotional support for both himself and his partner. The patient needs reassurance that confidentiality will be maintained.

- Men often do not feel comfortable discussing their problems with others because of society's expectations of a man's sexual abilities.
- The man may experience and demonstrate isolation from support systems, and he may also lose self-esteem, which can eventually lead to loss of role functions.
- In conjunction with treatment, it often becomes necessary to provide counseling and therapy for the couple to establish realistic expectations and develop meaningful communication patterns.

Nurses are in a unique position of conducting routine health assessments on men seeking any form of medical treatment. It provides an opportunity to ask not only general health questions but also those seldom asked sexual function ones. Given the opportunity, most men do not hesitate to answer these questions when they know that someone cares and can provide them with answers.

ESOPHAGEAL CANCER

Definition/Description
Squamous cell carcinoma is the most common form of esophageal cancer. Compared to portions of Asia in which the rate of esophageal cancer is extremely high, the incidence is low in Western societies. The incidence of squamous cell carcinoma of the esophagus is higher in men and African-Americans and increases with age. Because esophageal cancer is rarely diagnosed in the early stages, the 5-year prognosis is poor.

Pathophysiology
The cause of esophageal cancer is unknown. Possible predisposing factors are cigarette smoking, excessive alcohol intake, chronic trauma, poor oral hygiene, and spicy foods. Other risk factors include exposure to asbestos and metals and a low intake of fresh fruits and vegetables.
- The malignant tumor usually appears as an ulcerated lesion. It may have advanced to this stage before symptoms appear.
- The majority of tumors are located in the middle and lower portions of the esophagus with the tumor penetrating the muscular layer and even extending outside the esophageal wall.
- Tumor obstruction of the esophagus occurs in the later stages.

Clinical Manifestations
The onset of symptoms is usually late in relation to the extent of the tumor.
- Progressive dysphagia is the most common symptom and may be expressed as a substernal feeling that food is not passing. Initially dysphagia occurs only with meat, then with soft foods, and eventually with liquids.
- Pain develops later and is described as occurring in the substernal, epigastric, or back areas and usually increases with swallowing. The pain may radiate to the neck, jaw, ears, and shoulders.
- If the tumor is in the upper third of the esophagus, symptoms such as sore throat, choking, and hoarseness may occur. Weight loss is fairly common.
- When esophageal stenosis is severe, regurgitation of blood-flecked esophageal contents is common.

Complications may include hemorrhage from cancer eroding through the esophagus and into the aorta. Esophageal perforation into the lung or trachea may also develop. The liver and lung are common metastatic sites.

Diagnostic Studies

- Barium swallow with fluoroscopy may demonstrate esophageal narrowing at the tumor site.
- Esophagoscopy with biopsy is needed to make a definitive diagnosis.
- Endoscopic ultrasonography detects tumor invasion into the muscle layer.
- Bronchoscopic examination detects malignant involvement of the trachea.
- CT scan and MRI assess the extent of the disease.

Collaborative Care

Treatment depends on the location of the tumor and whether metastasis has occurred. The best treatment results have been obtained with a combination of surgery and radiation. Chemotherapeutic agents (cisplatin [Platinol] and 5-fluorouracil [5-FU]) in combination with radiation are currently under investigation.

If the tumor is in the cervical section (upper third) of the esophagus, radiation is usually indicated (see Radiation Therapy, p. 681). A tumor in the lower third of the esophagus is usually resected surgically. Dilation may be used to relieve dysphagia and allow for improved nutrition.

- Palliative therapy consists of restoration of the swallowing function and maintenance of nutrition and hydration. Obstruction can be relieved by dilation, stent placement, or both. Laser therapy or vaporization of the tumor by means of endoscopy may be used in combination with dilation.

Nutritional therapy. After esophageal surgery, parenteral fluids are given. When fluids are allowed after bowel sounds have returned, 30 to 60 ml of water are given hourly, with gradual progression to small, frequent, bland meals. The patient should be in an upright position to prevent fluid regurgitation. Symptoms of food intolerance include vomiting and abdominal distention. A gastrostomy may be performed for the purpose of feeding the patient and reducing aspiration.

Nursing Management

Goals

The patient with esophageal cancer will have relief of symptoms including pain and dysphagia, achieve optimal nutritional intake, understand the prognosis of the disease, and experience a quality of life appropriate to disease progression.

Nursing Diagnoses

- Altered nutrition: less than body requirements *related to* dysphagia, weakness, and radiation therapy
- Pain *related to* tumor

- Anxiety *related to* diagnosis of cancer, uncertain future, and poor prognosis
- Anticipatory grieving *related to* diagnosis of life-threatening malignancy
- Altered health maintenance *related to* lack of knowledge of the disease process and therapeutic regimen, unavailability of a support system, and chronic debilitating disease

Nursing Interventions

Preoperative care should focus on general preoperative teaching and preparation including meticulous oral care, information about chest tubes (if a thoracic approach is used), IV lines, nasogastric (NG) tube, gastrostomy feeding, turning, coughing, and deep breathing.

Postoperative care should include assessment of drainage; maintenance of the NG tube; oral and nasal care; prevention of respiratory complications by turning, coughing, and deep breathing, with incentive spirometry every 2 hours; and placing the patient in a semi-Fowler's position to prevent gastric reflux.

Many patients require long-term follow-up care after surgery for esophageal cancer. The patient may undergo radiation treatment following surgery. The patient needs encouragement and assistance in maintaining adequate nutrition. The patient may need a permanent feeding gastrostomy. The patient usually has fears and anxieties about a diagnosis of cancer.

- The nurse should know what the doctor has told the patient regarding the prognosis and then provide appropriate counseling. Some communities have resource groups consisting of persons with cancer who can serve as support systems.
- Referral to a home health nurse may be necessary for continued care of the patient (e.g., gastrostomy teaching and follow-up wound care.)

▼ **Patient Teaching**

- Health counseling needs to focus on the elimination of smoking and excessive alcohol intake.
- Maintenance of good oral hygiene and dietary habits (intake of fresh fruits and vegetables) may also be helpful.
- Having the patient obtain treatment of esophageal problems, such as Barrett's esophagus, is helpful because this is considered a premalignant condition.
- The patient should be encouraged to have regular physical examinations and seek medical attention for any esophageal problems, especially dysphagia.

FIBROCYSTIC BREAST CHANGES

Definition/Description
Fibrocystic changes in the breast constitute the most frequently occurring benign breast disorder. These changes include the development of excess fibrous tissue, hyperplasia of the epithelial lining of the
mammary ducts, proliferation of mammary ducts, and cyst formation.
Fibrocystic changes occur most frequently in women between 35 and
50 years of age but often begin in women as young as 20 years of age.

Pathophysiology
- The cause of fibrocystic changes is thought to be heightened responsiveness of breast parenchyma and stroma to circulating
  estrogens and progesterones.
- Fibrocystic changes produce pain by nerve irritation from connective tissue edema and by fibrosis from nerve pinching.
- Masses or nodularities can appear in both breasts and are often
  found in the upper, outer quadrants; they usually occur bilaterally.
- Characteristics of women affected include those with premenstrual abnormalities, nulliparous women, women with a history of
  spontaneous abortion, nonusers of oral contraceptives, and
  women with early menarche and late menopause.
- Fibrocystic changes often exacerbate in the premenstrual phase
  and subside after menstruation.

Clinical Manifestations
Manifestations of fibrocystic breast changes include one or more
palpable lumps that are usually round, well delineated, and freely
movable within the breast. There may be accompanying discomfort
ranging from tenderness to pain.
- The lump usually increases in size and perhaps in tenderness
  before menstruation. Cysts may enlarge or shrink rapidly.
- Nipple discharge associated with fibrocystic breasts is often
  milky, watery-milky, yellow, or green.
- Pain and nodularity often increase over time but tend to subside
  after menopause unless high doses of estrogen replacement are
  used.

Nursing and Collaborative Management
A wait of 7 to 10 days may be planned if the nodularity is recurrent
to note changes as the menstrual cycle changes. With the initial dis-
covery of a discrete mass in the breast, aspiration or surgical biopsy
may be indicated.

- An excisional biopsy should be done if no fluid is found on aspiration, if the fluid that is found is hemorrhagic, or if a residual mass remains.
- Surgery is performed in an office or day surgery unit under local anesthesia. Hyperplastic changes approximating the histologic appearance of carcinoma in situ (atypical hyperplasia) and a family history of breast cancer increases the probability of developing breast cancer.

Many types of treatment have been suggested for a fibrocystic condition. These approaches include diet (low-salt diet, restriction of methylxanthines such as coffee and chocolate), therapeutic measures (analgesics, danazol [Danocrine], diuretics, hormone therapy, antiestrogen therapy), and surgical procedures (subcutaneous mastectomy). The benefit of most of these treatments has not been proven.

▼ **Patient Teaching**
The role of the nurse in the care of the patient with fibrocystic breast changes is primarily one of teaching. A woman should be told that she may expect recurrences of the cysts in one or both breasts until menopause, and that cysts may enlarge or become painful just before menstruation. Additionally, these women should be reassured that cysts do not "turn into" cancer.

- The woman with cystic changes should be encouraged to return regularly for follow-up examinations. She should also be taught breast self-examination (BSE) to self-monitor the problem. Any new lumps should be evaluated and changes in symptoms should be reported and investigated.

FLAIL CHEST

Definition/Description
Flail chest results from multiple rib fractures causing instability of the chest wall. Flail chest may occur with pneumothorax, hemothorax, and tension pneumothorax.

Pathophysiology
The chest wall cannot provide the bony structure necessary to maintain bellows action and ventilation. The affected (flail) area will move paradoxically to the intact portion of the chest during respiration. During inspiration the affected portion is sucked in, and during expiration it bulges out.

- This paradoxic chest movement prevents adequate ventilation of the lung in the injured area. The underlying lung may or may not have serious injury.

■ Associated pain and any underlying lung injury, giving rise to loss of compliance, will contribute to an alteration in breathing patterns and lead to hypoxia.

Clinical Manifestations

Flail chest is usually apparent on visual examination of the unconscious patient.

■ Manifestations include rapid, shallow respirations; cyanosis; and tachycardia.

■ A flail chest may not be initially apparent in the conscious patient as a result of splinting of the chest wall. The patient moves air poorly, and movement of the thorax is asymmetric and uncoordinated.

Diagnostic Studies

■ Auscultation of abnormal breath sounds
■ Crepitus of the rib
■ Chest x-ray and arterial blood gases (ABGs)

Collaborative Care

Initial therapy consists of adequate ventilation, humidified oxygen (O_2), and careful administration of crystalloid IV solutions. Definitive therapy is to reexpand the lung and ensure adequate oxygenation. Although many patients can be managed without the use of mechanical ventilation, a short period of intubation and ventilation may be necessary until the diagnosis of the lung injury is complete. Positive expiratory end pressure (PEEP) used with mechanical ventilation to improve oxygenation will maintain positive pressure in the lungs throughout the respiratory cycle. Lung parenchyma and fractured ribs will heal with time.

FRACTURE

Definition/Description

A fracture is a disruption or break in the continuity of the structure of the bone. Traumatic injuries account for the majority of fractures, although some fractures are secondary to a disease process (pathologic fractures). Fractures are described and classified according to (1) type, (2) communication or noncommunication with the external environment, and (3) location of the fracture.

Fractures are also described as stable or unstable. A *stable fracture* occurs when some of the periosteum is intact across the fracture and either external or internal fixation has rendered the fragments stationary. Stable fractures are usually transverse, spiral, or green-stick. An *unstable fracture* is grossly displaced during injury and is a site of poor fixation. Unstable fractures are usually comminuted (having several breaks in the bone) or oblique (having a slanted fracture of the shaft).

Clinical Manifestations

The patient's history indicates injury associated with numerous signs and symptoms, including immediate localized pain, decreased function, and inability to use the affected part. The patient guards and protects the part against movement. The fracture may not be accompanied by obvious bone deformity.

- Manifestations include edema and swelling, pain and tenderness, muscle spasm, deformity, ecchymosis, loss of function, and crepitation.

Complications

The majority of fractures heal without complications. If death occurs after a fracture, it is usually the result of damage to underlying organs and soft tissue or from complications of the fracture or injury. For a summary of the complications of fracture healing, see Table 59-4, Lewis and others, *Medical-Surgical Nursing,* edition 5, p. 1772.

- *Direct complications* include problems with bone union, avascular necrosis, and bone infection.
- *Indirect complications* are associated with blood vessel and nerve damage resulting in conditions such as compartment syndrome, venous thrombosis, fat embolism, and traumatic or hypovolemic shock. A discussion of these complications is in Lewis and others, *Medical-Surgical Nursing,* edition 5, p. 1785.
- Although most musculoskeletal injuries are not life-threatening, open fractures or fractures accompanied by severe blood loss and fractures that damage vital organs (such as the lung or bladder) are medical emergencies requiring immediate attention.

Stages of Fracture Healing

The bone goes through a reparative process of self-healing (called union) that occurs in the following stages:

1. *Fracture hematoma.* When a fracture occurs, bleeding and edema precede the development of a hematoma, which surrounds the ends of the fragments.
2. *Granulation tissue.* Active phagocytosis absorbs the products of local necrosis. The hematoma changes into granulation tissue (consisting of new blood vessels, fibroblasts, and osteoblasts), which produces a new bony substance called osteoid.
3. *Callus formation.* As minerals are deposited in the osteoid, it forms an unorganized network of bone called callus, which is

woven bone about the fracture parts. It usually begins to appear by the end of the first week after injury. Evidence of callus formation can be verified by x-ray.

4. *Ossification.* Ossification of the callus begins within 2 to 3 weeks postfracture and continues until the fracture has healed. During this stage the patient can be converted from skeletal traction to a cast or the cast can be removed to allow limited mobility.

5. *Consolidation.* As the callus continues to develop, the distance between bone fragments diminishes and eventually closes. This stage is called consolidation, and ossification continues. It can be equated with radiographic union.

6. *Remodeling.* Excess cells are absorbed and union is completed. Gradual return of the injured bone to its preinjury structural strength and shape occurs. Remodeling of bone is enhanced as it responds to physical stress. Initially stress is provided through exercise. Weight-bearing is gradually introduced.

Diagnostic Studies
- History and physical examination
- X-ray examination

Collaborative Care
The goals of treatment are (1) anatomic realignment of bone fragments, (2) immobilization to maintain realignment, and (3) restoration of function of the injured part.

Fracture Reduction
Manipulation or *closed reduction* is a nonsurgical, manual realignment of bones to their previous anatomic position. Traction and countertraction are manually applied to bone fragments to restore position, length, and alignment.
- Closed reduction is usually performed under local or general anesthesia. After reduction or manipulation the injured part is immobilized by casting, traction, external fixation, splints, or orthoses (braces) to maintain alignment until healing occurs.

Open reduction is correction of bone alignment through a surgical incision. It may include internal fixation of the fracture with the use of wire, screws, pins, plates, intramedullary rods, or nails.
- If open reduction and internal fixation (ORIF) are used, early initiation of range of motion of the joint is indicated.

Traction devices apply a pulling force on the fractured extremity and result in realignment. The two most common types of traction are *skin traction* and *skeletal traction.*
- *Skin traction* is generally used for short-term treatment (48 to 72 hours) until skeletal traction or surgery is possible. Tape, boots, or slings are applied directly to the skin to maintain

alignment, assist in reduction, and help diminish muscle spasms in the injured part.

■ *Skeletal traction,* generally in place for longer periods of time, is used to align injured bones and joints. It provides a long-term pull that keeps injured bones and joints aligned. (For common types of traction, see Table 59-6, Lewis and others, *Medical-Surgical Nursing,* edition 5, p. 1773.)

Fracture alignment depends on the correct positioning and alignment of the patient while traction forces remain constant. For extremity traction to be effective, forces must be pulling in the opposite direction *(countertraction)* to prevent the patient from sliding to the end or side of the bed.

■ Countertraction is commonly supplied by the patient's body weight or may be augmented by elevating the end of the bed.

Fracture Immobilization

External fixation of fractures is achieved by a cast or an external fixator. Casting is a common treatment after closed reduction has been performed. It allows the patient to perform many normal activities of daily living (ADLs) while providing sufficient immobilization to ensure stability (see Casts, p. 640).

An *external fixator* is a metallic device composed of metal pins that are inserted into the bone and attached to external rods to stabilize the fracture while it heals. It can be used to immobilize reduced fragments when the use of a cast or traction is not appropriate. The external fixator is attached directly to the bones by percutaneous pins. Assessment for pin loosening and infection is critical. Infection signaled by exudate, redness, tenderness, and pain may require removal of the device. *Internal fixation* devices are surgically inserted at the time of realignment. Examples of internal fixation devices include pins, plates, and screws. They are biologically inert devices (made of titanium or stainless steel, for example) that are used to realign and maintain bony fragments. Proper alignment is evaluated by x-ray studies at regular intervals.

Maintenance traction is initiation or continuation of traction and countertraction. A continuous pulling force can be applied directly to the bone with wires and pins *(skeletal traction)* or can be applied indirectly by weights that are attached to the skin with adhesive straps or boots *(skin traction).*

Nursing Management

Goals

The patient with a fracture will have no associated complications, obtain satisfactory pain relief, and achieve maximal rehabilitation potential.

See NCP 59-1 for the patient with a fracture, Lewis and others, *Medical-Surgical Nursing,* edition 5, p. 1780.

Nursing Diagnoses/Collaborative Problems

- Pain *related to* edema, movement of bone fragments, and muscle spasms
- Risk for infection *related to* disruption of skin integrity and presence of environmental pathogens secondary to open fracture or external fixation pins
- Activity intolerance *related to* prolonged immobility
- Risk for peripheral neurovascular dysfunction *related to* nerve compression
- Risk for impaired skin integrity *related to* immobility and presence of a cast
- Ineffective management of therapeutic regimen *related to* lack of knowledge regarding muscle atrophy, exercise program, and cast care
- Potential complication: fat embolism *related to* fracture of a long bone

Nursing Interventions

Patients with fractures may be treated in an emergency department or physician's office and released to home care, or the patient may require hospitalization. Specific nursing measures depend on the type of treatment used and setting in which the patient is placed.

Preoperative management. If surgical intervention is required to treat the fracture, patients will need preoperative preparation. In addition to the usual preoperative nursing measures, the nurse should inform patients of the type of immobilization device that will be used and the expected activity limitations.

- Proper skin preparation is an important part of preoperative preparation. The aim of skin preparation is to clean the skin and remove debris and hair to reduce the possibility of infection.
- The patient must be assured that all needs will be met by the nursing staff until the patient can again meet his or her own needs. Assurance that pain medication will be available if needed is often beneficial.

Postoperative management. Frequent neurovascular assessments of the affected extremity are necessary to detect subtle changes. Any pain or limitations of movement or activity related to turning, positioning, and extremity support should be monitored closely.

- Pain and discomfort can be minimized through proper alignment and positioning.
- Dressings or casts should be carefully observed for any overt signs of bleeding, drainage, or pressure. A significant increase in the size of the drainage area should be reported.
- If a wound drainage system is in place, the patency of the system and the volume of drainage should be assessed at least once each shift. Whenever the contents of a drainage system

are measured or emptied, the nurse should use sterile technique to avoid contamination.

If the patient is immobilized as a result of the fracture, the nurse must plan care to prevent constipation and renal calculi

- Constipation can be prevented by physical activity, maintenance of a high fluid intake, and a diet high in bulk and roughage. If these measures are not effective in maintaining the patient's normal bowel pattern, stool softeners, laxatives, or suppositories may be necessary. Maintaining a regular time for elimination despite bed rest is effective in promoting regularity.

- Renal calculi can develop as a result of bone demineralization caused by immobilization. Unless contraindicated, a fluid intake of 2500 ml/day is recommended. Cranberry juice or ascorbic acid (500 mg/day) may be recommended to acidify the urine and prevent calcium precipitation.

Rapid deconditioning of the circulatory system can occur as a result of bed rest resulting in orthostatic hypotension. These effects can be diminished by permitting the patient to sit on the side of the bed, allowing the lower limbs to dangle over the bedside, and by performing standing transfers, unless these measures are contraindicated.

- When the patient is allowed to increase activity, careful evaluation should be made to assess for orthostatic hypotension.

▼ **Patient Teaching**

Because many fractures are cast in an outpatient setting, the patient often requires only a short hospitalization or none at all. Therefore patient education is an important nursing responsibility to prevent complications. In addition to specific instructions for cast care (see Casts, p. 640) and recognition of complications, the nurse should encourage the patient to contact the clinic or care provider should questions arise. The nurse should validate patient understanding of these instructions before discharge from the clinic or hospital.

For further information on rehabilitation management of fractures, see Lewis and others, *Medical-Surgical Nursing,* edition 5, p. 1783, and also the specific types of fractures discussed in this *Companion.*

FRACTURE, HIP

Definition/Description

Hip fractures are common in older adults. A hip fracture may be expected to occur more frequently in women than in men older than 65 years because of osteoporosis. It is estimated that 14% to 36% of patients who experience a hip fracture will die within 1 year of the injury because of medical complications caused by the fracture or the resulting immobility. Sixty percent do not regain their preinjury level of ambulation.

- Fractures that occur within the capsule are called *intracapsular* fractures. Intracapsular fractures are further identified by a name taken from their specific location: subcapital, transcervical, and basilar neck. These fractures are often associated with osteoporosis and minor trauma.
- *Extracapsular* fractures occur below the capsule and are termed *intertrochanteric* if they occur in a region between the greater and lesser trochanter. They are termed *subtrochanteric* if they occur in the region below the trochanter. Extracapsular fractures are usually caused by severe direct trauma or a fall.

Clinical Manifestations

Manifestations of a hip fracture are external rotation, shortening of the affected extremity, and severe pain and tenderness in the region of the fracture site. Displaced femoral neck fractures cause serious disruption of the blood supply to the femoral head, which can result in *avascular necrosis.*

Complications associated with femoral neck fracture include nonunion, avascular necrosis, and degenerative arthritis. As a result of an intertrochanteric fracture, the affected leg may be shortened.

Collaborative Care

Surgical repair is the preferred method of managing intracapsular and extracapsular hip fractures. Surgical treatment permits the patient to be out of bed sooner and decreases the major complications associated with immobility. Initially the affected extremity may be temporarily immobilized by either Buck's or Russell's skin traction until the patient's physical condition is stabilized and surgery can be performed. Traction also helps relieve painful muscle spasms.

- Intracapsular fractures are usually repaired with the use of a hip prosthesis. Extracapsular fractures are usually pinned. The principles of patient care for these procedures are similar.
- The intracapsular fracture is slow to heal because of interruptions in blood supply. When avascular necrosis appears imminent, the surgeon may elect to resect the femoral head and neck and insert a femoral-head prosthesis. A variety of devices in the forms of compression screws and plates, nails, and pins are available to the surgeon for the purpose of repairing a hip fracture by pinning.

Nursing Management

Preoperative management. Because older adults are most prone to hip fractures, chronic health problems (e.g., diabetes mellitus [DM], hypertension) must often be considered when planning treatment. Surgery may be delayed for a brief time until the patient's general health is stabilized.

- Before surgery, severe muscle spasms that may increase pain can be managed by appropriate analgesics or muscle relaxants, comfortable positioning unless contraindicated, and properly adjusted traction if it is being used.
- The patient should know the method and frequency for exercising the unaffected leg and both arms. The patient should also be shown how to use the trapeze bar and opposite siderail to assist in changing positions. Practices for getting out of bed and transferring to a chair should be discussed and demonstrated.
- The family should be informed about the patient's weight-bearing status after surgery. Plans for discharge should be discussed, and arrangements should be initiated well before the actual discharge date.

Postoperative management. The initial management of a patient following surgical repair of a hip fracture is similar to that for any older surgical patient and includes monitoring vital signs and intake and output, supervising respiratory activities such as deep breathing and coughing, administering pain medication cautiously, and observing the dressing and incision for signs of bleeding and infection. Specific nursing interventions for the patient with a fracture of the hip are described in NCP 59-2 for the patient with a fracture, Lewis and others, *Medical-Surgical Nursing,* edition 5, p. 1791.

In the early postoperative period there is potential for neurovascular impairment. The nurse should assess the patient's toes for ability to move, weakness, warmth and pink color, sensation and absence of paresthesia, distal pulses, capillary refill, and edema.

- Edema is alleviated by elevation of the leg whenever the patient is in a chair.
- Pain resulting from poor alignment of the affected extremity can be prevented by keeping pillows (or an abductor splint) between the knees when the patient is turning to either side. Sandbags and pillows are also used to prevent external rotation and adduction.

Ambulation usually begins the first or second postoperative day. The nurse needs to monitor the patient's ambulation status for proper crutch walking or use of the walker. The patient must be able to use crutches or a walker before discharge.

If the hip fracture has been treated by insertion of a femoral-head prosthesis, measures to prevent dislocation must always be used (Table 30).

- The patient and family must be fully aware of positions and activities that predispose the patient to dislocation (>90 degrees of

Table 30	Patient and Family Teaching Guide: Femoral-Head Prosthesis

Do Not
Force hip into >90 degrees of flexion*
Force hip into adduction
Force hip into internal rotation
Cross legs
Put on own shoes or stockings until 8 wk after surgery without
    adaptive device (e.g., longhandled shoehorn or stocking-helper)
Sit on chairs without arms to aid rising to a standing position*

Do
Use toilet elevator on toilet seat*
Place chair inside shower or tub and remain seated while washing
Use pillow between legs for first 8 wk after surgery when lying on
    "good" side or when supine*
Keep hip in neutral, straight position when sitting, walking, or lying*
Notify surgeon if severe pain, deformity, or loss of function occurs*
Inform dentist of presence of prosthesis before dental work so that
    prophylactic antibiotics can be given

*These precautions may also apply after a hip pinning.

flexion, adduction, or internal rotation). Many daily activities may
reproduce these positions (e.g., putting on shoes and socks, crossing legs or feet while seated, assuming side-lying position incor-
rectly, standing up or sitting down while the body is flexed relative to the chair, sitting on low seats—especially low toilet seats).

- Until the soft tissue surrounding the hip has healed sufficiently
  to stabilize the prosthesis, these activities must be avoided,
  usually for at least 6 weeks.
- Sudden severe pain, a lump in the buttock, limb shortening,
  and extreme external rotation indicate prosthesis dislocation.
  This requires a closed reduction or open reduction to realign
  the femoral head in the acetabulum.

The nurse should place a large pillow between the patient's legs
when turning, keep leg abductor splints on the patient except when
bathing, avoid extreme hip flexion, and avoid turning the patient on
the affected side until it is approved by the surgeon.

If the hip fracture is treated by pinning, dislocation precautions
are not necessary. The patient is usually encouraged to be out of bed
on the first postoperative day. Weight-bearing on the involved extremity varies.

The nurse must assist both the patient and family in adjusting to the restrictions and dependence imposed by the hip fracture. Depression can easily occur, but creative nursing care and awareness of the problem can do much to prevent it.

- The patient and family may need to be informed about community referral services that can assist in the postdischarge rehabilitation phase.
- Hospitalization averages 4 days. Patients frequently require care in a skilled nursing facility or rehabilitation facility for a few weeks prior to returning home. Recovery can take up to a year.

FRACTURE, HUMERUS

Fractures involving the shaft of the humerus are a common injury among young and middle-aged adults. Clinical manifestations are an obvious displacement of the humeral shaft, shortened extremity, abnormal mobility, and pain.

- Major complications associated with fracture of the humerus are radial nerve injury and vascular injury to the brachial artery as a result of laceration, transection, or muscle spasm.

Treatment for a fracture of the humerus depends on the location and displacement of the fracture.

- Treatment may include a hanging arm cast, shoulder immobilizer, or the sling and swathe, which is a type of immobilization that prevents glenohumeral movement.
- Skin or skeletal traction may also be used for purposes of reduction and immobilization.

When these devices are used, the head of the bed should be elevated to assist gravity in reducing the fracture. The arm should be allowed to hang when the patient is sitting and standing.

Nursing care should include measures to protect the axilla and prevent skin maceration by placing lightly powdered absorption pads in the axilla and changing them twice daily or as needed.

- During the rehabilitative phase an exercise program geared toward improving strength and motion of the injured extremity is extremely important. This should include assisted motion of the hands and fingers. The shoulder can also be exercised to prevent stiffness if the fracture is stable.

FRACTURE, PELVIS

Pelvic fractures are usually caused by vehicular accidents, although older adult patients may sustain this injury from a fall. Pelvic fractures may cause serious intraabdominal injuries such as colon laceration, paralytic ileus, hemorrhage, and rupture of the urethra or bladder. This type of injury accounts for up to 20% of the mortality from fractures.

- Pelvic fractures are diagnosed and classified by x-ray. They may range from simple undisplaced fractures to more serious fracture dislocations with the potential for serious complications.
- Physical examination demonstrates local swelling, tenderness, deformity, unusual pelvic movement, and ecchymosis. The neurovascular status of the lower extremities and the manifestations of associated injuries should be assessed.

Treatment depends on the severity of the injury. Bed rest for stable pelvic fractures is maintained from a few days to 6 weeks. More complex fractures may be treated with pelvic sling traction, skeletal traction, hip spica casts, external fixation, open reduction, or a combination of these methods. Internal fixation of a pelvic fracture may be necessary if the fracture is displaced.

- Extreme care in handling or moving the patient is important to prevent serious injury from a displaced fracture fragment. Because a pelvic fracture can damage other organs, assessment of bowel and urinary tract function and distal neurovascular status are important in the early nursing activities for this patient.
- The patient should be turned only when it is specifically ordered by the physician. Back care is provided while the patient is raised from the bed, either by independent use of the trapeze or with adequate assistance.
- Weight-bearing on the affected side should be avoided until healing is complete.
- If the pelvic fracture is undisplaced, the patient is usually allowed to ambulate using a walker or crutches to distribute the weight-bearing between the upper and lower extremities.

FRACTURE, RIB

Rib fractures are the most common type of chest injury resulting from trauma. Ribs 4 through 9 are most commonly fractured because they are the least protected by the chest muscles. If the fractured rib is splintered or displaced, it may damage the pleura and lungs.

Manifestations include pain (especially on inspiration) at the site of injury. The individual splints the affected area and takes shallow breaths to decrease the pain. Because the individual is reluctant to take deep breaths and cough, atelectasis may develop because of decreased ventilation.

The goal of treatment is to decrease the pain so that the patient can breathe adequately to promote good chest expansion.

- Intercostal nerve blocks with local anesthesia can be used to provide pain relief. The nerves of the affected ribs and the two intercostal nerves above and below the injured rib are also blocked. The effect of anesthesia lasts for a period of hours to days. It needs to be repeated as necessary to provide pain relief.
- Strapping the chest with tape or using a binder is not common practice. Most physicians believe that these measures should be avoided because they reduce lung expansion and predispose the individual to atelectasis.
- Narcotic drug therapy must be individualized and used with caution because these drugs can depress respirations.

GASTRITIS

Definition/Description
Gastritis is an inflammation of the gastric mucosa and one of the most common problems affecting the stomach. Gastritis may be *acute* or *chronic* and *diffuse* or *localized.* Chronic gastritis can be further classified as type A (fundal) and type B (antral).

Pathophysiology
Gastritis is the result of a breakdown in the normal gastric mucosal barrier. The mucosal barrier normally protects the stomach tissue from autodigestion by acid and the enzyme pepsin. When the barrier is broken, acid diffuses back into the mucosa. This allows hydrochloric (HCl) acid to enter and increase the secretion of pepsinogen with subsequent release of histamine from mast cells. There is increased mucosal damage by HCl acid and pepsin.

- The combined result of these occurrences is tissue edema, loss of plasma into the gastric lumen with disruption of capillary walls, and possible hemorrhage.

Causes of gastritis are listed in Table 31.

Chronic gastritis may result from repeated episodes of acute gastritis. Chronic exposure to the causes of gastritis will also result in the eventual loss of viable mucosal tissue.

- Chronic gastritis, in particular *type A,* may be an autoimmune disorder. Autoimmune atrophic gastritis is associated with an increased risk of gastric malignancy.

Table 31	Causes of Gastritis
Aspirin	Physiologic stress
Nonsteroidal antiinflammatory drugs (NSAIDs)	Shock
	Sepsis
Corticosteroid drugs	Burns
Alcohol	Psychologic stress
Helicobacter pylori	Renal failure (uremia)
Staphylococcus organisms	Spicy, irritating food
	Trauma
Bile and pancreatic secretions	Nasogastric (NG) suction
Smoking	Large hiatal hernia

- *Type B* gastritis primarily involves the stomach antrum. The most common cause of type B gastritis is *Helicobacter pylori,* which promotes the breakdown process of the gastric mucosal barrier. *H. pylori* has also been correlated with other gastric disorders, including gastric and duodenal ulcers and possibly gastric cancer.
- Progressive gastric atrophy from chronic alterations in the mucosal barrier cause chief and parietal cells to die. As the number of acid-secreting parietal cells decreases with atrophy of gastric mucosa, *hypochlorhydria* (decreased acid secretion) or *achlorhydria* (lack of acid secretion) occurs.

Clinical Manifestations

- Symptoms of *acute gastritis* include anorexia, nausea and vomiting, epigastric tenderness, and a feeling of fullness. Hemorrhage is commonly associated with alcohol abuse and at times may be the only symptom. Acute gastritis is self-limiting, lasting from a few hours to a few days, with complete healing of mucosa expected.
- Manifestations of *chronic gastritis* are similar to those for acute gastritis. Some patients have no symptoms directly associated with the gastric lesion. However, when the acid-secreting cells are lost or do not function as a result of atrophy, the source of intrinsic factor is lost and cobalamin (vitamin B_{12}) cannot be absorbed in the ileum.

Diagnostic Studies

A diagnosis of gastritis is frequently delayed or completely missed because symptoms are nonspecific.

- Endoscopic examination with biopsy is necessary to obtain a definitive diagnosis.
- Serum antibodies to *H. pylori* help determine if *H. pylori* is present.
- Urine and fecal tests for *H. pylori.*
- A specific analysis of gastric tissue for the presence of *H. pylori* may be performed.
- Complete blood count (CBC) may demonstrate anemia from blood loss.
- Stools are tested for occult blood.
- A gastric analysis demonstrates the amount of HCl acid present, with achlorhydria being a common sign of severe atrophic gastritis.
- Serum tests for antibodies to parietal cells and intrinsic factor (IF) may be performed.
- Cytologic examination is done to rule out gastric carcinoma.

Collaborative Care

Elimination of the cause and preventing or avoiding it in the future are generally all that is needed to treat *acute gastritis.* The plan of care is supportive and similar to that described for nausea and vomiting.

- During the acute phase, bed rest, nothing by mouth (NPO), and IV fluids may be prescribed. Fluids and electrolytes lost through vomiting and occasional diarrhea are replaced. In severe cases a nasogastric (NG) tube may be used, either for lavage of the precipitating agent from the stomach or with suctioning to keep the stomach empty and free of noxious stimuli.
- Acute gastritis with hemorrhage is treated with blood transfusions and fluid replacement.
- Clear liquids are resumed when acute symptoms have subsided, with gradual reintroduction of solid, bland foods.
- Antiemetics are given for nausea and vomiting. Antacids are used for relief of abdominal discomfort, and histamine (H_2)-receptor antagonists such as ranitidine (Zantac) or cimetidine (Tagamet) will reduce gastric HCl acid secretion.
- Once *H. pylori* is diagnosed, antibiotic therapy is initiated.

Treatment of *chronic gastritis* focuses on evaluating and eliminating the specific cause.

- Currently, double and triple antibiotic combinations are used to eradicate infection with *H. pylori.*
- For the patient with pernicious anemia, regular injections or intranasal use of cobalamin are needed.
- An individualized bland diet and the use of antacids are recommended.
- Smoking is contraindicated in all forms of gastritis.
- The patient may have to adapt to lifestyle changes and strictly adhere to medication regimens. An interdisciplinary team approach in which the physician, nurse, dietitian, and pharmacist provide consistent information and support may increase patient success in making these alterations.

Nursing Management
Goals
The patient with gastritis will experience minimal or no symptoms of gastritis, no recurrent episodes of acute gastritis, and achieve an optimal pattern of gastric functioning relative to the disease stage.

Nursing Diagnoses
The nursing diagnoses listed for the patient with nausea and vomiting are also applicable in gastritis (see Nausea and Vomiting, p. 408).

Nursing Interventions
- Dehydration can occur rapidly in severe gastritis accompanied by vomiting. Keeping the patient on NPO status while monitoring IV fluids is essential.

- If hemorrhage is considered likely, frequently checking vital signs and testing vomitus for blood are indicated.
- Elimination of the cause of gastritis results in rapid improvement in the patient's condition. Identification of the causative agent is important to prevent future gastric irritation.

The majority of patients with gastritis receive care in the home, and chronic management may be necessary for extended periods of time. A bland diet consisting of six small feedings a day and the use of an antacid after meals helps the patient maintain normal gastric function.

▼ **Patient Teaching**
- The patient with gastritis should be encouraged to avoid causative factors and to follow a prescribed diet and medication regimen. Because the incidence of gastric cancer is higher in patients with a history of chronic gastritis, especially atrophic gastritis, close medical follow-up should be stressed.
- The patient who has gastric atrophy may need to have cobalamin therapy included in the plan of care.

GASTROENTERITIS

Gastroenteritis is an inflammation of the mucosa of the stomach and small intestine. The condition may be attributed to bacterial toxins, bacterial or viral invasion, chemical toxins, or miscellaneous conditions such as food allergies or drug reactions. Most cases are self-limiting and do not require hospitalization. However, older adults and chronically ill patients may be unable to consume sufficient fluids orally to compensate for fluid loss.

Clinical manifestations include nausea, vomiting, diarrhea, abdominal cramping, and distention. Fever, leukocytosis, and blood or mucus in the stool may also be present.

Until vomiting has ceased, the patient should be on nothing by mouth (NPO) status. If dehydration has occurred, IV replacement of fluids may be necessary. As soon as they can be tolerated, fluids containing glucose and electrolytes (e.g., Pedialyte) should be given. Accurate monitoring of intake and output is important for successful replacement of lost fluid.

If the causative agent is identified, appropriate antibiotic, antimicrobial, or antiinfective medication is given. Strict medical asepsis and enteric precautions should be instituted when indicated. Symptomatic nursing care is given for nausea, vomiting, and diarrhea (see Nausea and Vomiting, p. 408 and Diarrhea, p. 200). The nurse should assess complaints of pain, vomiting, and diarrhea because gastroenteritis is often confused with appendicitis.

- The patient should be instructed in the importance of proper food handling and preparation of food to prevent infections, such as *salmonellosis* and *trichinosis.*
- The importance of rest and increased fluid intake as symptomatic treatment measures for gastroenteritis should be stressed.
- To allay the patient's apprehension, the nurse should explain that gastroenteritis usually runs an acute course with no sequelae.

GASTROESOPHAGEAL REFLUX DISEASE

Definition/Description
Gastroesophageal reflux disease (GERD) is not a disease but a syndrome produced by conditions that result in the reflux of gastric secretions into the esophagus. Predisposing conditions include hiatal hernia, incompetent lower esophageal sphincter (LES), decreased esophageal clearance, and decreased gastric emptying.

Pathophysiology
In GERD there is confirmed evidence of the reflux of gastric contents into the lower portion of the esophagus. Acidity of the gastric secretions results in esophageal irritation and inflammation (esophagitis).

One of the primary factors in GERD is an incompetent LES, which is defined by a lack of high pressure in the distal portion of the esophagus. Gastric contents are then able to move from an area of higher pressure (the stomach) to an area of lower pressure (the esophagus) when the patient is in a supine position or intraabdominal pressure is increased (see Hiatal Hernia, p. 305).

Clinical Manifestations
- *Heartburn (pyrosis),* caused by irritation of the esophagus by gastric hydrochloric (HCl) acid and pepsin, is the most common clinical manifestation. Heartburn is described as a burning, tight sensation that appears intermittently beneath the lower sternum and spreads upward to the throat or jaw.
- *Regurgitation* (the effortless return of material from the stomach into the esophagus or mouth) is a fairly common manifestation of an incompetent LES. It is often described as hot, bitter, or sour liquid coming into the throat or mouth.
- Other symptoms include feelings of a lump in the throat or of food stopping, dysphagia, and bleeding.

- Respiratory complications, including bronchospasm or laryngospasm, may occur because of the movement of gastric contents into the upper airway.

Complications
Complications of GERD are related to the effects of gastric acid on the esophageal mucosa. As a result of repeated gastric acid exposure, there may be scar tissue formation and decreased distensibility of the esophagus resulting in dysphagia. Esophageal metaplasia (Barrett's syndrome) may also occur.
- The potential for pulmonary complications (pneumonia) exists secondary to aspiration of gastric contents into the pulmonary system.

Diagnostic Studies
- Barium swallow to determine protrusion of gastric cardia
- Radionucleotide tests for esophageal clearance rate and reflux of gastric contents
- Esophagoscopy to determine LES incompetence and extent of inflammation, scarring, and strictures
- Biopsy and cytologic specimens for differential diagnosis
- Esophageal motility studies to measure esophagus motility and LES pressure
- pH studies to detect acid in normally alkaline esophagus

Collaborative Care
A four-phase management approach is often used. Phase 1 is lifestyle modification (see Tables 39-8 and 39-9, Lewis and others, *Medical-Surgical Nursing,* edition 5, pp. 1093-1094). Phase 2 involves drug therapy. Phase 3 is intensified drug intervention, and phase 4 is antireflux surgery.
  Drug therapy includes:
- Antacids to relieve heartburn
- Histamine (H_2)-receptor blockers (e.g., ranitidine [Zantac], cimetidine [Tagamet]) to decrease gastric acid production
- Cisapride (Propulsid) a serotonin antagonist, to increase LES pressure and promote healing
- Omeprazole (Prilosec), an antisecretory drug, to decrease HCl acid secretion and facilitate the healing of erosive reflux esophagitis
- Cholinergic drugs (e.g., Urecholine) to increase LES pressure, improve esophageal clearance, and increase gastric emptying
- Sucralfate (Carafate), an antiulcer drug, which has cytoprotective properties
  Surgical therapy may be necessary if conservative therapy fails, a hiatal hernia is present, or complications such as stenosis, chronic

esophagitis, and bleeding exist. The objective of surgery is to restore gastroesophageal integrity (see Nursing and Collaborative
Management, Hiatal Hernia, p. 306).

Nutritional therapy includes a diet high in protein and low in fats.
Foods that decrease LES pressure, such as chocolate, peppermint,
coffee, and tea, should be avoided because they cause reflux. Milk
products should be avoided, especially at bedtime, because milk increases gastric acid secretion.

- Small, frequent meals are advised to prevent stomach overdistention. The patient should avoid late meals and nocturnal
  snacking.
- Weight reduction is recommended if the patient is obese.

Nursing Management

Nursing care for the patient who is having acute symptoms consists
mainly of teaching and encouraging the patient to follow the necessary
regimen. The nurse should ensure that the head of the bed is elevated
to approximately 30 degrees (usually on 4- to 6-inch blocks) and that
the patient does not lie down during the first 2 to 3 hours after eating.

- Instruct the patient about possible medication side effects and
  to avoid factors that cause reflux.
- Smoking causes an almost immediate drop in LES pressure.
  The patient may need to be referred to other members of the
  health care team or to community resources for assistance in
  stopping smoking. If stress seems to bring on symptoms, measures to cope with stress should be discussed.
- Emphasis is placed on teaching and encouraging the patient to
  follow the necessary regimen.
- Additionally, the nurse should elevate the head of bed, instruct
  the patient not to lie down for 2 to 3 hours after eating, and help
  the patient to understand what factors affect and prevent GERD.

GIGANTISM AND ACROMEGALY

Definition/Description

Gigantism and acromegaly are rare disorders characterized by soft
tissue and bony overgrowth due to overproduction of growth hormone (GH), which is usually caused by a benign pituitary adenoma
(tumor). Prognosis depends on the patient's age at onset, age when
treatment is initiated, and tumor size. Usually bone growth can be
arrested and soft-tissue hypertrophy can be reversed. However,
sleep apnea and diabetic and cardiac complications may continue
in spite of treatment.

Clinical Manifestations

Gigantism results when the onset of GH overproduction occurs before the closure of the epiphyses, while the long bones are still capable of longitudinal growth. Onset usually occurs in early childhood but may occur at puberty.

- These children may grow as tall as 8 feet and weigh over 300 pounds. Affected children usually die in early adulthood unless treated.

Acromegaly is the more common abnormality caused by GH excess. Symptoms begin insidiously in the third and fourth decades of life, and both genders are affected equally. When the problem develops after epiphyseal closure, bones increase in thickness and width.

- Physical features include enlargement of hands, feet, and paranasal and frontal sinuses and deformities of the spine and mandible. Enlargement of soft tissue (e.g., tongue, skin, abdominal organs) causes speech difficulties and hoarseness, coarsening of facial features, sleep apnea, and abdominal distention.
- Persons with acromegaly may exhibit hypertension, cardiomegaly, hepatomegaly, peripheral neuropathy, left ventricular hypertrophy, proximal muscle weakness, and joint pain.
- The enlarged pituitary can exert pressure on the surrounding structures, leading to visual disturbances and headaches. Because GH increases free fatty acids levels in the blood, the patient is predisposed to atherosclerosis. The hormone also antagonizes the action of insulin and can cause hyperglycemia.

Diagnostic Studies

- Plasma GH and somatomedin C (insulin-like growth factor) levels
- GH response to oral glucose challenge
- CT scan and MRI for further evaluation and tumor localization

Collaborative Care

The therapeutic goal in gigantism and acromegaly is to return GH levels to normal. This is accomplished by surgery, radiation, drug therapy, or a combination of the three.

- *Surgery* is the usual treatment and offers the best hope for a cure, especially for microadenomas (<10 mm). Surgery is most commonly accomplished with the transsphenoidal approach, in which an incision is made in the inner aspect of the upper lip and gingiva. The goal of this surgery is to remove only the GH-secreting adenoma.
- *External radiation* normalizes GH levels in most patients, although it may be months to years before GH levels return to normal. Hypopituitarism is a common sequela that often requires replacement therapy.

- *Stereotactic radiosurgery* (gamma surgery) may be applied to small, surgically inaccessible pituitary tumors. This procedure consists of radiation delivered to a single site from multiple angles and can be used to occlude blood vessels feeding the tumor, thereby starving it.
- *Drug therapy* is accomplished with bromocriptine (Parlodel), a dopamine agonist, or with octreotide, a somatostatin analogue that reduces GH levels to within the normal range. The GH-lowering effects of these drugs are seldom complete or permanent, and they are often used as adjuncts to other therapies or to reduce tumor size before surgery.

Nursing Management

The nurse should assess for manifestations of abnormal tissue growth and physical size in each patient. Assessment of children includes evaluation of growth and development.

- Accelerated growth, especially if >5 to 6 inches (>12 to 15 cm) per year and if inconsistent with familial patterns, constitutes cause for medical referral. Adults should be questioned about increases in hat, ring, glove, and shoe size.
- The patient should be carefully monitored for hyperglycemia and cardiovascular symptoms such as angina pectoris, hypertension, and congestive heart failure (CHF).

Surgical Care

The individual treated surgically must be prepared before surgery for postoperative care. The patient should be instructed to avoid vigorous coughing, sneezing, and straining at stool to prevent cerebrospinal fluid leakage from the point at which the sella turcica was entered.

After surgery in which a *transsphenoidal approach* has been used, the head of the patient's bed should be elevated at a 30-degree angle at all times. This avoids pressure on the sella turcica and decreases postoperative headaches.

- Mild analgesia is given for headaches. The nurse should perform mouth care every 4 hours to keep the surgical area clean and free of debris and to promote patient comfort. Tooth brushing should be avoided for at least 10 days to prevent disrupting the suture line and creating discomfort.
- Any clear nasal drainage should be sent to the laboratory to be tested for glucose as an indicator of cerebrospinal fluid leakage. Complaints of persistent and severe generalized or supraorbital headaches may indicate cerebrospinal fluid leakage into the sinuses.

If *stereotactic radiosurgery* is used, patients are usually moved from the specialized radiation center to the neurosurgical nursing unit for overnight observation. Vital signs, neurologic status, and fluid volume status must be carefully monitored.

- Possible complications include increased headaches, nausea and vomiting, and discomfort at the pin sites. The patient with a history of seizures is at increased risk for seizures for 24 hours postprocedure.
- Anterior and posterior pin sites should be cleaned with hydrogen peroxide and covered with clean dressings.
- A common postoperative occurrence is transient diabetes insipidus (DI) (see Diabetes Insipidus, p. 187) because of the loss of antidiuretic hormone (ADH). If DI develops and ingestion of free water and non-salty fluids do not allow the patient to keep up with urinary water losses, IV fluids are indicated.

If a *hypophysectomy* is performed, the patient may exhibit signs of DI immediately after surgery because of the loss of ADH. Vasopressin (VP) (Pitressin) is given as needed if the urine output exceeds 800 to 900 ml over 2 hours or if the urine specific gravity is less than 1.005.

- Permanent ADH, cortisol, and thyroid hormone replacements may be needed. Patient education is necessary when replacements of these hormones are given.
- Hypopituitarism causes infertility because of deficient sex hormones secondary to the loss of gonadotropins. If an individual with deficient follicle-stimulating hormone (FSH) and luteinizing hormone (LH) wishes to have children, these hormones can be replaced, with a possible restoration of fertility.
- The need for continued drug therapy reduces the patient's perception of independence and requires considerable emotional adjustment.

GLAUCOMA

Definition/Description

Glaucoma is a group of disorders characterized by increased intraocular pressure (IOP), optic nerve damage, and peripheral visual field loss. Glaucoma may occur congenitally, as a primary disease, or secondary to other ocular or systemic conditions. Glaucoma is the leading cause of blindness among African-Americans.

Pathophysiology

Increased IOP results when the rate of aqueous production (inflow) is greater than aqueous reabsorption (outflow). If the pressure remains elevated, permanent visual damage may begin. Outflow of aqueous humor can be decreased by several mechanisms.

- In *primary open-angle glaucoma (POAG)*, aqueous outflow is decreased in the trabecular meshwork. The increased pressure affects the nerve tissue of the optic disc, causing ischemia, and the patient begins to lose peripheral vision.
- In *primary angle-closure glaucoma (PACG)*, the lens usually bulges forward due to age-related changes, blocking aqueous outflow. This condition can be acute, subacute, or chronic.
- In *secondary glaucoma,* increased IOP results from other ocular or systemic conditions that may block the outflow channels in some way, such as the inflammatory process.

Clinical Manifestations

- PAOG develops slowly with no symptoms of pain or pressure. The patient usually does not notice gradual visual field loss until peripheral vision is severely compromised (tunnel vision).
- Acute angle-closure glaucoma causes definite symptoms of sudden, excruciating pain in or around the eye and can be accompanied by nausea and vomiting. Visual symptoms include seeing colored halos around lights, blurred vision, and ocular redness. The acute pressure rise may cause corneal edema, giving the cornea a frosted appearance.
- Manifestations of subacute or chronic angle-closure glaucoma appear gradually. The patient who has had a previous unrecognized episode of subacute angle-closure glaucoma may report a history of blurred vision, colored halos around lights, ocular redness, or eye or brow pain.

Diagnostic Studies

- IOP with tonometry
- Visual acuity measurement and visual field perimetry
- In open-angle glaucoma, slit-lamp microscopy reveals a normal angle. In angle-closure glaucoma, a markedly narrow or flat anterior chamber angle, an edematous cornea, and a fixed, moderately dilated pupil are noticed.
- Ophthalmoscopy (direct and indirect) for optic disc cupping

Collaborative Care

If not recognized and treated, glaucoma may cause blindness that could have been prevented in most patients. The primary focus of therapy is to keep the IOP low enough to prevent the patient from developing severe and permanent visual loss. Specific therapies vary with the type of glaucoma.

- In open-angle or chronic glaucoma, initial drug therapy can include β-adrenergic receptor blocking agents, adrenergic agents, cholinergic agents (miotics), and carbonic anhydrase inhibitors.

- Surgical management may include argon laser trabeculoplasty, trabeculectomy, cyclocryotherapy, and implant.
- Acute angle-closure glaucoma is an ocular emergency that requires immediate management, including topical cholinergic and hyperosmotic agents with laser peripheral iridotomy or surgery iridectomy.
- Secondary glaucoma is managed by treating the underlying problem and using antiglaucoma drugs.

Nursing Management

Nursing management focuses on the chronicity of this disease and the fact that visual impairment is preventable in most patients.

Goals

The patient with glaucoma will have no progression of visual impairment, understand the disease process and therapeutic rationales, comply with all aspects of therapy (including medication administration and follow-up care), and have no postoperative complications.

Nursing Diagnoses

- Pain *related to* pathophysiologic process and surgical correction
- Noncompliance *related to* the inconvenience and side effects of glaucoma medications
- Risk for injury *related to* visual acuity deficits
- Self-care deficits *related to* visual acuity deficits

Nursing Interventions

The patient with acute angle-closure glaucoma requires immediate medication to lower the IOP. This patient may be uncomfortable, and nursing comfort interventions may include darkening the environment, applying cool compresses to the patient's forehead, and providing a quiet and private space. Most surgical procedures for glaucoma are outpatient procedures.

- The patient needs encouragement to follow therapy recommendations, including information about the disease processes, normal course of condition, and treatment options, which includes the rationale underlying each option.

See NCP 20-1 for the patient following eye surgery, Lewis and others, *Medical-Surgical Nursing,* edition 5, p. 457.

▼ Patient Teaching

- It is important to educate the patient and family about the risk of glaucoma. In addition, stress the importance of early detection and treatment in preventing visual impairment.
- The patient should know that the incidence of glaucoma increases with age and that a comprehensive ophthalmic examination is invaluable in identifying persons with glaucoma or at risk for developing glaucoma.
- The patient with glaucoma needs information about prescribed antiglaucoma agents.

GLOMERULONEPHRITIS

Glomerulonephritis is a bilateral inflammation of renal glomeruli due to immunologic processes. Two types of antibody-induced injury can initiate glomerular damage.

- In the first type, antibodies have specificity for antigens within the glomerular basement membrane (GBM). The mechanism that causes a person to develop autoantibodies against the GBM is not known.
- In the second type of immune process, antibodies react with circulating nonglomerular antigens and are randomly deposited as immune complexes along the GBM. Bacterial products appear to be important in poststreptococcal glomerulonephritis as well as in endocarditis. Viral agents have been recognized in certain cases of glomerulonephritis that develop after hepatitis and measles.
- All forms of immune complex disease are characterized by an accumulation of antigen, antibody, and complement in the glomeruli, which can result in tissue injury and inflammation.

Clinical manifestations of glomerulonephritis include varying degrees of hematuria (ranging from microscopic to gross) and urinary excretion of various formed elements, including red blood cells (RBCs), white blood cells (WBCs), and some granular casts. Proteinuria, elevated blood urea nitrogen (BUN), and elevated serum creatinine levels are other manifestations.

In most cases, recovery from the acute illness is complete. If progressive involvement occurs, the result is destruction of renal tissue and marked renal insufficiency.

- The patient's history provides important information related to glomerulonephritis. It is necessary to assess exposure to drugs, immunizations, microbial infections, and viral infections such as hepatitis.
- It is also important to evaluate the patient for more generalized conditions involving immune disorders, such as systemic lupus erythematosus and systemic progressive sclerosis (scleroderma).

G

GLOMERULONEPHRITIS, ACUTE POSTSTREPTOCOCCAL

Definition/Description

Acute poststreptococcal glomerulonephritis (APSGN) develops 5 to 21 days after an infection of the pharynx or skin by certain nephrotoxic strains of group A β-hemolytic streptococci (e.g., streptococcal sore throat, impetigo). Antibodies are produced to the streptococcal antigen and the antigen-antibody complexes are deposited in the glomeruli. Complement activation causes an inflammatory reaction.

More than 95% of patients with APSGN recover completely or improve rapidly with conservative management. Prognosis for adults is less favorable than for children. Chronic glomerulonephritis develops in 5% to 15% of the affected persons, and irreversible renal failure occurs in less than 1% of patients.

Clinical Manifestations

Manifestations appear as a variety of signs and symptoms, which may include generalized body edema, hypertension, oliguria, hematuria with a smoky or rusty appearance, and proteinuria. Fluid retention occurs as a result of decreased glomerular filtration.

- Edema initially appears in low-pressure tissues, such as the eyes (periorbital edema), but later progresses to involve the total body as ascites or peripheral edema in the legs.
- Smoky urine is indicative of bleeding in the upper urinary tract. The degree of proteinuria varies with the severity of the glomerulonephropathy.
- Hypertension results from increased extracellular fluid volume.
- The patient may have abdominal or flank pain. At times the patient has no symptoms, and the problem is found on routine urinalysis.

Diagnostic Studies

- Urinalysis will reveal significant numbers of erythrocytes. If erythrocyte casts are present, acute glomerulonephritis is highly suggested. Proteinuria may be mild to severe.
- Complete blood count (CBC), BUN, serum creatinine, and albumin assess the extent of renal impairment.
- Decreased complement levels indicate an immune-mediated response.
- Antistreptolysin titer demonstrates an immune response to streptococcus.
- Renal biopsy (if indicated) may confirm the presence of the disease.

Collaborative Care

Management focuses on symptomatic relief.

- Rest is recommended until the signs of glomerular inflammation (proteinuria, hematuria) and hypertension subside.
- Edema is treated by restricting sodium and fluid intake and by administering diuretics.
- Severe hypertension is treated with antihypertensive drugs.
- Dietary protein intake may be restricted if there is evidence of an increase in nitrogenous wastes (e.g., elevated BUN).
- Antibiotics should be given only if streptococcal infection is still present.
- Corticosteroids and cytotoxic drugs have not been shown to be of value.

Nursing Management

One of the most important ways to prevent the development of APSGN is to encourage early diagnosis and treatment of sore throats and skin lesions. If streptococci are found in the culture, treatment with appropriate antibiotic therapy (usually penicillin) is essential. The patient needs to be encouraged to take the full course of antibiotics to ensure that the bacteria have been eradicated.

- Good personal hygiene is an important factor in preventing the spread of cutaneous streptococcal infections.
- An important nursing measure is helping the patient plan adequate rest to allow the kidneys to heal. The patient may need assistance in the management of fluid and dietary restrictions.

GLOMERULONEPHRITIS, CHRONIC

Chronic glomerulonephritis is a syndrome that reflects the end stage of glomerular inflammatory disease. Most types of glomerulonephritis and nephrotic syndrome can eventually lead to chronic glomerulonephritis.

Chronic glomerulonephritis is characterized by proteinuria, hematuria, and the slow development of the uremic syndrome as a result of decreasing renal function. Chronic glomerulonephritis does not usually follow an acute course; it progresses insidiously toward renal failure over a few years to as many as 30 years.

- Chronic glomerulonephritis is often found coincidentally when an abnormality on a urinalysis or elevated BP is detected. It is quite common to find that the patient has no recollection or history of acute nephritis or any renal problems. A renal biopsy may be performed to determine the exact cause and nature of the glomerulonephritis. Ultrasound and CT scan may be used as diagnostic measures.

Treatment is supportive and symptomatic. Hypertension and urinary tract infections (UTIs) should be treated vigorously. Protein and phosphate restrictions may slow the rate of progression of renal failure (see Renal Failure, Chronic, p. 496).

GONORRHEA

Definition/Description

Overall cases of gonorrhea have been declining since 1975. Strains of gonorrhea resistant to penicillin, tetracycline, or both account for 30% of all cases.

- Teenagers and young adults account for 25% to 40% of all gonorrhea cases reported. Most states have enacted laws that permit examination and treatment of minors without parental consent.

Pathophysiology

Gonorrhea is caused by *Neisseria gonorrhoeae,* a gram-negative diplococcus. Mucosa with columnar epithelium is susceptible to gonococcal infection. This tissue is present in the genitalia (urethra in men, cervix in women), rectum, and oropharynx.

- The disease is spread by direct physical contact with an infected host, usually during sexual activity.
- Neonates can develop a gonococcal infection after passage through an infected birth canal.
- The incubation period is 3 to 4 days. The disease confers no immunity to subsequent reinfection.
- Gonococcal infection elicits an inflammatory response, which, if left untreated, leads to the formation of fibrous tissue and adhesions. This fibrous scarring is subsequently responsible for many complications such as strictures and tubal abnormalities, which can lead to tubal pregnancy, chronic pelvic inflammatory disease (PID), and infertility.

Clinical Manifestations

Men. The initial site of infection is usually the urethra.

- Symptoms of urethritis consist of dysuria and a profuse, purulent urethral discharge developing 2 to 5 days after infection.
- Men generally seek medical assistance early in the disease because their symptoms are usually obvious and distressing. It is very unusual for men with gonorrhea to be asymptomatic.

Women. Most women who contract gonorrhea are asymptomatic or have minor symptoms that are often overlooked, making it possible for them to remain a source of infection.

- A few women may complain of vaginal discharge, dysuria, or frequency of urination. Changes in menstruation may be a symptom, but these changes are often disregarded by the woman.
- After the incubation period, redness and swelling occur at the site of contact, which is usually the cervix or urethra. A purulent exudate often develops with a potential for abscess formation.
- The disease may remain local or can spread by direct tissue extension to the uterus, fallopian tubes, and ovaries. Although the vulva and vagina are uncommon sites for a gonorrheal infection, they may become involved when little or no estrogen is present, such as in prepubertal girls and postmenopausal women.

Anorectal gonorrhea may be present, particularly in homosexual men, and is usually caused by anal intercourse. Gonococcal proctitis in women probably results from rectal coitus as well as contamination from infected vaginal secretions.

- Most patients with rectal infections have no significant symptoms. A small percentage of individuals develop gonococcal pharyngitis resulting from orogenital sexual contact. When the gonococcus can be demonstrated by culture, individuals of either gender are infectious to their sexual partners.

Complications

Because men often seek treatment early in the course of the disease, they are less likely to develop complications. Complications that do occur in men are prostatitis, urethral strictures, and sterility from orchitis or epididymitis.

Because women who are free of symptoms seldom seek treatment, complications are more common and usually constitute the reason for seeking medical attention. PID, bartholinian abscess, ectopic pregnancy, and infertility are the main complications in women.

- A small percentage of infected persons, mainly women, may develop a disseminated gonococcal infection (DGI). In disseminated infection the appearance of skin lesions, fever, arthralgia, or arthritis usually causes the patient to seek medical help.

Diagnostic Studies

- For men, a presumptive diagnosis of gonorrhea is made if there is a history of sexual contact with an infected individual followed within a few days by a urethral discharge.

- Cultures for *N. gonorrhoeae* with Gram-stained smears of ure-thral and endocervical exudate. Cultures of the discharge or secretion can provide definitive diagnosis after incubation for 24 to 48 hours.
- Deoxyribonucleic acid (DNA) amplification techniques, such as polymerase chain reaction (PCR), hold promise for testing of genital secretions and urine in the near future.

Collaborative Care

A history of sexual contact with a partner known to have gonorrhea is considered good evidence for the presence of gonorrhea. Because of a short incubation period and high infectivity, treatment is insti-tuted without awaiting culture results, even in the absence of signs or symptoms.

Treatment of gonorrhea in the early stage is curative. Tradition-ally the drug of choice has been penicillin. As a result of resistant strains of *N. gonorrhoeae,* ceftriaxone (Rocephin), a penicillinase-resistant cephalosporin, has become part of the treatment plan. The high frequency (up to 45%) of coexisting chlamydial and gonococ-cal infections has led to the addition of doxycycline to the treatment regimen. Patients with existing syphilis are likely to be cured by the same drugs.

- All sexual contacts of patients with gonorrhea must be treated to prevent reinfection after resumption of sexual re-lations. The "ping-pong" effect of reexposure, treatment, and reinfection can cease only when infected partners are treated simultaneously.
- The patient should be counseled to abstain from sexual inter-course and alcohol during treatment. Sexual intercourse allows the infection to spread and can retard complete healing as a re-sult of vascular congestion. Alcohol has an irritating effect on the healing urethral walls.
- Men should be cautioned against squeezing the penis to look for further discharge.
- Follow-up examination and reculture should be done at least once after treatment, usually in 4 to 7 days.
- Relapse, reinfection, and complications should be treated appropriately.

Nursing Management: Sexually Transmitted Diseases
See Chlamydial Infection, p. 127.

GOUT

Definition/Description

Gout is characterized by recurrent attacks of acute arthritis in association with increased levels of serum uric acid. In *primary gout* a hereditary error of purine metabolism leads to overproduction or retention of uric acid

Primary gout occurs predominantly in middle-aged men and is very rare in premenopausal women. Frequency of hyperuricemia is increased in families of patients with primary gout. *Secondary gout* may be related to another acquired disorder such as obesity, hyperlipidemia, or hypertension, or may be the result of medications known to inhibit uric acid excretion.

Pathophysiology

Uric acid is the major end product of purine catabolism and is primarily excreted by the kidneys. Thus hyperuricemia may be the result of increased purine synthesis, decreased renal excretion, or both.

- About half the patients with primary gout produce excessive amounts of uric acid. Although high dietary intake of purine has little effect on uric acid levels, it is clear that hyperuricemia may result from prolonged fasting or excessive drinking because of increased production of ketones, which then inhibit the normal renal excretion of uric acid.

Clinical Manifestations

In the acute phase, gouty arthritis may occur in one or more joints. Affected joints may appear dusky or cyanotic and are extremely tender. Inflammation of the great toe *(podagra)* is the most common joint involved. Other joints affected are the midtarsal, ankle, knee, and wrist joints and the olecranon bursa.

- Acute gouty arthritis is usually precipitated by events such as trauma, surgery, alcohol ingestion, or systemic infection. Onset of symptoms is usually rapid, with swelling and pain peaking within several hours, often accompanied by a low-grade fever.
- Individual attacks usually subside, treated or untreated, in 2 to 10 days. The affected joint returns entirely to normal, and patients are often free of symptoms between attacks.

Chronic gout is characterized by multiple joint involvement and deposits of sodium urate crystals *(tophi)*. These are typically seen in the synovium, subchondral bone, olecranon bursa, and vertebrae; along the tendons; and in the skin and cartilage. Tophi are rarely present at the time of the initial attack and are generally noted only many years after the onset of the disease.

The severity of gouty arthritis is variable. The clinical course may consist of infrequent mild attacks or multiple severe episodes associated with a slowly progressive disability.

Complications

Complications of chronic inflammation may result in joint deformity. Destruction of the cartilage may predispose the joint to secondary osteoarthritis. Tophaceous deposits may be large and unsightly and may perforate overlying skin, producing draining sinuses that often become secondarily infected. Excessive uric acid excretion may lead to urinary tract stone formation. Pyelonephritis associated with intrarenal sodium urate deposits and obstruction may contribute to renal disease.

Diagnostic Studies

- Joint aspiration with the presence of monosodium urate monohydrate crystals in the synovial fluid establishes the diagnosis.
- Serum uric acid levels are elevated.
- Twenty-four–hour urine collection for uric acid levels determines whether the patient undersecretes or overproduces uric acid.

Collaborative Care

The management of gout has several goals. The first is to terminate an acute attack. This is accomplished by the use of an antiinflammatory agent such as colchicine. Future attacks are prevented by a maintenance dose of colchicine, weight reduction if necessary, avoidance of alcohol and high purine foods, and the use of drugs to reduce the serum urate concentration. Treatment is also aimed at preventing the formation of uric acid kidney stones and other associated conditions such as hypertriglyceridemia and hypertension.

Drug Therapy

Acute gouty arthritis is treated with one of three types of antiinflammatory agents: colchicine, nonsteroidal antiinflammatory agents (NSAIDs), or corticosteroids. Corticosteroids should be reserved for cases in which colchicine or NSAIDs are contraindicated or ineffective.

- Aspirin inactivates the effect of uricosurics, resulting in urate retention, and should be avoided while patients are taking probenecid (Benemid) and other uricosuric drugs. Acetaminophen can be used safely if analgesia is required.
- Adequate urine volume must be maintained to prevent precipitation of uric acid in the renal tubules. Allopurinol (Zyloprim), which blocks the production of uric acid, may control the

serum level. It is particularly useful in patients with uric acid stones or renal impairment, in whom uricosuric drugs may be ineffective or dangerous.

Nutritional Therapy

Dietary restrictions may include limiting the use of alcohol and foods high in purine. However, medication can generally control the situation without necessitating these limitations. Obese patients should be instructed in a weight-reduction program.

Nursing Management

Nursing intervention is directed at supportive care of the inflamed joints.

- Bed rest may be appropriate, with the affected joints properly immobilized. Limitation of motion and the degree of pain should be assessed.
- Special care is taken to avoid causing pain to an inflamed joint by careless handling. Involvement of a lower extremity may require the use of a cradle or footboard to protect the painful area from the weight of bed clothes.

▼ **Patient Teaching**

The patient and family should understand that hyperuricemia and gouty arthritis are chronic problems that can be controlled with careful adherence to a treatment program.

- Thorough explanations should be given concerning the importance of drug therapy and the need for periodic determination of serum uric acid levels.
- The patient should be able to demonstrate knowledge of precipitating factors that may cause an attack, including overindulgence in caloric intake, purines and alcohol; starvation (fasting); medication use (e.g., aspirin, diuretics); and major medical events (e.g., surgery, myocardial infarction [MI]).

GUILLAIN-BARRÉ SYNDROME

Definition/Description

Guillain-Barré syndrome is an acute, rapidly progressing, and potentially fatal form of polyneuritis. It is also called *postinfectious polyneuropathy* and *ascending polyneuropathic paralysis.* This disorder affects the peripheral nervous system, resulting in edema and inflammation of the affected nerves and a loss of myelin. With adequate supportive care, 85% of these patients will recover completely.

Pathophysiology

The etiology is unknown, but it is believed to be a cell-mediated immunologic reaction directed at the peripheral nerves. The syndrome is frequently preceded by immune system stimulation from a viral illness, trauma, surgery, viral immunization (e.g., swine flu vaccine), HIV, or lymphoproliferative neoplasms. These stimuli are thought to cause an alteration in the immune system, resulting in sensitization of T lymphocytes to the patient's myelin and subsequent myelin damage. Demyelination occurs and the transmission of nerve impulses is stopped or slowed down. Muscles innervated by the damaged peripheral nerves undergo denervation and atrophy.

- In the recovery phase, remyelination occurs slowly and returns in a proximal to distal pattern; lymphocytes are basically normal and return to complete functioning after the illness.

Clinical Manifestations

Symptoms usually develop 1 to 3 weeks after an upper respiratory or gastrointestinal infection.

- Weakness of the lower extremities (evolving more or less symmetrically) occurs over hours to days to weeks, usually peaking about day 14. Distal muscles are more severely affected.
- *Paresthesia* (numbness and tingling) is frequent, and paralysis usually follows in the extremities.
- Hypotonia and areflexia are common, persistent symptoms.
- Objective sensory loss is variable, with deep sensitivity more affected than superficial sensations.
- Autonomic nervous system dysfunction is usually seen in patients with severe muscle involvement and respiratory muscle paralysis. The most dangerous autonomic dysfunctions include orthostatic hypotension, hypertension, and abnormal vagal responses (bradycardia, heart block, and asystole).
- Other autonomic dysfunctions include bowel and bladder dysfunction, facial flushing, and diaphoresis.
- Patients may also have syndrome of inappropriate antidiuretic hormone (SIADH) secretion (see Syndrome of Inappropriate Antidiuretic Hormone, p. 550).
- The progression of Guillain-Barré syndrome to include the lower brainstem involves the facial, abducens, oculomotor, hypoglossal, trigeminal, and vagus cranial nerves. This involvement manifests itself through facial weakness, extraocular eye movement difficulties, dysphagia, and paresthesia of the face.
- Pain is a common finding; the pain can be categorized as paresthesias, muscular aches and cramps, and hyperesthesias. Pain appears to be worse at night. Narcotics may be indicated for those experiencing severe pain. Pain may lead to a decrease in appetite and interfere with sleep.

The most serious complication is respiratory failure, which occurs as paralysis progresses to the nerves that innervate the thoracic area. Respiratory infections or urinary tract infections (UTIs) may occur. Fever is generally the first sign of infection, and treatment is directed at the infecting organism. Immobility from the paralysis can cause problems such as paralytic ileus, muscle atrophy, deep vein thrombosis, pulmonary emboli, and orthostatic hypotension.

Diagnostic Studies
Diagnosis is based primarily on patient history and clinical signs.
- Cerebrospinal fluid is normal or has a low protein content initially, but after 7 to 10 days shows a greatly elevated protein level (700 mg/dl [7 g/L]).
- Electromyographic (EMG) and nerve conduction studies are markedly abnormal (showing reduced nerve conduction velocity) in affected extremities.

Collaborative Care
Management is aimed at supportive care, particularly ventilatory support, during the acute phase.
- Plasmapheresis is used in the first 2 weeks of Guillain-Barré syndrome. In patients with severe disease treated within 2 weeks of onset, a reduction in the length of stay, a decreased length of time on a ventilator, and a decreased time required to resume walking have all been observed.
- IV administration of high-dose immunoglobulin has been as effective as plasmapheresis and has the advantage of immediate availability and increased safety. Because of the ease of administering immunoglobulin, it is now being used more frequently than plasmapheresis.
- Corticosteroids and adrenocorticotropic hormone (ACTH) are used to suppress the immune response but appear to have little effect on the disease prognosis or duration.
- Monitoring BP and cardiac rate and rhythm is also important during the acute phase because transient cardiac arrhythmias have been reported. Autonomic dysfunction is common and usually takes the form of bradycardia. Orthostatic hypotension secondary to muscle atony may occur in severe cases.
- Vasopressor agents and volume expanders may be needed to treat low BP.

Nutritional intake is compromised during the acute phase. The patient may experience difficulty swallowing because of cranial nerve involvement.
- Mild dysphagia can be managed by placing the patient in an upright position and flexing the head forward during feeding. For more severe dysphagia, tube feedings may be required.

G

Later in the course of the disease, motor paralysis or weakness will affect the ability to self-feed.

- The patient's nutritional status, including body weight, serum albumin levels, and calorie counts, needs to be evaluated at regular intervals.

Nursing Management

Goals

The patient with Guillain-Barré syndrome will maintain adequate ventilation, be free from aspiration, be free of pain or have pain controlled, maintain an acceptable method of communication, maintain adequate nutritional intake, and return to usual physical functioning.

Nursing Diagnoses

- Risk for aspiration *related to* dysphagia
- Pain *related to* paresthesias, muscle aches and cramps, and hyperesthesias
- Impaired verbal communication *related to* intubation or paralysis of the muscles of speech
- Inability to sustain spontaneous ventilation *related to* disease process resulting in respiratory muscle paralysis
- Fear *related to* uncertain outcome and seriousness of the disease
- Self-care deficits *related to* inability to use muscles to accomplish activities of daily living (ADLs)

Nursing Interventions

The objective of care is to support the body systems until the patient recovers. Respiratory failure and infection are serious threats.

- Monitoring vital capacity and arterial blood gases (ABGs) is essential. A tracheostomy or endotracheal intubation may be done so that the patient can be mechanically ventilated (see Tracheostomy, p. 686 and Artificial Airways: Endotracheal Tubes, p. 668).
- Whether the patient has an endotracheal tube or tracheostomy, meticulous suctioning technique is needed to prevent infection. Thorough bronchial hygiene and chest physiotherapy help to clear secretions and prevent respiratory deterioration.
- If fever develops, sputum cultures should be obtained to identify whether the respiratory tract is the source of the pathogen. Appropriate antibiotic therapy is then initiated.

A communication system must be established with the use of the patient's available abilities. This is extremely difficult if the disease progresses to involvement of cranial nerves; at the peak of a severe episode the patient may be incapable of communicating.

- The nurse must explain all procedures before doing them and reassure the patient that muscle function will return to some part of the body so that his or her needs and desires can be communicated.

Urinary retention is common for a few days. Intermittent catheterization is preferred to an indwelling catheter to avoid UTIs. However, for the acutely ill patient receiving a large volume of fluids (>2.5 L/day), indwelling catheterization may be safer to reduce overdistention of a temporarily flaccid bladder and to prevent vesicoureteral reflux.

Physical therapy is indicated early to help prevent problems related to immobility. Passive range-of-motion (ROM) exercises and attention to body position help maintain function and prevent contractures.

Nutritional needs must be met in spite of possible problems associated with gastric dilation, paralytic ileus, and aspiration potential if the gag reflex is lost.

- The nurse should note drooling and other difficulties with secretions, which may be indicative of an inadequate gag reflex.
- Initially tube feedings or parenteral nutrition may be used to ensure adequate caloric intake. Fluid and electrolyte therapy must be monitored carefully to prevent electrolyte imbalances.

G

HEAD INJURY

Definition/Description

Head injury includes any trauma to the scalp, skull, or brain. The term *head trauma* refers primarily to craniocerebral trauma, which includes any alteration in consciousness no matter how brief. The majority of deaths after a head injury occur immediately after the injury, either from the direct head trauma or massive hemorrhage and shock. Deaths occurring within a few hours of the trauma are caused by progressive worsening of the head injury or from internal bleeding. Immediate notation of changes in neurologic status, together with surgical intervention, is critical in the prevention of deaths at this point. Deaths occurring 3 weeks or more after the injury result from multisystem failure.

Types of Head Injuries

Scalp lacerations. These are the most minor of the head traumas. The major complication associated with scalp laceration is infection.

Skull fractures. These frequently occur with head trauma. Fractures may be closed or open, depending on the presence of a scalp laceration or extension of the fracture into the air sinuses or dura.

- Type and severity of a skull fracture depend on the velocity, momentum, and direction of the injuring agent, and the site of impact. Specific manifestations of a skull fracture are generally associated with the location of the injury (see Table 54-9, Lewis and others, *Medical-Surgical Nursing,* edition 5, p. 1624).

Major potential complications are intracranial infections and hematoma as well as meningeal and brain tissue damage.

Minor head trauma

- *Concussion* is a sudden transient head injury associated with a disruption in neural activity and a change in the level of consciousness (LOC). The patient may not lose total consciousness. Signs include a brief disruption in the LOC, amnesia for the event (retrograde amnesia), and headache. Manifestations are generally of short duration.
- *Postconcussion syndrome* is seen anywhere from 2 weeks to 2 months after the concussion. Symptoms include persistent headache, lethargy, behavior changes, decreased short-term memory, and changes in intellectual ability.

Although a concussion is generally considered benign and usually resolves spontaneously, the symptoms may be the beginning of a more serious, progressive problem. At the time of discharge it is important to give the patient and family instructions for observation and accurate reporting of symptoms or changes in neurologic status.

Major head trauma. Contusions and lacerations are injuries which involve severe brain trauma. Contusions and lacerations are generally associated with closed injuries.

- A *contusion* is a bruising of brain tissue with a potential for the development of areas of necrosis, pulping infarction, hemorrhage, and edema. A contusion frequently occurs at the site of a fracture. Bleeding around the contusion site is generally minimal, and blood is reabsorbed slowly. Neurologic assessment demonstrates focal findings and a generalized disturbance in the LOC. Seizures are a common complication.
- *Lacerations* involve actual tearing of brain tissue and occur frequently in compound fractures and penetrating injuries. Tissue damage is severe, and surgical repair of the laceration is impossible because of the texture of the brain tissue. If bleeding is deep into the brain parenchyma, focal and generalized signs are noted.

When major head trauma occurs, many delayed responses are seen, including hemorrhage, hematoma formation, seizures, and cerebral edema (see Increased Intracranial Pressure, p. 343, and Seizure Disorders, p. 520)

- Prognosis is generally poor for the person with a large intracerebral hemorrhage. Subarachnoid hemorrhage and intraventricular hemorrhage can also occur secondary to head trauma.

Complications

Epidural hematoma. An epidural hematoma results from bleeding between the dura and inner surface of the skull. An epidural hematoma is a neurologic emergency and is usually associated with a linear fracture crossing a major artery in the dura, causing a tear. It can have a venous or arterial origin.

- Venous epidural hematomas are associated with a tear of the dural venous sinus and develop slowly.
- With arterial hematomas, the middle meningeal artery lying under the temporal bone is frequently torn. Because this is an arterial hemorrhage, the hematoma develops rapidly.

Manifestations typically include unconsciousness, with a brief lucid interval followed by a decrease in the LOC. Other symptoms may be headache, nausea and vomiting, or focal findings. Rapid surgical intervention is needed to prevent cerebral herniation.

Subdural hematoma. A subdural hematoma occurs from bleeding between the dura mater and the arachnoid layer of the meningeal covering of the brain. A subdural hematoma usually results from injury to the brain substance and its parenchymal vessels. Because a subdural hematoma is usually venous in origin, the hematoma is much slower to develop a mass large enough to produce symptoms. Subdural hematomas may be acute, subacute, or chronic (see Table 54-10, Lewis and others, *Medical-Surgical Nursing,* edition 5, p. 1627).

H

- An *acute subdural hematoma* manifests signs within 48 hours of the injury. Manifestations are similar to those associated with brain tissue compression in increased intracranial pressure (ICP) (see Increased Intracranial Pressure, p. 343). The patient appears drowsy and confused, and the ipsilateral pupil dilates and becomes fixed.
- A *subacute subdural hematoma* usually occurs within 2 to 14 days of the injury. Failure to regain consciousness may point to this possibility.
- A *chronic subdural hematoma* develops over weeks or months after a seemingly minor head injury. Peak incidence is in the sixth and seventh decades of life when a larger subdural space is available as a result of brain atrophy. The presenting complaints are focal symptoms, rather than signs of increased ICP.

Diagnostic Studies
- Skull x-rays to rule out skull fracture.
- CT scan and MRI to determine craniocerebral trauma.
- Positron emission therapy (PET) and evoked potential studies assist in diagnosis and differentiation of head injuries.
- Transcranial Doppler studies measure cerebral blood flow and velocity.

Collaborative Care
Emergency management of the patient with head injury includes measures to prevent secondary injury by treating cerebral edema and managing increased ICP (see Table 54-11, Lewis and others, *Medical-Surgical Nursing,* edition 5, p. 1627). The principal treatment of head injuries is timely diagnosis and surgery if necessary. For the patient with a concussion or contusion, observation and management of increased ICP are primary management strategies.

- The treatment of skull fractures is usually conservative. For depressed fractures and fractures with loose fragments, a craniotomy is necessary to elevate depressed bone and remove free fragments. If large amounts of bone are destroyed, the bone may be removed *(craniectomy)* and a cranioplasty will be needed at a later time (see the section on cranial surgery, Lewis and others, *Medical-Surgical Nursing,* edition 5, p. 1633).
- In cases of acute subdural and epidural hematomas the blood must be removed. A craniotomy is generally performed to visualize the bleeding vessels so that bleeding can be controlled. Burr hole openings may be used in an emergency for more rapid decompression, followed by a craniotomy to stop all bleeding. A drain is generally placed postoperatively for several days to prevent any reaccumulation of blood.

Nursing Management

Goals

The patient with an acute head injury will maintain adequate cerebral perfusion; remain normothermic; be free from pain, discomfort, fever, and infection; and attain maximal motor and sensory function.

Nursing Diagnoses

- Altered cerebral tissue perfusion *related to* interruption of cerebral blood flow associated with cerebral hemorrhage, hematoma, and edema
- Hyperthermia *related to* increased metabolism, infection, and loss of cerebral integrative function secondary to possible hypothalamic injury
- Sensory/perceptual alterations *related to* cerebral injury and intensive care unit environment
- Pain *related to* headache and nausea and vomiting
- Impaired physical mobility *related to* decreased LOC and treatment-imposed bed rest
- Risk for infection *related to* environmental contamination secondary to open wound

Nursing Interventions

One of the best ways to prevent head injuries is to prevent car and motorcycle accidents.

- The nurse can be active in campaigns that promote driving safety and can speak to driver education classes regarding the dangers of unsafe driving and of driving after drinking alcohol.
- The wearing of seat belts in cars and the use of helmets for riding on motorcycles are the most effective measures for increasing survival after accidents.
- Parents should be educated in the proper use of car seats and restraints for their young children.
- The nurse should also teach younger children about safety precautions for bicycle riding, skateboarding, and contact sports.

Acute nursing care may initially consist only of observation for changes in neurologic status. This action is important because the patient's condition may deteriorate rapidly, necessitating emergency surgery.

- The nurse should explain the need for frequent neurologic assessments to both the patient and family.
- Behavioral manifestations associated with head injury can result in a frightened, disoriented patient who is combative and resists help.
- Restraints should be avoided if possible because they often produce agitation, which further increases ICP. A family member may be available to stay with the patient and thus prevent increasing anxiety and fear.

H

The Glasgow Coma Scale (GCS) is useful in assessing the level of arousal (see Glasgow Coma Scale, p. 720). Indications of a deteriorating neurologic state, such as a decreasing LOC or lessening of motor strength, should be reported.

Much of the nursing care for the brain-injured patient relates to the unconscious state and increased ICP (see Increased Intracranial Pressure, Nursing Management, p. 346).

- Loss of the corneal reflex may necessitate administering lubricating eye drops, taping the eyes shut, or suturing the eyelids to prevent abrasion.
- Periorbital ecchymosis and edema disappear spontaneously, but cold and, later, warm compresses provide comfort and hasten the process.
- Diplopia can be relieved by use of an eye patch.
- If cerebrospinal fluid (CSF) rhinorrhea or otorrhea occurs, the nurse should inform the physician immediately. A loose collection pad may be placed under the nose or over the ear. The patient should be cautioned not to sneeze or blow the nose.
- Nausea and vomiting may be a problem and can be alleviated by antiemetic medication.
- Headache can usually be controlled with aspirin or small doses of codeine.

If the patient's condition deteriorates, intracranial surgery may be necessary. A Burr hole or craniotomy may be indicated, depending on the underlying injury. The patient is often unconscious before surgery, making it necessary for a family member to sign the consent form for surgery. This is a difficult and frightening time for the patient's family and requires sensitive nursing management. Suddenness of the situation makes it especially difficult for the family to cope.

Once the condition has stabilized, the patient is usually transferred for postacute rehabilitation management. As with any craniocerebral problem, there may be chronic problems related to motor and sensory deficits, communication, memory, and intellectual functioning.

- Many of the principles of nursing management of the patient with a stroke are appropriate (see Cerebrovascular Accident, p. 109). With time and patience, many of the chronic problems subside or disappear. Outward appearance is not a good indicator of how well the patient will function in the home or work environment.

Progressive recovery may continue for 6 months or more before a plateau is reached and a prognosis for recovery can be made. Specific nursing management depends on the residual deficits. In all cases the family must be given special consideration. They need to understand what is happening, and they must be taught appropriate interaction patterns.

- The family often has unrealistic expectations of the patient as the coma begins to recede. The nurse needs to prepare the family for the emergence of the patient from coma and must explain that the process of awakening often takes several weeks.
- Family members, particularly spouses, go through role transition as the role changes from one of spouse to that of caregiver.

HEAD AND NECK CANCER

Definition/Description

Head and neck cancer represents about 5% of all cancer cases, with more men than women diagnosed, generally after age 50. Although specific causes of head and neck cancer are not known, well-known risk factors include prolonged use of tobacco and alcohol, exposure to various chemicals, and infection with the Epstein-Barr virus.

Clinical Manifestations

Early signs of upper airway cancers vary with tumor location. Cancer of the oral cavity may be a painless growth in the mouth, an ulcer that does not heal, or a change in the fit of dentures. Pain is a late symptom that may be aggravated by acidic food.

Cancers of the oropharynx, hypopharynx, and supraglottic larynx rarely produce early symptoms and are usually diagnosed in later stages.

- The patient may complain of persistent unilateral sore throat or *otalgia* (ear pain). Hoarseness may be a symptom of early laryngeal cancer. Some patients experience a change in voice quality or what may feel like a lump in the throat.
- There may be thickening of the normally soft and pliable oral mucosa.
- *Leukoplakia* (white patch) or *erythroplakia* (red patch) may be seen and should be noted for later biopsy. Both leukoplakia and carcinoma in situ (localized to a defined area) may precede invasive carcinoma by many years.
- Late stages of head and neck cancer have easily detectable signs and symptoms including pain, dysphagia, decreased mobility of the tongue, airway obstruction, and cranial neuropathies.

Diagnostic Studies

- If lesions are suspected, upper airways may be examined using a indirect laryngoscopy. A flexible nasopharyngoscope may also be used.

- A CT scan or MRI may be performed to detect local and regional spread.
- Multiple biopsy specimens are obtained to determine the extent of the disease.

Collaborative Care

Using diagnostic information obtained, a decision will be made about the stage of the disease based on tumor size (T), number and location of involved nodes (N), and extent of metastasis (M). TNM staging classifies the disease as stage I to stage IV and guides treatment (see Table 11, p. 79).

- Approximately one third of patients have stage I or II highly confined lesions at diagnosis. These patients can undergo surgery or radiation therapy with the goal of cure. In stage III or IV disease, fewer than 30% of patients are cured.
- More advanced disease is managed with a combination of surgery and radiation therapy or just surgery.
- Advanced lesions are managed by a total laryngectomy in which the entire larynx and preepiglottic region are removed and a permanent tracheostomy is performed (see Tracheostomy, p. 686). Radical neck dissection frequently accompanies total laryngectomy. Depending on the extent of involvement, extensive dissection and reconstruction may be performed.

Nutritional Therapy

The patient will likely return from the operating room (OR) with a nasogastric (NG) tube in place. Initially the tube is used for gastric decompression and then later for tube feedings. It is the responsibility of the nurse to assess correct placement and function of the tube.

- Gastric distention may lead to vomiting, aspiration, stress on the suture line, or wound contamination.
- The patient who undergoes extensive surgical procedures may require tube feedings to maintain nutrition until healing is sufficient to permit oral intake (see Tube Feedings, p. 689).

Nursing Management

Goals

The patient with head or neck cancer will have a patent airway, no spread of cancer, no complications related to therapy, adequate nutritional intake, minimal to no pain, and appropriate communication methods.

See NCP 25-6 for the patient having total laryngectomy or radical neck surgery, Lewis and others, *Medical-Surgical Nursing,* edition 5, p. 604.

Nursing Diagnoses

- Impaired verbal communication *related to* removal of vocal cords

- Anxiety *related to* lack of knowledge regarding surgical procedure, pain management, and prevention of complications
- Ineffective airway clearance *related to* difficulty expectorating sputum and presence of tracheostomy tube
- Altered tissue perfusion *related to* tissue edema and disruption of lymphatic and vascular drainage
- Altered nutrition: less than body requirements *related to* dysphagia, edema, surgical procedure, and presence of a NG tube

Nursing Interventions

Development of head and neck cancer is closely related to personal habits, primarily prolonged tobacco and alcohol use. The nurse should include information about these risk factors in health teaching.

- If cancer has been diagnosed, smoking cessation is still important because the patient who continues to smoke during radiation therapy has lower rates of response and survival.

The nurse is in a key position to detect early signs of head and neck cancer. Early detection is critical. Early symptoms are often not reported because the patient does not know their significance or fears the consequences. The patient and family must be taught about the type of therapy to be performed and care required. This teaching should include (1) changes as a result of radiation therapy or surgical intervention, (2) the duration of changes, (3) changes in voice and ability to the eat, (4) alternate methods of speech, (5) self-help groups and community resources, and (6) emotional adjustments to be anticipated. It is essential to include the patient and significant other in all aspects of teaching and care.

Preoperative care for radical neck surgery must include information about expected changes in speech after surgical intervention. The nurse or speech pathologist should demonstrate means of communicating without speech. This assists in decreasing patient anxiety about what to anticipate after surgery.

The primary concern of postoperative care is airway management. The patient will be placed in a semi-Fowler's position to decrease edema and tension on the suture lines. Vital signs should be monitored frequently because of the risk of hemorrhage and respiratory compromise. Immediately after surgery, the postlaryngectomy patient requires frequent suctioning because secretions or saliva cannot be swallowed.

- If the patient develops mucous plugs or very thick secretions, a 3 to 5 ml bolus of normal saline should be instilled into the airway to loosen secretions enough for the patient to clear the airway either through coughing or suctioning.
- Patency of drainage tubes should be monitored every 4 hours for 24 hours to ensure that they are properly removing serous drainage. After the drainage tubes are removed, the area should

be closely monitored to detect any swelling. If fluid continues to accumulate, aspiration may be necessary.

A speech therapist or speech pathologist should meet with the patient to discuss voice restoration. The International Association of Laryngectomees, an association of laryngectomy patients, focuses on assisting patients to reestablish speech. Local groups, called "Lost Cord Clubs," identify members who can visit the patient, preferably preoperatively.

▼ **Patient Teaching**
- Since the patient with a laryngectomy no longer breathes through the nose, the ability to smell smoke and food may be lost. Advise the patient to install smoke detectors in the home. It is important for food to be colorful, attractively prepared, and nutritious, since taste may also be diminished.
- Instruct the patient on resumption of exercise, recreation, and sexual activity when able. Most patients can return to work 1 to 2 months after a laryngectomy.
- Loss of speech, loss of the ability to taste and smell, inability to produce audible sounds (including laughing and weeping), and presence of a permanent tracheal stoma that produces undesirable mucus are often overwhelming to the patient. The nurse can help by allowing verbalization of feelings and conveying acceptance.
- Encouraging the patient to participate in self-care activities is an important part of rehabilitation.
- If pain is a problem, a pain control regimen for comfort should be identified with the patient. A referral should be made to a hospice, if indicated.

HEADACHE

Definition/Description

Headaches are one of the most common types of pain experienced by humans. Of all persons with headache, the majority have functional headaches, such as benign migraine or tension-type; the remainder have organic headaches caused by significant intracranial or extracranial disease.

Headaches are classified based on the characteristics of the headache and facial pain.
- Primary classifications include tension-type, migraine, and cluster headaches. Characteristics of these headaches are shown in Table 56-1, Lewis and others, *Medical-Surgical Nursing,* edition 5, p. 1673.

Tension-Type Headache

Tension-type headaches have been called muscle contraction, tension, psychogenic, and rheumatic headaches. It is the most common type of headache and is also considered the most difficult to treat. This type of headache is related to increased pain sensitivity; the exact etiology remains obscure.

Clinical manifestations. There is no *prodrome* (early manifestation of impending disease) in tension-type headache. The pain is usually bilateral, occurring most often in the back of the neck. It usually does not interfere with sleep. The pain is often described as a tight, squeezing, bandlike pressure. It is sustained, chronic, dull, and persistent.

■ Headaches may occur intermittently for weeks, months, or years. Many patients have a combination of migraine and tension-type headaches with features of both headaches occurring simultaneously.

■ Patients with migraine headaches may experience tension-type headaches between migraine attacks.

Diagnostic studies. Careful history taking is the most important diagnostic tool. Electromyography (EMG) may reveal sustained contraction of the neck, scalp, or facial muscles, but many patients may not show increased muscle tension with this test. If tension-type headache is present during physical examination, increased resistance to passive movement of the head and tenderness of head and neck may be present.

Migraine Headache

Migraine headache is a benign, recurring headache characterized by unilateral or bilateral pain, a triggering event or factor, strong family history, and manifestations associated with neurologic and autonomic nervous system dysfunction. For some individuals migraine headaches begin in childhood or adolescence. A family history of migraine can be found in 65% of patients with migraine. In many cases, migraine headaches have no known precipitating events. However, for other patients, the headache may be precipitated by stress, bright lights, menstruation, alcohol, or certain foods such as chocolate or cheese.

Pathophysiology. Although the exact etiology of migraine headaches is not known, recent evidence suggests that neurologic, vascular, and chemical factors are involved.

The neurogenic model of migraine implies that a stimulus can trigger the trigeminovascular system (the trigeminal nerve and its connections to meningeal blood vessels) resulting in inflammation of the blood vessels and vasodilation, resulting in headache.

■ The *aura* of migraine is associated with "spreading depression," a wave of oligemia (diminished cerebral blood flow) beginning in the occipital lobe and spreading forward in the brain.

Clinical manifestations. *Migraine without aura* is the most common type of migraine headache. The prodrome is not sharply defined, and it can involve psychic disturbances, GI upset, and changes in fluid balance. The prodrome may precede the headache phase by several hours or days. The headache itself may last several hours or days.

Migraine with aura occurs in only 10% of migraine headache episodes. The sharply defined aura may last 10 to 30 minutes before the start of the headache and may include sensory dysfunction (e.g., visual field defects, tingling or burning sensations, or paresthesias), motor dysfunction (e.g., weakness or paralysis), dizziness, confusion, and loss of consciousness. The classic preheadache symptom is the perception of flashing lights in one quadrant of the visual field. This type of migraine headache usually peaks in 1 hour and may last several hours.

Other clinical manifestations that occur in migraine with and without aura are generalized edema, irritability, pallor, nausea and vomiting, and sweating. During the headache phase, patients with migraine tend to "hibernate;" that is, they seek shelter from noise, light, odors, people, and problems. The headache is described as a steady, throbbing pain that is synchronous with the pulse.

Diagnostic studies. Diagnosis of migraine headache is usually made from the history. Neurologic and other diagnostic examinations are often normal.

Cluster Headache

Cluster headache is one of the most severe forms of head pain. Cluster headache occurs less frequently than migraine and is more frequent in men than in women. Onset is usually between the ages of 30 and 60 years.

Pathophysiology. Neither the cause nor pathophysiology of cluster headache is fully known. The vasodilation that occurs in the affected part of the face is extracranial with the trigeminal nerve implicated in the production of pain. Activation of this nerve causes release of substance P and other vasoactive substances, which cause vasodilation, stimulation of afferent pain fibers, and neurogenic inflammation.

Periodicity and clocklike regularity of cluster headaches indicate a dysfunction of the biologic clock mechanisms of the hypothalamus. These headaches can also be triggered by alcohol ingestion.

Clinical manifestations. The headache has an abrupt onset, usually without a prodrome. It peaks in 5 minutes and lasts 30 to 90 minutes. It is not uncommon for this type of headache to start at night, awakening the patient after a few hours of sleep. The headache may recur several times a day over a period of several days, with each cluster lasting 2 to 3 months.

- It usually affects the upper face, periorbital region, and the forehead on one side of the face and head. The headache may not recur for months or years.
- The patient may also exhibit conjunctivitis, increased lacrimation (tearing), and nasal congestion on the side of the headache. A partial Horner's syndrome (constriction of the pupil and ptosis [drooping] of the eyelid on the affected side) may be seen.
- The headache is described as deep, steady, and penetrating, but not throbbing.
- Unlike the patient with migraine who seeks isolation and quiet, the patient with a cluster headache paces the floor, cries out, may do bizarre things, and resents being touched.
- The patient with a cluster headache does not experience the systemic manifestations that accompany a migraine headache, such as nausea or vomiting.

Diagnostic studies. Diagnosis is primarily based on the history. However, a CT scan, MRI, or cerebral angiography may be performed to rule out an aneurysm, tumor, or infection.

Collaborative Care: Headaches

If no systemic underlying disease is found, therapy is directed toward the functional type of headache. Table 32 summarizes current therapies for symptomatic and prophylactic relief of headaches. These therapies can include meditation, yoga, biofeedback, and muscle relaxation training.

H

Drug Therapy

Tension-type headache. Drug treatment usually involves a nonnarcotic analgesic (e.g., aspirin, acetaminophen) used alone or in combination with a sedative, a muscle relaxant, a tranquilizer, or codeine. Many of these drugs have potentially dangerous side effects.

Migraine headache. Drug treatment is aimed at terminating or decreasing the symptoms of the attack. Many people with mild or moderate migraine can obtain relief with aspirin or acetaminophen. Ergotamine (Ergomar) is often used when simple analgesics do not relieve the headache. Other drugs that may relieve migraine headache include butalbital with aspirin or acetaminophen (Fiorinal, Fioricet), isometheptene with acetaminophen and dichloralphenazone (Midrin), and in certain cases, narcotics.

- Drugs that affect serotonin have also been found to be beneficial. Methysergide (Sansert) produces vasoconstriction, which is useful in the prevention of migraine headaches. Serotonin receptor agonists, which are selective for vascular serotonin receptors, produce vasoconstriction and are used for management of acute migraine headaches. These drugs include sumatriptan (Imitrex), zolmitriptan (Zomig), naratriptan (Amerge), and rizatriptan (Maxalt).

Table 32   Collaborative Therapy: Headache

	Tension-type headache	Migraine headache	Cluster headache
Symptomatic	Nonnarcotic analgesics (aspirin, acetaminophen, ibuprofen) Analgesic combinations (butalbital, Fiorinal) Muscle relaxants	Nonnarcotic analgesics (aspirin, acetaminophen, ibuprofen) Serotonin receptor agonist (sumatriptan [Imitrex], zolmitriptan [Zomig], naratriptan [Amerge], rizatriptan [Maxalt]) α-Adrenergic blockers (ergotamine tartrate [Ergomar]) Vasoconstrictors (isometheptene [Midrin])	α-Adrenergic blockers (ergotamine tartrate) Vasoconstrictors Oxygen

Prophylactic		
Tricyclic antidepressants (doxepin [Sinequan], amitriptyline [Elavil])	β-Adrenergic blockers (propranolol)	... tartrate)
β-Adrenergic blockers (propranolol [Inderal])	Serotonin antagonists* (methysergide [Sansert])	Serotonin antagonists (methysergide)
Biofeedback	Antidepressants (amitriptyline, imipramine)	Corticosteroids (prednisone)
Muscle relaxation training	Calcium channel blockers (verapamil [Isoptin])	Lithium
Psychotherapy	Antiseizure drugs (valproate [Depakene])	Calcium channel blockers (verapamil)
	Biofeedback	Antiseizure drugs
	Yoga	
	Meditation	
	Electric counterstimulation	

*Only for patients suffering from one or more severe headaches per week.

H

- β-Blockers (e.g., propranolol [Inderal]), tricyclic antidepressants, calcium channel blockers, clonidine (Catapres), thiazides, and other antihypertensive drugs may be used prophylactically for very severe or frequent migraine headaches.

Cluster headache. Because these headaches occur suddenly, often at night, and are not long lasting, drug therapy is not as useful as it is for other types of headache. Prophylactic medications may include verapamil (Isoptin), lithium, ergotamine, divalproex (Depakote), or nonsteroidal antiinflammatory drugs (NSAIDs). Acute treatment of cluster headache is inhalation of 100% oxygen (O_2) delivered at a rate of 7 to 9 L/minute for 15 to 20 minutes, which may relieve headache by causing vasoconstriction. Sumatriptan is also effective in treating acute cluster headache.

Nursing Management: Headaches
Goals
The patient with a headache will have reduced or no pain, experience increased comfort and decreased anxiety, demonstrate an understanding of triggering events and treatment strategies, and use positive coping strategies to deal with chronic pain.

See NCP 56-1 for the patient with headache, Lewis and others, *Medical-Surgical Nursing,* edition 5, p. 1677.

Nursing Diagnoses
- Pain *related to* headache
- Sleep pattern disturbance *related to* pain
- Anxiety *related to* lack of knowledge of etiology and treatment of headache
- Hopelessness *related to* chronic pain, alteration of lifestyle, and ineffective treatment modalities

Nursing Interventions
Headaches may result from an inability to cope with daily stresses. The most effective therapy may be to help patients examine their lifestyle, recognize stressful situations, and learn to cope with them more appropriately. Precipitating factors can be identified, and ways of avoiding them can be developed. Daily exercise, relaxation periods, and socializing can be encouraged, since each can help decrease the recurrence of headache.

- The nurse can suggest alternative ways of handling the pain of headache through techniques such as relaxation, meditation, yoga, and self-hypnosis. Massage and moist hot packs to the neck and head can help a patient with tension-type headaches.
- The patient should learn about medications prescribed for prophylactic and symptomatic treatment of headache and should

be able to describe the purpose, action, dosage, and side effects of the medication.

- For the patient whose headaches are triggered by food, dietary counseling may be provided. The patient is encouraged to eliminate foods that may provoke headaches (e.g., chocolate, alcohol, excessive caffeine, cheese, fermented foods, monosodium glutamate).

▼ **Patient Teaching**

A teaching guide for the patient with a headache is provided in Table 33.

Table 33	Patient Teaching Guide: Headache

The patient with headaches should be taught to do the following:
1. Avoid factors that can trigger a headache. Triggers can include:
   - Foods containing amines (cheese, chocolate), nitrates (meats, including hot dogs), vinegar, onions, fermented or marinated foods
   - Monosodium glutamate
   - Caffeine
   - Nicotine
   - Ice cream
   - Alcohol (particularly red wine)
   - Emotional stress
   - Fatigue
   - Medications such as ergot-containing medicines and monoamine oxidase inhibitors
2. Be able to describe the purpose, action, dosage, and side effects of medications taken
3. Self-administer sumatriptan subcutaneously if prescribed
4. Utilize stress reduction techniques such as relaxation
5. Exercise regularly
6. Keep a diary or calendar of headaches and possible precipitating events
7. Contact the health care provider if the following occur:
   - Symptoms become more severe, last longer than usual, or are resistant to medication
   - Nausea, vomiting, change in vision, or fever occur with the headache
   - Problems with medications

H

HEAT-RELATED INJURIES

Heat-related injuries are a failure of the thermoregulatory mechanisms to compensate for exposure to increased ambient temperatures. Strenuous activities in hot or humid environments, clothing that interferes with perspiration, high fevers, and preexisting illnesses predispose individuals to heat stress. Effects can be mild (heat rash and heat edema) or severe (heat exhaustion and heat stroke). Heat stress is a leading cause of death in athletes.

- Specific heat injuries are heat rash, heat syncope, heat edema, heat cramps, heat exhaustion, and heat stroke.

Heat rash. Heat rash (miliaria or prickly heat) is a fine, red, papular rash that occurs on the torso, neck, and skin folds. The rash occurs when sweat ducts are obstructed and become inflamed, which does not allow sweat excretion to occur.

- The rash usually occurs in warm weather but has also been reported in cold weather due to constrictive clothing.

Heat syncope. Heat syncope is associated with prolonged standing and heat exposure. Manifestations include dizziness, orthostatic hypotension, and syncope. Inadequate vasomotor tone associated with aging places the elderly at greater risk for heat syncope.

Heat edema. Heat edema is swelling of the hands, feet, and ankles, usually in individuals not acclimated to the environment, as a result of prolonged standing or sitting. Swelling usually resolves in days with rest, elevation, and support hose.

- Diuretics are not recommended as this condition is usually self-limiting.

Heat cramps. Heat cramps refers to severe cramping in large muscle groups fatigued by heavy work. Cramps are brief, intense, and tend to occur during a rest after exercise or heavy labor. They are usually seen in healthy, acclimatized athletes with adequate fluid intake. Profuse sweating and ingestion of water or other salt-poor solutions deplete sodium and lead to hyponatremia.

- Cramps resolve rapidly with rest and oral or parenteral replacement of sodium and water. Elevation, gentle massage, and analgesia minimize pain.
- Education of the patient should emphasize the inclusion of salt replacement during heavy exercise in a hot, humid environment. Commercially prepared electrolyte solutions such as Gatorade are recommended.

Heat exhaustion. Heat exhaustion is prolonged exposure to heat over hours or days. Heat exhaustion is usually seen in people who have engaged in strenuous exercise in hot, humid weather. Heat exhaustion is characterized by fatigue, lightheadedness, nausea, vomiting, diarrhea, and feelings of impending doom.

- The patient will exhibit tachypnea, hypotension, tachycardia, and an elevated body temperature.
- Additional manifestations include dilated pupils, mild confusion, profuse diaphoresis, and ashen color.

Treatment begins with placement of the patient in a cool area and the removal of constrictive clothing. Oral fluid and electrolyte replacement is initiated unless the patient is nauseated. Salt tablets are not recommended due to potential gastric irritation and hypernatremia. Intravenous 0.9% normal saline solution is initiated when oral solutions are not tolerated. A moist sheet placed over the patient decreases core temperature.

- Hospital admission is considered for the elderly, chronically ill, or those who do not improve within 3 to 4 hours.

Heat stroke. Heat stroke (hyperthermia) is the most serious heat-related injury and has a high risk of mortality. For the risk factors associated with heat-related emergencies, see Table 64-9, Lewis and others, *Medical-Surgical Nursing,* edition 5, p. 1965. The patient presents with a core temperature >105° F (>40.6° C), altered mentation, an absence of perspiration, circulatory collapse, and hot, dry, ashen skin. Prognosis is related to age, health, and the length of exposure.

- Heat stroke is common during periods of prolonged heat (>3 days) with accompanying high humidity. Fluid and electrolytes become depleted and blood vessels dilate, which results in increased cardiac output (CO). Eventually the sweat glands stop functioning; when sweating ceases, core temperature increases rapidly.

Treatment focuses on the rapid reduction of core temperature and the treatment of subsequent complications. Administration of 100% oxygen (O_2) compensates for the patient's hypermetabolic state. Fluid resuscitation with 1 or 2 L of 0.9% normal saline solution over the first 4 hours is usually adequate. See Table 64-10 for the emergency management of hyperthermia, *Medical-Surgical Nursing,* p. 1966.

- Conventional cooling methods include tepid water mist, fans, and ice packs to the head, groin, axillae, and neck. Ice baths, alcohol rubs, and antipyretics should not be used. Ice water lavage, cold water peritoneal dialysis, and cardiopulmonary bypass are used in extreme cases of hyperthermia. More aggressive cooling techniques are implemented when conventional techniques fail. Ice water immersion is not recommended since the massive peripheral vasoconstriction that occurs can interfere with cooling. Cooling blankets are used.
- Cooling efforts are complicated by shivering because the associated muscle activity increases core temperature. Intravenous chlorpromazine (Thorazine) is the drug of choice to suppress shivering.

H

- Aggressive temperature reduction should continue until core temperature reaches 102° F (38.8° C).
- Additional therapy includes corticosteroid therapy with methylprednisolone for cerebral edema and mannitol when urinary output is less than 0.5 ml/kg/hr.
- Muscle breakdown associated with hypothermia leads to myoglobinuria, which places the kidneys at risk. Urine should be carefully monitored for color, amount, pH, and hemoglobin.

HEMOPHILIA

Definition/Description

Hemophilia is a hereditary bleeding disorder caused by defective or deficient coagulation factors. The two major forms of hemophilia that can occur in mild to severe forms are hemophilia A (classic hemophilia, factor VIII deficiency) and hemophilia B (Christmas disease, factor IX deficiency). Von Willebrand disease is a related disorder involving a congenitally acquired deficiency of the von Willebrand coagulation protein.

Hemophilia A is the most common form of hemophilia, comprising about 80% of all cases. Von Willebrand disease is considered the most common congenital bleeding disorder in humans, with estimates as high as 1 in 100 persons.

Deficiency and inheritance patterns of these three forms of inherited coagulopathies are compared in Table 34.

Clinical Manifestations and Complications

Clinical manifestations and complications related to hemophilia include (1) slow, persistent, prolonged bleeding from minor trauma and small cuts; (2) delayed bleeding after minor injuries (the delay may be several hours or days); (3) uncontrollable hemorrhage after dental extractions or irritation of the gingiva with a hard bristle toothbrush; (4) epistaxis, especially after a blow to the face; (5) GI bleeding from ulcers and gastritis; (6) hematuria from genitourinary (GU) trauma and splenic rupture resulting from falls or abdominal trauma; (7) ecchymoses and subcutaneous (SC) hematomas; (8) neurologic signs such as pain, anesthesia, and paralysis, which may develop from nerve compression caused by hematoma formation; and (9) hemarthrosis (bleeding into the joints), which may lead to joint deformity severe enough to cause unresolvable crippling (commonly in knees, elbows, shoulders, hips, and ankles).

- All manifestations relate to bleeding. Any bleeding episode in persons with hemophilia may result in death from hemorrhage.

Table 34	Comparison of Hemophilic States	
Disorder	**Deficiency**	**Inheritance pattern**
Hemophilia A	Factor VIII	Recessive sex-linked, transmitted by female carriers, displayed almost exclusively in men
Hemophilia B	Factor IX	Recessive sex-linked, transmitted by female carriers, displayed almost exclusively in men
von Willebrand disease	vWF and platelet dysfunction	Autosomal dominant, seen in both sexes Recessive (in severe forms of the disease)

vWF, von Willebrand factor.

- Before 1986 donated blood and blood products were not tested for the HIV antibody. As a result, many persons with hemophilia became seropositive for HIV infection transmitted via cryoprecipitates and factor concentrates.
- The development of hepatitis C in hemophilia patients was also common for many years because of a lack of available testing to detect it and the use of pooled blood products. Hepatitis C antibody screening is now routinely done on all donated blood and blood products.

Diagnostic Tests
- Partial prolonged thromboplastin time (PTT) due to deficiency in any intrinsic clotting system factor.
- Prolonged bleeding time in von Willebrand disease because of structurally defective platelets; bleeding time is normal in hemophilia A and B because platelets are not affected.
- Factor assays will reveal reduction of factor VIII in hemophilia A, vWF in von Willebrand disease, and reduction of factor IX in hemophilia B.

Collaborative Care
The goal of management is to prevent and treat bleeding. Therapy for persons with hemophilia or von Willebrand disease focuses on maintaining adequate blood levels of the deficient clotting factors. This goal is achieved by assessing clinical manifestations, determining

the blood levels of the involved factors, and administering the necessary factors when needed.

- Replacement of deficient clotting factors is the primary means of supporting patients with hemophilia. In addition to treating acute crises, replacement therapy may be given before surgery and dental care as a prophylactic measure. Cryoprecipitate is commonly used and primarily contains factor VIII and fibrinogen.
- Most patients with hemophilia A use factor VIII concentrate, which is prepared from multiple donors and supplied as a lyophilized powder.
- For mild hemophilia or certain subtypes of von Willebrand disease, desmopressin acetate (DDAVP), a synthetic analog of vasopressin, may be used to stimulate an increase in factor VIII and vWF. This drug acts on endothelial cells to cause the release of vWF, which subsequently binds with factor VIII, thus increasing their concentrations. Beneficial effects (e.g., decreased bleeding time) of DDAVP, when administered IV, are seen within half an hour and can last more than 12 hours.

The most common problem with acute management is starting factor replacement therapy too late and stopping it too soon. Generally, minor bleeding episodes should be treated for at least 72 hours. Surgery and traumatic injuries may need support for 10 to 14 days. Because of the short half-life of the factors, regular intermittent or continuous infusions have been used to manage bleeding episodes or expected surgical procedures. Chronically, the development of inhibitors to the factor products has occurred and requires individualized expert patient management.

Nursing Management

Because of the hereditary nature of hemophilia, referral for genetic counseling is essential when considering preventive measures. This is especially important today since persons with hemophilia are living longer and reaching an age when reproduction is possible.

Nursing interventions for acute bleeding episodes focus on controlling the bleeding and include the following:

1. Stop the topical bleeding as quickly as possible by applying direct pressure or ice, packing the area with Gelfoam or fibrin foam, and applying topical hemostatic agents such as thrombin.
2. Administer the specific coagulation factor concentrate as ordered.
3. When joint bleeding occurs, it is important to totally rest the involved joint in addition to administering antihemophilic factors. The joint may be packed in ice. Analgesics are given to reduce severe pain; aspirin should never be used. As soon as the bleeding ceases, encourage mobilization of the affected area through range-of-motion (ROM) exercises and physical

therapy. Actual weight-bearing is avoided until all swelling has resolved and muscle strength has returned.

4. Manage life-threatening complications that may develop as a result of hemorrhage. Examples include prevention or treatment of airway obstruction from hemorrhage into the neck and pharynx, as well as early assessment and treatment of intracranial bleeding.

Quality and length of life may be significantly affected by the patient's knowledge of the illness and how to live with it. The nurse must provide ongoing assessment of the patient's adaptation to the illness. Psychosocial support and assistance should be available as needed.

▼ **Patient Teaching**

■ The patient with hemophilia must be taught to recognize disease-related problems and to learn which can be resolved at home and which require hospitalization. Immediate medical attention is required for severe pain or swelling of a muscle or joint that restricts movement or inhibits sleep and for a head injury, a swelling in the neck or mouth, abdominal pain, hematuria, melena, and skin wounds in need of suturing.

■ Daily oral hygiene must be performed without causing trauma.

■ The patient should understand how to prevent injuries. The patient can learn to participate in noncontact sports (e.g., golf) and wear gloves when doing household chores to prevent cuts or abrasions from knives, hammers, and other tools.

■ The patient should wear a medical-alert tag to ensure that health care providers know about the hemophilia in case of an accident.

■ The patient needs information about routine follow-up care, and compliance with scheduled visits must be assessed.

■ A reliable person can be taught to self-administer some of the factor replacement therapies at home. With the exception of intranasal DDAVP, this will require providing instructions regarding venipuncture and infusion techniques.

H

HEMORRHOIDS

Definition/Description

Hemorrhoids are dilated hemorrhoidal veins that may be internal (occurring above the internal sphincter) or external (occurring outside the external sphincter). They occur in all age groups and appear in affected persons periodically. Manifestations of hemorrhoids include bleeding, pruritus, prolapse, and pain.

Pathophysiology

Hemorrhoids develop when the flow of blood through the veins of the hemorrhoidal plexus is impaired. Hemorrhoids may be caused by many factors, including pregnancy, prolonged constipation, straining in an effort to defecate, heavy lifting, prolonged standing and sitting, and portal hypertension.

- *Internal hemorrhoids* may become constricted and painful. They are the most common cause of bleeding with defecation. The amount of blood lost at one time may be small but may lead to iron deficiency anemia over time.
- *External hemorrhoids* are reddish blue and seldom bleed or cause pain unless a vein ruptures. If blood clots in external hemorrhoids, they are said to be thrombosed.

Diagnostic Studies

Hemorrhoids are diagnosed by inspection, digital examination, proctoscopy, or examination with a flexible sigmoidoscope.

Collaborative Care

Therapy should be directed toward the causes of the condition and the patient's symptoms. A high-fiber diet and increased fluid intake will prevent constipation and reduce straining. Ointments such as Nupercaine, creams, suppositories, and impregnated pads that contain antiinflammatory agents (e.g., hydrocortisone) or astringents and anesthetics (e.g., witch hazel, benzocaine, pramoxine) may be used to shrink mucous membranes and relieve discomfort. Stool softeners may be ordered to keep stools soft, and sitz baths may be ordered to relieve pain.

Application of ice packs for a few hours, followed by warm packs, may be used for thrombosed hemorrhoids. Another treatment involves the use of a sclerosing solution, such as 5% phenol in oil, or a combined solution of quinine and urea may be injected into the submucous tissue surrounding the hemorrhoids, causing a fibrosing and shrinking of supporting tissues.

Internal hemorrhoids may be ligated with a rubber band. The constrictive effect impairs circulation, and the tissue becomes necrotic, separates, and sloughs off. There is some local discomfort with this procedure, but no anesthetic is required.

- A *hemorrhoidectomy* (surgical excision of hemorrhoids) is indicated when there is prolapse, excessive pain or bleeding, or large hemorrhoids. Surgical removal may be done by cautery, clamp, or excision.

Nursing Management

Conservative nursing care includes teaching measures to prevent constipation, avoidance of prolonged standing or sitting, proper use of over-the-counter medications available for hemorrhoidal symptoms, and instructions on when to seek medical care for symptoms (e.g., excessive pain and bleeding, prolapsed hemorrhoids).

- Pain is a common problem after a hemorrhoidectomy. The nurse must be aware that although the procedure is minor, the pain is severe, and narcotics are usually given initially.
- Sitz baths are started 1 to 2 days after surgery. A sponge ring in the sitz bath helps relieve pressure on the area. Initially the patient should not be left alone because of the possibility of weakness or fainting.
- Packing may be inserted into the rectum to absorb drainage. A T-binder may hold the dressing in place. If packing is inserted, it usually is removed the first or second postoperative day. The nurse should assess for rectal bleeding. The patient may be embarrassed when the dressing is changed, and privacy should be provided.
- A stool softener such as dioctyl sodium sulfosuccinate (Colace) is usually ordered the first few postoperative days. If the patient does not have a bowel movement within 2 to 3 days, an oil retention enema is given.
- The patient usually dreads the first bowel movement and often resists the urge to defecate. Pain medication may be given before the bowel movement to reduce discomfort.

▼ **Patient Teaching**
- Discharge teaching includes the importance of diet, care of the anal area, symptoms of complications (especially bleeding), and avoidance of constipation and straining.
- Sitz baths are recommended for 1 to 2 weeks
- The physician may order a stool softener to be taken for a time.
- Regular checkups are important in the prevention of any further problems.

Hemorrhoids may recur. Occasionally anal strictures develop and dilation is necessary.

HEPATITIS, VIRAL

Definition/Description

Hepatitis is an inflammation of the liver. Acute viral hepatitis is the most common cause of hepatitis. The types of infectious viral hepatitis are A, B, C (formerly called posttransfusion non-A, non-B), D, and E. Viral hepatitis is a major public health concern in the United States.

- Noninfectious hepatitis may also be caused by drugs and other chemicals. Rarely, hepatitis is caused by bacteria such as streptococci, salmonellae, and *Escherichia coli*.

Etiology

Viral hepatitis can be caused by one of five viruses: A, B, C, D, and E. Other viruses known to damage the liver include cytomegalovirus, Epstein-Barr virus, herpesvirus, coxsackievirus, and rubella virus.

- The only definitive way to distinguish the various forms of viral hepatitis is by the presence of the antigens and the subsequent development of antibodies to them. Outbreaks of hepatitis are consistently caused by the hepatitis A virus.
- Approximately 50% of viral hepatitis cases in American adults are hepatitis B, 20% are hepatitis C, and 30% are hepatitis A. Table 35 lists the characteristics of hepatitis viruses.
- Infection with each virus provides immunity to that virus (homologous immunity). However, the patient can still develop another type of viral hepatitis. For a more complete description of each hepatitis virus, see Lewis and others, *Medical-Surgical Nursing,* edition 5, p. 1192.

Pathophysiology

The pathophysiologic changes in the various types of viral hepatitis are similar. Hepatitis involves widespread inflammation of liver tissue.

- Liver cell damage consists of hepatic cell degeneration and necrosis. There is proliferation and enlargement of the Kupffer cells. Inflammation of the periportal areas may interrupt bile flow. Cholestasis may occur.
- Liver cells regenerate in an orderly manner, and if no complications occur, they should resume normal appearance and function during convalescence.
- Circulating immune (antigen-antibody) complexes activate the complement system. Manifestations of this activation are rash, angioedema, arthritis, fever, and malaise. Glomerulonephritis and vasculitis have also been found secondary to immune complex disease.

Clinical Manifestations

A large number of patients, especially the younger ones, have no symptoms. Manifestations of viral hepatitis may be classified into three phases: (1) preicteric or prodromal phase, (2) icteric phase, and (3) posticteric or convalescent phase.

- *Preicteric phase* precedes jaundice and lasts from 1 to 21 days. This is the period of maximal infectivity for hepatitis A.

Table 35   Characteristics of Hepatitis Viruses

	Incubation period	Mode of transmission	Sources of infection and spread of disease	Infectivity
Hepatitis A virus (HAV)	15-50 days (average 28)	Fecal-oral (fecal contamination and oral ingestion)	Crowded conditions; poor personal hygiene; poor sanitation; contaminated food, milk, water, and shellfish; persons with subclinical infections; infected food handlers; sexual contact	Most infectious during 2 wk before onset of symptoms; infectious until 1-2 wk after symptoms start
Hepatitis B virus (HBV)	45-180 days (average 56-96)	Percutaneous (parenterally)/permucosal exposure to blood or blood products; Sexual contact; Perinatal transmission; Human bile	Contaminated needles, syringes, and blood products; sexual activity with infected partners; asymptomatic carriers; Tattoo/body piercing, bites	Before and after symptoms appear; infectious for 4-6 mo; in carriers, continues for patient's lifetime

Continued

H

Table 35   Characteristics of Hepatitis Viruses—cont'd

	Incubation period	Mode of transmission	Sources of infection and spread of disease	Infectivity
Hepatitis C virus (HCV)	14-180 days (average 56)	Percutaneous (parenteral)/permucosal exposure to blood or blood products High-risk sexual contact Perinatal contact	Blood and blood products, needles and syringes, sexual activity with infected partners	1-2 wk before symptoms; continues during clinical course; indefinitely with carriers
Hepatitis D virus (HDV)	2-26 weeks HBV must precede HDV; chronic carriers of HBV are always at risk	Can cause infection only together with HBV; routes of transmission same as for HBV	Same as HBV	Blood is infectious at all stages of HDV infection
Hepatitis E virus (HEV)	15-64 days (average 26-42 days in different epidemics)	Fecal-oral Outbreaks associated with contaminated water supply in developing countries	Contaminated water; poor sanitation; found in Asia, Africa, and Mexico; not common in the United States and Canada	Not known; may be similar to HAV

Hepatitis B patients who are hepatitis B core antigen (HBcAg)–positive can be infective for years. GI symptoms include anorexia, nausea, and abdominal (right upper quadrant) discomfort. Other symptoms include malaise, headache, weight loss, fever, urticaria, arthralgias, and skin rashes.

- *Icteric phase* lasts 2 to 4 weeks and is characterized by jaundice. Jaundice results when bilirubin diffuses into the tissues. The urine may darken because of excess bilirubin being excreted by the kidneys. GI symptoms remain, and the liver is usually enlarged and tender. Pruritus is sometimes present.
- The convalescent stage of the *posticteric phase* begins as jaundice is disappearing and lasts weeks to months, with an average of 2 to 4 months. During this period the patient's major complaints are malaise and easy fatigability. Hepatomegaly remains for several weeks. Relapses may occur, and the disappearance of jaundice does not mean the patient has totally recovered.

Additional considerations include:

- Not all patients with viral hepatitis have jaundice. This is referred to as *anicteric hepatitis* and occurs more frequently in children. A high percentage of persons with hepatitis A virus (HAV) are anicteric and do not have symptoms.
- There is some slight variation in manifestations between the types of hepatitis. In hepatitis A the onset is more acute and the symptoms are usually mild, flulike manifestations. In hepatitis B the onset is more insidious and the symptoms are usually more severe. There may be fewer GI symptoms. In hepatitis C the majority of cases are mild or asymptomatic.

H

Complications

Most patients with acute hepatitis A and B recover completely with no complications.

- *Chronic persistent hepatitis* is the most common complication of viral hepatitis. It is characterized by a delayed convalescent period. It is usually benign and is accompanied by fatigue and hepatomegaly. However, no treatment is required. Liver function tests may remain abnormal for several years.
- *Chronic active hepatitis* is characterized by the persistence of signs and symptoms of hepatitis and abnormal liver function tests for more than 6 months. Chronic active hepatitis is seen in hepatitis B and C; it is only seen in patients with hepatitis D if they also have hepatitis B. Hepatitis B surface antigen (HBsAg) persists longer than 6 months in approximately 10% of patients with hepatitis B. It is distinguished from chronic persistent hepatitis by liver biopsy. The ongoing process of liver necrosis may progress to cirrhosis.

- *Fulminant viral hepatitis* is a clinical syndrome that results in severe impairment or necrosis of liver cells and potential liver failure. Fulminant viral hepatitis develops in a small percentage of patients. The disorder may occur as a complication of hepatitis B or C, particularly hepatitis B accompanied by infection with hepatitis D virus (HDV). Toxic reactions to drugs and congenital metabolic disorders may also cause fulminant hepatitis and fulminant liver failure. Hepatocellular failure with death usually occurs.

Diagnostic Studies

Liver function tests show significant abnormalities, especially elevated liver enzymes.

Hepatitis serology:

1. *Virus A.* Anti-HAV (immunoglobulin M [IgM] and immunoglobulin G [IgG]) for HAV.
2. *Virus B.* HBsAg for active hepatitis B virus (HBV). Hepatitis Be antigen (HBeAg) indicates high infectivity and is present in acute, active infection.
   Anti-HBsAg indicates immunity to hepatitis B; also is a marker for response to hepatitis B vaccine.
   Anti-HBc IgM indicates acute infection with hepatitis B.
   Anti-HBc IgG indicates previous infection.
3. *Virus C.* Anti-hepatitis C virus (anti-HCV) is a marker for acute or chronic infection for HCV.
4. *Virus D.* Anti-HDV indicates coexisting infection with HBV.
5. *Virus E.* Anti-hepatitis E virus (HEV) serologic tests are being developed.

Collaborative Care

There is no specific treatment for viral hepatitis. Most patients can be managed at home. Emphasis is on measures to rest the body and assist the liver in regenerating. Adequate nutrients and rest seem to be most beneficial for healing and liver cell (hepatocyte) regeneration. Dietary emphasis is on a well-balanced diet that the patient can tolerate.

- The degree of rest ordered depends on symptom severity; usually alternating periods of activity with rest is adequate.
- There are no specific drug therapies for the treatment of acute viral hepatitis. Corticosteroid therapy is controversial. Supportive drug therapy may include antiemetics, such as dimenhydrinate (Dramamine) or trimethobenzamide (Tigan).
- α-Interferon (an antiviral or immune-modulating drug) has been approved to treat hepatitis B and C. It is primarily used in the treatment of chronic hepatitis. The efficacy of α-interferon is greater in the treatment of HBV than HCV infections.

- Immune globulin (IG) is used in the prevention and modification of viral hepatitis.
- IG is effective for hepatitis A if given up to 2 weeks after exposure. It provides temporary passive immunity. IG is recommended in cases of exposure to hepatitis A from close (household or day care center) contact in persons who are not positive for anti-HAV and for travelers to foreign countries with high endemic levels of hepatitis A.
- IG for hepatitis B (HBIG) is used for one-time exposure (e.g., needle stick, contact of mucous membrane with infectious material).

Immunization with hepatitis A vaccine or hepatitis B vaccine is the most effective method of preventing HAV and HBV infection. Recommendations of the Centers for Disease Control and Prevention's (CDC) Immunization Practices Advisory Committee include making hepatitis B vaccine a part of routine vaccination schedules for all newborns and adolescents.

An important measure in assisting hepatocytes to regenerate is adequate nutrition. No special diet is required. However, a diet high in carbohydrates and proteins with a low fat content is usually recommended.

Nursing Management

Goals

The patient with viral hepatitis will have relief of discomfort, be able to resume normal activities, and return to normal liver function without complications.

See NCP 41-1 for the patient with viral hepatitis, Lewis and others, *Medical-Surgical Nursing,* edition 5, p. 1200.

Nursing Diagnoses

- Altered nutrition: less than body requirements *related to* anorexia, nausea, and altered metabolism of nutrients by liver
- Activity intolerance *related to* fatigue and weakness
- Ineffective management of therapeutic regimen *related to* lack of knowledge of follow-up care
- Body-image disturbance *related to* stigma of having a communicable disease, change in appearance (jaundice), and possible alterations in lifestyle (alcohol consumption, drug use, restriction of sexual activity) and roles

Nursing Interventions

Viral hepatitis is a community health problem. The nurse must assume a significant role in the control and prevention of this disease.

Hepatitis A. The mode of transmission is fecal-oral. Preventive measures include personal and environmental hygiene and health education to promote good sanitation.

- Handwashing is essential and is probably the most important precaution. Health teaching should include careful handwashing after bowel movements and before eating.

Hepatitis B. Control and prevention of hepatitis B focuses on the identification of possible exposure via percutaneous and sexual transmission.

- The nurse must be aware of the groups at increased risk of contracting hepatitis B and teach methods to reduce the risks. Groups at increased risk include patients receiving frequent transfusions or hemodialysis, workers in hemodialysis units and blood chemistry laboratories, IV drug users, persons with multiple sexual partners, prison inmates, and the household and sexual partners of HBV carriers.
- Good hygienic practices, including handwashing and the use of gloves when expecting contact with blood, are important. A condom is advised for sexual intercourse, and the partner should be vaccinated. Razors, toothbrushes, and other personal items should not be shared. Close contacts of the patient with hepatitis B who are HBsAg negative and antibody negative should be vaccinated.

Hepatitis C. Risk factors for HCV infection include IV drug use, high-risk sexual behavior, tatooing, needle-stick accidents, hemophilia, and hemodialysis. Primary measures to prevent hepatitis C are the screening of blood, organ, and tissue donors; the use of infection control measures; and the modification of high-risk sexual behavior.

When a patient develops hepatitis, it is important to assess for jaundice. The patient's response to rest and activity should also be assessed. Diversional activities may help, and the patient should be assisted in understanding the temporary nature of symptoms, especially sexual abstinence, during the period of communicability.

- The nurse should try to determine whether there is something that appeals to the patient with anorexia. Small, frequent meals may be preferable to three large ones and may also help prevent nausea.
- The patient should be assessed for manifestations indicative of complications, including bleeding tendencies with increasing prothrombin time values, symptoms of encephalopathy, or markedly abnormal liver function tests

▼ **Patient Teaching**
- Teach the patient and family about preventive measures and how to prevent transmission to other family members. The patient should know what symptoms need to be reported to the physician.
- Stress the importance of regular follow-up for at least 1 year after the diagnosis of hepatitis. Because relapses are fairly common with hepatitis B and C, the patient should be instructed

about the symptoms of recurrence. Alcohol should be avoided for 1 year because it is detoxified in the liver and may interfere with recovery.

- The patient with hepatitis B should be instructed to use condoms when engaging in sexual intercourse until tests for HBsAg are negative.
- A patient who remains positive for HbsAg is a carrier and should never be a blood donor.
- The patient who is receiving α-interferon for the treatment of hepatitis B or C requires education regarding the medication. α-Interferon needs to be administered by intramuscular (IM) or subcutaneous (SC) injection; thus the patient or a family member needs to be taught how to administer the drug.

HERNIA

Definition/Description
A hernia is a protrusion of a viscus through an abnormal opening or a weakened area in the wall of the cavity in which it is normally contained. A hernia may occur in any part of the body, but it usually occurs within the abdominal cavity.

- If the hernia can be placed back into the abdominal cavity, it is known as *reducible*. The hernia can be reduced by manipulation, or it can occur without manipulation when the person lies down.
- If the hernia cannot be placed back into the abdominal cavity, it is known as *irreducible* or *incarcerated*. In this situation intestinal flow may be obstructed. When the hernia is irreducible and the intestinal flow and blood supply are obstructed, the hernia is strangulated. The result is an acute intestinal obstruction.

Types
The types of hernias include inguinal, femoral, umbilical, and ventral (incisional).

- *Inguinal* hernia is the most common type of hernia and occurs at the point of weakness in the abdominal wall where the spermatic cord in men and the round ligament in women emerge. An inguinal hernia is more common in men. When the protrusion escapes through the inguinal ring and follows the spermatic cord or round ligament, it is termed an *indirect* hernia. When it escapes through the posterior inguinal wall, it is a *direct* hernia.
- *Femoral hernia* occurs when there is a protrusion through the femoral ring into the femoral canal. It becomes strangulated easily and occurs more frequently in women.

- *Umbilical hernia* occurs when the rectus muscle is weak or the umbilical opening fails to close after birth. It is found most commonly in children.
- *Ventral,* or *incisional, hernias* occur due to a weakness of the abdominal wall at the site of a previous incision. It is found most commonly in patients who are obese, who have had multiple surgical procedures in the same area, or who have had inadequate wound healing because of poor nutrition or infection.

Clinical Manifestations

A hernia commonly occurs over the involved area when the patient stands or strains. There may be some discomfort as a result of tension; severe pain occurs if the hernia becomes strangulated. In this situation, the clinical manifestations of a bowel obstruction, such as vomiting, crampy abdominal pain, or distention, are found. Diagnosis is based on history and physical examination findings.

Collaborative Care

Surgery is the treatment of choice for hernias to prevent the possible complication of strangulation. Surgical repair of a hernia is known as a *herniorrhaphy.* The reinforcement of the weakened area with wire, fascia, or mesh is known as a *hernioplasty.* When there is strangulation, necrosis and gangrene may develop if immediate care is not given. Bowel resection of the involved area or a temporary colostomy may be needed to treat a strangulated hernia.

Nursing Management

Some patients with hernias may wear a truss, which is a pad placed over the hernia and held in place with a belt. The truss is worn to keep the hernia from protruding. If a patient wears a truss, the nurse should check for skin irritation caused by continual rubbing of the truss.

After a hernia repair, the patient may have difficulty voiding. Therefore the nurse should observe for a distended bladder.

- Scrotal edema is a painful complication after inguinal hernia repair. A scrotal support with application of an ice bag may help relieve pain and edema.
- Coughing is not encouraged, but deep breathing and turning should be done. If the patient needs to cough or sneeze, the incision should be splinted during coughing, and sneezing should be done with mouth open.
- After discharge the patient may be restricted from heavy lifting or physical activities for 6 to 8 weeks.

HERPES, GENITAL

Definition/Description
There are two different strains of herpes simplex virus (HSV) that cause infection.

- HSV type 1 (HSV-1) generally causes infection above the waist, involving the gingivae, dermis, upper respiratory tract, and central nervous system (CNS).
- HSV type 2 (HSV-2) most frequently involves the genital tract and perineum (i.e., locations below the waist).

However, either strain of HSV can cause disease on the mouth or genitals. When a person is infected with HSV, the virus usually persists within the individual for life. The incubation period ranges from 1 to 45 days with an average of 6 days.

- About 500,000 people a year contract genital herpes. Most people (80%) infected with HSV are asymptomatic or unaware of their infection.

Pathophysiology
In the course of primary infection, HSV is established in the sensory nerve ganglion innervating the primary site. Upon activation, the virus travels down the nerve axon to the skin or mucous membranes. Additional sexual contact is not necessary for a recurrence of HSV infection. The recurrent infection produces a syndrome similar to but less intense than the primary infection.

Because HSV is readily inactivated at room temperature and by drying, airborne and fomitic spread have not been documented as a significant means of transmission. The virus enters through the mucous membranes or breaks in the skin during contact with an infected person. There does not appear to be any period of time when viral transmission is not possible once primary HSV-2 infection has occurred. Women with recurrent symptomatic genital herpes shed the virus up to 1% of the time even when no visible lesions are present.

Clinical Manifestations
A patient with a primary HSV-2 infection initially complains of burning or tingling at the site of inoculation. Vesicular lesions, which may occur on the penis, scrotum, vulva, perineum, perianal region, vagina, or cervix, contain large quantities of infectious viral particles. The lesions rupture and form shallow, moist ulcerations. Finally, crusting and epithelialization of the erosions occur.

- Primary infections tend to be associated with local inflammation and pain accompanied by systemic manifestations of fever, headache, malaise, myalgia, and regional lymphadenopathy.

H

- Urination may be painful, caused by the urine touching active lesions. Retention may occur as a result of HSV urethritis or cystitis.
- A purulent vaginal discharge may develop with HSV cervicitis.
- In women, the duration of symptoms is longer with a greater frequency of complications.

Many HSV-2 infections, both primary and secondary, are asymptomatic. Therefore transmission of genital herpes can occur by means of sexual contact with an excretor of the virus who is free of symptoms.

After the first infection, HSV-2 establishes latency in the sacral ganglia and may be reactivated periodically. Recurrent attacks occur in about 50% to 80% of all persons during the year following the primary episode. Stress, sexual activity, sunburn, and fever tend to trigger recurrence. Many patients can predict a recurrence by noticing early symptoms of tingling, burning, and itching at the site where lesions eventually arise. Symptoms of recurrent episodes are less severe, and the unilateral lesions heal within 8 to 12 days. With time, recurrent lesions generally occur less frequently.

Complications

Although most infections are relatively benign, complications of genital herpes may involve the CNS, causing aseptic meningitis and lower motor neuron damage.

- Neuron damage may result in atonic bladder, impotence, and constipation.
- The most common complication is autoinoculation of the virus to extragenital sites such as fingers (whitlow), lips, and breasts.

Diagnostic Studies

- Diagnosis is usually based on the patient's symptoms and history.
- Viral isolation by tissue culture from active lesions confirms diagnosis.
- Serologic methods for identification of specific antibody to the glycoprotein G component of HSV.

Collaborative Care

The skin lesions of genital herpes heal spontaneously unless secondary infection occurs. Symptomatic treatments, such as good genital hygiene and the wearing of loose-fitting cotton undergarments, should be encouraged. The lesions should be kept clean and dry to ensure complete drying of the perineal area; women may use a hair dryer set on a cool setting.

- Frequent sitz baths may soothe the area and reduce inflammation. Pain may require a local anesthetic such as lidocaine (Xylocaine) or systemic analgesics such as codeine and aspirin.

- Barrier forms of contraception, especially condoms, used during asymptomatic periods, decrease the transmission of the disease. When lesions are present, the patient should avoid sexual activity altogether as even barrier protection is not satisfactory in eliminating disease transmission.
- Acyclovir (Zovirax), famciclovir (Famvir), and valacyclovir (Valtrex) inhibit herpetic viral replication. They are also prescribed for primary infections or suppression of frequent recurrences (more than six episodes per year). Although not a cure, these drugs shorten the duration of viral shedding and healing time of genital lesions and suppress 75% of recurrences with daily use. Continued use of oral acyclovir for up to 5 years is safe and effective but should be interrupted after 1 year to assess the patient's rate of recurrent episodes. IV acyclovir is reserved for severe or life-threatening infections.

Nursing Management: Sexually Transmitted Diseases
See Chlamydial Infection, p. 127.

HIATAL HERNIA

Definition/Description

Hiatal hernia is a herniation of a portion of the stomach into the esophagus through an opening (or hiatus) in the diaphragm. It is also referred to as diaphragmatic hernia or esophageal hernia. Hiatal hernias are more common in older adults and occur more frequently in women than in men.

Hiatal hernias are classified into two types:

- A *sliding hernia* occurs at the junction of the stomach and esophagus and is located above the hiatus of the diaphragm. It "slides" into the thoracic cavity through the diaphragm hiatal opening when the patient is supine and usually goes back into the abdominal cavity when the patient is standing upright. This is the most common type of hiatal hernia.
- A *paraesophageal* or *rolling hernia* occurs at the esophagogastric junction where the fundus and greater curvature of the stomach roll up through the diaphragm to form a pocket alongside the esophagus.

Pathophysiology

The actual cause of hiatal hernia is unknown. Many factors may contribute to the development of hiatal hernia, including structural changes, such as weakening of the muscles in the diaphragm around the esophagogastric opening. Factors that increase intraabdominal pressure, including obesity, pregnancy, ascites, intense physical exertion, and heavy lifting on a continual basis, may also contribute to the development of a hiatal hernia. In some cases, congenital weakness is a contributing factor.

Clinical Manifestations

Signs and symptoms frequently mimic gallbladder disease, peptic ulcer disease, or angina. However, some patients with hiatal hernia have no symptoms.

- The reflux and discomfort described are associated with position, occurring soon or several hours after lying down. Bending over may cause a severe burning pain, which is usually relieved by sitting or standing. Large meals, alcohol, and smoking may precipitate pain.
- Nocturnal attacks are common, especially if the person has eaten before going to sleep.

Complications may include problems such as hemorrhage from erosion, stenosis, ulcerations of the herniated portion of the stomach, strangulation of the hernia, and regurgitation with tracheal aspiration.

Diagnostic Studies

- Barium swallow may show gastric mucosa protrusion through the esophageal hiatus.
- Esophagoscopy is useful to determine incompetence of the lower esophageal sphincter (LES) and whether gastric reflux is present.
- pH monitoring of gastric and esophageal secretions; acidic gastric contents in the lower esophagus.
- Motility (manometry) studies may be done to determine pressure gradients.

Nursing and Collaborative Management

Conservative management includes the administration of antacids and antisecretory agents, elimination of constricting garments, avoidance of lifting and straining, and elimination of alcohol and smoking. Elevation of the bed on 4- to 6-inch blocks assists gravity in maintaining the stomach in the abdominal cavity and also helps prevent reflux and tracheal aspiration. If obese, the patient is encouraged to lose weight.

Surgical therapy may include *valvuloplasties* or *antireflux* procedures.

- There are three slightly varied surgical procedures: the Nissen fundoplication, the Hill gastroplexy, and the Belsey fundoplication. These three surgical procedures are all variations of fundoplication, which involves the "wrapping" of the fundus of the stomach around the lower portion of the esophagus in varying degrees.

- These procedures reduce the hernia, provide an acceptable LES pressure, and prevent movement of the gastroesophageal junction. They are effective in preventing reflux in 90% of all patients.
- The Nissen fundoplication procedure is being performed laparoscopically with increasing frequency.

Postoperative care focuses on the prevention of respiratory complications, the maintenance of fluid and electrolyte balance, and the prevention of infection.

- Respiratory complications can occur in a patient treated by an abdominal approach because of the high abdominal incision. Coughing and deep breathing are essential to reexpand the lungs.
- Patient should receive only IV fluids until peristalsis returns; the need to maintain accurate intake and output records and observe for fluid and electrolyte imbalances is important.

▼ **Patient Teaching**

After successful surgical intervention, there should be no symptoms of gastric reflux.

- The patient should be instructed to report symptoms such as heartburn and regurgitation. In the early postoperative period there is usually mild dysphagia caused by edema, but it should resolve.
- The patient should be told to report persistent dysphagia, epigastric fullness, and bloating. Immediately after the surgical procedure, the patient cannot voluntarily vomit or belch; this may cause bloating and abdominal discomfort.
- Emphasize with patient that a normal diet can be resumed within 6 weeks and that the patient should avoid foods that are gas forming. Food should be thoroughly chewed.

H

HODGKIN'S DISEASE

Definition/Description

Hodgkin's disease, which makes up 15% of all lymphomas, is a malignant condition characterized by proliferation of abnormal, giant, multinucleated cells called Reed-Sternberg cells, which are located in the lymph nodes. The disease has a bimodal age-specific incidence, occurring most frequently in persons from 15 to 35 years of age and above 50 years of age. In adults, it is twice as prevalent in men as in women.

Pathophysiology

Although the cause of Hodgkin's disease remains unknown, several key factors are thought to play a role in its development. The main interacting factors include infection with the Epstein-Barr virus, genetic predisposition, and exposure to occupational toxins.

In Hodgkin's disease the normal structure of the lymph nodes is destroyed by hyperplasia of monocytes and macrophages. The disease is believed to arise in a single location (it originates in the lymph nodes in 90% of patients) and then spread along adjacent lymphatics. It eventually infiltrates other organs, especially the lungs, spleen, and liver. In about two thirds of patients the cervical lymph nodes are the first to be affected.

Clinical Manifestations

The initial sign is most often an enlargement of the cervical, axillary, or inguinal lymph nodes. The enlarged nodes are not painful unless pressure is exerted on adjacent nerves.

- The patient may notice weight loss, fatigue, weakness, fever, chills, tachycardia, or night sweats. A group of initial findings, including fever, night sweats, and weight loss (referred to as *B symptoms*), correlates with a worse prognosis.
- Generalized pruritus without skin lesions may develop. Cough, dyspnea, stridor, and dysphagia may all reflect mediastinal node involvement.
- In more advanced disease there is hepatomegaly and splenomegaly. Anemia results from increased destruction as well as decreased production of erythrocytes. Intrathoracic involvement may lead to superior vena cava syndrome. Enlarged retroperitoneal nodes may cause palpable abdominal masses or interfere with renal function.
- Jaundice may result from liver involvement.
- Spinal cord compression leading to paraplegia may occur with extradural involvement.

Diagnostic Studies

- Peripheral blood analysis often reveals microcytic hypochromic anemia; neutrophilic leukocytosis (15,000 to 28,000/μl [15 to 28 $\times$ 10^9/L]), which may be associated with lymphopenia; and an increased platelet count.
- Other blood studies may show hypoferremia caused by excessive iron uptake by the liver and spleen, elevated alkaline phosphatase from liver and bone involvement, hypercalcemia from bone involvement, and hypoalbuminemia.
- Excisional lymph node biopsy offers a definitive diagnosis. If removed, an enlarged peripheral lymph node can be examined histologically for the presence of Reed-Sternberg cells.

- Bone marrow biopsy is performed as an important aspect of staging.
- Chest x-rays, radioisotope studies, and CT scans may show mediastinal lymphadenopathy, renal displacement caused by retroperitoneal node enlargement, abdominal lymph node enlargement, and liver, spleen, bone, and brain infiltration.
- Lymphangiography, a radiographic dye study that uses blue dye injected into the lymphatic system, assesses the lymph nodes and lymph vessels. This test can also visualize retroperitoneal structures.

Collaborative Care

Treatment decisions are made based on the stage of the disease. Radiation therapy given over 4 to 6 weeks can cure 95% of patients with stage I or stage II disease. Combination chemotherapy is used in some early stages in patients believed to have resistant disease or at increased risk for relapse. Stage IIIA disease is treated with both radiotherapy and chemotherapy (see Radiation Therapy, p. 681, and Chemotherapy, p. 643). The role of radiation as a supplement to chemotherapy in stages III and IV varies depending on the disease sites.

Advances in treatment now enable some stage IIIB and stage IV diseases to be cured with high-dose chemotherapy and bone marrow or peripheral stem cell transplantation. Intensive chemotherapy with or without the use of bone marrow transplantation and hematopoietic growth factors is the treatment of choice for advanced Hodgkin's disease (stages IIIB and IV).

Nursing Management

Nursing care for Hodgkin's disease is largely based on managing pancytopenia and other side effects of therapy.

- Because the survival of patients with Hodgkin's disease depends on their response to treatment, supporting the patient through the immunosuppressive state is extremely important.
- Psychosocial considerations are just as important as they are with leukemia (see Leukemia, p. 360). Although the prognosis for Hodgkin's disease is better than that for many forms of cancer or leukemia, patients must still be helped to deal with all of the physical, psychologic, social, and spiritual consequences of their disease.
- Evaluation of patients for long-term effects of therapy are important because delayed consequences of the disease and treatment may not be apparent for many years.

HUMAN IMMUNODEFICIENCY VIRUS INFECTION

Definition/Description
Human immunodeficiency virus (HIV) infection follows a highly individualized course from the time of infection to the clinical manifestations of acquired immunodeficiency syndrome (AIDS). More than 29 million people worldwide are infected with HIV. AIDS is the final phase of a chronic, progressive immune function disorder caused by HIV.

Pathophysiology
HIV is a fragile virus that can be transmitted from human to human through infected blood, semen, vaginal secretions, and breast milk. Sexual contact with an infected partner is the most common method of transmission. A HIV-infected individual can transmit HIV to others starting a few days after the initial infection. The ability to transmit HIV is lifelong because HIV has no noninfectious state.

HIV is a ribonucleic acid (RNA) virus. RNA viruses are called retroviruses because they replicate in a "backward" manner, going from RNA to deoxyribonucleic acid (DNA). Like all viruses, HIV is an obligate parasite; it cannot replicate unless it is in a living cell. HIV can infect several types of human cells; predominately infected are CD4+ T cells (lymphocytes). Immunosuppression leads to the development of infections and cancers.

Clinical Manifestations
Acute retroviral syndrome (the development of HIV antibodies or seroconversion) is frequently accompanied by a flulike or mononucleosis-like syndrome of fever, lymphadenopathy, pharyngitis, headache, malaise, nausea, and a diffuse rash.

- Symptoms generally occur 1 to 3 weeks after the initial infection and last for 1 to 2 weeks. CD4+ T cell counts will fall temporarily during this time but will quickly return to baseline. In most people these symptoms are mild and may be mistaken for a cold or flu.

In *early HIV infection* the patient is generally healthy but has some vague symptoms, including fatigue, headache, low grade fever, and night sweats.

Early symptomatic disease occurs toward the end of early HIV infection and before a diagnosis of AIDS. The CD4+ T cell count drops below 500 to 600 cells/μL and early symptomatic disease develops.

- Symptoms can include constitutional problems such as persistent fever, recurrent drenching night sweats, chronic diarrhea, headaches, and fatigue. Other problems that may occur include localized infections (oropharyngeal candidiasis, shingles, oral hairy leukoplakia), lymphadenopathy, and neurologic manifestations (myopathy and aseptic meningitis).

A diagnosis of AIDS cannot be made until the HIV-infected patient meets the case definition criteria established by the Centers for Disease Control and Prevention (CDC), which include the development of at least one of these additional criteria:

1. CD4$^+$ lymphocyte count below 200/μL
2. Development of an opportunistic infection (see Table 13-1, Lewis and others, *Medical-Surgical Nursing,* edition 5, p. 245)
3. Development of an opportunistic cancer (e.g., Kaposi's sarcoma)
4. Wasting syndrome (defined as a loss of 10% or more of ideal body mass)
5. Development of dementia

Diagnostic Studies

- Highly sensitive enzyme immunoassay (EIA) or enzyme-linked immunosorbent assay (ELISA) detects serum antibodies that bind to HIV antigens.
- Western blot or immunofluorescence assay (IFA) more specifically confirms HIV.
- CD4$^+$ T cell count to monitor the progression of the infection.
- White blood cell (WBC) count, red blood cell (RBC) count, and platelets decrease with the progression of HIV.

Collaborative Care

HIV infection management focuses on monitoring the disease progression and immune function, preventing the development of opportunistic diseases, initiating and monitoring antiretroviral therapy, detecting and treating opportunistic diseases, managing symptoms, and preventing complications of treatment.

Drugs that have been approved to treat HIV infection decrease HIV replication and may delay disease progression. These drugs include zidovudine (AZT, ZDV, Retrovir), didanosine (ddl, Videx), zalcitabine (ddC, HIVID), stavudine (d4T, Zerit), lamivudine (3TC, Epivir), and nevirapine (Viramune). Antiretroviral agents used in HIV infection are described in Table 13-7, Lewis and others, *Medical-Surgical Nursing,* edition 5, p. 261.

Opportunistic diseases and debilitating problems associated with HIV can be delayed or prevented through prophylactic interventions, including pneumococcal and hepatitis B vaccines, low-dose acyclovir (Zovirax) for herpes simplex viral infection, isoniazid (INH) for tuberculosis (TB) if reactive purified protein derivative (PPD) skin test is present, trimethoprim-sulfamethoxazole (TMP-SMX) inhalation for *Pneumocystis carinii,* rifabutin (Mycobutin) for *Mycobacterium avium* complex, ganciclovir (Cytovene) for *Cytomegalovirus,* and nutritional support.

Nursing Management

Goals

The patient with HIV infection will comply with the medical regimen; prevent opportunistic diseases; not transmit HIV to others; maintain or develop healthy, supportive relationships; come to terms with issues related to disease, death, and spirituality; and maintain activities and productivity for as long as possible. Goals will change as new treatment protocols develop and as HIV disease progresses.

Nursing Diagnoses

- Pain *related to* neuropathy, arthralgia, lymphadenopathy, and opportunistic infections
- Anxiety *related to* multiple physical, emotional, and economic changes and losses
- Altered thought processes *related to* hypoxemia, fever, dehydration, and neurologic changes
- Altered nutrition: less than body requirements *related to* anorexia, impaired swallowing, oral lesions, fever, fatigue, and depression
- Risk for activity intolerance *related to* chronic HIV infection, stress, anemia, and malnutrition
- Diarrhea *related to* opportunistic infections and tube feeding intolerance
- Impaired gas exchange *related to* pulmonary infection, hypoxemia, anemia, ineffective cough, anxiety, and pain

Nursing Interventions

The initial nursing focus is to prevent infection. In the absence of a vaccination for HIV, education and behavioral changes are the only effective prevention tools.

- Encourage the early detection of HIV infection, including pre- and post-test counseling as the patient awaits the results of HIV antibody testing.
- Intervention after detection should focus on the early recognition of symptoms, opportunistic diseases, and psychosocial problems.

Useful interventions for HIV-infected patients include nutritional support to maintain lean mass, tobacco- and drug-use cessation interventions, moderation or elimination of alcohol intake, regular exercise, stress reduction, avoiding exposure to new infectious agents, mental health counseling, and involvement in support groups.

- Facilitating empowerment is particularly important because the individual with HIV infection often experiences losses, including an overwhelming feeling of loss of control.

- Symptomatic patient care includes education and treatment for diarrhea, fatigue, wasting syndrome, and AIDS-dementia complex.
- The focus of terminal care is patient comfort, facilitation of emotional and spiritual issues, and helping significant others deal with grief and loss.

▼ **Patient Teaching**

Emphasis is placed on the prevention of HIV infection and on risk-reducing activities related to sexual intercourse, drug use, and occupational exposure. Once infected, the focus is on education and counseling to prevent further virus transmission.

- Educate the patient and family about symptoms to report to ensure early recognition and treatment (see Table 13-18 for a patient teaching guide, Lewis and others, *Medical-Surgical Nursing,* edition 5, p. 262).
- Teach about the actions and common side effects of drug therapy; provide a written list of medications with times, dosages, and possible side effects to promote safe drug use (see Table 13-17 for a patient teaching guide on the use of antiretroviral drugs, *Medical-Surgical Nursing,* p. 261).
- Teach and encourage the use of alternate methods of pain relief.
- Teach energy conservation measures and the use of assistive devices to increase safety and decrease fatigue.
- Discuss infection control measures with the patient, family, and visitors.
- Provide information about support groups and community resources.

HUNTINGTON'S DISEASE

Definition/Description

Huntington's disease (HD) is a genetically transmitted, autosomal dominant disorder that affects both men and women of all races. The offspring of a person with this disease have a 50% risk of inheriting it. Like Parkinson's disease, the pathology of HD involves the basal ganglia and the extrapyramidal system. However, instead of a deficiency of dopamine (DA), HD involves a deficiency of the neurotransmitters acetylcholine (ACh) and gamma-aminobutyric acid (GABA). The net effect is an excess of DA, which leads to symptoms opposite those of Parkinson's disease.

Clinical manifestations typically appear between the ages of 35 and 45 years and are characterized by abnormal and excessive involuntary movements *(chorea)*. These are writhing, twisting movements of the face, limbs, and body that get worse as the disease progresses.

- Facial movements involving speech, chewing, and swallowing are affected; this may cause aspiration and malnutrition. The gait deteriorates and ambulation eventually becomes impossible. Perhaps the most devastating deterioration is in mental functioning, including symptoms of intellectual decline, emotional lability, and psychotic behavior.
- Death usually occurs 10 to 20 years after the onset of symptoms.

Diagnosis in the past was based on family history and clinical symptoms. However, since the gene for HD has been discovered, one can now be tested for the presence of the gene. People who are asymptomatic but who have a positive family history of HD face the dilemma of whether or not to get tested. If the test is positive, the person will develop HD, but when and to what extent the disease develops cannot be determined.

Because there is no cure, collaborative care is palliative. Antipsychotic, antidepressant, and antichorea medications are prescribed and have some benefit. However, they do not alter the course of the disease. This disease presents a great challenge to health care professionals.

The goal of nursing care is to provide the most comfortable environment possible for the patient and family by maintaining physical safety, treating physical symptoms, and providing emotional and psychologic support.

- Because of the choreic movements, caloric requirements are high. Patients may require as high as 4,000 to 5,000 cal/day to maintain body weight. As the disease progresses, meeting caloric needs becomes a greater challenge when the patient has difficulty swallowing and holding the head still. Depression and mental deterioration can also compromise nutritional intake.

HYPERPARATHYROIDISM

Definition/Description

Hyperparathyroidism is a condition involving increased secretion of parathyroid hormone (PTH). PTH helps regulate calcium and phosphate levels by stimulating bone resorption, renal tubular reabsorption of calcium, and activation of vitamin D.

Hyperparathyroidism is classified as primary, secondary, or tertiary.

- *Primary hyperparathyroidism* is due to an increased secretion of PTH leading to disorders of calcium, phosphate, and bone metabolism. Excessive concentrations of circulating PTH usually lead to hypercalcemia and hypophosphatemia. The most common cause is a benign pituitary neoplasm or a single adenoma (80% of cases). Previous head and neck radiation are predisposing factors for adenoma development.
- *Secondary hyperparathyroidism* is a compensatory response to conditions that induce or cause hypocalcemia, the main stimulus of PTH secretion. These conditions include vitamin D deficiencies, malabsorption, chronic renal failure, and hyperphosphatemia.
- *Tertiary hyperparathyroidism* occurs when there is hyperplasia of the parathyroid glands and a loss of negative feedback from circulating calcium levels. This causes autonomous secretion of PTH even with normal calcium levels. It is observed in the patient who has had a kidney transplant after a long period of dialysis treatment for chronic renal failure.

Pathophysiology
Increased PTH has a multisystem effect (see Table 47-10, Lewis and others, *Medical-Surgical Nursing,* edition 5, p. 1429).
- In the bones, decreased bone density, cyst formation, and general weakness can occur as a result of the effect of PTH on osteoclastic and osteoblastic activity.
- In the kidneys, excess calcium cannot be reabsorbed, which leads to hypercalciuria. This urinary calcium, along with a large amount of urinary phosphate, can lead to calculi formation. PTH stimulates the synthesis of a form of vitamin D, which increases GI absorption of calcium.

Clinical Manifestations
Hyperparathyroidism has varying symptoms, including weakness, loss of appetite, constipation, increased need for sleep, and shortened attention span.
- Major signs include loss of calcium from the bones (osteoporosis), broken bones, and kidney stones (nephrolithiasis). Neuromuscular abnormalities are characterized by muscle weakness, particularly in proximal muscles of the lower extremities.

Complications include renal failure, pancreatitis, collapse of vertebral bodies, cardiac changes, and long bone and rib fractures.

Diagnostic Studies
- Radioimmunoassay measurement of PTH, which is elevated
- Serum calcium levels elevated with decreased phosphorus levels

- Urine calcium, serum chloride, serum uric acid, and serum creatinine elevated
- Serum amylase (if pancreatitis present) and alkaline phosphatase (if bone disease present) both elevated

Collaborative Care

The treatment objectives are to relieve the symptoms and prevent complications caused by excess PTH. The choice of therapy depends on the urgency of the clinical situation, the degree of hypercalcemia, the underlying disorder, and the status of renal and hepatic function.

- Parathyroid tumors should be removed surgically. The parathyroids occasionally lie in ectopic sites such as the mediastinum. Generally, a single gland is removed if an adenoma is the cause of hyperparathyroidism. When cancer is the cause, all of the parathyroids are removed.
- If symptoms are mild, or if the patient is elderly or at increased surgical risk from other health problems, a conservative management approach is used. This includes an annual examination with tests for serum PTH, calcium, phosphorus, and alkaline phosphatase levels and renal function; x-rays to assess for metabolic bone disease; and measurement of urinary calcium excretion.

Additional measures include maintenance of a high fluid intake, a moderate calcium intake, and phosphorus supplementation, unless contraindicated by an increased risk for urinary calculi formation.

Drug Therapy

Plicamycin (Mithracin), an antihypercalcemic agent, lowers serum calcium within 48 hours. However, because of toxic side effects, its use is limited to patients with metastatic parathyroid carcinoma and severe bone disease. Estrogen or progestin therapy can reduce serum and urinary calcium levels in postmenopausal women and may retard demineralization of the skeleton.

- In severe hyperparathyroidism, normal saline is given IV to correct fluid volume deficit and promote calcium excretion. Furosemide (Lasix) is given orally or IV to decrease renal tubular reabsorption of calcium.

Nursing Management
Goals

The patient with hyperparathyroidism will maintain a satisfactory activity level, keep a consistently high fluid intake, not experience any serious complications related to the disease or its treatment, maintain a positive self-image, and accept and comply with the long-term nature of the problem

See NCP 47-3 for the patient with hyperparathyroidism, Lewis and others, *Medical-Surgical Nursing,* edition 5, p. 1432.

Nursing Diagnoses

- Activity intolerance *related to* muscle weakness and fatigue
- Sensory/perceptual alterations *related to* slowed mentation, depression, and drowsiness
- Body image disturbance *related to* weight loss, weakness, fatigue, and mental status changes
- Altered nutrition: less than body requirements *related to* anorexia and nausea
- Risk for injury *related to* possible fractures from decreased bone density and joint contractures from improper body alignment
- Constipation *related to* dehydration and inactivity

Nursing Interventions

If surgery is performed, close monitoring of the patient's vital signs is required. Other aspects of care are similar to those after thyroidectomy (see Hyperthyroidism, p. 329).

The major postoperative complications are tetany and fluid and electrolyte disturbances. Tetany is usually apparent early in the postoperative period but may develop over several days. Mild tetany, characterized by an unpleasant tingling of the hands and around the mouth, may be present but should abate without problems. If tetany becomes more severe (e.g., muscular spasms or laryngospasms develop), IV calcium may be given.

- Strict monitoring of intake and output is necessary to evaluate fluid status.
- Calcium, potassium, phosphate, and magnesium levels are assessed frequently.
- Mobility is encouraged to promote bone calcification.
- If surgery is not performed, treatment to relieve symptoms and prevent complications is carried out.

▼ **Patient Teaching**

- The nurse can assist the patient with hyperparathyroidism to adapt the meal plan to his or her lifestyle. A referral to a dietitian may be useful.
- Since immobility can aggravate bone loss, the nurse can assist the patient in implementing an exercise program and identifying places, such as shopping malls and YMCAs, to exercise safely.
- The patient should be encouraged to keep annual appointments. All tests being performed should be explained. The patient should also be instructed in the symptoms of hypocalcemia or hypercalcemia and when to report these should they occur.

H

HYPERSENSITIVITY REACTIONS

Definition/Description

The classification of hypersensitivity reactions may be done according to the source of the antigen, time sequence (immediate or delayed), or the basic immunologic mechanisms causing the injury.

- Four types of hypersensitivity reactions exist; Types I, II, and III are immediate and are examples of humoral immunity, while Type IV is a delayed hypersensitivity reaction and is related to cell-mediated immunity. Table 36 presents a summary of the four types of hypersensitivity reactions.

Type I: anaphylactoid reactions. These occur *only* in susceptible persons who are highly sensitized to specific allergens. IgE antibodies, produced in response to the allergen, attach to mast cells and basophils. On first exposure to the allergen, immunoglobulin E (IgE) antibodies are produced. On subsequent exposures, the allergen links with IgE bound to mast cells or basophils and triggers degranulation of the cells. In this process, mediators (e.g., histamine, serotonin) are released, which then attack target organs, causing clinical allergy symptoms.

- These reversible effects include smooth muscle contraction, increased vascular permeability, vasodilation, hypotension, increased secretion of mucus, and itching.
- The capacity to become sensitized to an allergen appears to be inherited.
- Clinical manifestations of an anaphylactoid reaction depend on whether the mediators remain local or become systemic. When mediators remain localized, a cutaneous response called the *wheal-and-flare reaction* occurs. This reaction is characterized by a pale wheal containing edematous fluid surrounded by a red flare from hyperemia. The reaction occurs in minutes or hours and is usually not dangerous.

Anaphylactic shock (anaphylaxis) occurs when mediators are released systemically (e.g., after the injection of a drug or an insect sting). The reaction occurs within minutes and is life threatening because of airway obstruction and vascular collapse. Initial symptoms include edema and itching at the site of exposure to the allergen. Within minutes, shock manifested by rapid, weak pulse; hypotension; dilated pupils; dyspnea; and cyanosis may occur. This is compounded by bronchial edema and angioedema. Death will occur if emergency treatment is not initiated (see Allergic Disorders, Nursing and Collaborative Management, p. 15). Allergens leading to anaphylactic shock in hypersensitive persons may include drugs (e.g., penicillin),

Table 36 Types of Hypersensitivity Reactions

	Type I Anaphylactic	Type II Cytotoxic	Type III Immune complex–mediated	Type IV Delayed-hypersensitivity
Antigen	Exogenous pollen, food, drugs, dust	Cell surface of RBCs Basement membrane	Extracellular fungal, viral, bacterial	Intracellular or extracellular
Antibody involved	IgE	IgG IgM	IgG IgM	None
Complement involved	No	Yes	Yes	No
Mediators of injury	Histamine SRS-A	Complement lysis Neutrophils	Neutrophils Complement lysis	Lymphokines T-cytotoxic cells Monocytes/macrophages Lysosomal enzymes
Examples	Allergic rhinitis Asthma	Transfusion reaction Goodpasture's syndrome	Serum sickness Systemic lupus erythematosus Rheumatoid arthritis	Contact dermatitis Tumor rejection Transplant rejection
Skin test	Wheal and flare	None	Erythema and edema in 3 to 8 hours	Erythema and edema in 24 to 48 hours (e.g., TB test)

IgE, Immunoglobulin E; *IgG*, immunoglobulin G; *IgM*, immunoglobulin M; *RBCs*, red blood cells; *SRS-A*, slow-reacting substance of anaphylaxis; *TB*, tuberculosis.

H

insect venom, animal serum (e.g., tetanus antitoxin), foods (e.g., nuts), and treatments (e.g., blood products).

Allergic rhinitis or *hay fever* is the most common type I hypersensitivity reaction. It may occur year round (perennial allergic rhinitis), or it may be seasonal (seasonal allergic rhinitis).

- Airborne substances such as pollen or dust are the primary cause of allergic rhinitis. Perennial allergic rhinitis may be caused by dust, molds, and animal dander. Seasonal allergic rhinitis is commonly caused by trees, weeds, or grasses.
- Target areas affected are the conjunctiva of the eyes and the mucosa of the upper respiratory tract. Symptoms include nasal discharge, sneezing, lacrimation, mucosal swelling with airway obstruction, and pruritus around the eyes, nose, throat, and mouth (see Lewis and others, *Medical-Surgical Nursing,* edition 5, p. 219).

Atopic dermatitis is a chronic, inherited skin disorder characterized by exacerbations and remissions. It is caused by several environmental allergens that are difficult to identify. Skin lesions are generalized and involve vasodilation of the blood vessels, resulting in interstitial edema with vesicle formation.

Urticaria (hives) is a cutaneous lesion that can occur as a reaction to systemic allergens. It is characterized by transient wheals (pink, raised, edematous, pruritic areas) that vary in size and shape and may occur throughout the body. Urticaria develops rapidly after exposure to an allergen and may last minutes or hours. Histamine causes localized vasodilation (erythema), transudation of fluid (wheal), and flaring. Internal urticaria is characterized by edema in internal organs (see the section on urticaria, Lewis and others, *Medical-Surgical Nursing,* edition 5, p. 220).

Type II: cytotoxic and cytolytic reactions. These involve the direct binding of immunoglobulin G (IgG) or immunoglobulin M (IgM) antibodies to an antigen on the cell surface. Antigen-antibody complexes activate the complement system, which mediates the reaction. Cellular tissue is rapidly destroyed in one of two ways: activation of the complement cascade resulting in cytolysis or enhanced phagocytosis.

- Target cells frequently destroyed in type II reactions are erythrocytes, platelets, and leukocytes. Pathophysiologic disorders characteristic of type II reactions include ABO- and Rh-incompatibility transfusion reaction, autoimmune and drug-related hemolytic anemias, leukopenias, thrombocytopenias, erythroblastosis fetalis (hemolytic disease of the newborn), and Goodpasture's syndrome.

Type III: immune-complex reactions. These involve antigens combining with immunoglobulins (IgG and IgM classes) to form complexes that are too small to be effectively removed by the mononuclear phagocyte system. Therefore the complexes deposit in tissue or small blood vessels. They cause the fixation of complement and the release of chemotactic factors that lead to inflammation and destruction of involved tissue. Type III reactions may be local or systemic and immediate or delayed.

- Manifestations depend on the number and location of complexes in the body.
- Common sites for deposit are the kidneys, skin, joints, lungs, and blood vessels.
- Severe type III reactions are associated with autoimmune disorders such as systemic lupus erythematosus, acute glomerulonephritis, and rheumatoid arthritis.

Type IV: delayed hypersensitivity reactions. These are called cell-mediated immune responses. The tissue damage in a type IV reaction is due to sensitized T lymphocytes attacking antigens or releasing cytokines. Macrophages and enzymes released by T lymphocytes are responsible for most of the tissue destruction. The delayed hypersensitivity response takes 24 to 48 hours. Examples of this response include contact dermatitis; hypersensitivity reactions to bacterial, fungal, and viral infections; and transplant rejections. Some drug sensitivity reactions are also in this category.

Contact dermatitis is a reaction that occurs when skin is exposed to haptens. The haptens easily penetrate the skin to combine with epidermal proteins. The hapten-carrier substance then becomes antigenic.

On subsequent exposure to the hapten, a sensitized person develops eczematous skin lesions within 48 hours. The most common haptens encountered are metal compounds (e.g., nickel, mercury); rubber compounds; catechols present in poison ivy, poison oak, and sumac; cosmetics; and some dyes.

- In acute contact dermatitis the skin lesions appear erythematous and edematous and are covered with papules, vesicles, and bullae. The involved area is very pruritic but may also burn or sting.
- When contact dermatitis becomes chronic, the lesions resemble atopic dermatitis because they are thickened, scaly, and lichenified.

H

HYPERTENSION

Definition/Description

Hypertension is a sustained elevation in BP. The diagnosis of hypertension is confirmed in the adult when systolic pressure is ≥140 mm Hg and/or diastolic pressure is ≥90 mm Hg on at least three occasions over several weeks. In the United States, 50 million people either have elevated BP or are taking antihypertensive medication. High BP is one of the major risk factors for coronary artery disease (CAD) and is the most significant risk factor for cerebrovascular disease.

- Classification of hypertension according to stages is described in Table 37.

The etiology of hypertension can be classified as primary (essential) or secondary. Primary (essential) hypertension accounts for 95% of all cases of hypertension, with the onset usually between the ages of 31 and 50 years. Although the exact cause of essential hypertension is unknown, several contributing factors, including greater than ideal body weight, diabetes mellitus (DM), sedentary lifestyle, increased sodium intake, and excessive alcohol intake, have been identified.

Pathophysiology

The hemodynamic hallmark of hypertension is persistently increased systemic vascular resistance (SVR). This persistent elevation in SVR may come about in various ways. There is probably no single cause of *primary hypertension*. It is multifactorial in origin and only some of the factors have been identified. However, risk factors have been identified that are known to be related to the development of primary hypertension or contribute to the disease (Table 38).

Secondary hypertension is elevated BP with a specific cause that can often be corrected by surgery or medication. If a person below age 20 or over age 50 suddenly develops hypertension, especially if it is severe, a secondary cause should be suspected. Causes of secondary hypertension include (1) coarctation or congenital narrowing of the aorta; (2) renal diseases, such as renal artery stenosis and parenchymal disease; (3) endocrine disorders, such as Cushing's syndrome and hyperaldosteronism; (4) neurologic disorders, such as brain tumors, quadriplegia, and head injury; (5) medications, such as sympathetic stimulants, monoamine oxidase (MAO) inhibitors taken with tyramine-containing foods, estrogen replacement therapy, oral contraceptive pills, and nonsteroidal antiinflammatory drugs (NSAIDs); and (6) pregnancy-induced hypertension.

Clinical Manifestations

Hypertension is often called the "silent killer" because it is frequently asymptomatic until it becomes severe and target disease has occurred. A patient with severe hypertension may experience a variety of symptoms secondary to the effects on blood vessels in the various organs and tissues or to the increased workload of the heart. These secondary symptoms include fatigue, reduced activity tolerance, dizziness, palpitations, angina, and dyspnea.

Table 37	Classification of Blood Pressure for Adults Aged 18 Years and Older*		

	Blood pressure (BP), mm Hg		
Category	**Systolic**		**Diastolic**
Optimal**	<120	and	<80
Normal	<130	and	<85
High-normal	130-139	or	85-89
Hypertension***			
Stage 1	140-159	or	90-99
Stage 2	160-179	or	100-109
Stage 3	≥180	or	≥110

From US Department of Health and Human Services: *The sixth report of the Joint National Committee on Detection, Evaluation, and Treatment of High Blood Pressure (JNC-VI)*, Washington, DC, 1997, National Institutes of Health.

*Not taking antihypertensive drugs and not acutely ill.

**Optimal BP with respect to cardiovascular risk is <120/80 mm Hg. However, unusually low readings should be evaluated for clinical significance.

***Based on the average of two or more readings taken at each of two or more visits after an initial screening. When systolic and diastolic BPs fall into different categories, the higher category should be selected to classify the individual's BP status. For example, 160/92 should be classified as stage 2 hypertension, and 174/120 should be classified as stage 3 hypertension. Isolated systolic hypertension is defined as systolic BP ≥140 mm Hg and diastolic BP <90 mm Hg and staged appropriately (e.g., 170/82 mm Hg is defined as stage 2 isolated systolic hypertension).

NOTE: In addition to classifying stages of hypertension based on average BP levels, the clinician should specify the presence or absence of target-organ disease and additional risk factors. This specificity is important for risk classification and treatment.

The most common complications of hypertension are target organ diseases, including hypertensive heart disease (CAD and congestive heart failure [CHF]), cerebrovascular disease, peripheral vascular disease, nephrosclerosis, and retinal damage.

Coronary artery disease and congestive heart failure. Hypertension is a major risk factor for CAD and CHF. The hypertensive patient is more susceptible to silent ischemia, unrecognized myocardial infarction (MI), and sudden cardiac death (see Coronary Artery Disease, p. 170). CHF occurs when the heart can no longer

Table 38	Risk Factors in Primary Hypertension
Age	BP rises progressively with increasing age. Elevated BP is present in approximately 50% of people over 65 years of age.
Sex	Hypertension is more prevalent in men in young adulthood and early middle age. After age 55, hypertension is more prevalent in women.
Race	Incidence of hypertension is twice as great in African-Americans as in Caucasians.
Family history	Level of BP is strongly familial. Risk of hypertension increases for those with a close relative who has hypertension.
Obesity	Weight gain is associated with increased frequency of hypertension. The risk is greatest with central abdominal obesity.
Cigarette smoking	Smoking greatly increases the risk of cardiovascular disease. Hypertensives who smoke are at even greater risk.
Excess dietary sodium	High sodium intake can contribute to hypertension in some patients and can decrease the efficacy of certain antihypertensive medications.
Elevated serum lipids	Elevated levels of cholesterol and triglycerides are primary risk factors in atherosclerosis. Hyperlipidemia is more common in hypertensives.
Alcohol	Excessive alcohol intake is strongly associated with hypertension. Hypertensive patients should limit their daily intake of ethanol to 1 oz.
Sedentary lifestyle	Regular physical activity can help control weight and reduce cardiovascular risk. Physical activity may decrease BP.
Diabetes mellitus (DM)	Hypertension is more common in diabetics. When hypertension and diabetes coexist, complications are more severe.
Socioeconomic status	Hypertension is more prevalent in lower socioconomic groups and among the less educated.
Stress	People exposed to repeated stress may develop hypertension more frequently than others. People who become hypertensive may respond differently to stress than those who do not become hypertensive.

BP, Blood pressure.

pump effectively against increasing resistance. Resistance to blood flow increases cardiac workload (see Congestive Heart Failure, p. 158).

Cerebrovascular disease. Hypertension is a major risk factor for stroke and atherosclerosis. As a result of hypertension, blood vessels become more rigid because of thickening of vessel walls and the replacement of smooth muscle tissue with fibrous tissue. The vessel is weakened by this process and tends to rupture more easily (see Cerebrovascular Accident, p. 109).

Peripheral vascular disease. As it does with other vessels, hypertension speeds up the process of atherosclerosis in peripheral blood vessels, leading to the development of aortic aneurysm, aortic dissection, and peripheral vascular disease. *Intermittent claudication* (ischemic muscle pain precipitated by activity and relieved with rest) is a classic symptom of peripheral vascular disease.

Nephrosclerosis. Hypertension is one of the leading risk factors for end-stage renal disease, especially in African-Americans. Some degree of renal dysfunction is usually present in the hypertensive patient, even one with a minimally elevated BP. This disorder is the result of ischemia caused by the narrowed lumen of intrarenal blood vessels. The gradual closure of arteries and arterioles leads to the destruction of glomeruli, atrophy of tubules, and eventual death of nephrons. These changes may eventually lead to renal failure. The earliest symptom of renal dysfunction is usually nocturia.

Retinal damage. The appearance of the retina provides important information about the severity of the hypertensive process. The retina is the only place in the body where the blood vessels can be directly visualized. Therefore retinal damage provides an indication of vessel damage in the heart, brain, and kidneys. Manifestations of severe retinal damage include blurring of vision, retinal hemorrhage, and loss of vision.

Diagnostic Studies

Measurements should be taken in both arms when initially evaluating a patient's BP. The average of at least two BP measurements (taken 2 to 5 minutes apart while the patient is sitting) should be used to determine if the patient should return for further evaluation. If the first two readings differ by more than 5 mm Hg, additional readings should be obtained. Basic laboratory studies are performed to evaluate target organ disease, determine overall cardiovascular risk, or establish baseline levels before initiating therapy.

- Routine urinalysis and blood urea nitrogen (BUN) and serum creatinine level screens for renal involvement
- Serum electrolytes, especially potassium (K^+) levels, to detect hyperaldosteronism and Cushing's syndrome
- Blood glucose (fasting, if possible) level to assess for DM

- Serum lipid profile, cholesterol, and triglyceride levels to assess for atherogenesis risk factors
- ECG to assess cardiac rhythm

Collaborative Care

The goal in treating a hypertensive patient is to reduce the overall cardiovascular risk factors and to control BP by the least intrusive means possible. Lifestyle modifications are indicated for all hypertensive patients. These modification measures include dietary changes, smoking cessation, regular exercise, and limitation of alcohol intake.

- Drug therapy is indicated for all patients with stage II or III hypertension that is not controlled by lifestyle changes.
- Periodic monitoring of BP is very important. After the BP has stabilized, it should be monitored every 3 to 6 months to ensure control.
- Diet therapy consists of sodium restriction, caloric restriction if the patient is overweight, and maintenance of K^+, calcium (Ca^{++}), and magnesium (Mg^+) intake. Restrict cholesterol and fat, and reduce weight if indicated. The patient should be advised to limit alcohol intake to 1 oz per day (the amount of alcohol in 2 oz of 100 proof whiskey, 8 oz of wine, or 24 oz of beer).
- Physical activity of moderate intensity, such as brisk walking, jogging, or swimming, can help control BP, promote relaxation, and decrease or control body weight. It is recommended that all adults engage in 30 minutes or more of moderate intense physical activity on most or (preferably) all days of the week. The patient with heart disease or other serious health problems needs a thorough examination, possibly including an ECG stress test, before beginning an exercise program.
- Cigarette smoking is a major risk factor for cardiovascular disease. The nicotine contained in tobacco causes vasoconstriction and increases BP in hypertensive people. Everyone, especially a hypertensive patient, should be strongly advised to avoid tobacco use.

Drug Therapy

The general goals of drug therapy are to achieve a BP of <130/85 in young adults with mild hypertension. In older adults with elevation of both systolic and diastolic BP, lowering BP to <140/90 mm Hg is desirable. The drugs currently available for treating hypertension have two main actions: reduction of systemic vascular resistance and decreasing the volume of circulating blood.

- Drugs used in treatment of hypertension include diuretics, β-adrenergic blocking agents, vasodilators, angiotensin converting enzyme (ACE) inhibitors, and calcium channel blockers. (See Table 31-8, Lewis and others, *Medical-Surgical Nursing,* edition 5, p. 827 for a description of antihypertensive drug therapy and p. 326 for drug recommendations for the stages of hypertension.)

Nursing Management

Goals

The patient with hypertension will achieve and maintain desired BP; understand, accept, and implement the therapeutic plan; and experience minimal or no unpleasant side effects of therapy.

Nursing Diagnoses/Collaborative Problems

- Altered health maintenance *related to* lack of knowledge of pathology, complications, and management of hypertension
- Anxiety *related to* complexity of therapeutic plan, possible complications, and lifestyle changes associated with hypertension
- Ineffective management of therapeutic regimen *related to* unpleasant side effects of medication, lack of knowledge and motivation, and inconvenient schedule for taking medications
- Potential complication: hypertensive crisis
- Potential complication: cerebrovascular accident
- Potential complication: coronary artery and peripheral vascular disease

Nursing Interventions

The nurse in routine screening settings is in an ideal position to assess for the presence of hypertension, identify risk factors for hypertension and CAD, and educate the patient regarding these conditions.

- Effort and resources should be focused on controlling BP in persons already identified as having hypertension; identifying and controlling BP in high-risk groups such as African-Americans, obese persons, and relatives of people with hypertension; and screening those with limited access to the health care system.

The patient with a severe and abruptly elevated BP, especially with significant target organ damage, may be hospitalized. The purpose of hospitalization is to lower BP, determine the underlying cause of hypertension, prevent or limit target organ damage, and treat the cause if it is secondary hypertension. The primary goal for the nurse at this stage of intervention is to assist in reducing BP and to begin patient education.

For the patient with severe hypertension, the BP should be monitored every 1 to 2 hours and then with decreasing frequency as the BP stabilizes. Antihypertensive drug therapy at this time may be given parenterally; this requires very frequent (every 2 to 3 minutes) BP checks. Careful monitoring of vital signs with hourly urine output provides information regarding the effectiveness of drugs and the patient's response to therapy.

- Frequent neurologic checks, including level of consciousness, pupillary size and reaction, movement of extremities, and reaction to stimuli, help to detect changes in patient condition. Cardiac, pulmonary, and renal systems should be monitored for decompensation (e.g., pulmonary edema, CHF, angina, and renal failure) caused by the severe elevation in BP.
- A patient with severe elevation of BP but without target organ damage may not require hospitalization. Allowing the patient to sit for 20 or 30 minutes in a quiet environment may significantly reduce BP. Oral drugs may then be instituted or adjusted.
- Additional nursing interventions include encouraging the patient to verbalize fears, answering questions concerning hypertension, and eliminating excess noise in the patient's environment.

▼ **Patient Teaching**

Patient and family education includes diet therapy, drug therapy, physical activity, and if appropriate, BP home monitoring and tobacco cessation.

Diet therapy. The patient and family, especially the member who prepares the meals, should be educated about sodium-restricted diets. They need to be instructed on reading the labels of over-the-counter drugs as well as packaged foods and health products to identify hidden sources of sodium. It is helpful to review the patient's normal diet and to identify foods high in sodium

Drug therapy. Side effects of antihypertensive drug therapy are common. The number or severity of side effects may be related to dosage, and it may be necessary to change the drug or decrease the dosage. Side effects are common and may be caused by an initial response to the drug. These effects may decrease with long-term use of the drug.

Physical activity. Generally, physical activity is more likely to be sustained if it is safe and enjoyable, fits easily into the daily schedule, and does not generate financial or social costs. Nurses can assist patients to increase their physical activity by identifying and communicating the need for increased activity, explaining the difference between physical activity and exercise, assisting in initiating activity, and following up appropriately.

Home BP monitoring. The patient should be assessed individually about the feasibility of being taught, or having a family member be taught, to take weekly BP readings at home once the BP is stabilized. Often, home BP measurement gives a more valid indication of BP because the patient is more relaxed.

Patient compliance. Active patient participation increases the likelihood of adherence to the treatment plan. Measures such as involving the patient in scheduling medications convenient to a daily routine, helping the patient link pill-taking with another daily activity, and involving family members (if necessary) help increase patient compliance.

- It is important to help the patient and family understand that hypertension is a chronic condition that cannot be cured but can be controlled with drug therapy, diet therapy, an exercise program, periodic evaluation, and other relevant lifestyle changes.

HYPERTHYROIDISM

Definition/Description
Hyperthyroidism is the sustained and increased synthesis and release of thyroid hormones by the thyroid gland. The most common form of hyperthyroidism is Graves' disease, followed by multinodular goiter. A *goiter* is an enlargement of the thyroid gland. *Thyrotoxicosis* is hypermetabolism that results from excess circulating levels of thyroxine (T_4), triiodothyronine (T_3), or both.

- The incidence of hyperthyroidism is greater in women, with the highest frequency in the 30 to 50 year old age group.
- Iodine deficiency is believed to predispose the patient to thyrotoxicosis and other thyroid diseases, with a greater incidence in iodine-poor geographic locations.

Types
Graves' disease (diffuse toxic goiter) is an autoimmune disease of unknown etiology marked by an increased production of thyroid hormone. Patients who are generally susceptible become sensitized to and develop antibodies against various antigens within the thyroid gland.

The hyperthyroidism and diffuse thyroid hyperplasia are caused by antibodies that attack thyroid tissue and thus stimulate hyperplasia. These antibodies, known as *thyroid-stimulating antibodies* (TSAbs), stimulate the thyroid-stimulating hormone (TSH) receptor and activate the production of thyroid hormones.

- The disease is characterized by remissions and exacerbations, with or without treatment. It may progress to destruction of thyroid tissue, causing hypothyroidism.
- Precipitating factors such as insufficient iodine supply, infections, and emotions may interact with genetic factors to cause Graves' disease.

Nodular goiters are characterized by small, discrete, autonomously functioning nodules that secrete thyroid hormone. If associated with hyperthyroidism, a nodule is termed *toxic*. There may be multiple nodules or a single nodule.

- The frequency of toxic multinodular goiter is highest in women in the sixth and seventh decades of life. There is usually a history of a preexisting simple goiter before the onset of demonstrable thyrotoxicosis.
- Manifestations are slower to develop and usually less severe than in Graves' disease.

Clinical Manifestations

The manifestations of hyperthyroidism are related to the effects of excess thyroid hormones. Manifestations are numerous and include arrhythmias, angina, fatigue, insomnia, weight loss, increased appetite, diarrhea, diaphoresis, goiter, intolerance to heat, and menstrual irregularities.

- *Exophthalmos (proptosis),* in which the eyeballs protrude from the orbits, is due to impaired venous drainage from the orbit leading to increased deposits of fat and fluid (edema) in the retroorbital tissues. This sign is seen in 20% to 40% of patients with Graves' disease. When the eyelids do not close completely, exposed corneal surfaces become dry and irritated. Serious consequences, such as corneal ulcers and eventual loss of vision, can occur.
- A patient with advanced disease may exhibit many symptoms, whereas a patient in the early stages of hyperthyroidism may only exhibit weight loss and increased nervousness. Table 47-4, Lewis and others, *Medical-Surgical Nursing,* edition 5, p. 1417, compares features of hyperthyroidism in young and older adult patients.

Complications

Thyrotoxic crisis (thyroid storm) is an acute but rare condition where all hyperthyroid manifestations are heightened. The cause is presumed to be stressors such as infection, trauma, or surgery in a patient with preexisting hyperthyroidism. It is potentially fatal, but death is rare when treatment is vigorous and initiated early.

- Manifestations include severe tachycardia, heart failure, shock, hyperthermia (up to 105.3° F [40.7° C]), restlessness, agitation, abdominal pain, nausea, vomiting, diarrhea, delirium, and coma.
- Measures must be taken to prevent death. Treatment is aimed at reducing circulating thyroid hormone levels by appropriate drug therapy. Therapy is directed at fever reduction, fluid replacement, and elimination or management of the initiating stressor(s).

Diagnostic Studies

- Serum TSH, T_4, T_3, free T_3 and T_4 levels, T_3 resin uptake, and radioactive iodine uptake.

- Thyrotropin-releasing hormone (TRH) stimulation test and thyroid scan.
- ECG may show tachycardia, atrial fibrillation, and alterations in P and T waves.
- Ophthalmologic examination.

Collaborative Care

The therapeutic goals are to block the adverse effects of thyroid hormones and stop their oversecretion. Therapy involves medication with antithyroid drugs and β-adrenergic receptor blockers, thyroid ablation with radioactive iodine, and subtotal thyroidectomy after adequate preparation.

Drug Therapy

Thiomides. The most commonly used antithyroid drugs are classified as thiomides; propylthiouracil (PTU) and methimazole (Tapazole) are the most commonly used drugs. These drugs inhibit the synthesis of thyroid hormones; PTU also blocks the peripheral conversion of T_4 to T_3.

- Indications for the use of antithyroid drugs include Graves' disease in the young patient, hyperthyroidism during pregnancy, and the need to make a patient euthyroid before surgery or irradiation.

Iodine. In large doses, iodine (e.g. Lugol's solution, potassium iodide) inhibits the synthesis of T_3 and T_4 and blocks the release of these hormones into circulation. Iodine decreases thyroid size and vascularity, making resection safer and easier. Administration of PTU, with iodine therapy added 10 days before surgery, is a common method for surgical preparation of a patient with hyperthyroidism.

β-Adrenergic blockers. Propranolol (Inderol) is the most frequently used β-adrenergic blocker. It relieves the symptoms of thyrotoxicosis that result from increased β-adrenergic receptor stimulation caused by excess thyroid hormones.

Radioactive iodine. Radioactive iodine limits thyroid hormone secretion by damaging or destroying thyroid tissue. This treatment is effective but often results in hypothyroidism.

Surgical Therapy

For thyroidectomy to be effective, approximately 90% of the thyroid tissue must be removed. If too much tissue is taken, the gland will not regenerate after surgery and hypothyroidism will develop. Occasionally the recurrent laryngeal nerve or parathyroid glands may be damaged during surgery.

Nutritional Therapy

The potential for nutritional deficits is high when an increased metabolic rate is present. A high-calorie diet (4000 to 5000 kcal/day) may be ordered to satisfy hunger and prevent tissue breakdown. This is accomplished with six full meals a day and snacks high in protein, carbohydrates, minerals, and vitamins, particularly vitamin A, thiamine, vitamin B_6, and ascorbic acid. Highly seasoned and high-fiber foods should be avoided because they stimulate the already hypermotile GI tract.

Nursing Management

Goals
The patient with hyperthyroidism will experience relief of symptoms, have no serious complications related to the disease or treatment, and comply with the therapeutic plan.

See NCP 47-1 for the patient with hyperthyroidism, Lewis and others, *Medical-Surgical Nursing,* edition 5, p. 1420.

Nursing Diagnoses
- Activity intolerance *related to* fatigue, exhaustion, and heat intolerance secondary to hypermetabolism
- Altered nutrition: less than body requirements *related to* hypermetabolism and inadequate diet
- Anxiety *related to* lack of knowledge about management and course of disease and hypermetabolism
- Risk for injury *related to* fine muscle tremors, fatigue, inattentiveness, and incoordination

Nursing Interventions
A restful, calm, quiet room should be provided because increased metabolism causes sleep disturbances. Provision of adequate rest may be a challenge because of the patient's irritability and restlessness.
- Interventions may include placing the patient in a cool room away from very ill patients and noisy, high-traffic areas; using light bed coverings and changing the linen frequently if the patient is diaphoretic; encouraging and assisting with exercise involving large muscle groups (tremors can interfere with small-muscle coordination) to allow the release of nervous tension and restlessness; and establishing a supportive, trusting relationship to help the patient cope with aggravating events and to lessen anxiety.

If exophthalmos is present, there is a potential for corneal injury. The patient may also have orbital pain. Interventions to relieve eye discomfort and prevent corneal ulceration include applying artificial tears to soothe and moisten conjunctival membranes, restricting salt, elevating the patient's head to reduce periorbital edema, and providing dark glasses to reduce glare and prevent irritation from smoke, air currents, dust, and dirt. If the eyelids cannot be closed, they should be lightly taped shut for sleep.
- To maintain flexibility, the patient should be taught to exercise intraocular muscles several times a day by turning the eyes in the complete range of motion.

Nursing Management: Patient Receiving Radioactive Iodine Therapy

Radioactive iodine therapy (ablation) is usually done on an outpatient basis and is the therapy of choice for adults beyond childbearing years. Because the usual therapeutic dose of iodine is only 7 to 10 millicurie (mCi), no radiation safety precautions are necessary.

- The patient should be instructed that radiation thyroiditis and parotiditis are possible and may cause dryness and irritation of the mouth and throat. Relief may be obtained with frequent sips of water, ice chips, or the use of a salt and soda gargle three to four times per day. Discomfort should subside in 3 to 4 days.
- Because of the high frequency of hypothyroidism after radioactive iodine therapy, the patient and significant others should be taught the symptoms of hypothyroidism and instructed to seek medical help if these symptoms occur.

Nursing Management: Patient Having Thyroid Surgery

When subtotal thyroidectomy is the treatment of choice, the patient must be adequately prepared to avoid postoperative complications.

- Preoperative teaching should include comfort and safety measures in which the patient can participate and the practice and importance of deep breathing and leg exercises. The patient should also be taught how to support the head manually while turning in bed to minimize stress on the surgery suture line. Range-of-motion (ROM) exercises of the neck should be practiced and the patient should be told that talking is likely to be difficult for a short time after surgery.
- The hospital room must be prepared before the patient's return from surgery. Oxygen, suction equipment, and a tracheostomy tray should be readily available.
- Recurrent laryngeal nerve damage leads to vocal cord paralysis. If there is paralysis of both cords, spastic airway obstruction will occur, requiring an immediate tracheostomy.
- Respiration may become difficult because of excess swelling of the neck tissue, hemorrhage, and hematoma formation.
- Laryngeal stridor (harsh, vibratory sound) may occur during respiration as a result of tetany, which occurs if the parathyroid glands are removed or damaged during surgery. To treat tetany, calcium salts should be readily available for IV administration.

After a thyroidectomy the nurse should do the following:

- Assess the patient every 2 hours for 24 hours for signs of hemorrhage or tracheal compression, such as irregular breathing, neck swelling, frequent swallowing, sensations of fullness at the incision site, choking, and blood on anterior or posterior dressings.

- Place the patient in a semi-Fowler's position and support the head with pillows, avoiding flexion of the neck and any tension on the suture lines.
- Monitor vital signs. Check for signs of tetany secondary to hypoparathyroidism (e.g., tingling of toes, fingers, or around the mouth; muscular twitching; apprehension) and by evaluating any difficulty in speaking and hoarseness.
- Control postoperative pain by giving medication.
- The neck incision should be lubricated and ROM exercises should be carried out three or four times daily to promote comfort and the return of the full range of motion.
- The appearance of the incision may be quite distressing; the patient can be reassured that the scar will fade in color and eventually look like a normal neck wrinkle.

▼ Patient Teaching

Follow-up care is important for the patient who has undergone thyroid surgery.

- Hormone balance should be monitored periodically to ensure normal function has returned.
- Caloric intake must be reduced substantially below the amount that was required before surgery to prevent weight gain.
- Adequate iodine is necessary to promote thyroid function, but excesses inhibit the thyroid. Seafood once or twice a week or the normal use of iodized salt should provide sufficient intake.
- Regular exercise helps stimulate the thyroid and should be encouraged.
- High environmental temperatures should be avoided because they inhibit thyroid regeneration.
- If a complete thyroidectomy has been performed, the patient needs instruction in lifelong thyroid replacement therapy.
- The patient should be taught the signs and symptoms of progressive thyroid failure and instructed to seek medical care if these develop.

HYPOPARATHYROIDISM

Definition/Description

Hypoparathyroidism is an uncommon condition characterized by inadequate circulating parathyroid hormone (PTH), which results in hypocalcemia. PTH resistance at the cellular level may also occur. This is caused by a genetic defect resulting in hypocalcemia in spite of normal or high PTH levels and is often associated with hypothyroidism and hypogonadism.

Pathophysiology

The most common cause of hypoparathyroidism is the accidental removal of parathyroids or damage to the vascular supply of the glands during neck surgery (e.g., thyroidectomy, radical neck surgery).

- Idiopathic hypoparathyroidism resulting from absence, fatty replacement, or atrophy of the glands is a rare disease that usually occurs early in life and may be associated with other endocrine disorders. Affected patients may have antiparathyroid antibodies.
- Hypomagnesemia is another cause of hypoparathyroidism. Hypomagnesemia, as seen in alcoholism or malabsorption, impairs PTH secretion and its action on bone and kidneys.

Clinical Manifestations

The clinical features of acute hypoparathyroidism are due to a low serum calcium level (see Table 47-10, Lewis and others, *Medical-Surgical Nursing,* edition 5, p. 1429).

Sudden decreases in calcium concentration give rise to a syndrome called *tetany.*

- This state is characterized by tingling of the lips, finger tips, and occasionally feet, and increased muscle tension leading to paresthesias and stiffness.
- Dysphagia, painful tonic spasms of smooth and skeletal muscles (particularly of the extremities and face), and laryngospasms are also present. *Chvostek's sign* (a facial muscle spasm when the face is tapped below the temple) and *Trousseau's sign* (a carpopedal spasm when arterial circulation is interrupted by applying a blood pressure cuff for 3 minutes) are usually positive.

Respiratory function may be severely compromised by accessory muscle spasm and laryngeal spasm–induced airway obstruction. Patients are usually anxious and apprehensive.

Diagnostic studies include decreased serum calcium and PTH levels and increased serum phosphate levels.

Collaborative Care

The main objectives of treatment are to treat tetany when present and to prevent long-term complications by maintaining normal calcium levels. Tetany is treated with IV infusion or slow push of calcium salts. Long-term therapy consists of administration of vitamin D and possibly supplemental calcium and oral phosphate binders.

- Emergency treatment of tetany requires administration of IV calcium. Calcium salts can cause hypotension and cardiac arrest; thus a slow IV push is required. For long-term management, oral calcium supplements may be prescribed.

- Specific hormone replacement of PTH is not used to treat hypoparathyroidism because of the expense and the need for parenteral administration.
- Vitamin D is used in chronic and resistant hypocalcemia to enhance intestinal calcium absorption and bone resorption. Preferred preparations are dihydrotachysterol (Hytakerol) and calcitriol (Rocaltrol). These drugs are more potent, raise calcium levels rapidly, and are quickly metabolized.

Nursing Management

Goals

The patient with hypoparathyroidism will develop no complications, such as tetany or arrhythmias, recognize the signs and symptoms of hypoparathyroidism and hyperparathyroidism, and comply with periodic assessment of calcium level.

Nursing Diagnoses/Collaborative Problem

- Impaired skin integrity *related to* dry, scaly skin
- Activity intolerance *related to* fatigue, weakness, and painful muscle cramps
- Altered thought processes *related to* personality and psychiatric changes and memory impairment
- Ineffective management of therapeutic regimen *related to* lack of knowledge regarding the signs and symptoms of calcium deficiency, calcium-rich foods and supplements, and chronic nature of the problem
- Potential complication: arrhythmias
- Potential complication: tetany

Nursing Interventions

If tetany or generalized muscle cramps develop, rebreathing may partially alleviate the symptoms. The patient who can cooperate should be instructed to breathe in and out of a paper bag or breathing mask. This reduces carbon dioxide excretion from the lungs and lowers body pH. Because an acidic environment enhances both solubility and the degree of ionization of calcium, ionized calcium is increased, temporarily relieving the hypocalcemia.

- IV calcium salts should be available at the bedside for the treatment of acute tetany. Calcium salts must be infused slowly because high blood levels can cause serious cardiac arrhythmias or cardiac arrest. The patient who has been digitalized is particularly vulnerable. ECG monitoring is indicated.
- Side rails should be padded as a seizure precaution. Patients should be kept in a nonstimulating environment, assisted with hygienic needs, and given support and encouragement until they are free of symptoms.

▼ Patient Teaching

The patient with hypoparathyroidism needs instruction in the management of long-term nutrition and drug therapy.

- A high-calcium meal plan includes foods such as dark green vegetables, soy beans, and tofu. The patient should be told that foods containing oxalic acid (e.g., spinach and rhubarb), phytic acid (e.g., bran and whole grains), and phosphorus reduce calcium absorption.
- Calcium supplements of at least 1 g/day for patients under 40 years of age and 2 g/day for patients more than 40 years of age are usually prescribed. These supplements are best administered 2 to 3 hours after meals. Calcium carbonate often leads to constipation and flatulence. Nursing interventions include providing stool softeners, adequate fluids, and fresh fruits.
- The patient should be instructed with written handouts about the signs and symptoms of hypocalcemia and hypercalcemia and about reporting these to a clinician as soon as possible if they occur.
- If manifestations of hypocalcemia occur, calcium supplementation should be increased. The need for lifelong treatment and health supervision should be stressed.
- Patient calcium levels should be monitored three to four times a year. Treatment modification is often necessary because hypercalcemia can develop.
- Thorough patient instruction and frequent serum calcium assessment should allow a normal life expectancy. The patient needs support and encouragement to continue with the regimen.

HYPOPITUITARISM

Definition/Description

Hypopituitarism is a rare disorder that involves a decrease in one or more of the anterior pituitary hormones. Primary hypofunction may be due to infections, autoimmune disorders, tumors, or destruction of the gland through radiation or surgical procedures. Failure to secrete growth hormone (GH) is the most common abnormality, followed by deficiencies of gonadotropins, thyroid-stimulating hormone (TSH), adrenocorticotropic hormone (ACTH), and prolactin.

The manifestations of hypopituitarism depend on the specific pituitary hormones that are lacking. Infertility may be caused by primary gonadal failure or may be the first indication of pituitary hypofunction (gonads lack tropic hormone stimulation).

Clinical Manifestations

Findings associated with pituitary hypofunction vary with the degree and speed of onset of pituitary dysfunction and are related to hyposecretion of the target glands.

- Symptoms are often nonspecific and commonly include weakness, fatigue, headache, sexual dysfunction, fasting hypoglycemia, dry and sallow skin, diminished tolerance for stress, and poor resistance to infection.
- In the adult, premature, fine wrinkling around the eyes and mouth is common.
- Psychiatric symptoms include apathy, mental slowness, and delusions.
- Orthostatic hypotension may occur.
- If a pituitary tumor exerts pressure on the optic chiasma, there may be asymmetric visual field changes. If the tumor is large, blindness in one or both eyes may occur.
- When pituitary hypofunction affects follicle-stimulating hormone (FSH) and luteinizing hormone (LH), sexual development is impaired and features remain childlike. FSH and LH deficiencies in the adult woman are first manifested as menstrual irregularities, diminished libido, and changes in secondary sex characteristics. Men with FSH and LH deficiencies experience testicular atrophy, loss of libido along with impotence, and decreased facial hair and muscle mass.

If hypopituitarism is not detected and treated, the patient eventually develops deficiencies of thyroid hormone and the adrenal corticosteroids. The latter deficiency causes a tendency toward shock and may result in an episode of acute adrenal insufficiency (refractory and life-threatening shock resulting from sodium and water depletion).

Collaborative Care

Treatment of hypopituitarism consists of surgery or radiation for tumor removal, permanent target gland hormone replacement, and nutritional therapy. Replacement therapy is carried out with corticosteroids, thyroid hormone, and sex hormones. Gonadotropins can sometimes restore fertility.

A primary nursing role in anterior pituitary insufficiency is the assessment and recognition of subtle signs and symptoms.

- The patient with hypopituitarism may first exhibit symptoms in stressful situations such as trauma or surgery. In addition, hypopituitarism may be detected in patients with complaints of a failure to grow, infertility, or amenorrhea.

HYPOTHYROIDISM

Definition/Description

Hypothyroidism usually results from insufficient circulating thyroid hormone as a result of a variety of abnormalities. Hypothyroidism may occur in infancy *(cretinism),* childhood, or adulthood. Although the typical patient with hypothyroidism is a woman over 50, the disease can occur at any age and in either sex.

Pathophysiology

Cretinism is caused by thyroid hormone deficiencies during fetal or early neonatal life. It can be caused by maternal iodine deprivation or congenital thyroid abnormalities.

In the adult, the most common cause of primary hypothyroidism is atrophy of the thyroid gland. This atrophy is the end result of both Hashimoto's thyroiditis and Graves' disease. These autoimmune diseases destroy the thyroid gland. Thyroid deficiency also occurs when pituitary thyroid-stimulating hormone (TSH) production is inadequate. Iatrogenic causes of hypothyroidism include surgical removal of the thyroid, destruction of thyroid gland by radiation, and surgical removal of the pituitary gland.

Clinical Manifestations

Manifestations of *cretinism* are defective physical development and mental retardation. Although affected infants usually appear normal at birth, cretinism should be suspected when there is a long gestational period and a large infant who fails to thrive.

In the adult, hypothyroidism is characterized by an insidious and nonspecific slowing of body processes; personality changes; fatigue; and lethargy. Mental changes include impaired memory, slowed speech, and somnolence. In addition, cold intolerance, hair loss, dry and coarse skin, brittle nails, muscle weakness and swelling, constipation, weight gain, and menorrhagia are common. Hypothyroid heart disease includes cardiomyopathy, pericardial effusion, and coronary atherosclerosis.

- Symptoms are so insidious that medical attention is seldom sought. The patient and family are often unaware of the changes. The severity of symptoms depends on the degree of thyroid hormone deficiency.
- The term *myxedema* is often used synonymously with hypothyroidism but actually connotes severe, long-standing hypothyroidism. Myxedema is the accumulation of hydrophilic mucopolysaccharides in the dermis and other tissues. This mucinous

H

edema causes the characteristic facies of hypothyroidism, including puffiness, periorbital edema, and masklike affect.

The mental sluggishness, drowsiness, and lethargy may progress gradually or suddenly to a notable impairment of consciousness or coma. This situation, termed *myxedema coma,* constitutes a medical emergency. Myxedema coma can be precipitated by infection, drugs (especially narcotics, tranquilizers, and barbiturates), exposure to cold, and trauma. It is characterized by subnormal temperature, hypotension, and hypoventilation. Vital functions must be supported, and IV thyroid hormone administered.

Diagnostic Studies

- Serum thyroxine (T_4), triiodothyronine (T_3), and T_3RU levels are low.
- Serum TSH levels help determine the cause of hypothyroidism. If high, the thyroid is diseased, and if low, the pituitary is diseased.
- ECG shows bradycardia and low voltage.
- Serum cholesterol is increased.
- Thyrotropin-releasing hormone (TRH) stimulation test will show an increase in TSH if the problem is hypothalamic dysfunction; no change in TSH suggests anterior pituitary dysfunction.

Collaborative Care

The therapeutic objective in hypothyroidism is the restoration of a euthyroid state as safely and rapidly as possible with hormone replacement therapy. Synthetic oral thyroxine (Synthroid, Levothroid, Noroxin) is the drug of choice to treat hypothyroidism. In the young, otherwise healthy patient, the maintenance replacement dose can be started at once. In the older adult patient and the person with compromised cardiac status, a small initial dose is recommended because the usual dose may increase myocardial oxygen (O_2) consumption. Any chest pain experienced by a patient starting thyroid replacement should be reported immediately, and ECG and serum cardiac enzyme tests must be performed. The dose is increased at 1- to 4-week intervals. It is important that the patient take replacement medication regularly.

- With treatment, striking transformations occur in both appearance and mental function. Most adults return to a normal state. Cardiovascular conditions and (occasionally) psychosis may persist despite corrections of the hormonal imbalance. Relapses occur if treatment is interrupted.

Nursing Management

Goals

The patient with hypothyroidism will experience relief of symptoms, maintain an euthyroid state, maintain a positive self-image, and comply with lifelong thyroid replacement therapy.

See NCP 47-2 for the patient with hypothyroidism, Lewis and others, *Medical-Surgical Nursing,* edition 5, p. 1427.

Nursing Diagnoses

- Altered comfort *related to* cold intolerance
- Altered thought processes *related to* diminished cerebral blood flow secondary to decreased cardiac output (CO)
- Activity intolerance *related to* decreased metabolic rate and mucin deposits in joints and interstitial spaces
- Constipation *related to* gastrointestinal hypomotility
- Altered nutrition: more than body requirements *related to* hypometabolism

Nursing Interventions

- Provide a comfortable, warm environment because of the patient's intolerance to cold.
- Take measures to prevent skin breakdown. Use soap sparingly and apply an emollient or lotion. An alternating-pressure mattress may be helpful.
- Avoid using sedatives. If they must be given, give the lowest possible dose and closely monitor mental status, level of consciousness, and respirations.
- Prevent constipation by gradually increasing exercise, increasing fiber in meal plan, administering stool softeners, and promoting regular bowel habits. Avoid enemas because they produce vagal stimulation, which can be hazardous to the patient with cardiac disease.
- For assessment of the patient's progress, vital signs, body weight, fluid intake and output, and visible edema should be monitored. Cardiac assessment is especially important because the cardiovascular response to the hormone determines the medication regimen.
- Energy level and mental alertness should be noted. These should increase within 2 to 14 days and continue to rise steadily to normal levels.

▼ **Patient Teaching**

Repeated patient education is imperative. Initially the hypothyroid patient needs more time than usual to comprehend all the necessary information.

- The need for lifelong drug therapy must be stressed. Signs and symptoms of hypothyroidism or hyperthyroidism that indicate hormone imbalance should be included in the teaching plan. It is sometimes difficult for the patient to recognize signs of overdosage or underdosage; therefore a family member or friend should be included in the teaching.
- The patient must be taught to contact a clinician immediately if signs of overdose such as orthopnea, dyspnea, rapid pulse, palpitations, nervousness, or insomnia appear.

- The patient with diabetes mellitus (DM) should test his or her capillary blood glucose at least daily because a return to the euthyroid state frequently increases insulin requirements.
- In addition, thyroid preparations potentiate the effects of other common drugs, such as anticoagulants, antidepressants, and digitalis compounds. The patient should be taught the toxic signs and symptoms of these medications and remain under close medical observation until stable.

INCREASED INTRACRANIAL PRESSURE

Definition/Description

Increased intracranial pressure (ICP) is a life-threatening situation that results from an increase in any or all of the three components of the skull: brain tissue, blood, and cerebrospinal fluid (CSF). Cerebral edema is an important factor related to increased ICP. Regardless of the cause (Table 39), cerebral edema results in an increase in tissue volume that has the potential for increased ICP. The extent and severity of the original insult are factors that determine the degree of cerebral edema.

Three types of cerebral edema—vasogenic, cytotoxic, and interstitial—have been identified. More than one type may be present from a single insult in the same patient.

- *Vasogenic cerebral edema* is the most common type of edema. It occurs mainly in the white matter and is attributed to changes in the endothelial linings of the cerebral capillaries.
- *Cytotoxic cerebral edema* results from a local disruption of the functional or morphologic integrity of the cell membranes and occurs most often in the gray matter. This type of edema develops from destructive lesions or trauma to brain tissue.
- *Interstitial cerebral edema* is the result of periventricular diffusion of ventricular CSF in a patient with uncontrolled hydro-

Table 39	Conditions Associated with Cerebral Edema
Mass Lesions	**Vascular Insult**
Neoplasm (primary and metastatic)	Infarct (thrombolic and embolic)
Abscess	Venous sinus thrombosis
Hemorrhage (intracerebral and extracerebral)	Anoxic and ischemic episodes
Head Injuries	**Toxic or Metabolic Encephalopathic Conditions**
Hemorrhage	Lead or arsenic intoxication
Contusion	Renal failure
Posttraumatic brain swelling	Liver failure
	Reye's syndrome
Brain Surgery	
Infections	

cephalus. It can also be caused by enlargement of the extracellular space as a result of systemic water excess (hyponatremia).

Pathophysiology

Increased ICP can be caused by many factors, including a mass lesion (e.g., hematoma), cerebral edema associated with brain tumors, hydrocephalus, head injury, or brain inflammation, or by metabolic insult. These insults may result in hypercapnia, cerebral acidosis, impaired autoregulation, and systemic hypertension, which promote the formation and spread of cerebral edema. This edema distorts brain tissue, further increasing ICP, which leads to even more tissue hypoxia and acidosis. (For an illustration of the progression of increased ICP, see Fig. 54-4, Lewis and others, *Medical-Surgical Nursing,* edition 5, p. 1613.)

Unless there is a reduction in ICP, brainstem compression occurs. As the intracranial mass continues to increase, herniation of the brain from one compartment to another can occur.

With brain displacement and herniation, ischemia and edema are further increased. Compression of the brainstem and cranial nerves may be fatal. Fig. 54-6, *Medical-Surgical Nursing,* p. 1615, illustrates the symptoms of supratentorial increased ICP from the early phase through herniation of the brain.

- Subtentorial and infratentorial herniations force the cerebellum and brainstem downward through the foramen magnum. If compression of the brainstem is unrelieved, respiratory arrest may occur.

Clinical Manifestations

Manifestations of increased ICP can take many forms, depending on the cause, location, and rate at which the pressure increase occurs. The earlier the condition is recognized and treated, the better the prognosis. Manifestations of increased ICP associated with supratentorial lesions include the following:

- *Change in the level of consciousness* (LOC). LOC is a sensitive and important indicator of the patient's neurologic status. The change in consciousness may be dramatic, as in coma, or subtle, such as a change in orientation or a decrease in the level of attention.
- *Change in vital signs.* Although the complex of increasing systolic pressure (widening pulse pressure), bradycardia with a full and bounding pulse, and irregular respiratory pattern (Cushing's triad) may be present, these symptoms often do not appear until ICP has been increased for some time. A change in body temperature may also be noted.
- *Ocular signs.* Compression of the oculomotor nerve (CN III) results in dilation of the pupil ipsilateral to the mass, sluggish or no response to light, an inability to move the eye upward, and

ptosis of the eyelid. A fixed, unilaterally dilated pupil is a neurologic emergency that indicates transtentorial brain herniation. Other cranial nerves may also be affected, with signs of blurred vision, diplopia, and changes in extraocular eye movements. Papilledema is also seen and is a nonspecific sign that is associated with longstanding increased ICP.

- *Decrease in motor function.* As ICP continues to rise, the patient manifests changes in motor ability. A contralateral hemiparesis or hemiplegia may be seen. If painful stimuli are used to elicit a motor response, the patient may exhibit a localization to the stimuli or a withdrawal from it. *Decorticate* (flexor) and *decerebrate* (extensor) posturing may also be elicited by noxious stimuli (see Fig. 54-7, Lewis and others, *Medical-Surgical Nursing,* edition 5, p. 1616).
- *Headache.* Although the brain itself is insensitive to pain, compression of other intracranial structures, such as the walls of arteries and veins and the cranial nerves, can produce headache. The headache is often continuous but is worse in the morning; straining or movement may accentuate the pain.
- *Vomiting.* Vomiting that is usually not preceded by nausea is often a nonspecific sign of increased ICP.

Diagnostic Studies

- MRI and CT scan
- Vital signs, neurologic checks, ICP measurements (via intraventricular catheter, subdural bolt, or epidural transducer)
- Skull, chest, and spinal x-ray studies
- Electroencephalogram (EEG), ECG, angiography
- Cerebral blood flow and velocity studies; positron emission tomography (PET)
- Laboratory studies, including complete blood count (CBC), coagulation profile, electrolytes, creatinine, arterial blood gases (ABGs), ammonia level, general drug and toxicology screen, and CSF protein

Collaborative Care

The goals of management are to identify and treat the underlying cause of increased ICP and to support brain function. A careful history is an important diagnostic aid that can direct the search for the underlying cause.

While the cause of increased ICP is being sought, the condition itself must be treated aggressively to interrupt the cycle. Ensuring adequate oxygenation to support brain function is the first step. An endotracheal tube or tracheostomy may be necessary to maintain adequate ventilation. It may be necessary to maintain the patient on a ventilator to ensure adequate oxygenation.

- If the condition is caused by a mass lesion, such as a tumor or hematoma, surgical removal of the mass is the best management (see Intracranial Tumors, p. 354).
- Nonsurgical intervention for the reduction of tissue volume related to cerebral tissue swelling and edema includes the use of diuretics, corticosteroids, and fluid restriction.

Drug Therapy

Drug therapy plays an important part in the management of increased ICP. Osmotic and loop diuretics are used to reduce the volume of brain water, and corticosteroids are used to control the cerebral edema. Osmotically active agents such as mannitol (Osmitrol), glycerol, and urea are used. Fluid and electrolyte status must be monitored when these drugs are used. Loop diuretics such as furosemide (Lasix) and ethacrynic acid (Edecrin) cause a decrease in CSF production, thus lowering ICP. Corticosteroids have been used extensively in the treatment of cerebral edema. Dexamethasone (Decadron) is the most commonly used corticosteroid to reduce vasogenic cerebral edema. High-dose barbiturates (e.g., pentobarbital [Nembutal] and thiopental [Pentothal]) are used to produce a decrease in cerebral metabolism and a subsequent decrease in increased ICP.

Nursing Management

Goals

The primary goals for the unconscious patient—with the assumption that ICP has increased or has the potential to increase—are to prevent secondary cerebral damage, maintain function, and prevent complications secondary to immobility and the decreased LOC.

See NCP 54-1 for the unconscious patient, Lewis and others, *Medical-Surgical Nursing,* edition 5, p. 1621.

Nursing Diagnoses

- Altered cerebral tissue perfusion *related to* cerebral tissue swelling
- Ineffective breathing pattern *related to* loss of central nervous system (CNS) integrative function and immobility
- Ineffective airway clearance *related to* unconsciousness and the inability to mobilize secretions
- Altered nutrition: less than body requirements *related to* hypermetabolism and inability to ingest food and fluids
- Impaired skin integrity *related to* nutritional deficit, self-care deficit, and immobility

Nursing Interventions

Maintenance of respiratory function. Maintenance of a patent airway is critical with increased ICP and is a primary nursing responsibility. As the LOC decreases, the patient is at increased risk of airway obstruction. Altered breathing patterns may become evident.

- Airway patency can be aided by keeping the patient lying on one side, with frequent position changes. Snoring sounds, which may indicate obstruction, should be noted. Accumulated secretions should be removed by suctioning. An oral airway facilitates breathing and provides an easier suctioning route in the comatose patient.

The nurse must use measures to prevent hypoxia and hypercapnia. Proper positioning of the head is important.

- Elevation of the head of the bed by 30 degrees enhances respiratory exchange and aids in decreasing cerebral edema.
- Suctioning and coughing can cause transient increases in ICP and decreases in the partial pressure of oxygen in arterial blood (PaO_2). Suctioning should be kept to a minimum.
- Abdominal distention can interfere with respiratory function and should be prevented. Insertion of a nasogastric tube to aspirate the stomach contents can prevent distention, vomiting, and possible aspiration.
- ABGs should be measured and evaluated regularly.
- Unless the patient is on ventilatory support, the use of narcotic sedatives and opiates should be evaluated on an individual basis. Besides depressing respirations, these agents can also cloud the patient's LOC. A narcotic that does not increase the ICP, depress respiration, or cloud the LOC should be selected to control pain.

Fluid and electrolyte balance. Fluid and electrolyte disturbances can have an adverse effect on ICP. IV fluids should be closely monitored. Intake and output, with insensible losses and daily weights taken into account, are important parameters in the assessment of fluid balance.

- Electrolyte determinations should be made daily. It is especially important to monitor glucose, sodium (Na^+), potassium (K^+), and serum osmolality. Urinary output is monitored for problems related to diabetes insipidus (DI) and syndrome of inappropriate antidiuretic hormone (SIADH) (see Diabetes Insipidus, p. 187 and Syndrome of Inappropriate Antidiuretic Hormone, p. 550).

Monitoring of intracranial pressure. Measurement of ICP is valuable in detecting the early rise of ICP and the patient's response to treatment. These methods are discussed in detail in Chapter 63, Lewis and others, *Medical-Surgical Nursing,* edition 5.

Body position. Patients should be maintained in the head-up position. The nurse must take care to prevent extreme neck flexion, which can cause venous obstruction and increased ICP. The bed should be positioned so that it lowers the ICP while maintaining cerebral perfusion pressure (CPP).

- Care should be taken to turn the patient with slow, gentle movements because rapid changes in position may increase ICP. Caution should be used to prevent discomfort in turning and positioning of the patient because pain or agitation also increases pressure. Increased intrathoracic pressure contributes to increased ICP; thus coughing, straining, and the Valsalva maneuver should be avoided.

Protection from injury and environment management. The patient with increased ICP and a decreased LOC needs protection from self-injury. Confusion, agitation, and the possibility of seizures can put the patient at risk of injury. Restraints should be used judiciously in the agitated patient. The patient can benefit from a quiet, nonstimulating environment. Touching and talking to the patient, even one who is in coma, is always an appropriate approach. The nurse needs to create a balance between sensory deprivation and sensory overload.

Psychologic considerations. Anxiety over the diagnosis and prognosis for the patient with neurologic problems can be distressing to the patient, family, and nursing staff. Short, simple explanations are appropriate and allow the patient and family to acquire the amount of information they desire. There is a need for support, information, and education of both patients and families that begins with the traumatic event and continues for years after the event.

- The nurse should assess the family members' desire and need to assist in providing care for the patient and allow for their participation as appropriate.

INFERTILITY

Definition/Description

Infertility is the inability to achieve pregnancy after at least 1 year of regular intercourse without contraception. Approximately 15% of couples in North America are involuntarily infertile. Evaluation and therapeutic measures can be invasive, expensive, and take a year or more, with only 50% eventually conceiving. Understandably, infertility can constitute a physical and emotional life crisis.

Etiology

- Female infertility can be due to anovulation, disorders of the hypothalamic-pituitary-ovary axis, tubal obstructions or dysfunctions such as endometriosis, and uterine or cervical factors such as leiomyomas.
- Male infertility can be due to disorders of the hypothalamic-pituitary-gonad (testes) system, disorders of the testes, or abnormalities of the ejaculatory system.

Risk factors include increasing age, tobacco and illicit drug use, extremes of exercise activity, severe dietary restrictions, and specific occupational and environmental exposures. The infertility risk for women ages 35 to 44 years is double the risk for women 30 to 34 years old. One third of women older than 35 who desire pregnancy will experience infertility.

Diagnostic Studies

After a detailed history is obtained and a general physical examination of the woman and man is performed to rule out any related medical or gynecologic disease, several basic tests can be performed. These include the following:

- *Women.* Ovulatory studies, tubal patency studies, and post-coital studies
- *Men.* Semen analysis, plasma testosterone, serum luteinizing hormone (LH) and follicle-stimulating hormone (FSH) levels, and testicular biopsy

Nursing and Collaborative Management

The management of infertility problems depends on the cause. If infertility is secondary to an alteration in ovarian function, supplemental hormone therapy to restore and maintain ovulation may be attempted. Drugs used to induce ovulation include clomiphene (Clomid), menotropins (Pergonal, Humegon), and bromocriptine (Parlodel).

- When a tubal blockage exists, the woman should be referred to a specialist to discuss surgery or in vitro fertilization. Chronic cervicitis and inadequate estrogenic stimulation are cervical factors causing infertility. Antibiotic therapy is indicated for cervicitis. Inadequate estrogenic stimulation is treated by the administration of estrogens.

When a couple has not succeeded in conceiving while under infertility management, another option is intrauterine insemination with the husband's or donor's sperm. If this technique does not succeed, *in vitro fertilization* (IVF) may be used. IVF is the removal of mature oocytes from the woman's ovarian follicle via laparoscopy, followed by fertilization of the ova with the partner's sperm in a Petri dish. When fertilization and cleavage have occurred, the resulting embryos are transferred into the woman's uterus. The procedure requires 2 to 3 days to complete and is used in cases of fallopian tube obstruction, oligospermia, and unexplained infertility.

Assisted reproductive technologies (ART) consist of IVF, gamete intrafallopian transfer (GIFT), zygote intrafallopian transfer (ZIFT), embryo cryopreservation, and donor gametes.

The nurse has a major responsibility for teaching and providing emotional support throughout the infertility testing and treatment period.

- Feelings of anger, frustration, sadness, and helplessness may heighten as more and more diagnostic tests are performed.

Infertility can generate great tension in a marriage as the couple exhausts their financial and emotional resources. Few insurance carriers cover the cost of infertility testing or the therapeutic measures associated with infertility.

- Recognizing and taking steps to deal with the psychologic and emotional factors that surface can assist the couple to better cope with the situation.
- Couples should be encouraged to participate in a support group for infertile couples as well as in individual therapy.

INFLAMMATORY BOWEL DISEASE

Crohn's disease and *ulcerative colitis* are immune-related disorders that are referred to as *inflammatory bowel disease* (IBD). These disorders are characterized by chronic, recurrent inflammation of the intestinal tract. For both conditions, clinical manifestations are varied, with periods of remission interspersed with episodes of acute inflammation. Both diseases can be debilitating.

Although there has been extensive research on the etiology of IBD, the cause of both ulcerative colitis and Crohn's disease remains unknown. Possible causes include (1) an infectious agent (e.g., virus, bacteria), because IBD produces mucosal changes in the colon similar to those of infectious diarrhea, although no consistent pathogen has been identified; (2) an autoimmune reaction due to the presence of other immune-related disorders, such as systemic lupus erythematosus, ankylosing spondylitis (AS), and erythema nodosum in patients with IBD; (3) food allergies (although this has not been substantiated); and (4) heredity (familial recurrences have been documented). There is a familial tendency for both Crohn's disease and ulcerative colitis.

See Ulcerative Colitis, p. 590 and Crohn's Disease, p. 172 for more detailed discussion.

INTESTINAL OBSTRUCTION

Definition/Description

Intestinal obstruction occurs when the intestinal contents cannot pass through the GI tract. The obstruction may be partial or complete. The causes of intestinal obstruction can be classified as mechanical or nonmechanical.

- *Mechanical obstruction* may be caused by an occlusion of the intestinal tract lumen. Most intestinal obstructions occur in the small intestine. Mechanical obstruction accounts for 90% of all intestinal obstructions. Adhesions can develop after abdominal surgery. Obstruction can occur within days of surgery or years later. Carcinoma is the most common cause of large bowel obstruction, followed by volvulus and diverticular disease.
- *Nonmechanical obstruction* may result from a neuromuscular or vascular disorder. *Paralytic ileus* is the most common form of nonmechanical obstruction. It occurs to some degree after any abdominal surgery. Other causes of paralytic ileus include inflammatory reactions (e.g., acute pancreatitis, acute appendicitis), electrolyte abnormalities, and thoracic or lumbar spinal fractures.

Pathophysiology

When fluid, gas, and intestinal contents accumulate proximal to the intestinal obstruction, distention occurs, and the distal bowel may collapse. As the fluid increases, so does the pressure in the lumen of the bowel. The increased pressure leads to an increase in capillary permeability and extravasation of fluids and electrolytes into the peritoneal cavity. Edema, congestion, and necrosis from impaired blood supply, and possible rupture of the bowel may occur. Retention of fluid in the intestine and peritoneal cavity can lead to a severe reduction in circulating blood volume and result in hypotension and hypovolemic shock.

- Strangulation and gangrene are likely to develop if treatment is not immediate. A strangulated obstruction occurs when the circulation to the obstructed intestine is impaired. This is the most dangerous form of obstruction because it may lead to necrosis of the intestine (incarcerated). It is most commonly caused by volvulus, hernias, or adhesions.

Clinical Manifestations

Manifestations vary, depending on the location of the intestinal obstruction, and include nausea, vomiting, abdominal pain, distention, inability to pass flatus, and obstipation.

- An obstruction located high in the small intestine produces rapid-onset, sometimes projectile vomiting with bile-containing vomitus. Vomiting from more distal obstructions of the small intestine is more gradual in onset. Vomitus may be orange-brown and foul smelling because of bacterial overgrowth. In some cases it may be feculent. Vomiting may be entirely absent in large bowel obstruction if the ileocecal valve is competent; otherwise, the patient may eventually vomit feculent material.

- Abdominal pain in high intestinal obstructions is usually relieved by vomiting. Persistent, colicky abdominal pain is seen with lower intestinal obstruction. A characteristic sign of mechanical obstruction is pain that comes and goes in waves. This is due to intestinal peristalsis trying to move bowel contents past the obstructed area. In contrast, paralytic ileus produces a more constant generalized discomfort. Strangulation causes severe, constant pain that is rapid in onset.
- Abdominal distention is a common manifestation of all intestinal obstructions. It is usually absent or minimally noticeable in high obstructions of the small intestine and greatly increased in lower intestinal obstructions. Abdominal tenderness and rigidity are usually absent unless strangulation or peritonitis has occurred.
- Auscultation of bowel sounds reveals high-pitched sounds above the area of obstruction. Audible borborygmi are often noted by the patient. The patient's temperature rarely rises above 100° F (37.8° C) unless strangulation or peritonitis has occurred.

Diagnostic Studies

- Abdominal x-rays are the most useful diagnostic aids. Upright and lateral abdominal x-rays show the presence of gas and fluid in the intestines. The presence of intraperitoneal air indicates perforation.
- Barium enemas are helpful in locating large intestinal obstructions.
- Sigmoidoscopy or colonoscopy may provide direct visualization of an obstruction in the colon.
- An elevated white blood cell (WBC) count may indicate strangulation or perforation; elevated hematocrit (Hct) values may reflect hemoconcentration; decreased hemoglobin (Hb) and Hct values may indicate bleeding from a neoplasm or strangulation with necrosis.
- Serum sodium, potassium (K^+), and chloride concentrations are decreased in small-bowel obstruction.
- Blood urea nitrogen (BUN) values may be increased due to dehydration.
- Stools should be checked for occult blood.

Collaborative Care

Treatment is directed toward decompression of the intestine by the removal of gas and fluid, correction and maintenance of fluid and electrolyte balance, and relief or removal of the obstruction.

- Nasogastric (NG) or nasointestinal tubes may be used to decompress the bowel. NG tubes should be inserted before surgery to empty the stomach and relieve distention. They are also used instead of nasointestinal tubes to treat partial or complete small bowel obstruction. (See Intestinal and Nasogastric Tubes, p. 668.)
- Sigmoidoscopy may successfully reduce a sigmoid volvulus.

■ Colon decompression catheters may be passed through partially obstructed areas via a colonoscope to decompress the bowel before surgery.

IV infusions that contain normal saline solution and K$^+$ should be given to maintain the fluid and electrolyte balance. Total parenteral nutrition (TPN) may be necessary in some cases to correct nutritional deficiencies, improve the patient's nutritional status before surgery, and promote postoperative healing.

Most mechanical obstructions are treated surgically. They may involve resecting the obstructed segment of bowel and anastomosing the remaining healthy bowel. Partial or total colectomy, colostomy, or ileostomy may be required when extensive obstruction or necrosis is present. Occasionally obstructions can be removed nonsurgically. A colonoscope can be used to remove polyps, dilate strictures, and remove and necrose tumors with a laser.

Nursing Management
Goals
The patient with an intestinal obstruction will have relief from the obstruction and a return to normal bowel function, experience minimal to no discomfort, and have normal fluid and electrolyte status.

Nursing Diagnoses
■ Pain *related to* abdominal distention and increased peristalsis
■ Fluid volume deficit *related to* a decrease in intestinal fluid reabsorption and the loss of fluids secondary to vomiting
■ Altered nutrition: less than body requirements *related to* intestinal obstruction and vomiting

Nursing Interventions
The patient should be monitored closely for signs of dehydration and electrolyte imbalance.

■ A strict intake and output record should be maintained. All vomitus and tube drainage should be included. IV fluids should be administered as ordered.
■ Serum electrolyte levels should be monitored closely. A patient with a high obstruction is more likely to have metabolic alkalosis; a patient with a low obstruction is at greater risk of metabolic acidosis.
■ A patient is often restless and constantly changes position to relieve the pain. Analgesics may often be withheld until the obstruction is diagnosed because they may mask other signs and symptoms and decrease intestinal motility.
■ The nurse should provide comfort measures, promote a restful environment, and keep distractions and visitors to a minimum.
■ Nursing care of the patient after surgery for an intestinal obstruction is similar to the care of the patient after a laparotomy (see Abdominal Pain, Acute, p. 3).

INTRACRANIAL TUMORS

Definition/Description

Tumors of the brain may be primary, arising from tissues (usually non-neural tissues) within the brain, or secondary, resulting from a metastasis from a malignant neoplasm elsewhere in the body. Brain tumors are generally classified according to the tissue from which they arise—either those arising inside the brain substance (e.g., gliomas, vascular tumors) or those arising outside the brain substance (e.g., meningiomas, cranial nerve tumors).

- Unless treated, all intracranial tumors eventually cause death from increasing tumor volume leading to increased intracranial pressure (ICP). (For a comparison of the major intracranial tumors, see Table 54-13, Lewis and others, *Medical-Surgical Nursing,* edition 5, p. 1630.)

Clinical Manifestations

Manifestations are generally caused by local destructive effects of the tumor, displacement of structures, obstruction of cerebrospinal fluid (CSF) flow, and the effects of edema and increased ICP on cerebral function. The appearance of manifestations depends on the location, size, and rate of tumor growth.

A wide range of clinical manifestations are associated with brain tumors. In some circumstances, a slight decrease in mental acuity may be the only symptom. In other cases there may be a dramatic event, such as a seizure, or increased ICP signs may be apparent.

- Manifestations may clearly indicate the location of the tumor by an alteration in the function controlled by the affected area (see Table 54-14, Lewis and others, *Medical-Surgical Nursing,* edition 5, p. 1631).

If the tumor mass obstructs the ventricles or occludes the outlet, ventricular enlargement *(hydrocephalus)* can occur. Surgical treatment is needed to relieve pressure and involves placement of a ventriculo-atrial or a ventriculoperitoneal shunt. The physician should be notified if signs of increased ICP, such as headache, blurred vision, vomiting without nausea, decreasing level of consciousness (LOC), or restlessness, occur. Signs of an infected shunt, such as high fever, persistent headache, and stiff neck, warrant investigation.

Diagnostic Studies

- MRI allows for detection of very small tumors.
- Cerebral angiography determines blood flow and localization of tumor.
- CT and brain scanning assist in tumor location.

■ Other useful diagnostic studies include skull x-rays, electroen-cephalogram (EEG), and positron emission tomography (PET).

Collaborative Care

Treatment goals are aimed at identifying the tumor type and location, removing or decreasing tumor mass, and preventing or managing increased ICP.

Surgical therapy is the preferred treatment for brain tumors (see the section on cranial surgery in Lewis and others, *Medical-Surgical Nursing*, edition 5, p. 1633). Surgical outcome depends on the type, size, and location of the tumor. Meningiomas and oligodendrogliomas can usually be completely removed, whereas more invasive gliomas and medulloblastomas can be only partially removed. Tumors located in deep central areas of the dominant hemisphere, posterior corpus callosum, or upper brainstem cause extensive neurologic damage and are considered inoperable. Surgery can reduce tumor mass, which decreases ICP and provides relief of symptoms with an extension of survival time.

Radiation therapy lengthens survival in patients with malignant gliomas, especially when it is combined with partial surgical re-moval. Patients with less-malignant tumors respond to radiation with a longer survival time and a decreased recurrence of tumor. Cerebral edema and rapidly increasing ICP may be a complication of radiation therapy, but they can be managed with high doses of corticosteroids (dexamethasone [Decadron], prednisone).

Normally the blood-brain barrier prohibits the entry of most drugs into brain parenchyma. Malignant brain tumors cause a breakdown of the blood-brain barrier in the tumor area, allowing chemothera-peutic agents to be used to treat the malignancy. Carmustine (BCNU) and lomustine (CCNU) are particularly effective in treating brain tumors. Other drugs being used include methotrexate and procar-bazine (Matulane). (See Radiation Therapy, p. 681, and Chemo-therapy, p. 643).

Brain tumors that cannot be totally removed may be treated with a combination of corticosteroids, surgery, radiation, and chemother-apy. Many techniques to control and treat brain tumors are under investigation, including radium implants into the tumor bed, local hyperthermia, and biologic therapy.

■ Although progress in treatment has increased the length and quality of survival of patients with gliomas, death is almost always inevitable.

Nursing Management
Goals

The patient with a brain tumor will maintain normal ICP, maxi-mize neurologic functioning, be free from pain and discomfort, and be aware of the long-term implications with respect to prognosis and cognitive and physical functioning.

Nursing Diagnoses/Collaborative Problems

- Altered cerebral tissue perfusion *related to* cerebral edema
- Pain (headache) *related to* cerebral edema and increased ICP
- Self-care deficits *related to* altered neuromuscular function secondary to tumor growth and cerebral edema
- Anxiety *related to* diagnosis and treatment
- Potential complication: seizures *related to* abnormal electrical activity of the brain
- Potential complication: increased ICP *related to* presence of tumor and failure of normal compensatory mechanisms

Nursing Interventions

Behavioral changes such as loss of emotional control, confusion, memory loss, and depression are often not perceived by the patient but can be very disturbing and frightening to the family. Assisting and supporting the family in understanding what is happening are very important roles for the nurse.

- The confused patient with behavioral instability can be a challenge. Close supervision of activity, use of side rails, judicious use of restraints, padding of rails, and a calm, reassuring approach are all essential care techniques.
- Minimization of environmental stimuli, creation of a routine schedule, and the use of reality orientation can be incorporated into the care plan for the confused patient.
- Motor and sensory dysfunctions are problems that interfere with the activities of daily living. Alterations in mobility must be managed, and the patient needs to be encouraged to provide as much self-care as physically possible. Self-image often depends on the patient's ability to participate in care within the limitations of the physical deficits.
- Motor (expressive) or sensory (receptive) dysphasias may occur. Disturbances in communication can be frustrating for the patient and may interfere with the nurse's ability to meet patient needs. Attempts should be made to establish a communication system that can be used by both the patient and staff.
- Nutritional intake may be decreased because of the patient's inability to eat, loss of appetite, or loss of desire to eat. Assessing the nutritional status of the patient and ensuring adequate nutritional intake are important aspects of care. The patient may need encouragement to eat or, in some cases, may have to be fed orally, parenterally, by gastrostomy or nasogastric (NG) tube, or by total parenteral nutrition (TPN) (see Tube Feedings, p. 689, and Total Parenteral Nutrition, p. 684).

The patient with a brain tumor who undergoes cranial surgery requires complex nursing care. (See the section on cranial surgery, Lewis and others, *Medical-Surgical Nursing,* edition 5, p. 1633).

IRRITABLE BOWEL SYNDROME

Definition/Description

Irritable bowel syndrome (IBS) is a symptom complex characterized by intermittent and recurrent abdominal pain associated with an alteration in bowel function (diarrhea or constipation). Other symptoms commonly found include abdominal distention, excessive flatulence, urge to defecate, and sensation of incomplete evacuation.

IBS is a common problem, affecting approximately 10% to 17% of the population in the United States. Stress, psychologic factors, and specific food intolerances have been identified as factors that precipitate IBS symptoms.

The key to accurate diagnosis is a thorough health history and physical examination. Emphasis should be on symptoms, past health history (e.g., psychosocial aspects including physical or sexual abuse), family history, and drug and dietary history. The health care provider should establish a trusting relationship with the patient.

- The patient needs reassurance that the symptoms are functional. The patient should be encouraged to verbalize concerns and anxiety.
- A diet containing at least 20 g per day of dietary fiber should be initiated. This may also include the addition of psyllium-containing products (e.g., Metamucil). The patient whose primary symptoms are abdominal distention and increased flatulence should be advised to eliminate common gas-producing foods such as broccoli and cabbage from the diet and to substitute yogurt for milk products if there is lactose intolerance.
- Anticholinergic agents, such as dicyclomine (Bentyl), may be helpful if taken before meals to alleviate the pain associated with the ingesting of food.
- For the patient with a high level of anxiety, a mild sedative or tranquilizer may be ordered but should be prescribed for only a short time. Additional therapies include relaxation and stress management techniques, although no single therapy has been found to be effective for all patients with IBS.

LACTASE DEFICIENCY

Definition/Description
Lactase deficiency is a condition in which intestinal lactase, the enzyme that breaks down lactose into two simple sugars (glucose and galactose), is deficient or absent.

Although *primary lactase deficiency* seems to be hereditary, milk intolerance may not become clinically evident until late adolescence or early adulthood. About 5% of the adult population has primary lactase deficiency, with the highest incidence found in African-Americans, Native Americans, Mexican-Americans, and individuals of Jewish descent.

Acquired lactase deficiency is often seen in GI diseases in which the mucosa has been damaged; these include ulcerative colitis, Crohn's disease, gastroenteritis, and sprue syndrome.

Clinical Manifestations
Symptoms of lactose intolerance include bloating, flatulence, crampy abdominal pain, and diarrhea. These symptoms may occur within half an hour to several hours after drinking a glass of milk or ingesting a milk product.

Diagnostic Studies
A lactose tolerance test can be performed to diagnose lactose intolerance. The patient is given 50 to 100 mg of lactose orally. Blood samples are drawn before the consumption of lactose and at 15-, 30-, 60-, and 90-minute intervals. Failure of the blood glucose level to increase more than 20 mg/dl is suggestive of lactase deficiency. An increase in hydrogen breath test after ingestion of lactose is found.

Nursing and Collaborative Management
Treatment consists of eliminating lactose from the diet by avoiding milk and milk products.
- A lactose-free diet is given initially and is gradually advanced to a low lactose diet as tolerated by the patient. The objective of care is to teach the importance of adherence to the diet. Many lactose-intolerant persons may not exhibit symptoms if lactose is taken in small amounts. In some persons, lactose may be tolerated better if taken with meals.
- The patient needs to be aware that milk, ice cream, cottage cheese, and cheese have a high lactose content.
- If the milk has been fermented (e.g., cultured buttermilk, yogurt, sour cream), the patient with low lactase levels may tolerate milk and milk products better.

- Lactase enzyme (Lactaid) is available commercially as an over-the-counter product. It is mixed with milk and breaks down the lactose before the milk is ingested.

LEIOMYOMAS (FIBROIDS)

Leiomyomas (fibroids, myomas, fibromyomas, fibromas) are the most common benign tumors of the female genital tract. By 30 years of age, 10% of Caucasian women and 30% of African-American women will have uterine leiomyomas.

The cause of leiomyomas is unknown. Leiomyomas appear to depend on ovarian hormones because they grow slowly during the woman's reproductive years and undergo atrophy after menopause. Leiomyomas consist of smooth muscle cells.

The majority of women with fibroids do not have symptoms. Of the women with leiomyomas who develop symptoms, the most common is menorrhagia. Although rarely experienced with leiomyomas, the pain is associated with an infection or twisting of the pedicle from which the tumor is growing. Dysmenorrhea and dyspareunia may occasionally occur.

Pressure on surrounding organs may result in rectal, bladder, and lower abdominal discomfort. Large tumors may cause a general enlargement of the lower abdomen. These tumors are sometimes associated with spontaneous abortion and infertility.

Diagnosis is based on the characteristic pelvic findings of an enlarged uterus distorted by nodular masses.

Treatment depends on the symptoms, age of the patient, her desire to bear children, and the location and size of the tumor(s). If the symptoms are minor, the health care provider may elect to follow the patient closely for a time.

- Persistent heavy menstrual bleeding causing anemia and large or rapidly growing fibroids are indications for surgery. Fibroids are removed by hysterectomy or myomectomy. A myomectomy is performed for women who wish to have children. In this case, only the fibroids are removed in order to preserve the uterus. Small fibroids may be removed using a hysteroscope and laser resection instruments.
- In cases of large leiomyomas, the treatment is hysterectomy. Gonadotropin-releasing hormone agonist (Lupron) may be used preoperatively to shrink the size of the leiomyomas.

L

LEUKEMIA

Definition/Description
Leukemia is a general term used to describe a group of malignant disorders affecting the blood and blood-forming tissues of the bone marrow, lymph system, and spleen. It results in an accumulation of dysfunctional cells because of a loss of regulation in cell division. Although often thought of as a disease of children, the number of adults affected with leukemia is 10 times that of children. Table 40 summarizes the relative incidence and features of the different types of leukemia.

Regardless of the specific type, there is generally no single causative agent in the development of leukemia. Most leukemias result from a combination of factors including genetic and environmental influences.

Classification
Acute leukemia is characterized by clonal proliferation of immature, undifferentiated hematopoietic cells (blasts). The most prominent characteristic of the neoplastic cell in acute leukemia is a defect in maturation beyond the myeloblast or promyelocyte level in *acute myelogenous leukemia* (AML) and the lymphoblast in *acute lymphocytic leukemia* (ALL). Acute leukemia has a rapid onset and requires immediate and aggressive intervention.

Chronic lymphocytic leukemia (CLL) is a neoplasm of activated B lymphocytes. CLL cells, which morphologically resemble mature, small lymphocytes of the peripheral blood, accumulate in large numbers in the bone marrow, blood, lymph nodes, and spleen. Many individuals in the early stages of CLL require no treatment. As the disease progresses, various treatments can be used to control symptoms.

Chronic myelogenous leukemia (CML) is a clonal stem cell disorder characterized by greatly increased myelopoiesis and the presence of the Philadelphia chromosome in 90% of patients. The chronic phase of CML can persist for 2 to 4 years and can usually be well controlled with treatment.

Hairy cell leukemia accounts for 2% of all adult leukemias and is a chronic disease of lymphoproliferation. This leukemia type predominantly involves B lymphocytes that infiltrate the bone marrow and spleen.

Clinical Manifestations
Manifestations of leukemia are varied (see Table 40). Essentially they relate to problems caused by bone marrow failure and the formation of masses composed of leukemic infiltrates. The patient is pre-

Table 40 Types of Leukemia

Type/incidence*	Age of onset	Clinical manifestations	Diagnostic findings
Acute myelogenous leukemia (AML)—33%	Increase in incidence with advancing age; peak incidence between 60-70 yr of age	Fatigue and weakness, headache, mouth sores, minimal hepatosplenomegaly and lymphadenopathy, anemia, bleeding, fever, infection, sternal tenderness	Low RBC count, Hb, Hct; low platelet count; low to high WBC count with myeloblasts; greatly hypercellular bone marrow with myeloblasts
Acute lymphocytic leukemia (ALL)—11%	Before 14 yr of age; peak incidence between 2-9 yr of age and also in older adults	Fever; pallor; bleeding; anorexia; fatigue and weakness; bone, joint, and abdominal pain; generalized lymphadenopathy; infections; weight loss; hepatosplenomegaly; headache; mouth sores; neurologic manifestations, including CNS involvement and ICP, secondary to meningeal infiltration	Low RBC count, Hb, Hct; low platelet count; low, normal, or high WBC count; transverse lines of rarefaction at ends of metaphysis of long bones on x-ray; hypercellular bone marrow with lymphoblasts; lymphoblasts also possible in CSF

CNS, Central nervous system; *CSF,* cerebrospinal fluid; *Hb,* hemoglobin; *Hct,* hematocrit; *ICP,* intracranial pressure; *RBC,* red blood cell; *WBC,* white blood cell.
*This is the incidence based on all types of leukemia; the number does not add up to 100% because approximately 16% of cases are unclassifiable.

Continued

L

Table 40 Types of Leukemia—cont'd

Type/incidence*	Age of onset	Clinical manifestations	Diagnostic findings
Chronic myelogenous leukemia (CML)— 15%	25-60 yr of age; peak incidence around 45 yr of age	No symptoms early in disease; fatigue and weakness, fever, sternal tenderness, weight loss, joint pain, bone pain, massive splenomegaly, increase in sweating	Low RBC count, Hb, Hct; high platelet count early, lower count later; increase in polymorphonuclear neutrophils, normal number of lymphocytes, and normal or low number of monocytes in WBC differential; low leukocyte alkaline phosphatase; presence of Philadelphia chromosome in 90% of patients
Chronic lymphocytic leukemia (CLL)— 25%	50-70 yr of age; rare below 30 yr of age; predominance in men	No symptoms usually; detection of disease often during examination for unrelated condition; chronic fatigue, anorexia, splenomegaly and lymphadenopathy, hepatomegaly	Mild anemia and thrombocytopenia with disease progression; increase in peripheral lymphocytes; increase in presence of lymphocytes in bone marrow

disposed to anemia, thrombocytopenia, and a decreased or increased number and decreased function of white blood cells (WBCs).

- Increased numbers of WBCs lead to infiltration and damage to the bone marrow, lymph nodes, spleen, and other organs, including the central nervous system (CNS).
- Leukemic infiltration leads to problems such as splenomegaly, hepatomegaly, lymphadenopathy, bone pain, meningeal irritation, and oral lesions.

Diagnostic Studies

The goal is to define the specific type of leukemia so that the appropriate treatment and prognosis can be determined.

- Peripheral blood evaluation and bone marrow examination are the primary methods of diagnosing and classifying the acute and chronic types of leukemia. (For these classifications, see Tables 29-25 and 29-26 in Lewis and others, *Medical-Surgical Nursing,* edition 5, p. 771.)
- Morphologic, histochemical, immunologic, and cytogenetic methods are all used to identify cell subtypes and the stage of development of leukemic cell populations.
- Studies such as lumbar puncture and CT scan can determine the presence of leukemic cells outside the blood and bone marrow.

Collaborative Care

Collaborative care includes remission induction with chemotherapeutic drugs and (sometimes) radiation therapy. (See Chemotherapy, p. 643 and Radiation Therapy, p. 681). Other considerations include regular examination of patients to evaluate their progress and supportive interventions to prevent disease and therapy complications (e.g., hemorrhage, infection).

- The nurse needs to understand the principles of cancer chemotherapy, including cellular kinetics, the use of multiple drugs rather than single agents, and the cell cycle (see Chemotherapy, p. 643).
- Corticosteroids and radiation therapy may have a role in therapy for the patient with leukemia. Total body radiation may be used to prepare a patient for bone marrow transplantation, or radiation may be restricted to certain areas (fields) such as the liver, spleen, or other organs affected by infiltrates.
- In ALL, prophylactic intrathecal methotrexate is given to decrease CNS involvement, which is common in this type of leukemia. When CNS leukemia does occur, cranial radiation is given. The use of biologic therapy in the treatment of leukemia is being investigated (see Lewis and others, *Medical-Surgical Nursing,* edition 5, p. 310).

L

Chemotherapeutic agents used to treat leukemia vary. The choice of drugs and the sequence of therapy depend on the preference of the oncologist and on current research findings.

Bone marrow transplantation (BMT) and *stem cell transplantation* are other forms of therapy used for patients with different forms of leukemia, including ALL, AML, and CML. In leukemia, the goal of transplant is to totally eliminate leukemia cells from the body using combinations of chemotherapy with or without total body radiation. This treatment also eradicates the patient's hematopoietic stem cells, which are then replaced with those of a human leukocyte antigen (HLA)–matched sibling or volunteer donor (allogeneic), an identical twin (syngeneic), or with the patient's own (autologous) stem cells that were removed (harvested) before the intensive therapy. (See the sections on BMT and peripheral stem cell transplantation in Lewis and others, *Medical-Surgical Nursing,* p. 312 and p. 774).

The primary complications of patients with allogeneic BMT are graft-versus-host disease (GVHD), relapse of leukemia (especially ALL), and infection (especially interstitial pneumonia). Because transplantation is highly toxic therapy, the patient must weigh the significant risks of treatment-related death or treatment failure (relapse) with the hope of cure.

Nursing Management

Goals
The patient with leukemia will understand and cooperate with the treatment plan, experience minimal side effects and complications associated with both the disease and its treatment, and feel hopeful and supported during the periods of treatment, remission, and/or relapse.

See NCPs 29-1, p. 740; 29-2, p. 759; and 29-3, p. 769, Lewis and others, *Medical-Surgical Nursing,* edition 5.

Nursing Diagnoses
Nursing diagnoses related to leukemia include those appropriate for anemia (see Anemia, p. 22), thrombocytopenia (see Thrombocytopenic Purpura, p. 570), and neutropenia (see the section on neutropenia in Lewis and others, *Medical-Surgical Nursing,* edition 5, p. 766).

Nursing Interventions
The nursing role during the acute phase of leukemia is extremely challenging because the patient has many physical and psychosocial needs. As with other forms of cancer, the diagnosis of leukemia can evoke great fear and be equated with death. The nurse has a special responsibility in helping patients and families deal with these feelings.

- The nurse must help the patient realize that although the future may be uncertain, one can have a meaningful quality of life while in remission or with disease control.

- Families need help in adjusting to the stress of the abrupt onset of serious illness (e.g., dependence, withdrawal, changes in role responsibilities, alterations in body image) and the losses imposed by the sick role. The diagnosis of leukemia often brings with it the need to make difficult decisions at a time of profound stress for the patient and family.

The nurse is an important advocate in helping the patient and family understand the complexities of treatment decisions as well as the expected side effects and toxicities. A patient may require isolation or may need to temporarily relocate to an appropriate treatment center. These situations can lead patients to feel deserted and isolated at a time when they need the most support.

- From a physical care perspective, the nurse is challenged to make assessments and plan care to help the patient deal with the side effects of chemotherapy. The potential life-threatening problems of bone marrow suppression (anemia, thrombocytopenia, neutropenia) require aggressive nursing interventions.
- The nurse must be knowledgeable about all of the drugs being administered. In addition, the nurse must know how to assess laboratory data reflecting the effects of the drugs. Patient survival and comfort during aggressive chemotherapy are significantly affected by the quality of nursing care.

▼ **Patient Teaching**

The patient and family must be educated to understand the importance of their continued diligence in disease management and the need for follow-up care.

- Assistance may be needed to reestablish various relationships that are a part of the patient's life. Friends and family may not know how to interact with the patient.
- Involving the patient in survivor networks, support groups, or services, such as CanSurmount and Make Today Count, may help the patient adapt to living with a life-threatening illness. Exploring resources in the community (e.g., American Cancer Society, Leukemia Society, Meals-on-Wheels, wheelchair taxis) may reduce the financial burden and feelings of dependence.

LIVER CANCER

L

Definition/Description

Although it is quite rate, the most common malignant tumor of the liver is a primary carcinoma. Some cases of hepatocellular carcinoma are associated with chronic hepatitis B or C. A high percentage of patients with primary liver cancer have cirrhosis of the liver, with men having a higher incidence than women.

The liver is a common site of metastatic growth due to its high rate of blood flow and extensive capillary network. Cancer cells in other parts of the body are commonly carried to the liver via the portal circulation. Primary liver tumors commonly metastasize to the lung.

- The prognosis for liver cancer is poor. The cancer grows rapidly, and death may occur within 4 to 7 months as a result of hepatic encephalopathy or massive blood loss from GI bleeding.

Clinical Manifestations
It is difficult to diagnose carcinoma of the liver. It is particularly difficult to differentiate it from cirrhosis in its early stages, since many of the clinical manifestations (e.g., hepatomegaly, weight loss, peripheral edema, ascites, portal hypertension) are similar.

Other common manifestations include dull abdominal pain in the epigastric or right upper quadrant region, jaundice, anorexia, nausea and vomiting, and extreme weakness.

Diagnostic Studies
Tests used to assist in the diagnosis of liver cancer are a liver scan, hepatic arteriography, endoscopic retrograde cholangiopancreatography (ERCP), and a liver biopsy. The test for α-fetoprotein (AFP) may be positive in hepatocellular carcinoma. AFP helps to distinguish primary cancer from metastatic cancer.

Nursing and Collaborative Management
Treatment is largely palliative. Surgical excision (lobectomy) is sometimes performed if the tumor is localized to one portion of the liver. Only 30% to 40% of patients have surgically resectable disease. Usually surgery is not feasible because the cancer is too far advanced when it is detected. Surgical excision offers the only chance for a cure of liver cancer. The management of liver cancer is very similar to that for cirrhosis (see Cirrhosis, p. 143). Chemotherapy may be used, but there is usually a poor response. Portal vein or hepatic artery perfusion with 5-fluorouracil (5-FU) may be attempted.

Nursing interventions focus on keeping the patient as comfortable as possible. Because the patient with liver cancer manifests the same problems as the patient with advanced liver disease, the nursing interventions discussed for cirrhosis of the liver apply (see Cirrhosis, p. 143, and Cancer, p. 97).

LOW BACK PAIN, ACUTE

Definition/Description
Low back pain is common and probably affects 80% of adults in the United States at least once during their lifetime. Risk factors associated with low back pain include smoking, stress, poor posture, lack of muscle tone, and excess weight. Jobs which require repetitive heavy lifting, vibration (e.g., jackhammer operator), and extended periods of driving are also associated with low back pain.

Pathophysiology
Pain in the lumbar region is a common problem because this area (1) bears most of the weight of the body, (2) is the most flexible region of the spinal column, (3) has nerve roots that are vulnerable to injury or disease, and (4) has an inherently poor biomechanical structure.

Low back pain is most often due to a musculoskeletal problem. Other causes such as metabolic, circulatory, gynecologic, urologic, or psychologic problems, which may refer pain to the lower back, must not be overlooked.

- The causes of low back pain of musculoskeletal origin include (1) acute lumbosacral strain, (2) instability of lumbosacral bony mechanism, (3) osteoarthritis of the lumbosacral vertebrae, (4) intervertebral disk degeneration, and (5) herniation of the intervertebral disk.

Clinical Manifestations
Acute low back pain is usually associated with some type of activity that causes undue stress on the tissues of the lower back. Often symptoms do not appear at the time of injury but develop later because of gradual buildup of paravertebral muscle spasms.

Few definitive diagnostic abnormalities are present with paravertebral muscle strain. The straight-leg raise test may produce pain in the lumbar area without radiation along the sciatic nerve.

Collaborative Care
If the muscle spasms are not severe, the patient may be treated on an outpatient basis with a combination of the following: analgesics, nonsteroidal antiinflammatory drugs (NSAIDs), muscle relaxants, and the use of a corset. A corset prevents rotation, flexion, and extension of the lower back.

- If the spasms and pain are severe, a period of rest at home may be necessary. Since paravertebral muscle spasms are worse when the patient is upright, bed rest is the main treatment for severe acute low back pain. At this time, gradually increasing activity is initiated.

- When the patient is comfortable on oral pain medication, a progressive physical therapy program is begun to regain flexibility and strength in the lower back structures.

If conservative treatment is ineffective and the cause of the pain is nerve root irritation, an epidural corticosteroid injection may be performed. Epidural corticosteroids have been shown to decrease pain, speed the return of function, and improve objective neurologic signs. Epidural injections typically consist of a series of one to three injections over a span of several days to several weeks.

Nursing Management
Goals
The patient with acute low back pain will have satisfactory pain relief, avoid constipation secondary to medication and immobility, learn back-sparing practices, and return to previous level of activity within prescribed restrictions.

See NCP 59-4 for the patient with low back pain, Lewis and others, *Medical-Surgical Nursing,* edition 5, p. 1805.

Nursing Diagnoses
- Pain *related to* herniated nucleus pulposus, muscle spasms, ineffective comfort measures, and progression of problem
- Impaired physical mobility *related to* pain
- Ineffective individual coping *related to* effects of pain on lifestyle
- Ineffective management of therapeutic regimen *related to* lack of knowledge regarding posture, body mechanics, and weight reduction
- Body-image disturbance *related to* impaired mobility and chronic pain

Nursing Interventions
Primary nursing responsibilities are to assist the patient to maintain activity limitations, promote comfort, and educate the patient about the disease process and exercise.

- Although actual muscle-strengthening exercises are often taught by the physical therapist, it is the nurse's responsibility to ensure that the patient understands the type and frequency of exercise prescribed, as well as the rationale for the program.
- The frustration, pain, and disability imposed on the patient with low back pain problems require emotional support and understanding care by the nurse.

A goal of management is to make an episode of acute low back pain an isolated incident. If the lumbosacral mechanism is unstable, repeated episodes can be anticipated. Intervention is aimed at strengthening the supporting muscles by exercise and the use of a corset to limit extremes of movement. In addition, weight reduction decreases the mechanical demands on the lower back.

▼ **Patient Teaching**

The nurse is a significant role model and teacher for patients with low back problems. The nurse should use proper body mechanics at all times. This should be a primary consideration when teaching transfer and turning techniques to patients and care providers. The nurse should assess the patient's use of body mechanics and offer advice when activities that could produce back strain are used (see Tables 59-17 and 59-18, Lewis and others, *Medical-Surgical Nursing,* edition 5, p. 1806-1807).

- Patients are advised to maintain an appropriate weight. Excess body weight places extra stress on the lower back and weakens the abdominal muscles that support the lower back.
- The position assumed while sleeping is also important in preventing low back pain. Sleeping in a prone position should be avoided because it produces excessive lumbar lordosis, placing excessive stress on the lower back. A firm mattress is recommended. The patient should sleep in either a supine or side-lying position with the knees and hips flexed to prevent unnecessary pressure on support muscles, ligamentous structures, and lumbosacral joints.

LOW BACK PAIN, CHRONIC

Definition/Description

Chronic low back pain is caused by degenerative disk disease, lack of physical exercise, obesity, structural and postural abnormalities, and systemic disease. Structural degeneration of the intervertebral disk results in degenerative disease manifested by low back pain. Degeneration can also occur in the cervical spine area. The degeneration results in intervertebral narrowing and a lessening of the efficiency of the intervertebral disks to act as shock absorbers. As stresses on the degenerated disk continue and eventually exceed the strength of the disk, herniation of the intervertebral disk may result, causing compression or tension on a lumbar or sacral spinal nerve root.

L

Clinical Manifestations

The most characteristic feature of a lumbar herniated intervertebral disk is back pain with associated buttock and leg pain along the distribution of the sciatic nerve *(radioculopathy).* (Manifestations based on the level of lumbar disk herniation are summarized in Table 59-19, Lewis and others, *Medical-Surgical Nursing,* edition 5, p. 1809.)

- Back or leg pain may be reproduced by raising the leg and flexing the foot at 90 degrees. Low back pain from other causes may not be accompanied by leg pain.
- The straight leg-raise may be positive.
- Reflexes may be depressed or absent, depending on the spinal nerve root involved, and paresthesia or muscle weakness in the legs, toes, or feet may be felt by the patient.
- If the disk ruptures in the cervical area, stiff neck, shoulder pain radiating to the hand, and paresthesias and sensory disturbances of the hand are evident.

Diagnostic Studies

- X-rays are done to note any structural defects.
- A myelogram, MRI, and CT scan are helpful in localizing the site of herniation. A diskogram may be necessary if other methods of diagnosis are unsuccessful.
- An electromyogram (EMG) of the lower extremities may determine the severity of nerve irritation caused by herniation.

Collaborative Care

Degenerative disk disease is managed conservatively with rest, limitation of extremes of spinal movement (corset), local heat or ice, ultrasound, transcutaneous electrical nerve stimulation (TENS), and nonsteroidal antiinflammatory drugs (NSAIDs). If herniation of the disk occurs, more aggressive treatment is indicated.

Conservative treatment sometimes results in a healing over of the herniated area with a decrease in the pain of nerve root irritation. Muscle relaxants may be used to decrease muscle spasms. Once symptoms subside, back-strengthening exercises are begun. Extremes of flexion and torsion are strongly discouraged.

- Most patients with herniated disks recover with a conservative treatment plan. However, if conservative treatment is unsuccessful, surgery may be indicated.

Surgical Therapy

A *diskectomy* may be performed to decompress the nerve root. It involves the partial removal of the lamina (posterior arch of the vertebra).

- *Microsurgical diskectomy* is a version of the standard diskectomy in which a surgeon uses a microscope to allow better visualization of the disk and disk space during surgery to aid in the removal of the herniated portion.
- A *percutaneous laser diskectomy* is a surgical procedure using a scope that is passed through the retroperitoneal soft tissues to the lateral border of the disk with the aid of fluoroscopy. Laser

therapy is performed on the herniated portion of the disk. Small stab wounds are used with minimal blood loss.

A *laminectomy* is the traditional and most common procedure performed. It involves the surgical excision of part of the lamina to gain access to all or part of the protruding disk and remove it.

A *spinal fusion* may be performed if an unstable bony mechanism is present. The spine is stabilized by creating an ankylosis (fusion) of contiguous vertebrae with a bone graft from the patient's fibula or iliac crest or from donated bone. If vertebral instability exists, metal fixation with rods, plates, or screws may be done at the time of spinal surgery to provide more stability and decrease vertebral motion.

Nursing Management
See the section on nursing management for Low Back Pain, Acute, p. 368.

LUNG CANCER

Definition/Description
Lung cancer is the leading cause of death in men and women who have malignant disease in the United States. The overall 5-year survival rate is 14%, which is the poorest prognosis for any cancer other than cancers of the pancreas, liver, and esophagus. The disease is found most frequently in persons 40 to 75 years of age.

Risk factors for lung cancer include cigarette smoking, inhaled carcinogens, and preexisting pulmonary diseases.

- Cigarette smoking as a chronic respiratory irritant is the greatest risk factor. Smoking is responsible for approximately 80% to 90% of all lung cancers. Cigarette smoking causes a change in the bronchial epithelium, which usually returns to normal when smoking is discontinued
- Inhaled carcinogens are another major risk factor. These include asbestos, radon, nickel, iron and iron oxides, uranium, polycyclic aromatic hydrocarbons, arsenic, and air pollution.
- The incidence of lung cancer correlates with the degree of urbanization and population density. One reason for this may be increased exposure to irritants and pollutants.
- Preexisting pulmonary diseases such as tuberculosis (TB), pulmonary fibrosis, bronchiectasis, and chronic obstructive pulmonary disease (COPD) are also possible risk factors. Chronic inflammatory conditions often precede cancer.

Pathophysiology

The pathogenesis of lung cancer is not well understood. More than 90% of cancers originate from epithelium of the bronchus (bronchogenic). They grow slowly, and it takes 8 to 10 years for a tumor to reach 1 cm in size, which is the smallest lesion detectable on x-ray. Lung cancers occur primarily in the segmental bronchi or beyond and have a preference for the upper lobes of the lungs.

Pathologic changes in the bronchial system show nonspecific inflammatory changes with hypersecretion of mucus, desquamation of cells, reactive hyperplasia of basal cells, and metaplasia of normal respiratory epithelium to stratified squamous cells. Primary lung cancers are often categorized into two broad types—*non–small cell lung cancer* and *small cell lung cancer.* Lung cancer metastasizes primarily by direct extension and via the blood circulation and lymph system. Common sites for metastasis are the liver, brain, bones, lymph nodes, and adrenal glands.

Clinical Manifestations

Manifestations are usually nonspecific, dependent on the type of primary lung cancer, and usually appear late in the disease process. Often, extensive metastasis occurs before symptoms become apparent.

- Persistent pneumonitis as a result of obstructed bronchi may be one of the earliest manifestations, causing fever, chills, and cough.
- A significant symptom that is often reported first is a persistent cough that may be productive of sputum. Blood-tinged sputum may be produced because of bleeding, but hemoptysis is not a common early symptom.
- Chest pain may be localized or unilateral and range from mild to severe.
- Dyspnea and an auscultatory wheeze may be present with bronchial obstruction.

Later manifestations may include nonspecific systemic symptoms such as anorexia, fatigue, weight loss, and nausea and vomiting. Hoarseness may be present as a result of involvement of the recurrent laryngeal nerve. Unilateral paralysis of the diaphragm, dysphagia, and superior vena cava obstruction may occur because of intrathoracic spread of malignancy. There may be palpable lymph nodes in the neck or axilla. Mediastinal involvement may lead to pericardial effusion, cardiac tamponade, and arrhythmias.

Paraneoplastic syndrome is caused by certain lung cancers, especially small cell lung cancers. The syndrome is characterized by various manifestations due to certain substances (e.g., hormones, antigens, and enzymes) produced by the tumor cells. Systemic manifestations may include hormonal syndromes (Cushing's syndrome,

syndrome of inappropriate antidiuretic hormone [SIADH]), neuro-muscular signs (peripheral neuropathy), dermatologic signs (dermato-myositis), vascular and hematologic signs (anemia, thrombophlebitis), and connective tissue disease (arthalgias, digital clubbing).

Diagnostic Studies

- Chest x-ray for diagnosis, evidence of metastasis, and presence of pleural effusion.
- CT and MRI scans for diagnosis, lymph node enlargement, and mediastinal involvement.
- Positron emission tomography (PET) scan for early detection and for staging and monitoring the effect of treatment.
- Additional diagnostic studies include sputum specimens, biopsy, bronchoscopy, pulmonary angiography, lung scans, and medi-astinoscopy.

Collaborative Care

Surgical therapy is usually the only hope for a cure for lung cancer. Unfortunately, detection is often so late that the tumor is no longer localized and is not amenable to resection. Small cell carcinomas usually have widespread metastasis at the time of diagnosis. There-fore surgery is usually contraindicated. Squamous cell carcinomas are more likely to be treated with surgery because they remain lo-calized, or if they metastasize they primarily do so by local spread. The type of surgery usually performed is a lobectomy (one or more lung lobes removed) or pneumonectomy (one entire lung removed).

Radiation therapy is used as a curative approach in the individual who has a resectable tumor but is considered a poor surgical risk. Adenocarcinomas are the most radioresistant type of cancer cell.

- Radiation is also done as a palliative procedure to reduce dis-tressing symptoms such as cough, hemoptysis, bronchial ob-struction, and superior vena cava syndrome (see Radiation Therapy, p. 681).

Chemotherapy may be used for nonresectable tumors or as an ad-juvant therapy to surgery in non–small cell lung cancer with distant metastases (see Chemotherapy, p. 643).

Nursing Management

Goals

The patient with lung cancer will have effective breathing pat-terns, adequate airway clearance, adequate oxygenation of tissues, and minimal to no pain.

Nursing Diagnoses

- Ineffective airway clearance *related to* increased tracheobron-chial secretions

L

- Anxiety *related to* lack of knowledge of diagnosis or unknown prognosis and treatments
- Pain *related to* pressure of tumor on surrounding structures and erosion of tissues
- Altered nutrition: less than body requirements *related to* increased metabolic demands, weakness, and anorexia
- Altered health maintenance *related to* lack of knowledge about the disease process and therapeutic regimen
- Ineffective breathing pattern *related to* decreased lung capacity

Nursing Interventions

When obtaining a health history, it is important to get information related to respiratory carcinogens. The patient should be asked about occupational exposure to carcinogens and excessive exposure to air pollution.

- A detailed history of cigarette smoking should also be obtained. This information should be used to evaluate the patient's risk for lung cancer and also to teach about early recognition of symptoms.
- Anyone with a history of exposure to respiratory carcinogens who has pneumonitis that persists for longer than 2 weeks in spite of antibiotic therapy should be evaluated for the possibility of lung cancer.

Another major responsibility of the nurse is to help patients and their families deal with the diagnosis of lung cancer. Patients may feel guilty about their cigarette smoking having caused the cancer and need to discuss this feeling with someone who has a nonjudgmental attitude. Questions regarding each patient's condition should be answered honestly. Additional counseling from a social worker, psychologist, or member of the clergy may be needed.

Specific care of the patient will depend on the treatment plan.

- Postoperative care for the patient having surgery is discussed in chapter 16, Lewis and others, *Medical-Surgical Nursing,* edition 5. Care of the patient undergoing radiation therapy and chemotherapy is discussed in chapter 14. The nurse has a major role in providing patient comfort, in teaching methods to reduce pain, and in assessing indications for hospitalization (see Cancer, p. 97).

▼ **Patient Teaching**

- For the individual who does have a smoking habit, efforts should be made to assist the smoker to stop smoking. Nicotine's addictive properties make quitting a difficult task and that requires much support.
- Discharge instructions for the patient who has had a surgical resection with an intent to cure should focus on manifestations of metastasis. The patient and family should be told to contact the physician if symptoms such as hemoptysis, dysphagia, chest pain, and hoarseness develop.

LYME DISEASE

Definition/Description
Lyme disease is a spirochetal infection caused by *Borrelia burgdorferi*. The disease is transmitted by the bite of an infected tick. It is the most common vector-borne disease in the United States. The peak season for human infection is during the summer months. Most cases occur in three U.S. endemic areas: (1) along the northeastern coast from Maryland to Massachusetts, (2) in the Midwestern states of Wisconsin and Minnesota, and (3) along the northwestern coast of northern California and Oregon.

Clinical Manifestations
The most characteristic sign is a skin lesion, *erythema migrans (EM)*, which occurs at the site of the tick bite in 80% of patients. This lesion begins as a red macule or papule that slowly expands to form a large round lesion with a bright red border and central clearing. The EM lesion is often accompanied by other acute symptoms, such as intermittent fever, headache, fatigue, stiff neck, and migratory joint and muscle pain.

- If not treated, Lyme disease can progress in several weeks or months to severe arthritis, atrioventricular conduction defects such as bradycardia or myocarditis, and neurologic abnormalities including meningitis, facial palsy, and radiculoneuropathy.
- Other illnesses are frequently misdiagnosed as Lyme disease, particularly chronic fatigue syndrome and fibromyalgia.

Diagnostic Studies
Diagnosis is based on the clinical manifestations, history of exposure in an endemic area, and a positive serologic test for *Borrelia burgdorferi*.

Nursing and Collaborative Management
Active lesions can be treated with antibiotic therapy. Oral doxycycline or amoxicillin is often effective in early-stage infection and in the prevention of later stages of the disease. More diffuse infection may require 20 to 30 days of therapy. IV ceftriaxone (Rocephin) is used for cardiac or neurologic abnormalities. Lyme disease arthritis usually responds to oral antibiotic therapy. New vaccines look promising for conferring immunity to Lyme disease.

- Public education for the prevention of Lyme disease is outlined in Table 60-9, Lewis and others, *Medical-Surgical Nursing*, edition 5, p. 1839.

L

MACULAR DEGENERATION, AGE-RELATED

Definition/Description

Age-related macular degeneration (AMD) is a retinal degenerative process involving the macula and resulting in varying degrees of central vision loss. AMD is the most common cause of uncorrectable vision loss in adults over 52 years of age.

Pathophysiology

Little is known about the etiology of AMD. Although it is clearly related to retinal aging, there is no explanation for the fact that not all aged retinas develop AMD and vision loss. The pathophysiologic mechanism may be an abnormal accumulation of waste material in the retinal pigment epithelium. Cigarette smokers have a significantly higher risk of developing AMD.

Clinical Manifestations

The hallmark sign of AMD is the appearance of drusen in the fundus. *Drusen* appears as yellowish exudates beneath the retinal pigment epithelium and represents localized or diffuse deposits of extracellular debris. The patient may complain of blurred vision, the presence of scotomas, or metamorphopsia (distortion of vision).

Diagnostic Studies

- Visual acuity measurement
- Ophthalmic examination to look for drusen and other changes in the fundus
- Amsler grid test to define the involved area and provide a baseline for future comparison
- Fundus photography and IV fluorescein angiography to further define the extent and type of degenerative disease

Nursing and Collaborative Management

There are no specific treatments for most patients with AMD. Laser treatment may help reduce visual loss in the patient with choroidal neovascularization. Laser treatment seals leakage in the neovascular area, preventing the progression of visual loss. However, in most cases of AMD laser treatment is not helpful.

- Vitamin, mineral, and other nutritional supplements (e.g., antioxidants) may slow or halt the progression of visual loss. Unfortunately, this therapy is also of questionable value.
- When no treatment is possible, or when treatment fails, the patient with AMD can benefit from low-vision aids, such as magnifying lenses and amplification lamps.

The permanent loss of central vision associated with AMD has significant psychosocial implications for nursing care. Nursing management of the patient with uncorrectable visual impairment is discussed in Lewis and others, *Medical-Surgical Nursing,* edition 5, p. 447, and is appropriate for the patient with AMD. It is especially important when caring for the patient to avoid giving them the impression that "nothing can be done" about their problem. While it is true that therapy will not recover lost vision (and is not even appropriate in most cases) much can be done to augment the remaining vision.

MALABSORPTION SYNDROME

Malabsorption results from the impaired absorption of fats, carbohydrates, proteins, minerals, and vitamins. Lactose intolerance is the most common malabsorption disorder, followed by inflammatory bowel disease, nontropical (celiac) and tropical sprue, and cystic fibrosis.

The stomach, small intestine, liver, and pancreas regulate normal digestion and absorption. Nutrients are broken down so that absorption can take place through the intestinal mucosa and nutrients can get into the bloodstream. If there is an interruption in this process at any point, malabsorption may occur.

- Malabsorptions can be caused by (1) biochemical or enzyme deficiencies, (2) bacterial proliferation, (3) disruption of small intestine mucosa, (4) disturbed lymphatic and vascular circulation, and (5) surface area loss.

The most common clinical manifestation of malabsorption is steatorrhea (fatty stools). Bulky, foul-smelling stools that float in water and are difficult to flush are characteristic of steatorrhea.

Diagnostic studies include qualitative examination of stool for fat (Sudan stain), a 72-hour stool collection for quantitative measurement of fecal fat, and the D-xylose absorption-excretion test. Additional breath test studies may include (1) the bile acid breath test to evaluate bile-salt malabsorption or malabsorption from bacterial overgrowth; (2) the triolein breath test, which measures carbon dioxide excretion after the ingestion of a radioactive triglyceride; and (3) the excretion of breath hydrogen after ingestion of lactose, which is a sensitive, specific, and noninvasive test for detection of lactase deficiency.

- A pancreatic secretin test may be performed to rule out pancreatic insufficiency.
- Endoscopy may be used to obtain a small bowel biopsy specimen for diagnosis.

M

- Radiographic studies of the esophagus, stomach, and small intestine may be indicated.

See the specific disorders of Crohn's Disease, p. 172, Cystic Fibrosis, p. 181, Lactase Deficiency, p. 358, Sprue, p. 547, and Ulcerative Colitis, p. 590.

MALIGNANT MELANOMA

Malignant melanoma is a tumor arising in cells producing melanin; these are usually the melanocytes of the skin. Melanoma has the ability to metastasize to any organ including the brain and heart. This is the deadliest form of skin cancer, and it is increasing at a faster rate worldwide than any other cancer.

The four types of cutaneous melanoma are *superficial spreading* (SSM), *lentigo maligna* (LMM), *acral-lentiginous* (ALM), and *nodular* (NM) *melanoma.*

- SSM often occurs on chronically sun-exposed areas such as the legs and upper back.
- LMM is commonly located on the face.
- ALM often appears as dark, irregular-shaped lesions on the soles, palms, mucous membranes, and terminal phalanges. ALM is more common in Asian-Americans and African-Americans.
- NM occurs more often in men and can be located anywhere on the body. It is the most frequently misdiagnosed melanoma because it resembles a blood blister or polyp.

Risk factors for melanoma include ultraviolet (UV) radiation; skin sensitivity; genetic, hormonal, and immunologic factors; and recreational lifestyle changes that lead to greater sun exposure. An abnormal mole pattern called *dysplastic nevus syndrome* (DNS) also places a person at increased risk for melanoma.

- Cutaneous melanoma is nearly 100% curable by excision if diagnosed when the malignant cells are restricted to the epidermis.
- The most important prognostic factor is tumor thickness (Breslow's classification) at the time of presentation.
- If spread to regional lymph nodes occurs, the patient has a 30% 5-year survival rate. If metastasis occurs, treatment is largely palliative.

Diagnosis is made by histologic examination of the excised lesion. Patients should consult their physician immediately if their moles or lesions show any of the clinical signs (ABCDs) of melanoma. The ABCDs of melanoma include **A**symmetry, **B**order (irregular or poorly circumscribed), **C**olor varied from one area to another, and

Diameter >6 mm. (See Fig. 22-5, Lewis and others, *Medical-Surgical Nursing,* edition 5, p. 504.)

The initial treatment is a wide surgical excision with a margin of normal skin. Subsequent treatment modalities such as chemotherapy, biologic therapy, chemoimmunotherapy, and radiation may be planned depending on the stage of the disease. Gene therapy is currently being examined as another treatment plan. (For a discussion of these therapies, see *Medical-Surgical Nursing,* p. 504.)

MALNUTRITION

Definition/Description

Malnutrition is an excess, deficit, or imbalance in the essential components of a balanced diet. Malnutrition is also described as undernutrition or overnutrition.

Pathophysiology

Protein-calorie malnutrition (PCM) is the most common form of undernutrition and can result from primary (poor eating habits) or secondary (alteration or defect in ingestion, digestion, absorption, or metabolism) factors.

The potential for developing malnutrition is increased with severe burns, chronic renal or liver disease, hemorrhage, and malabsorption syndrome. Nitrogen loss after severe injury or major surgery may be as much as 20 g/day. This is excreted as urea, creatine, and creatinine.

- In the early phase of starvation, the only use of protein is in its obligatory participation in cellular metabolism. Once carbohydrate stores (glycogen) are depleted, protein begins to be converted to glucose for energy.

Clinical Manifestations

- Malnutrition signs are evident in many body systems and include conjunctiva and cornea dryness; cavities, loose teeth, and discolored enamel; constant hunger, diarrhea, and flatulence; hepatomegaly; decreased BP; increased number of infections; and depression, confusion, and motor weakness.
- Major complications are related to delayed wound healing and increased susceptibility to infection.

Diagnostic Studies

- Serum albumin, prealbumin, and transferrin levels are decreased.
- Serum electrolytes are often elevated, especially potassium (K^+).

M

- Red blood cell (RBC) count and hemoglobin (Hb) levels are decreased and may indicate anemia.
- White blood cell (WBC) count and total lymphocyte count are decreased.
- Liver enzyme studies may be elevated.
- Serum levels of fat-soluble and water-soluble vitamins are often decreased.

Collaborative Care

Early management of uncomplicated PCM is usually achieved without hospitalization by means of a diet high in calories and protein and by close supervision. In severe PCM the patient may be hospitalized for correction of fluid and electrolyte imbalances and for infections secondary to a compromised immune system. Enteral feedings, both oral and tube, can be used to supplement the diet. In cases of severe PCM, total parenteral nutrition (TPN) may be initiated (see Tube Feedings, p. 689 and Total Parenteral Nutrition, p. 684).

Nursing Management
Goals

The patient with malnutrition will achieve weight gain, consume a specified number of calories a day (with a diet individualized for the patient), and have no adverse consequences related to malnutrition.

Nursing Diagnoses

- Altered nutrition: less than body requirements *related to* decreased ingestion, digestion, or absorption of food or to anorexia
- Feeding self-care deficit *related to* decreased strength and endurance, fatigue, and apathy
- Constipation or diarrhea *related to* poor eating patterns, immobility, or medication effects
- Risk for fluid volume deficit *related to* problems affecting access to or absorption of fluids
- Risk for impaired skin integrity *related to* poor nutritional state
- Noncompliance *related to* alteration in perception, lack of motivation, or incompatibility of regimen with lifestyle or resources
- Activity intolerance *related to* weakness, fatigue, and inadequate caloric intake

Nursing Interventions

The nurse must assess the patient's nutritional state as well as focus on the other physical problems of the patient. The incidence of nutritional deficiency, especially PCM, is high in hospitalized patients. It is important for the nurse to identify patients who are at risk, why they are at risk, and how to intervene appropriately.

- The nurse must have a thorough understanding of nutritional support and the rationale for it; a dietitian should assist with the plan of care.
- Any psychosocial problems should be assessed that may have led to an undernourished state.

▼ **Patient Teaching**
- Discuss with the patient and family the importance of high-caloric, high-protein foods. The family can be encouraged to bring the patient's favorite food while the patient is still hospitalized.
- Education for both the patient and family should include (1) the cause of the undernourished state and ways to avoid the problem in the future, (2) the need for continuous follow-up care if successful rehabilitation is to be accomplished, and (3) the importance of dietary change.
- The patient's understanding needs to be assessed and information provided by the dietitian should be reinforced whenever possible.

MENIÈRE'S DISEASE

Definition/Description
Menière's disease is an inner ear disease characterized by episodic vertigo, tinnitus, aural fullness, and fluctuating sensorineural hearing loss. Symptoms are incapacitating due to sudden, severe attacks of vertigo with nausea and vomiting.

Pathophysiology
The cause of the disease is unknown, but it results in an excessive accumulation of endolymph in the membranous labyrinth. The volume of endolymph increases until the membranous labyrinth ruptures, mixing high-potassium endolymph with low-potassium perilymph. These changes lead to degeneration of delicate vestibular and cochlear hair cells.

Clinical Manifestations
- Attacks of vertigo are sudden and often without warning. Attacks may be preceded by an aura consisting of a sense of fullness in the ear, increasing tinnitus, and a decrease in hearing.
- The patient complains of a whirling sensation and may experience the feeling of being pulled to the ground ("drop attacks").
- Autonomic symptoms include pallor, sweating, nausea, and vomiting.

M

- The duration of the attacks may be hours or days, and attacks may occur several times a year. The clinical course is highly variable.
- Low-pitched tinnitus may be present continuously in the affected ear or may be intensified during an attack.
- Hearing loss fluctuates, decreasing with each vertigo attack, eventually leading to permanent hearing loss.

Diagnostic Studies

- Audiogram demonstrates mild, low frequency hearing loss.
- Vestibular test indicates imbalances.
- Glycerol test supports the diagnosis if hearing improvement is obtained.
- Neurologic testing is done to rule out central nervous system (CNS) disease.

Nursing and Collaborative Management

During an acute attack, antihistamines, anticholinergics, and benzodiazepines can be used as labyrinth suppressants. Acute vertigo is treated symptomatically with bed rest, sedation, and antiemetics or drugs for motion sickness. Diazepam (Valium) and Antivert (Bonamine plus nicotinic acid) are commonly used to reduce the dizziness. Most patients respond to the prescribed medications but must learn to live with the unpredictability of the attacks.

During an acute attack a patient needs reassurance that the condition is not life-threatening. The nurse should focus on providing only essential care, as motion aggravates vertigo.

- Siderails should be up and the bed in low position if the patient is in bed. Avoid the use of lights and TV, which exacerbate symptoms. Have an emesis basin available because vomiting is common. Assist with ambulation because unsteadiness remains after an attack.
- Inform the patient that severe tinnitus and vertigo may exist for days to weeks after the attack.

Management between attacks may include vasodilators, diuretics, antihistamines, avoidance of caffeine and nicotine, and a low-sodium diet.

With frequent incapacitating attacks and reduced quality of life, surgical therapy is indicated. Surgical options include endolymphatic shunt, vestibular nerve section, and labyrinth ablation. Careful management can decrease the possibility of progressive sensorineural loss in many patients.

MENINGITIS

Definition/Description

Meningitis is an acute inflammation of the pia mater and arachnoid membrane surrounding the brain and spinal cord. Meningitis usually occurs in the fall, winter, or early spring and is often secondary to viral respiratory disease. *Staphylococcus pneumoniae* causes about 30% of the cases. Children under 6 years of age, older adults, and persons who are debilitated are more often affected than the general population. See Table 29, p. 215, for a comparison of meningitis and encephalitis.

Pathophysiology

Organisms usually gain entry to the central nervous system (CNS) through the upper respiratory tract or bloodstream, but they may enter by direct extension from penetrating wounds of the skull or through fractured sinuses in basal skull fractures.

The inflammatory response to the infection tends to increase cerebrospinal fluid (CSF) production with a moderate increase in pressure. The purulent secretion produced quickly spreads to other areas of brain through the CSF.

- All patients must be observed closely for manifestations of increased intracranial pressure (ICP), which is a result of swelling around the dura, increased CSF volume, and endotoxins produced by the bacteria (see Increased Intracranial Pressure, p. 343).

Clinical Manifestations

Fever, severe headache, nausea, vomiting, and nuchal rigidity (resistance to flexion of the neck) are key signs.

- A positive Kernig's sign, a positive Brudzinksi's sign, photophobia, a decreased level of consciousness (LOC), and signs of increased ICP may also be present.
- If the infecting organism is a meningococcus, a skin rash is common and petechiae may be seen.
- Seizures occur in 20% of all cases of meningitis.
- Coma is associated with a poor prognosis and occurs in 5% to 10% of patients with bacterial meningitis.

Complications

In bacterial meningitis, cranial nerve dysfunction, which usually disappears within a few weeks, often occurs with cranial nerves III, IV, VI, VII, or VIII.

- Cranial nerve irritation can have serious sequelae; the optic nerve (CN II) is compressed by increased ICP. Papilledema is often present, and blindness may occur.

M

- When the oculomotor (CN III), trochlear (CN IV), and abducens (CN VI) nerves are irritated, ocular movements are affected. Ptosis, unequal pupils, and diplopia are common.
- Irritation of the trigeminal nerve (CN V) is evidenced by sensory losses and loss of the corneal reflex, with irritation of the facial nerve resulting in facial paresis. Irritation of the vestibulocochlear nerve (CN VIII) causes tinnitus, vertigo, and deafness.
- Hemiparesis, dysphasia, and hemianopsia may also occur, with these signs resolving over time.
- Acute cerebral edema may occur with bacterial meningitis, causing seizures, optic nerve palsy, bradycardia, hypertensive coma, and death.
- Hearing loss may be permanent after bacterial meningitis, but it is not a complication of viral meningitis.
- A complication of meningococcal meningitis is the *Waterhouse-Friderichsen syndrome*. The syndrome is manifested by petechiae, disseminated intravascular coagulation (DIC), and adrenal hemorrhage.

Diagnostic Studies

- Analysis of CSF includes (1) cultures to identify the causative organism, (2) protein levels (often elevated; are even higher in bacterial meningitis), (3) glucose concentration (decreased in bacterial meningitis), and (4) gross examination (purulent and turbid in bacterial meningitis).
- Skull x-rays may detect infected sinuses.
- CT scan may reveal increased ICP or hydrocephalus.

Collaborative Care

A rapid diagnosis based on a history and physical examination is crucial because the patient is usually in a critical state when health care is sought. When meningitis is suspected, antibiotic therapy is instituted after the collection of specimens for cultures, even before the diagnosis is confirmed. Penicillin, ampicillin, and a third-generation cephalosporin (ceftriaxone or cefotaxime) are the drugs of choice.

Nursing Management

Goals

The patient with meningitis will have a return to maximal neurologic functioning, resolution of the infection, and a decrease in pain and discomfort.

See NCP 54-3 for the patient with an inflammatory condition of the brain, Lewis and others, *Medical-Surgical Nursing,* edition 5, p. 1640.

Nursing Diagnoses/Collaborative Problems

- Sensory/perceptual alterations *related to* decreased LOC
- Pain *related to* headache, muscle and joint aches, and malaise

- Hyperthermia *related to* infection and abnormal temperature regulation by the hypothalamus from increased ICP
- Ineffective management of therapeutic regimen *related to* possible sequelae of condition
- Potential complication: seizure activity *related to* cerebral irritation
- Potential complication: increased ICP *related to* presence of infectious exudate and increased production of CSF

Nursing Interventions

The prevention of respiratory infections through vaccination programs for pneumococcal pneumonia and influenza should be supported by the nurses. In addition, early and vigorous treatment of respiratory and ear infections is important. Persons who have close contact with anyone who has meningitis should be given prophylactic antibiotics.

The patient with meningitis is acutely ill. The fever is high and resistant to aspirin, and head pain is severe. Irritation of the cerebral cortex may result in seizures with changes in mental status and a LOC dependent on the level of ICP.

- Assessment of vital signs, neurologic evaluation, fluid intake and output, and evaluation of lung fields and skin should be performed at regular intervals. These should be reassessed at frequent intervals based on the patient's condition.
- Head and neck pain secondary to movement requires attention. Codeine provides some pain relief without undue sedation for most patients. A darkened room and cool cloth over the eyes relieves the discomfort of photophobia. For the delirious patient, additional low lighting may be necessary to decrease hallucinations.
- All patients suffer some degree of mental distortion and hypersensitivity and may be frightened and misinterpret the environment. Every attempt should be made to minimize environmental stimuli and the resulting exaggerated perception.

If seizures occur, protective measures should be taken. Antiseizure medications are administered as ordered. Problems associated with increased ICP need to be managed (see Increased Intracranial Pressure, p. 343). Restraints should be avoided. Padded siderails with sheets tied to the four corners to keep the patent from getting out of bed may be used to prevent injury. The presence of a familiar person at the bedside has a calming effect.

Fever must be vigorously managed because it increases cerebral edema and the frequency of seizures. Aspirin or acetaminophen may be used to reduce fever. However, if the fever is resistant to aspirin or acetaminophen, more vigorous means are necessary. The automatic cooling blanket is the most efficient. If a cooling blanket is

M

not available, tepid sponge baths with water may be effective. Because high fever greatly increases the metabolic rate, the patient should be assessed for dehydration and adequacy of intake. Supplemental feedings to maintain adequate nutritional intake via tube or oral feedings may be necessary.

- In most cases, meningitis no longer requires isolation, with the exception of meningococcal meningitis.

In the recovery period, good nutrition should be stressed with an emphasis on a high-protein, high-caloric diet in small, frequent feedings.

- Muscle rigidity may persist in the neck and backs of the legs. Progressive range-of-motion (ROM) exercises and warm baths are useful. Activity should be gradually increased as tolerated, but adequate bed rest and sleep should be encouraged. Quiet activities that are based on an assessment of individual interests should be encouraged to prevent boredom.

- Residual effects are uncommon in meningococcal meningitis but pneumococcal meningitis can result in sequelae such as dementia, epilepsy, deafness, hemiplegia, and hydrocephalus. Vision, hearing, cognitive skills, and motor and sensory abilities should be assessed after recovery with appropriate referrals as indicated.

- Throughout the acute and recovery periods the nurse should be aware of the anxiety and stress experienced by individuals close to the patient. The family needs to be supported and involved in care as much as possible.

MONONUCLEOSIS

Definition/Description

Mononucleosis, often referred to as "mono" or the "kissing disease," is a benign, self-limiting disease characterized by lymph node enlargement, lymphocytosis, and elevated temperature. Peak incidence occurs between 14 and 18 years of age. It may occur in isolated cases or in epidemics.

- Although benign, the disease may incapacitate patients because of the extreme fatigue associated with it.

Pathophysiology

Mononucleosis is caused by Epstein-Barr virus (EBV), a type of herpesvirus, which is primarily transmitted in saliva. The virus grows rapidly in B lymphocytes and oropharyngeal epithelial cells.

Once exposed, susceptible patients manifest symptoms of the disease after a 4- to 8-week incubation period. Symptoms evolve gradually, intensifying as the disease becomes apparent.

- In the United States and Canada, 50% of the population have experienced a primary EBV infection by adolescence. These early infections are usually mild, nonspecific, and clinically inapparent. By adulthood, most individuals have antibodies to EBV.

Clinical Manifestations

Prodromal symptoms of headache, fatigue, malaise, chills, puffy eyelids, anorexia, arthralgia, and a distaste for smoking cigarettes (if the person smokes) may occur.

- As the disease becomes more acute, most patients have a triad of symptoms, including fever, painful lymph node enlargement (especially cervical, axillary, and groin nodes), and sore throat. The sore throat may be severe enough to cause dysphagia.
- If the spleen is enlarged by massive lymphocyte infiltration, pain will occur in the left upper quadrant.

Infectious mononucleosis is a self-limiting disease in the majority of cases, rarely lasting more than 2 to 3 weeks. The most persistent symptom is malaise. It is rare for significant complications to develop from mononucleosis.

- Problems that may occur include pneumonia, neurologic changes (e.g., encephalitis), splenic rupture, hepatitis, thrombocytopenia, hemolytic anemia, airway obstruction, pericarditis, Guillain-Barré syndrome, and Bell's palsy.

Diagnostic Studies

- Initially, the white blood cell (WBC) and differential cell counts are normal, but within a week, leukocytosis will occur. There is an increase in lymphocytes and monocytes.
- A "monospot" test is used to determine heterophilic antibodies. Specificity for mononucleosis is limited with the "monospot" test because cytomegalovirus, adenovirus, and toxoplasmosis may also produce heterophilic antibodies.
- Immunoglobulin M (IgM) antibodies to EBV are diagnostic of a primary EBV infection
- Liver function studies may be used to determine liver involvement

Nursing and Collaborative Management

There is no specific therapy for patients with mononucleosis. Patients need to rest for 2 to 3 weeks and get adequate nutrition and fluids. Fever and sore throat can be treated with acetaminophen. Isolation procedures are not required because mononucleosis is minimally con-

M

tagious in adults. Antibiotics have not proved useful unless the throat culture is positive for β-hemolytic streptococci. Corticosteroids may be used to treat airway obstruction, hemolytic anemia, and thrombocytopenia.

- Recovery is gradual and malaise may occur intermittently for some time.

Nursing interventions are most appropriate when the disease is actually present. Helping the patient comply with the prescribed rest may prove challenging if fatigue is negligible. Saline solution mouthwashes may ease sore throat pain. The nurse needs to be observant for the development of complications.

- For the patient with splenomegaly, the nurse must emphasize the need to avoid any possible activities that can lead to splenic rupture. For example, the patient should avoid Valsalva's maneuver with bowel movements, and abdominal trauma from lifting or from sports must be avoided until the splenic enlargement resolves.
- After 2 to 3 weeks, the patient can usually return to a normal lifestyle. If mononucleosis occurs in older adults, complications may be more common and the complete disease may take longer to resolve.

MULTIPLE MYELOMA

Definition/Description

Multiple myeloma, or plasma cell myeloma, is a condition in which neoplastic plasma cells infiltrate the bone marrow and destroy bone. The incidence of multiple myeloma is about 2 to 3 per 100,000 people, which is a rate similar to that of Hodgkin's disease or chronic lymphocytic leukemia. The disease is twice as common in men as in women and usually develops after 40 years of age.

Pathophysiology

There are many hypotheses regarding the etiology of multiple myeloma, including chronic inflammation, chronic hypersensitivity reactions, and viral influences, but no actual cause has been identified.

- The disease process involves the excessive production of plasma cells that infiltrate the bone marrow and produce abnormal and excessive amounts of immunoglobulins, usually G, A, D, and E (IgG, IgA, IgD, and IgE). The abnormal immunoglobulin is known as myeloma protein.
- Plasma cell production of excessive and abnormal amounts of cytokines (IL-4, IL-5, IL-6) also contributes to the pathologic process of bone destruction.

- Ultimately, plasma cells destroy bone and invade the lymph nodes, liver, spleen, and kidneys.

Clinical Manifestations
Multiple myeloma develops slowly and insidiously.

- The patient often does not manifest symptoms until the disease is advanced, at which time skeletal pain is the major symptom. Pain in the pelvis, spine, and ribs is common.
- Diffuse osteoporosis develops as the myeloma protein destroys more bone. Osteolytic lesions are seen in the skull, vertebrae, and ribs. Vertebral destruction can lead to vertebral collapse with compression of the spinal cord, which requires emergency measures (e.g., radiation, surgery, chemotherapy) to prevent paraplegia.
- Loss of bone integrity can lead to the development of pathologic fractures.
- Bony degeneration causes calcium loss from bones, resulting in hypercalcemia. Hypercalcemia may cause renal, GI, or neurologic changes such as polyuria, anorexia, and confusion.
- Cell destruction contributes to the development of hyperuricemia, which, along with the high protein levels caused by the myeloma protein, can result in renal failure from renal tubular obstruction and interstitial nephritis from uric acid precipitates.
- The patient may display symptoms of anemia, thrombocytopenia, and granulocytopenia, all of which are related to the replacement of normal bone marrow elements with plasma cells.

Diagnostic Studies
- High serum protein may be present as evidenced by an "M" spike on serum electrophoresis.
- Pancytopenia, hyperuricemia, hypercalcemia, and elevated creatinine may be found.
- An abnormal globulin known as *Bence Jones protein* is found in the urine of patients with multiple myeloma.
- Radiologic studies, including bone scans, are done to establish the degree of bone involvement. The studies identify diffuse bony lesions, demineralization, and osteoporosis in affected skeletal areas.
- Bone marrow analysis shows significantly increased numbers of plasma cells.

Collaborative Care
The therapeutic approach involves managing both the disease and its symptoms, because with treatment the chronic phase of multiple myeloma may last for more than 10 years.

M

Ambulation and adequate hydration are used to treat hypercalcemia, hyperuricemia, and dehydration. Weight-bearing helps the bones reabsorb some calcium, and fluids dilute calcium and prevent protein precipitates from causing renal tubular obstruction.

Control of pain is another goal of collaborative care. Analgesics, orthopedic supports, and localized radiation help to reduce skeletal pain. Chemotherapy is used to reduce the number of plasma cells (see Chemotherapy, p. 643). Corticosteroids may be added because they exert an antitumor effect in some patients. Radiotherapy is used for its palliative effect on localized lesions (see Radiation Therapy, p. 681).

- Drugs may be used to treat the complications of multiple myeloma. For example, allopurinol (Zyloprim) may be given to reduce hyperuricemia, and IV furosemide (Lasix) promotes renal excretion of calcium. Calcitonin and pamidronate (Aredia) may be used to treat moderate to severe hypercalcemia.

Nursing Management

Maintaining adequate hydration is a primary nursing consideration to minimize problems from hypercalcemia. Fluids are administered to attain an urinary output of 1.5 to 2 L per day. This may require an intake of 3 to 4 L. In addition, weight-bearing helps bones to reabsorb some of the calcium, and corticosteroids may augment the excretion of calcium.

Once chemotherapy is initiated, uric acid levels increase because of the increased cell destruction. Hyperuricemia must be resolved by ensuring adequate hydration and using allopurinol.

- Because of the potential for pathologic fractures, the nurse must be careful when moving and ambulating the patient. A slight twist or strain in the wrong area (e.g., weak area in patient's bones) may be sufficient to cause a fracture.

Pain management requires innovative and knowledgeable nursing interventions. If radiotherapy is used to diminish pain from localized myeloma lesions, appropriate skin care techniques must be used. Mild analgesics, such as nonsteroidal antiinflammatory drugs (NSAIDs), acetaminophen, or acetaminophen with codeine, may be more effective than stronger analgesics in diminishing bone pain. Braces, especially for the spine, may also help control pain.

- The patient's psychosocial needs require sensitive, skilled management. As with leukemia (see Leukemia, p. 360), it is important to help the patient and significant others adapt to changes fostered by chronic illness and to adjust to the losses related to the disease process.
- The way in which patients and families deal with confronting death may be affected by the manner in which they have learned to accept and live with the chronic nature of the disease.

MULTIPLE SCLEROSIS

Definition/Description

Multiple sclerosis (MS) is a chronic, progressive, degenerative disorder of the CNS. It is considered an autoimmune disease with the onset usually between 15 and 50 years of age. Women are affected more often than men.

MS primarily affects Caucasian persons of northern European descent. The incidence of MS is highest in temperate climates (between 45 and 65 degrees of latitude), such as those found in Europe, Canada, and the northern United States, as compared to tropical regions. It is also associated with the place of birth; an individual born and raised in one of the regions listed above who moves to a warmer climate (nearer the equator) after 15 years of age carries the same risk of MS as others in the country of origin.

- It is not known exactly how many people have MS. Currently it is thought that there are approximately 250,000 to 350,000 people in the United States with MS as diagnosed by a physician. Approximately 200 new cases are diagnosed each week.

Pathophysiology

The cause of MS is unknown, although research findings suggest MS is related to infectious (viral), immunologic, and genetic factors and perpetuated as a result of intrinsic factors (e.g., faulty immunoregulation). Susceptibility to MS appears to have an inherited tendency; first-, second-, and third-degree relatives of patients with MS are at a slightly increased risk. Possible precipitating factors include infection, physical injury, emotional stress, and pregnancy.

MS is characterized by chronic inflammation, demyelination, and gliosis (scarring) in the central nervous system (CNS). The primary neuropathologic condition is an immune-mediated inflammatory demyelinating process which some believe may be triggered by a virus in genetically susceptible individuals.

- Activated T cells responding to environmental triggers (e.g., infection) enter the CNS in increased numbers. These T cells, in conjunction with astrocytes, disrupt the blood-brain barrier. Oligodendrocytes are damaged, resulting in demyelination. Monocytes are recruited and cause further cell damage.
- The disease process consists of the loss of myelin, the disappearance of oligodendrocytes (cells that make myelin), and the proliferation of astrocytes. These changes result in characteristic plaque formation, or *sclerosis,* with plaques scattered throughout multiple regions of the CNS.

M

- As the disease progresses, the myelin is totally disrupted and is replaced by glial scar tissue, which forms hard, sclerotic plaques in multiple regions of the CNS. Without myelin, nerve impulses slow down, and with the destruction of nerve axons, impulses are totally blocked, resulting in a permanent loss of function.

Clinical Manifestations

Because the onset is often insidious and gradual, with vague symptoms that occur intermittently over months or years, the disease may not be diagnosed until long after the onset of the first symptom.

- Because the disease process has a spotty distribution in the CNS, signs and symptoms vary over time. The disease is characterized by chronic progressive deterioration in some persons and by remissions and exacerbations in others.
- Some patients have severe, long-lasting symptoms early in the course of the disease while others may experience only occasional and mild symptoms for several years after onset. The average life expectancy after the onset of symptoms is more than 25 years.

Common signs and symptoms include motor, sensory, cerebellar, and emotional problems.

- Motor symptoms include weakness or paralysis of the limbs, trunk, or head; diplopia; and spasticity of muscles.
- Sensory symptoms include numbness and tingling, patchy blindness *(scotomas),* blurred vision, vertigo, tinnitus, and decreased hearing.
- Cerebellar signs include nystagmus, ataxia, dysarthria, and dysphagia.
- Bowel and bladder function can be affected if the sclerotic plaque is located in the areas of the CNS that control elimination. Problems usually involve constipation and a spastic (uninhibited) bladder.
- Sexual dysfunction occurs in many persons. Physiologic impotence may result from spinal cord involvement in men. Women may experience decreased libido, difficulty with orgasmic response, painful intercourse, and decreased vaginal lubrication.
- Although intellectual functioning generally remains intact, emotional stability may be affected. Persons may experience anger, depression, or euphoria. Signs and symptoms are aggravated or triggered by physical and emotional trauma, fatigue, and infection.

Death usually occurs because of the infectious complications (e.g., pneumonia) of immobility or because of unrelated disease; suicide is occasionally a cause.

Diagnostic Studies

Because there is no definitive diagnostic test for MS, the diagnosis is based primarily on the history and clinical manifestations. Laboratory tests are adjuncts to the clinical examination.

- Cerebrospinal fluid (CSF) analysis may show an increase in immunoglobulin G (IgG) or a high number of lymphocytes and monocytes.
- Evoked response testing results are often delayed due to decreased nerve conduction from the eye and ear to the brain.
- MRI may detect sclerotic plaques.

Collaborative Care

Because there is no cure for MS, collaborative care is aimed at treating the disease process and providing symptomatic relief. The disease process is treated with drugs, and the symptoms are controlled with a variety of medications and other therapy.

- Spasticity is primarily treated with antispasmodic drugs. However, surgery (e.g., neurectomy, rhizotomy, cordotomy) or dorsal-column electrical stimulation may be required.
- Intention tremor that becomes unmanageable with medication is sometimes treated by stereotactic surgery on the thalamus.
- Neurologic dysfunction sometimes improves with physical therapy and speech therapy.

Drug Therapy

Adenocorticotropic hormone (ACTH), methylprednisolone, and prednisone are helpful in treating acute exacerbations. Immunosuppressive drugs, such as azathioprine (Imuran), cyclosporine, and cyclophosphamide (Cytoxan), have produced some beneficial effects in patients with severe and relapsing MS. Interferon β-1b (Betaseron) for patients with exacerbating and remitting MS has decreased the number of relapses and the number of new lesions seen on MRI scan. This was the first drug aimed at controlling the disease rather than the symptoms. Two newer drugs are now available. Interferon β-1a (Avonex) is similar to interferon β-1b in efficacy. Glatiramer acetate (Copaxone), formerly know as copolymer-1, is unrelated to interferon but has also been shown to decrease the number of relapses in MS.

Nutritional Therapy

A nutritious, well-balanced diet is essential. Although there is no standard prescribed diet, a high protein diet with supplementary vitamins is often advocated. A diet high in roughage may help relieve constipation.

Nursing Management

Goals

The patient with MS will maximize neuromuscular function, maintain independence in activities of daily living (ADLs) for as long as possible, optimize psychosocial well-being, adjust to the illness, and reduce the factors that precipitate exacerbations.

See NCP 56-3 for the patient with multiple sclerosis, Lewis and others, *Medical-Surgical Nursing,* edition 5, p. 1692.

Nursing Diagnoses

- Altered urinary elimination *related to* sensorimotor deficits and inadequate fluid intake
- Risk for impaired skin integrity *related to* immobility, sensorimotor deficits, and inadequate nutrition
- Sensory/perceptual alterations *related to* visual disturbances
- Sexual dysfunction *related to* neuromuscular deficits
- Constipation *related to* immobility, inadequate fluid intake, inadequate fiber and roughage, and neuromuscular impairment
- Self-care deficits *related to* muscle spasticity and neuromuscular deficits
- Impaired physical mobility *related to* muscle weakness or paralysis and muscle spasticity
- Altered family processes *related to* changing family roles, potential financial problems, and fluctuating physical condition

Nursing Interventions

The patient with MS should be aware of triggers that may cause exacerbations or worsening of the disease. Exacerbations of MS are triggered by infection (especially upper respiratory infections), trauma, childbirth, stress, fatigue, and climactic changes. The nurse should help the patient identify particular triggers and develop ways to avoid them or minimize their effects.

The most common reasons for hospitalization are for a diagnostic workup and for treatment of an acute exacerbation of complications such as bladder and pulmonary dysfunction.

- During the diagnostic phase the patient needs reassurance that even though there is a tentative diagnosis of MS, certain diagnostic studies must be made to rule out other neurologic disorders. The patient with recently diagnosed MS may need assistance with the grieving process.
- During an acute exacerbation the patient is often immobile and confined to bed for 2 to 3 weeks. The focus of nursing intervention at this phase is to prevent the hazards of immobility, such as respiratory and urinary tract infections (UTIs) and pressure ulcers.

▼ **Patient Teaching**

Patient education should focus on building a general resistance to illness. This includes avoiding fatigue, extremes of heat and cold, and exposure to infection.

- It is important to teach the patient to achieve a good balance of exercise and rest, eat nutritious and well-balanced meals, and avoid the hazards of immobility (contractures and pressure sores).

- Patients should know their treatment regimens, the side effects of medications and how to watch for them, and drug interactions with over-the-counter medications.
- Increasing dietary fiber may help some patients achieve regularity in bowel habits.
- Inform patients to avoid extreme heat such as hot baths.
- Inform patients of the National Multiple Sclerosis Society in the United States and of its local chapters, which offer a variety of services to meet the needs of patients with MS.

MYASTHENIA GRAVIS

Definition/Description
Myasthenia gravis (MG) is a disease of the neuromuscular junction characterized by fluctuating weakness of certain skeletal muscle groups. Women are affected slightly more often than men, although among patients with both thymoma (tumor of the thymus) and MG (which accounts for 15% to 20% of all persons with MG), the majority are men over the age of 50. Peak age at onset in women is 20 to 30 years.

Pathophysiology
MG is caused by an autoimmune process that results in the production of antibodies directed against the acetylcholine (ACh) receptors. A reduction in the number of ACh receptor sites at the neuromuscular junction prevents ACh molecules from attaching to the receptors and stimulating muscle contraction. Anti-ACh receptor antibodies are detectable in the serum of most patients with MG. Thymic tumors are found in about 15%-20% of all patients with MG.

- Although a viral infection is suspected as precipitating an attack, a single specific cause for all MG cases has not been found.

Clinical Manifestations
The primary feature of MG is easy fatigability of skeletal muscle during activity. Strength is usually restored after a period of rest. The muscles most often involved are those used for moving the eyes and eyelids, chewing, swallowing, speaking, and breathing. The muscles are generally the strongest in the morning and become exhausted with continued activity. By the end of the day, muscle fatigue is prominent.

- In more than 90% of cases, the eyelid muscles or extraocular muscles are involved. Facial mobility and expression can be

M

impaired. There may be difficulty in chewing and swallowing food. Speech is affected, and the voice often fades during long conversations.

- No other signs of neural disorder accompany MG; there is no sensory loss, reflexes are normal, and muscle atrophy is rare.

The course of the disease is highly variable. Some patients may have short-term remissions, others may stabilize, and others may have severe progressive involvement. Restricted ocular myasthenia, usually seen only in men, has a good prognosis.

- Exacerbations and the initial onset of MG can be precipitated by emotional stress, pregnancy, temperature extremes, hypokalemia, and the ingestion of drugs with neuromuscular blocking properties.

Complications result from muscle weakness in areas that affect swallowing and breathing. Aspiration, respiratory insufficiency, and respiratory infection are the major complications. An acute exacerbation of this type is sometimes called *myasthenic crisis.*

Diagnostic Studies

- The simplest test is to have the patient look upward for 2 to 3 minutes. If the problem is MG, there will be an increased droop of the eyelids, so that the person can barely keep the eyes open. After a brief rest, the eyes can open again.
- Electromyogram (EMG) may show a decremental response to repeated stimulation of the hand muscles, indicative of muscle fatigue.
- The Tensilon test reveals improved muscle contractility after an IV injection of the anticholinesterase agent edrophonium chloride (Tensilon chloride).

Collaborative Care

Major therapies are anticholinesterase drugs, alternate-day corticosteroids, immunosuppressants, and plasmapheresis. Because the thymus gland appears to enhance the production of ACh receptor antibodies, removal of the thymus gland results in improvement in a majority of patients. Plasmapheresis removes anti-ACh receptor antibodies. Plasmapheresis can provide short-term improvement in symptoms and is indicated for patients in crisis or in preparation for surgery when corticosteroids need to be avoided.

- Acetylcholinesterase is the enzyme responsible for the breakdown of ACh in the synaptic cleft. Acetylcholinesterase inhibitors will prolong the action of ACh and facilitate the transmission of impulses at the neuromuscular junction. Neostigmine (Prostigmin) and pyridostigmine (Mestinon) are the most successful drugs of this group.

- Because of the autoimmune nature of MG, corticosteroids (specifically prednisone) are used to suppress immunity. Cytotoxic drugs such as azathioprine (Imuran) and cyclophosphamide (Cytoxan) may also be used for immunosuppression.

Nursing Management

Goals

The patient with MG will have a return of normal muscle endurance, avoid complications, and maintain a quality of life appropriate to disease course.

Nursing Diagnoses

- Ineffective breathing pattern *related to* intercostal muscle weakness
- Impaired verbal communication *related to* weakness of the larynx, lips, mouth, pharynx, and jaw
- Altered nutrition: less than body requirements *related to* dysphagia, weakness, and inability to prepare food or feed self
- Sensory/perceptual alterations *related to* ptosis, decreased eye movements, and dysconjugate gaze
- Activity intolerance *related to* muscle weakness and fatigability
- Body image disturbance *related to* an inability to maintain usual lifestyle and role responsibilities

Nursing Interventions

The patient who is admitted to the hospital usually has a respiratory tract infection or is in acute myasthenic crisis. Nursing care is aimed at maintaining adequate ventilation, continuing drug therapy, and watching for side effects of therapy. The nurse must be able to distinguish cholinergic from myasthenic crisis because the causes and treatment of the two differ greatly (see Table 56-20, Lewis and others, *Medical-Surgical Nursing,* edition 5, p. 1702).

- As with other chronic illnesses, care focuses on the neurologic deficits and their impact on daily living.
- A balanced diet that can be chewed and swallowed easily should be prescribed. Semisolid foods may be easier to eat than solids or liquids. Scheduling doses of medications so that peak action is reached at mealtime may make eating less difficult.
- Diversional activities that require little physical effort and match the interests of the patient should be arranged.

▼ Patient Teaching

Education should focus on the importance of following the medical regimen, potential adverse reactions to specific drugs, planning activities of daily living (ADLs) to avoid fatigue, the availability of community resources, and the complications of the disease and therapy (crisis conditions) and what to do about them.

- Contact with the Myasthenia Gravis Society or an MG support group may be very helpful and should be explored.

M

MYOCARDIAL INFARCTION

Definition/Description
A myocardial infarction (MI) occurs when ischemic intracellular changes become irreversible and necrosis results. Angina as a result of ischemia causes reversible cellular injury, and infarction is the result of sustained ischemia, causing irreversible cellular death.

Prehospital mortality in patients with acute MI is approximately 30% to 50%. Mortality among patients who reach the hospital is about 5%. Most of these deaths occur within the first 3 to 4 days.

Pathophysiology
Cardiac cells can withstand ischemic conditions for approximately 20 minutes before cellular death (necrosis) begins. Contractile function of the heart stops in the areas of myocardial necrosis. The degree of altered function depends on the area of the heart involved and the size of the infarct. Most infarcts involve the left ventricle. A *transmural MI* occurs when the entire thickness of the myocardium in a region is involved. A *subendocardial (nontransmural) MI* exists when the damage has not penetrated through the entire thickness of the myocardial wall.

- Infarctions are described by the area of occurrence as anterior, inferior, lateral, or posterior wall infarctions. Common combinations of areas are the anterolateral or anteroseptal MI. An inferior MI is also called a diaphragmatic MI.
- The degree of preestablished collateral circulation also determines the infarction's severity. In an individual with a history of coronary artery disease, adequate collateral channels may have been established that provide the area surrounding the infarction site with blood supply and oxygen (O_2).

The body's response to cell death is the inflammatory process. Within 24 hours, leukocytes infiltrate the area. Enzymes are released from the dead cardiac cells. Proteolytic enzymes from neutrophils and macrophages remove all necrotic tissue by the second or third day. Collagen matrix that will eventually form scar tissue is laid down.

- The necrotic zone is identifiable by ECG changes within 4 to 10 days and by technetium scanning 24 to 72 hours after the onset of symptoms.
- At 10 to 14 days after a MI, the beginning scar tissue is still weak. The myocardium is considered to be especially vulnerable to increased stress because of the unstable state of the healing heart wall.

- By 6 weeks after a MI, scar tissue has replaced necrotic tissue. At this time, the injured area is said to be healed. The scarred area is often less compliant than the surrounding fibers. This condition may be manifested by uncoordinated wall motion, ventricular dysfunction, or pump failure.

Clinical Manifestations

Severe, immobilizing, and persistent chest pain not relieved by rest or nitrate administration is the hallmark of a MI. The pain is caused by inadequate O_2 supply to the myocardium. Persistent and unlike any other pain, it is usually described as a heaviness, tightness, or constriction.

- Common locations are substernal or retrosternal, radiating to the neck, jaw, and arms or to the back. It may occur while the patient is active or at rest, asleep or awake, and commonly occurs in the early morning hours.
- The pain usually lasts for 20 minutes or more and is described as more severe than anginal pain. It may be located atypically in the epigastric area. The patient may have taken antacids without relief.
- Some patients may not experience pain but may have "discomfort," weakness, or shortness of breath.

Additional manifestations may include nausea and vomiting, diaphoresis, and vasoconstriction of peripheral blood vessels. On physical examination, the patient's skin is ashen, clammy, and cool (cold sweat). Fever occurs within the first 24 hours (up to 100.4° F [38° C]), and may continue for 1 week. BP and pulse rate are also elevated initially. BP then drops, with decreased urine output, lung crackles, hepatic engorgement, and peripheral edema. Jugular veins may be distended with obvious pulsations.

Complications

Arrhythmias are the most common complication after an MI. Arrhythmias are caused by any condition that affects the myocardial cell's sensitivity to nerve impulses, such as ischemia, electrolyte imbalances, and sympathetic nervous system stimulation. The intrinsic rhythm of the heartbeat is disrupted, causing either a very fast heart rate (HR) (tachycardia), a very slow HR (bradycardia), or an irregular beat. Life-threatening arrhythmias occur most often with anterior wall infarction, pump failure, and shock. Complete heart block is seen in massive infarction (see Arrhythmias, p. 54).

- Ventricular fibrillation, a common cause of sudden death, is a lethal arrhythmia that most often occurs within the first 4 hours after the onset of pain. Premature ventricular contractions (PVCs) may precede ventricular tachycardia and fibrillation. Ventricular arrhythmias need immediate treatment.

M

Congestive heart failure (CHF) occurs when the pumping power of the heart has diminished. It is common to see some degree of left ventricular dysfunction in the first 24 hours after a MI.

- Depending on the severity and extent of the injury, CHF occurs initially with subtle signs such as slight dyspnea, restlessness, agitation, or slight tachycardia. Jugular vein distention from right-sided heart failure, crackles in the lungs, and the presence of an S_3 or S_4 heart sound may be found.

Cardiogenic shock occurs when inadequate oxygen and nutrients are supplied to the tissues because of severe left ventricular failure. Cardiogenic shock occurs in 10% to 15% of patients hospitalized with acute MI and has a high mortality rate.

Papillary muscle dysfunction may occur if the infarcted area includes or is adjacent to these structures.

- Papillary muscle dysfunction causes mitral valve regurgitation, which increases the volume of blood in the left atrium. Papillary muscle rupture is a severe complication causing massive mitral valve regurgitation, which results in dyspnea, pulmonary edema, and decreased cardiac output (CO).

Ventricular aneurysm results when the infarcted myocardial wall becomes thinned and bulges out during contraction. Ventricular aneurysms are identified by bulges seen on x-ray, echocardiogram, fluoroscopy, or persistent, long-term ST segment changes on an ECG.

- The patient with a ventricular aneurysm may experience intractable CHF, arrhythmias, and angina. Ventricular aneurysms also harbor thrombi, cause arrhythmias, and promote left ventricular dysfunction.

Acute pericarditis is an inflammation of the visceral or parietal pericardium, or both, and may result in cardiac compression, lowered ventricular filling and emptying, and cardiac failure. It may occur 2 to 3 days after a acute MI. Chest pain, which may vary from mild to severe, is aggravated by inspiration, coughing, and movement of the upper body. The pain may radiate to the back and down to the left arm and may be relieved by sitting in a forward position.

- Assessment of the patient may reveal a friction rub over the pericardium with fever also present. A diagnosis of pericarditis can be made with serial 12-lead ECGs.

Additional complications include pulmonary embolism and Dressler syndrome (antigen-antibody reaction to necrotic myocardium and right ventricular infarction).

Diagnostic Studies

Three noninvasive diagnostic parameters are used to determine whether a person has sustained an acute MI.

- Patient's history of pain, risk factors, and health history

- 12-lead ECG consistent with acute MI (ST-T wave elevations >1 mm or more in two contiguous leads)
- Serial measurement of troponin and myocardial serum enzymes, including creatine kinase (CK), lactic dehydrogenase (LDH), and aspartate aminotransferase (AST)

Other diagnostic measures can include an initial chest x-ray to assess cardiac size and pulmonary congestion, leukocytosis, radionucleotide imaging to assess coronary blood flow, and technetium pyrophosphate scanning which can localize areas of acute necrosis.

Collaborative Care

Initial management of the patient with MI is best accomplished in a cardiac care unit (CCU), where constant monitoring is available. Arrhythmias may be detected by nurses trained in continuous ECG monitoring techniques. An IV route is established to provide an accessible means for emergency drug therapy. Morphine sulfate or meperidine (Demerol) may be given IV for relief of pain. O_2 is usually administered by nasal cannula at a rate of 2 to 4 L/min. A continuous IV infusion of lidocaine may be given prophylactically to prevent ventricular fibrillation, which is the greatest threat to life after a MI.

- Vital signs are taken frequently during the first few hours after admission and monitored closely thereafter. Bed rest and limitation of activity are usually instituted initially, with a gradual increase in activity.
- A pulmonary artery catheter and intraarterial line may be used to accurately monitor intracardiac, pulmonary artery, and systolic arterial pressures in complicated MI so that the most effective treatment in the acute phase can be determined.
- Thrombolytic therapy is the standard of practice in the treatment of acute MI. The goal is to salvage as much myocardial muscle as possible. The most commonly used thrombolytics are tissue plasminogen activator (tPA), streptokinase, and urokinase. To be of the most benefit, thrombolytics must be given as soon as possible, preferably within the first 6 hours after the onset of pain. Contraindications and complications with thrombolytic therapy are described in Lewis and others, *Medical-Surgical Nursing,* edition 5, p. 866.

Surgical intervention can include a percutaneous transluminal coronary angioplasty (PTCA) which may be performed in the patient exhibiting signs of cardiogenic shock or in the patient in which thrombolytic therapy was unsuccessful. Coronary artery bypass graft (CABG) surgery may be a treatment choice in a select group of patients with acute MI.

M

Drug therapy may include IV nitroglycerin, antiarrhythmic drugs, morphine sulfate, positive inotropic drugs, β-adrenergic blockers, calcium channel blockers, angiotensin-converting enzyme (ACE) inhibitors, and stool softeners.

Nursing Management

Goals

The patient with a MI will experience relief of pain, have no progression of MI, receive immediate and appropriate treatment, cope effectively with associated anxiety, cooperate with the rehabilitation plan, and decrease risk factors.

See NCP 32-1 for the patient with myocardial infarction, Lewis and others, *Medical-Surgical Nursing,* edition 5.

Nursing Diagnoses

- Pain *related to* lactic acid production from myocardial ischemia and altered myocardial O_2 supply
- Altered cardiac tissue perfusion *related to* myocardial damage, ineffective CO, and potential pulmonary congestion
- Anxiety *related to* present status and unknown future, possible lifestyle changes, pain, and perceived threat of death
- Activity intolerance *related to* fatigue secondary to decreased CO and poor lung and tissue perfusion
- Ineffective management of therapeutic regimen *related to* lack of knowledge of disease process, rehabilitation, home activities, diet, and medications
- Anticipatory grieving *related to* actual or perceived losses secondary to cardiac condition

Nursing Interventions

Acute interventions include the initial CCU stay (1 to 2 days) and the rest of the hospitalization (4 to 6 days). Priorities for nursing interventions in the initial phase of recovery after MI include pain assessment and relief, physiologic monitoring, promotion of rest and comfort, alleviation of stress and anxiety, and understanding of the patient's emotional and behavioral reactions. Proper management of these priorities decreases the O_2 needs of a compromised myocardium. In addition, the nurse needs to institute measures to avoid the hazards of immobility while encouraging rest.

- Morphine should be given as needed to eliminate or reduce chest pain. The nurse should instruct the patient to rate the pain on a scale of 1 to 10 to assist in the assessment and treatment of pain.
- The nurse should be trained in ECG interpretation so that arrhythmias causing further deterioration of the cardiovascular status can be identified and eliminated.
- In addition to frequent vital signs, intake and output should be evaluated at least once a shift, and a physical assessment

should be carried out to detect deviations from the patient's baseline parameters; included are the assessment of lung and heart sounds and an inspection for evidence of fluid retention (e.g., distended neck veins, hepatic engorgement).

- Assessment of the patient's oxygenation status is helpful, especially if the patient is receiving O_2. The nares also should be checked for irritation or dryness (see Oxygen Therapy, p. 676).
- It is important to plan nursing and therapeutic actions to ensure adequate rest periods free from interruption.
- Anxiety is present in all patients in various degrees. The nurse's role is to identify the source of anxiety and assist the patient in reducing it. If the patient is afraid of being alone, a family member should be allowed to sit quietly by the bedside or to check in with the patient frequently. If a source of anxiety is fear of the unknown, the nurse should explore these concerns with the patient and help with appropriate reality testing.

The phases of cardiac rehabilitation are outlined in Table 41. The patient must realize that recovery takes time. Resumption of physical activity after MI is slow and gradual. However, with appropriate and adequate supportive care, recovery is more likely to occur. For a sample rehabilitation program, see Table 32-21 in Lewis and others, *Medical-Surgical Nursing*, edition 5, p. 877.

Table 41	Phases of Cardiac Rehabilitation

Phase I—Time when patient is in the CCU. Activity level depends on severity of MI; patient may rest in bed or chair; attention focuses on management of pain, anxiety, arrythmias, and cardiogenic shock

Phase II—Time from transfer from the CCU to discharge from hospital. Resumption of activities begins to the point of self-care at the time of discharge; information giving and teaching are appropriate at this time

Phase III—Time of convalescence at home. Patient and family examine and possibly restructure lifestyles and roles; exercise program begins, commonly a walking program, which progresses daily during first week and then weekly; patient undergoes exercise treadmill test at about 8 wk to determine workload of recovering myocardium

Phase IV—Time of recovery and maintenance. Involvement with the community rehabilitation program for physical training and fitness continues

CCU, Cardiac care unit; *MI,* myocardial infarction.

M

▼ Patient Teaching

Teaching begins with the CCU nurse and progresses through the staff nurse to the home health nurse. Careful assessment of the patient's learning needs helps the nurse to set goals and objectives that are realistic.

- In addition to teaching the patient and family what they want to know, there are several types of information that are considered essential in achieving maximum health. A teaching plan for the patient with MI should include the content in Table 42.
- Anticipatory guidance involves preparing the patient and the family for what to expect in the course of recovery and rehabilitation. By learning what to expect during treatment and recovery, the patient gains a sense of control over his or her life.
- The patient should be taught the parameters within which to exercise and how to check pulse rate. The patient should be told the maximum HR that should be present at any point. If the HR exceeds this level or does not return to the rate of the resting pulse within a few minutes, the patient should stop. The patient should be instructed to stop exercising if pain or dyspnea occurs.
- Because of the short hospitalization, it is critical to give the patient specific guidelines for activity and exercise so that overexertion will not occur. It is helpful to stress that when the patient "listens to what the body is saying" uncomplicated recovery should proceed.

Table 42	Patient Teaching Guide: Myocardial Infarction

- Anatomy and physiology of the heart and vessels
- Cause and effect of atherosclerosis
- Definition of terms (e.g., CAD, angina, MI, sudden death, CHF)
- Signs and symptoms of angina and MI and reasons they occur
- Healing after infarction
- Identification of risk factors (see Table 32-4, Lewis and others, *Medical-Surgical Nursing*, edition 5, p. 848)
- Rationale for tests and treatments, including ECG, blood tests, angiography and monitoring, rest, diet, and medications
- Appropriate expectations about recovery and rehabilitation (anticipatory guidance)
- Measures to take to promote recovery and health
- Importance of the gradual, progressive resumption of activity

CAD, Coronary artery disease; *CHF*, congestive heart failure; *ECG*, electrocardiogram; *MI*, myocardial infarction.

- It is important to include sexual counseling for cardiac patients and their partners. Reading material on resumption of sexual activity may be presented to the patient to facilitate discussion. The nurse should return to clarify and explain as necessary.

MYOCARDITIS

Definition/Description
Myocarditis is a focal or diffuse inflammation of the myocardium which has been associated with a variety of etiologic agents. Viruses are the most common etiologic agent in the United States and Canada, with a predominance of ribonucleic acid (RNA) viruses (coxsackievirus A and B), echovirus, influenza A and B, and mumps. Certain medical conditions such as metabolic disorders and collagen-vascular diseases (e.g., systemic lupus erythematosus) may also precipitate myocarditis.

- Myocarditis is frequently associated with acute pericarditis, particularly when it is caused by coxsackievirus B strains or echoviruses.

Pathophysiology
The pathophysiology of myocarditis is poorly understood because there is usually a period of several weeks after the initial infection before the development of the manifestations of myocarditis. Immunologic mechanisms may play a role in the development of myocarditis. The majority of infections are benign, self-limiting, and subclinical, although viral myocarditis in pregnant women may be virulent.

Clinical Manifestations
The clinical features for patients with myocarditis are variable, ranging from a benign course without any overt manifestations to severe heart involvement or sudden death. Fever, fatigue, malaise, myalgias, pharyngitis, dyspnea, lymphadenopathy, and GI complaints are early systemic manifestations of the viral illness.

- Early cardiac manifestations appear 7 to 10 days after viral infection and include pericardial chest pain with an associated friction rub. Cardiac symptoms (S_3, crackles, jugular venous distention, and peripheral edema) may progress to CHF, including pericardial effusion, syncope, and possibly ischemic pain.
- The majority of individuals with myocarditis recover spontaneously. Occasionally, acute myocarditis progresses to chronic dilated cardiomyopathy.

M

Diagnostic Studies

Laboratory findings are often inconclusive, with the presence of mild to moderate leukocytosis and atypical lymphocytes, elevated viral titers (virus is generally only present in tissue and fluid samples during the initial 8 to 10 days of illness), increased erythrocyte sedimentation rate, and elevated levels of enzymes such as the transaminases, creatine kinase (CK), and lactic dehydrogenase (LDH).

- ECG changes are often nonspecific and reflect associated pericardial involvement, including diffuse ST-segment abnormalities. Arrhythmias and conduction disturbances may be present.
- Histologic confirmation is possible through endomyocardial biopsy. A biopsy done during the initial 6 weeks of acute illness is most diagnostic because this is the period in which lymphocytic infiltration and myocyte damage indicative of myocarditis are present.
- Special myocardial imaging techniques may also be used in the diagnostic evaluation of myocarditis.

Collaborative Care

A specific therapy for myocarditis has yet to be established and usually consists of managing associated cardiac decompensation.

- Digoxin is often used to treat ventricular failure because it improves myocardial contractility and reduces ventricular rate. Digoxin should be used cautiously in patients with myocarditis because of the increased sensitivity of the heart to the adverse effects of this drug and the potential toxicity with minimal doses.
- Oxygen (O_2) therapy, bed rest, restricted activity, and maintenance of standby emergency equipment are general supportive measures.

Immunosuppression therapy with agents such as prednisone, azathioprine (Imuran), and cyclosporine has been used on a limited basis to reduce myocardial inflammation and to prevent irreversible myocardial damage. Administration of immunosuppressive agents is recommended only during the postinfectious stage of the disease, approximately 10 days after the onset of initial symptoms. If used early in the course of viral myocarditis, these drugs can actually increase tissue necrosis.

- The use of corticosteroids remains controversial because of the associated serious side effects and lack of clear documentation for their efficacy.

Nursing Management

Interventions focus on an assessment for the signs and symptoms of congestive heart failure (CHF) and instituting measures to decrease the cardiac workload (e.g., use of semi-Fowler's position, spaced activity and rest periods, and provisions for a quiet environment). Prescribed medications that increase the heart's contractility and decrease the preload, afterload, or both are administered. Careful monitoring and evaluation of the patient taking these medications is necessary.

The patient may be anxious about the diagnosis of myocarditis, recovery from myocarditis, and therapy. Nursing measures include assessing the level of anxiety, instituting measures to decrease anxiety, and keeping the patient and family informed about therapeutic measures.

The patient who receives immunosuppressive therapy may have additional problems of alterations in immune response with the potential for infection and complications related to the therapy. Guidelines for care include monitoring for complications and providing the patient with a clean, safe environment according to proper infection control standards.

M

NAUSEA AND VOMITING

Definition/Description

Nausea and vomiting are the most common manifestations of GI diseases. Although each symptom can occur independently, they are closely related and usually treated as one problem. They are also found in a wide variety of conditions unrelated to GI disease. These include pregnancy, infectious diseases, central nervous system (CNS) disorders (e.g., meningitis), cardiovascular problems (e.g., myocardial infarction [MI], congestive heart failure [CHF]), side effects of drugs (e.g., digitalis, antibiotics), metabolic disorders (e.g., uremia), and psychologic factors (e.g., stress, fear).

Nausea is a feeling of discomfort in the epigastrium with a conscious desire to vomit. Anorexia usually accompanies nausea and is brought on by unpleasant stimulation involving any of the five senses. Generally, nausea occurs before vomiting and is characterized by contraction of the duodenum and by the slowing of gastric motility and emptying.

Vomiting is the forceful ejection of partially digested food and secretions from the upper GI tract. It occurs when the gut becomes overly irritated, excited, or distended. Vomiting can be a protective mechanism to rid the body of spoiled or irritating foods and liquids.

Pathophysiology

The vomiting center in the brainstem coordinates the multiple components involved in vomiting. Neural impulses reach the vomiting center via afferent pathways through branches of the autonomic nervous system. Visceral receptors for these afferent fibers are located in the GI tract, kidneys, heart, and uterus. When stimulated, these receptors relay information to the vomiting center, which initiates the vomiting reflex.

In addition, the chemoreceptor trigger zone (CTZ) located in the brain responds to chemical stimuli of drugs and toxins. Once stimulated (by motion sickness, for example), the CTZ transmits impulses to the vomiting center.

Emotion, stress, unpleasant sights and odors, and pain can also trigger vomiting. Severe nausea and vomiting may also be caused by a metabolic crisis. For example, nausea and vomiting are frequently associated with uremia, hyperthyroidism, hyperparathyroidism and hypoparathyroidism, diabetic acidosis, Addison's disease, and hypertensive crisis.

Clinical Manifestations

Signs of severe or prolonged nausea and vomiting include rapid dehydration with essential electrolytes (e.g., potassium [K^+]) lost. As vomiting persists, there may be severe electrolyte imbalances, loss of extracellular fluid (ECF) volume, decreased plasma volume, and eventual circulatory failure. Weight loss may occur in a short time.

Diagnostic Studies

- Abdominal x-rays or upper GI findings.
- Serum electrolytes can be altered; hypokalemia is a common electrolyte abnormality.
- Decreased urine output and concentrated urine (e.g., increased specific gravity).

Collaborative Care

The goals of management are to determine and treat the underlying cause of nausea and vomiting and to provide symptomatic relief. Determining the cause is often difficult because nausea and vomiting are manifestations of many conditions of the GI tract and of disorders of other body systems. The amount, frequency, character (e.g., projectile), content (e.g., feces, bile, blood), and color of vomitus (e.g., red, "coffee ground") help to determine the etiology

Antiemetic medications are used with caution until the cause of the vomiting is determined. These may include scopolamine, chlorpromazine (Thorazine), diphenhydramine (Benadryl), metoclopramide (Reglan), promethazine (Phenergan), and ondansetron (Zofran).

The patient with severe vomiting requires IV fluid therapy with electrolyte replacement until he or she is able to tolerate oral intake. In some cases a nasogastric (NG) tube and suction are used to decompress the stomach. Once symptoms have subsided, oral nourishment beginning with clear liquids is started. As the condition improves, a diet high in carbohydrates and low in fat is preferred.

Nursing Management

Goals

The patient with nausea and vomiting will experience minimal or no nausea and vomiting, have normal electrolyte levels, and return to a normal pattern of fluid balance and nutrient intake.

See NCP 39-1 for the patient with nausea and vomiting, Lewis and others, *Medical-Surgical Nursing,* edition 5, p. 1091.

Nursing Diagnoses

- Nausea *related to* multiple etiologies
- Fluid volume deficit *related to* prolonged nausea and vomiting
- Anxiety *related to* lack of knowledge of etiology of the problem, treatment plan, and follow-up care
- Risk for altered nutrition: less than body requirements *related to* nausea and vomiting

Nursing Interventions

Until a diagnosis is confirmed, the patient is kept on nothing by mouth (NPO) status and given IV fluids. A NG tube may be necessary for persistent vomiting.

- The environment should be quiet, free of noxious odors, and well ventilated.
- Cleansing the face and hands with a cool washcloth and providing mouth care between episodes increase the person's comfort level. When the symptoms occur, all foods and medications should be stopped until the acute phase is past.

With prolonged vomiting, interventions include accurate intake and output with vital signs, assessment for dehydration, proper positioning to prevent aspiration, and observation for changes in comfort and mentation.

▼ **Patient Teaching**

- Instruct the patient to take several deep breaths and prevent sudden changes in position to decrease stimulation of the vomiting center.
- Provide explanations for diagnostic tests and procedures.
- The patient and family may need instructions on how to deal successfully with the unpleasant sensations of nausea, discussion of methods for preventing nausea and vomiting, and strategies to maintain fluid and nutritional intake during periods of nausea.
- When food is identified as the precipitating cause of nausea and vomiting, help the patient with problem solving. What food was it? When was it eaten? Has this food caused problems in the past? Is anyone else in the family sick?

NEPHROTIC SYNDROME

Definition/Description

Nephrotic syndrome describes a clinical course of increased glomerular membrane permeability, which is responsible for a massive urinary excretion of protein. The causes of nephrotic syndrome include primary glomerular disease (glomerulonephritis), infections (e.g., hepatitis, streptococcus), neoplasms (e.g., Hodgkin's disease), allergens (e.g., bee sting, drugs), and multisystem diseases (e.g., diabetes mellitus [DM]).

Pathophysiology and Clinical Manifestations

Diminished plasma oncotic pressure from the decreased serum proteins stimulates hepatic lipoprotein synthesis, which results in hyperlipidemia. Fat bodies (fatty casts) commonly appear in the urine.

Immune responses, both humoral and cellular, are altered in nephrotic syndrome. As a result, infection is a major cause of morbidity and mortality.

Hypercoagulability with thromboembolism is potentially the most serious complication of nephrotic syndrome. The renal vein is the most commonly involved site for thrombus formation. Pulmonary emboli occur in about 40% of nephrotic patients with thrombosis.

- Endocrine and skeletal abnormalities may occur, including hypocalcemia, blunted calcemic response to parathyroid hormone, hyperparathyroidism, and osteomalacia.

Collaborative Care

The goals of treatment are to relieve edema and cure or control the primary disease. Management of edema includes the cautious use of angiotensin converting enzyme (ACE) inhibitors, nonsteroidal antiinflammatory drugs (NSAIDs), low-sodium intake (2 to 3 g/day), and a low to moderate protein diet (0.5 to 0.6 g/kg/day).

- Treatment of hyperlipidemia is frequently unsuccessful. However, treatment with lipid-lowering agents, such as colestipol (Colestid) and lovastatin (Mevacor), may result in moderate decreases in serum cholesterol levels.
- Corticosteroids and cyclophosphamide (Cytoxan) may be used for the treatment of severe cases. Prednisone has been effective in some persons with membranous glomerulonephritis, proliferative glomerulonephritis, and lupus nephritis.
- Management of DM and the treatment of edema are the only measures used for nephrotic syndrome related to DM

Nursing Management

The major focus of care is related to edema. It is important to assess edema by weighing the patient daily, accurately recording intake and output, and measuring abdominal girth or extremity size. Comparing this information daily provides the nurse with a tool for assessing the effectiveness of treatment. Edematous skin needs careful cleaning. Trauma should be avoided and the effectiveness of diuretic therapy must be monitored. The person is often ashamed of their edematous appearance and may need support in dealing with an altered body image.

The patient has the potential to become malnourished from the excessive loss of protein in the urine. Maintaining a low to moderate protein diet that is also low in sodium is not always easy. The patient is usually anorexic; serving small, frequent meals in a pleasant setting may encourage better dietary intake.

- Because the patient is susceptible to infection, measures should be taken to avoid exposure to persons with known infections.

NEUROGENIC BLADDER

Neurogenic bladder is a general term referring to any bladder dysfunction resulting from a central nervous system (CNS) neurologic disorder. There are numerous causes of this condition, including such problems as CNS tumors, cerebrovascular accidents, multiple sclerosis (MS), diabetic neuropathy, and spinal cord injury.

A person with a neurogenic bladder may have problems with urgency, frequency, incontinence, inability to urinate, and obstruction-like symptoms. Long-term problems include the formation of calculi, urinary tract infection (UTI), and progressive deterioration in renal function.

A simple way to classify neurogenic dysfunction is to identify whether there is a failure to store, failure to empty, or both problems, and whether the dysfunction is of the bladder or urethra. Either or both problems lead to urinary tract damage if left untreated. The type of dysfunction usually depends on whether the problem affects the brain or spinal cord (e.g., cerebral centers, suprasacral spinal cord, or sacral cord area).

- Lesions in the brain or upper spinal cord usually cause hyperreflexic symptoms, whereas lesions in the sacral cord cause arreflexia. Detrusor sphincter dyssynergia (the bladder and sphincter contract at the same time) is often associated with lesions in the suprasacral spinal cord. (For further information, see Chapter 57 in Lewis and others, *Medical-Surgical Nursing,* edition 5, p. 1737).

NON-HODGKIN'S LYMPHOMA

Non-Hodgkin's lymphomas (NHLs) are a heterogenous group of malignant neoplasms of the immune system that affect all ages. They are classified according to different cellular and lymph node characteristics (see Table 29-33, Lewis and others, *Medical-Surgical Nursing,* edition 5, p. 781). NHLs can originate outside the lymph nodes, and the method of spread can be unpredictable. The majority of patients have widely disseminated disease at the time of diagnosis.

A variety of clinical presentations and courses are recognized from indolent to rapidly progressive disease. Common names for different types of NHL include Burkitt's lymphoma, reticulum cell sarcoma, and lymphosarcoma.

Although there is no hallmark feature in NHL, all NHLs involve lymphocytes arrested in various stages of development. The primary clinical manifestation is painless lymph node enlargement. Because the disease is usually disseminated when diagnosed, other symptoms will be present depending on where the disease has spread (e.g., hepatomegaly with liver involvement).

- Patients with high-grade lymphomas may have lymphadenopathy and constitutional ("B") symptoms such as fever, night sweats, and weight loss. The peripheral blood is usually normal, but some lymphomas may occur in a "leukemic" phase.

Diagnostic studies for NHL resemble those used for Hodgkin's disease. Lymph node biopsy establishes the cell type and pattern. Staging, as described for Hodgkin's disease, is used to guide therapy.

The treatment for NHL involves radiotherapy and chemotherapy (see Radiation Therapy, p. 681 and Chemotherapy, p. 643). Indolent lymphomas have a naturally long course but are more difficult to effectively treat. Ironically, aggressive lymphomas are more responsive to treatment and more likely to be cured.

- Radiotherapy alone may be effective for the treatment of stage I disease, but a combination of radiation therapy and chemotherapy is used for other stages. Initial chemotherapy uses alkylating agents such as cyclophosphamide (Cytoxan) and chlorambucil (Leukeran).
- High-dose chemotherapy with peripheral blood stem cell or bone marrow transplantation (BMT) is commonly used. Biologic therapies, such as α-interferon, interleukin-2, and tumor necrosis factor, are also being investigated for the treatment of NHL.

OBESITY

Definition/Description

Obesity is the most common nutritional problem in the United States. Among adults 20 years and older, 33% of men and 36% of women are overweight. The calculated body mass index (BMI), a clinical index of obesity, classifies individuals with a BMI of 25 to 29.9 kg/m^2 as overweight and those with values of 30 kg/m^2 or more as obese. Obese persons have a higher rate of hypertension, gout, degenerative joint disease, diabetes mellitus (DM), stroke, breast cancer, sleep apnea, and menstrual problems.

Pathophysiology

Many factors have been identified as critical elements in the development and maintenance of obesity. Environmental and genetic factors are considered important. Children of obese parents tend to be obese and obesity tends to affect several persons within a family. Evidence of a genetic component is suggested in studies of twin and adoptive children.

- Obesity may be modulated by a variety of factors including energy intake, level of habitual physical activity, resting metabolic rate, and the tendency to store ingested energy in the form of lean or fat tissue.

It is hypothesized that the hypothalamus has a set point for energy balance, above which energy conservation becomes increasingly less efficient and below which energy conservation becomes increasingly more efficient.

- This homeostatic mechanism accounts for the fact that most adults keep their weight remarkably constant, despite large swings in energy input and expenditure.
- It could also account for why the obese person tends to remain overweight no matter what dietary regimen is followed.
- An emotional tendency to overeat beyond satiety is also powerful for some persons.

Complications

Medical problems of obesity are numerous and frequently include cardiovascular and respiratory signs such as dyspnea on exertion, paroxysmal nocturnal dyspnea, orthopnea, drowsiness, and somnolence. There is an increased risk for polycythemia, which results in occluded vessels, sluggish vessel flow, varicose veins, hypertension, and increased heart size. Pickwickian syndrome or obesity hypoventilation leads to chronic hypercapnia with cyanosis, dyspnea, edema, and somnolence.

Impaired glucose tolerance is common with obesity and leads to type 2 DM. Gallstones may occur with increased serum cholesterol and triglyceride levels. Excessive weight on multiple joints contributes to degenerative joint disease.

- Long-standing emotional and social problems may lead to a poor self-esteem and body image.

Diagnostic Studies

- The presence of obesity is commonly calculated by BMI, standardized height-weight charts, anthropometric measurements, or hip-to-waist ratio.
- Liver function, fasting glucose and triglyceride levels, and low- and high-density lipoprotein cholesterol levels assess the cause and effects of obesity.

Assessment of etiologic factors includes testing for hypothyroidism, hypothalamic tumors, Cushing's syndrome, hypogonadism (in men), and polycystic ovarian disease (in women).

Collaborative Care

When no organic cause can be found for obesity, it should be considered a chronic, complex illness. Any supervised plan of care should be directed at:

- Successful weight loss, requiring a short-term energy deficit
- Successful weight control, requiring long-term behavioral changes

A multipronged approach should be taken with attention to dietary intake, physical activity, behavioral-cognitive modification, and perhaps drug therapy. The only effective method of treating primary obesity is to restrict dietary intake so that intake is below energy requirements. The most sensible approach is to follow a well-balanced, low-calorie diet.

- The addition of exercise is especially important in producing and maintaining weight loss.

Surgical therapy for treating morbid obesity may include:

- Lipectomy (adipectomy) to remove unsightly adipose folds
- Liposuction for cosmetic purposes and not weight reduction
- Gastrointestinal surgeries such as vertical banded gastroplasty and Roux-en-Y gastric bypass to reduce gastric capacity

Nursing Management
Goals

The patient with obesity should achieve and maintain weight loss to a specified level, modify eating habits, and participate in a regular physical activity program.

Nursing Diagnoses

- Altered nutrition: more than body requirements *related to* excessive intake in relation to metabolic need and decreased activity
- Impaired physical mobility *related to* excessive body weight
- Social isolation *related to* alterations in physical appearance and perceived unattractiveness
- Risk for impaired skin integrity *related to* alterations in nutritional state (obesity), immobility, excess moisture, and multiple skin folds
- Ineffective breathing pattern *related to* decreased lung expansion from obesity
- Noncompliance *related to* an alteration in perception or lack of motivation
- Body image disturbance *related to* deviation from the usual or expected body size and the inability to lose or retain weight loss

Nursing Interventions

When assessing the obese patient, the nurse needs to consider several different types of questions, such as the following:

- What is the psychologic importance of food to the patient?
- Is the patient's food intake influenced by hunger?
- Does the taste and appearance of food or other physical factors in the environment stimulate the patient to eat?
- Is there an emotional problem that stimulates the patient to eat?
- Are there any stressors influencing the patient's eating patterns?

Preoperative care for gastric surgery includes planning for special needs such as large-size blood pressure cuff; oversized bed and chair; reinforced trapeze bar; meat or freight scales for weighing; and special gowns.

Postoperative care and teaching emphasizes the administration of pain medications, facilitating patient respiratory efforts (elevating the head of the bed; turning, coughing, and deep breathing), monitoring the abdominal wound for healing, and monitoring nasogastric (NG) tube patency.

- Anticipate and recognize several potential psychologic problems after surgery. Some patients express guilt feelings concerning the fact that the only way they could lose weight was by surgical means rather than by the "sheer willpower" of reduced dietary intake. The nurse should be ready to provide support so that this patient does not dwell on negative feelings.
- Discharge teaching includes the importance of a diet high in protein and low in carbohydrates, fat, and roughage, with six small feedings daily, and prompt recognition of complications such as anemia, diarrhea, vitamin deficiencies, and psychiatric problems, especially episodes of depression.

- The nurse needs to reinforce physical activity programs and cognitive training such as self-help support groups or professional counseling.

ORAL CANCER

Definition/Description

Carcinoma of the oral cavity may occur on the lips or anywhere within the mouth (e.g., tongue, floor of mouth, buccal mucosa, hard palate, soft palate, pharyngeal walls, or tonsils). Carcinoma of the lips has the most favorable prognosis of any of the oral tumors, as lip lesions are more apparent to the patient than other oral lesions and are usually diagnosed earlier.

- Oral cancer is more common after 40 years of age, with 60 being the average age at onset. The 5-year survival for all stages of cancer of the oral cavity and pharynx is 53%.

Pathophysiology

Although the cause of oral cancers is not definitive, there are a number of predisposing factors including constant overexposure to ultraviolet (UV) radiation from the sun, tobacco use (cigar, cigarette, pipe, snuff), excessive alcohol intake, and chronic irritation, such as from a jagged tooth or poor dental care. A positive history of the use of tobacco and alcohol, in the past or currently, is the most significant etiologic factor.

Clinical Manifestations

Common manifestations include leukoplakia, erythroplasia, ulcerations, a sore spot, and a rough area felt with the tongue.

- *Leukoplakia,* called "white patch" or "smoker's patch," is a whitish precancerous lesion on the mucosa of the mouth or tongue that results from chronic irritations such as smoking. The patch becomes keratinized (hard and leathery) and is sometimes described as hyperkeratosis.
- *Erythroplasia (erythroplakia),* which is seen as a red velvety patch on the mouth or tongue, is also considered a precancerous lesion.
- Cancer of the lip appears as an indurated, painless lip ulcer.
- The first sign of carcinoma of the tongue is an ulcer or area of thickening. Soreness or pain of the tongue may occur, especially on eating hot or highly seasoned foods. Some patients experience limitation of movement of the tongue. Later symptoms of cancer of the tongue include increased salivation, slurred speech, dysphagia, toothache, and earache.

- Approximately 30% of patients with oral cancer present with an asymptomatic neck mass.

Diagnostic Studies

- Biopsy of suspected lesion with cytologic examination for definitive diagnosis
- Oral exfoliative cytology and toluidine blue test to screen for oral cancer
- CT and MRI scans for metastases

Collaborative Care

Management usually consists of surgery, radiation, chemotherapy, or a combination of these. Surgery remains the most effective treatment, especially for removing the central core of the tumor. Many of the operations are radical procedures involving extensive resections. Various surgical procedures may be performed, including hemiglossectomy (removal of half the tongue), glossectomy (removal of the entire tongue), and radial neck dissection. A tracheostomy (see Tracheostomy, p. 686) is commonly done with radical neck dissection to prevent airway obstruction.

Chemotherapy and radiation are used together when the lesions are more advanced or involve several structures of the oral cavity. Chemotherapy may also be used when surgery and radiation fail or as the initial therapy for smaller tumors (see Chemotherapy, p. 643).

Palliative treatment may be indicated when the prognosis is poor, the cancer is inoperable, or the patient decides against mutilating surgery. These treatments may include gastrostomy and analgesic medication. Frequent suctioning becomes necessary when swallowing difficulties occur.

Nursing Management

Goals

The patient with oral cancer will have a patent airway, be able to communicate, have adequate nutritional intake to promote wound healing, and have relief of pain and discomfort.

Nursing Diagnoses

- Altered nutrition: less than body requirements *related to* oral pain, difficulty swallowing, surgical resection, and radiation treatment
- Altered nutrition: less than body requirements *related to* oral pain, difficulty chewing and swallowing, and surgical resection
- Pain *related to* the tumor
- Anxiety *related to* a diagnosis of cancer, an uncertain future, and the potential for disfiguring surgery
- Altered health maintenance *related to* a lack of knowledge of the disease process and therapeutic regimen and the unavailability of a support system

Nursing Interventions

The nurse has a significant role in the early detection and treatment of carcinoma of the oral cavity. Inspection of a patient's oral cavity to detect suspicious lesions should be included in a routine physical examination.

Preoperative care for the patient who is having radical neck dissection involves consideration of the patient's physical and psychosocial needs (see NCP 25-6 for the patient with a radical neck dissection, Lewis and others, *Medical-Surgical Nursing,* edition 5, p. 604.) Special preparation emphasizes oral hygiene.

Postoperative care focuses on the maintenance of a patent airway, including tracheostomy care and observing for signs of respiratory distress.

- Oral hygiene decreases the probability of infection, with the patient needing proper positioning to prevent aspiration (lying on the side or supine with the head turned to one side). The dressing should be observed for signs of hemorrhage or infection.
- Malnourishment delays wound healing; tube feedings may be started with surgery.
- The patient may need alternate forms of communication such as chalkboard or pad and pencil.
- Allow for personal verbalization of feelings regarding surgery. Obtain a psychiatric referral for prolonged or severe depression.
- Facial disfigurement and other mutilating aspects of radical head and neck surgery may have a major long-term impact on the patient's body image and lifestyle, which may include learning to swallow again, altered physical appearance, taste and sensation changes, speech therapy, and reconstruction.

▼ **Patient Teaching**

- Teach correct oral hygiene and dental care and encourage the patient to seek preventive dental care.
- Educate the patient about predisposing factors.
- Instruct the patient to examine the mouth and to recognize the danger signals of oral cancer. If any of these signals are present, the patient should be instructed to visit a doctor. Danger signals are as follows:
  1. Unexplained pain or soreness in the mouth
  2. Unusual bleeding from the oral cavity
  3. Dysphagia
  4. Swelling or a lump in the neck
  5. Any ulcerative lesion that does not heal within 2 to 3 weeks
- In the postoperative period, provide information about measures to help improve appearance, such as wearing clothes with high collars and wearing accessories that draw attention away from the neck.

- Answer questions about the patient's body image honestly and assure the patient of his or her self-worth.

The patient is often discharged with a tracheostomy and gastrostomy tube. The patient and family need to be taught how to manage these tubes and who to call if there are problems. Initially, home health care may be needed to evaluate the family or the patient's ability to perform self-care activities.

OSTEOARTHRITIS

Definition/Description

Osteoarthritis (OA), also known as degenerative joint disease, is a slowly progressive disorder of the mobile joints, particularly weight-bearing articulations; it is characterized by the degeneration of articular cartilage. The spectrum of disease severity is wide—ranging from annoying and uncomfortable symptoms to significantly disabling disease.

OA may occur as a primary idiopathic or secondary disorder. The cause of primary OA is unknown. Although both are influenced by multiple factors (e.g., metabolic, genetic, chemical), secondary OA has an identifiable precipitating event, such as previous trauma, infection, or a congenital deformity, that is believed to predispose the person to later degenerative changes.

The most significant risk factor for OA is age. It is estimated that nearly one third of all adults have x-ray evidence of degenerative joint disease, with the incidence increasing to 60% to 80% by age 60. OA is more common in adult men than in women and is generally distributed throughout the peripheral and central joints.

Pathophysiology

Degenerative changes over time cause the normally smooth, white, translucent joint cartilage to become yellow and opaque with rough surfaces and areas of *malacia* (softening). As the cartilage breaks down, fissures may appear and fragments of cartilage become loose. Secondary inflammation of the synovial membrane may follow.

Deterioration of the cartilage is an active process. Deoxyribonucleic acid (DNA) synthesis, which is normally absent in adult articular cartilage, is active in OA tissue and appears to be directly proportional to the disease severity.

- Specific predisposing factors such as excessive use of or stress on a joint accelerate osteoarthritic changes.
- Genetic factors influence the development of Heberden's nodes.

- Other factors that influence the development of OA include congenital structural defects (e.g., Legg-Calvé-Perthes disease), metabolic disturbances (e.g., diabetes mellitus [DM]), repeated intraarticular hemorrhage (e.g., hemophilia), neuropathic arthropathies, and inflammatory and septic arthritis.

Clinical Manifestations

Constitutional symptoms such as fatigue or fever are not present in OA. Other organ involvement is absent as well, which is an important differentiation between OA and inflammatory joint disorders such as rheumatoid arthritis (Table 43).

Joints. Articular manifestations are related to the joint involved. The patient has pain on motion and weight-bearing that is generally relieved by rest. In advanced disease, sleep may be disrupted by night pain. Increasing pain is accompanied by progressive loss of function. Overall body coordination and posture may be affected as a result of the pain and loss of mobility. Advanced disease is complicated by gross deformity and *subluxation* (partial dislocation) caused by deterioration of cartilage, collapse of subchondral bone, and extensive bony overgrowth.

- Joints are usually affected asymmetrically. The joints most frequently involved are the distal and first interphalangeal joint(s) of the fingers, hips, knees, and lower lumbar and cervical vertebrae.

Nodules. Heberden's nodes are common, particularly in women with primary OA. These nodes are reactive bony overgrowths located at the distal interphalangeal joints. *Bouchard's nodes,* seen less commonly in OA, involve the proximal interphalangeal joints. Heberden's nodes and Bouchard's nodes may present with redness, swelling, tenderness, and aching. They often begin in one finger and spread to others. Although there is usually no significant loss of function, people are often distressed by the resulting disfigurement of their hands.

Hips. OA of the hips may be extremely disabling. Congenital or structural abnormalities are frequent causes. Sitting down is difficult, as is rising from a chair when the hips are lower than the knees. Eventually, the loss of motion range is significant, with marked limitation of extension and internal rotation.

Knees. Softening of the posterior surface of the patella (chondromalacia patellae) is seen most commonly in young people. Degeneration of the weight-bearing surfaces of the femoral and tibial condyles is usually seen in older women and is associated with limitation of motion, crepitus, and flexion deformity

Vertebral column. OA in the spine may produce localized symptoms of stiffness and pain. Herniation of the degenerating intervertebral disks causes muscle spasm or radicular pain.

Table 43   Comparison of Rheumatoid Arthritis and Osteoarthritis

Parameter	Rheumatoid arthritis	Osteoarthritis
Age	Young and middle-aged	Usually >40 yr of age
Gender	Female more often than male	Same incidence
Weight	Weight loss	Usually overweight
Illness	Systemic manifestations	Local joint manifestations
Affected joints	PIPs, MCPs, MTPs, wrists, elbows, shoulders, knees, hips, cervical spine	DIPs, first CMCs, thumbs, first MTPs, knees, spine, hips; asymmetric, one or more joints
	Usually bilateral	
Effusions	Common	Uncommon
Nodules	Present	Heberden's nodes
Synovial fluid	Inflammatory	Noninflammatory
X-rays	Osteoporosis, narrowing, erosions	Osteophytes, subchondral cysts, sclerosis
Anemia	Common	Uncommon
Rheumatoid factor	Positive	Negative
Sedimentation rate	Elevated	Normal except in erosive osteoarthritis

CMC, Carpometacarpal; *DIP,* distal interphalangeal; *MCP,* metacarpophalangeal; *MTP,* metatarsophalangeal; *PIP,* proximal interphalangeal.

Diagnostic Studies

- In late disease, x-rays of the involved joints show joint space narrowing, bony sclerosis, spur formation, and in some cases subluxation.
- Erythrocyte sedimentation rate (ESR) is normal except in instances of erosive OA, when moderate elevation may be noted.
- Synovial fluid aspirated from an involved joint may be increased in volume but is clear yellow and viscous. Fluid analysis reveals little or no sign of inflammation.

Collaborative Care

There are no specific therapies for managing OA. Therapy is aimed at pain control, prevention of progression and disability, and restoration of joint function. Once the diagnosis is confirmed, the patient should be assured that OA is likely to remain confined to a few joints and does not generally cause crippling. However, if joint destruction is extensive and pain is severe, surgery may be an option.

Drug Therapy

Acetaminophen—1 g up to four times daily—is now recommended as a first-line therapy. Topical agents such as capsaicin cream may be used alone or with acetaminophen. Low-dose ibuprofen may be also used.

Nonsteroidal antiinflammatory drugs (NSAIDs) at full dosages are a second-line therapy. Misoprostol (Cytotec) is used when NSAID-induced gastropathy is a concern. A new generation of NSAIDs, including celecoxib (Celebrex) and rofecoxib (Vioxx), have fewer GI side effects than traditional NSAIDs.

- Intraarticular injections of corticosteroids are used to treat a symptomatic flare. Systemic use of corticosteroids should be avoided because it may accelerate the disease process.

Nutritional Therapy

There is no specific diet except for one that maintains optimal health. If a patient is overweight, a weight-reduction program becomes an important part of the total treatment plan. Body weight is magnified five times through the hips and three times through the knees. Heavy thighs lead to malalignment at the knee, increasing wear on the medial aspect.

Nursing Management

Goals

The patient with OA will balance rest and activity, use joint protection measures to improve activity tolerance, modify the home and work environment to include work-saving and joint-protecting assistive devices, use pharmacologic and nonpharmacologic pain management techniques to achieve satisfactory pain control, and perform range-of-motion (ROM), muscle-strengthening, and aerobic exercises regularly.

Nursing Diagnoses

- Pain *related to* physical activity and lack of knowledge of pain self-management techniques
- Sleep pattern disturbance *related to* pain
- Impaired physical mobility *related to* weakness, stiffness, and pain on ambulation
- Self-care deficit *related to* joint deformity and pain with activity
- Altered nutrition: more than body requirements *related to* intake in excess of energy output
- Self-esteem disturbance *related to* changing social and work roles

Nursing Interventions

Prevention of primary OA is not possible; however, preventive education may include the elimination of excessive strain on the joints by a reduction of occupational and recreational hazards and nutritional counseling for weight reduction. Community education may include the proper body mechanics of lifting and good posture. Athletic instruction and physical fitness programs should include safety measures that protect and reduce trauma to the joint structures.

The person is most troubled by pain, stiffness, limitation of function, and the frustration of coping with these physical difficulties on a daily basis. The older adult may believe that OA is an inevitable part of the aging process and that nothing can be done to ease the discomfort and related disability.

- The hospital or home health nurse should assist the patient with activities of daily living (ADLs) as necessary and help the patient plan rest periods during the day. The patient needs sufficient time to move stiff, painful joints, especially when arising in the morning or after any period of sustained inactivity. Proper body alignment should be maintained at all times.
- Safety measures in the home and work environment are important. These measures include removing scatter rugs, providing rails at the stairs and bathtub, using night-lights, and wearing well-fitting supportive shoes. Assistive devices such as canes, walkers, elevated toilet seats, and grab bars reduce joint load and promote safety.
- Splints may be prescribed to rest and stabilize painful or inflamed joints. Soft collars and cervical traction may be used at home for cervical OA. Stiff, painful hands can be relieved by warm water soaking, contrast baths, or paraffin. If swelling is more diffuse, stretch gloves can be worn at night to provide relief.
- Sexual counseling helps the patient and loved one to enjoy physical closeness by learning to adapt positions, alter timing, and increase awareness of the partner's needs.
- Nonpharmacologic techniques such as meditation, relaxation, and transcutaneous electric nerve stimulation (TENS) are particularly

suited to chronic pain management. The nurse should be open to helping the patient and family to develop creative new approaches to pain relief.

■ Assist the patient and family to overcome feelings of helplessness and encourage active participation in managing chronic symptoms. The correct combination of joint protection, exercises (ROM, isotonic, and isometric), heat and cold therapy, and medication can restore self-esteem and improve physical functioning. Benefits exist with an aerobic exercise program such as walking or aquatics.

▼ **Patient Teaching**

Education is an important nursing responsibility that should be carried out regardless of patient setting.

■ Teaching should include information about the nature and treatment of the disease, pain management, correct posture and body mechanics, correct use of assistive devices such as a cane or walker, principles of joint protection and energy conservation, and a therapeutic exercise program.

■ The nurse needs to assist the patient in developing long-term strategies to manage OA.

■ Home care goals must be individualized to meet the patient's needs. Family and social supports should be included in goal setting and education.

OSTEOMALACIA

Osteomalacia is an uncommon disorder of adult bone associated with vitamin D deficiency, which results in decalcification and softening of bone. This disease is the same as rickets in children except that the epiphyseal growth plates are closed in the adult.

■ Vitamin D is required for absorption of calcium from the intestines. Insufficient vitamin D intake can interfere with the normal mineralization of bone, causing failure or insufficient calcification of bone, which results in bone softening, bone pain, and deformities.

Etiologic factors include lack of exposure to ultraviolet (UV) rays, GI malabsorption, chronic diarrhea, pregnancy, and kidney disease.

The most common clinical feature is persistent skeletal pain, especially upon weight-bearing. Other manifestations include low back pain, progressive muscular weakness, weight loss, and progressive deformities of the spine (kyphosis) or extremities. Fractures are common and demonstrate delayed healing.

Laboratory findings include decreased serum calcium or phosphorus levels and elevated serum alkaline phosphatase. X-ray examination may demonstrate the effects of generalized bone demineralization, especially a loss of calcium in the bones of the pelvis and the presence of associated bone deformity.

- Looser's transformation zones (ribbons of decalcification in bone found on x-ray) are diagnostic of osteomalacia. Significant osteomalacia may exist without demonstrable X-ray changes.

Collaborative care is directed toward the correction of the underlying cause. Vitamin D (cholecalciferol) is usually supplemented, and the patient often shows a dramatic response. Calcium and phosphorus intake may also be supplemented.

See Paget's Disease, p. 437.

OSTEOMYELITIS

Definition/Description
Osteomyelitis is an infection of bone caused by direct or indirect invasion by an organism. In children the long bones are most commonly affected whereas the vertebrae are more commonly affected in adults. The course and virulence of osteomyelitis are influenced by the blood supply to the affected bone.

Pathophysiology
Direct entry results from contamination as a result of an open fracture or surgical implementation. *Indirect* inoculation results from a blood-borne infection from a distant site such as teeth, infected tonsils, or furuncles. The most common infecting organism is *Staphylococcus aureus.*

After gaining entrance to the bone, the bacteria lodge in an area of the bone (usually the metaphysis) in which circulation is slow. Bacteria grow, resulting in an increase in pressure that eventually leads to ischemia and vascular compromise. Once ischemia occurs, the bone dies.

Sequestra (areas of devitalized bone) form havens for bacteria, and chronic osteomyelitis develops. Sequestra enlarge and serve as a source of bacteria for spread to other sites, including the lungs and brain. Unless resolved naturally or surgically, the necrotic sequestrum may develop a sinus tract, resulting in chronic wound drainage.

Clinical Manifestations

Acute osteomyelitis refers to the initial infection or an infection of less than 1 month in duration. Manifestations of acute osteomyelitis are both systemic and local.

- Systemic manifestations include fever, night sweats, chills, restlessness, nausea, and malaise.
- Local manifestations include severe pain in the bone that is unrelieved by rest and worsens with activity; swelling, tenderness, and warmth at the infection site; and restricted movement of the affected part.
- Later signs include drainage from the sinus tracts to the skin and fracture site.

Chronic osteomyelitis refers to a bone infection that persists for longer than 4 weeks or an infection that has failed to respond to the initial course of antibiotic therapy. Chronic osteomyelitis can represent either a continuous, persistent problem or a process of exacerbations and quiescence. It results from inadequately treated acute osteomyelitis.

- Pus accumulates, causing ischemia of the bone. Over time, granulation tissue turns to scar tissue. This avascular scar tissue provides an ideal site for bacterial growth and is impenetrable to antibiotics.

Diagnostic Studies

- Wound culture determines the causative organism. A bone or tissue biopsy is the definitive way to determine the causative agent.
- Blood cultures of sequestrum are frequently positive for the presence of organisms.
- An elevated leukocyte count and sedimentation rate may also be found.
- Radionuclide bone scans can help establish the diagnosis.
- MRI and CT scans may be used to help identify the boundaries of the infection.

Collaborative Care

Vigorous antibiotic therapy is the treatment of choice for *acute osteomyelitis* as long as ischemia has not yet occurred. Wound cultures or a bone biopsy should be taken before antibiotic therapy is initiated so that specific antibiotic therapy can be determined. If antibiotic therapy is not started early, surgical debridement and decompression are necessary to relieve pressure within the bone and prevent ischemia. Some type of immobilization for the affected part is usually indicated.

Treatment for *chronic osteomyelitis* includes the surgical removal of poorly vascularized tissue and dead bone as well as the extended use of antibiotics. After surgical debridement, the wound may be closed and a suction irrigation system for removal of any devitalized tissues is inserted. Intermittent or constant irrigation of the affected bone with antibiotics may be initiated. Ciprofloxacin (Cipro) and ofloxacin (Floxin) are effective agents for treating osteomyelitis. IV therapy may be started in the hospital and continued in the home. Hyperbaric oxygen (O_2) therapy may be used as an adjunctive therapy where available.

- Skin and bone grafting may be necessary if destruction is extensive. If infection and bone destruction are extensive, then amputation of the extremity may be necessary to preserve life or improve the quality of life (see Amputation, p. 623).

Nursing Management

Goals

The patient with osteomyelitis will have satisfactory pain and fever control, not experience any complications associated with osteomyelitis, cooperate with the treatment plan, and maintain a positive outlook on the disease outcome.

See NCP 59-3 for the patient with osteomyelitis, Lewis and others, *Medical-Surgical Nursing,* edition 5, p. 1797.

Nursing Diagnoses/Collaborative Problems

- Hyperthermia *related to* infection
- Pain *related to* inflammatory process secondary to infection
- Ineffective individual coping *related to* isolation, hospitalization, immobility, and uncertain outcome
- Ineffective management of therapeutic regimen *related to* lack of knowledge regarding long-term management of osteomyelitis
- Impaired physical mobility *related to* pain, immobilization devices, and weight bearing limitations
- Potential complication: pathologic fracture of involved bone *related to* presence of weakened necrotic bone

Nursing Interventions

Patients with artificial implants such as a total joint replacement or metallic bone implants should be educated about methods to prevent osteomyelitis. Some physicians recommend prophylactic doses of antibiotics for procedures such as teeth cleaning, colonoscopy, or vaginal exams.

For the patient with osteomyelitis the involved extremity should be handled carefully to avoid excessive manipulation, which increases pain and could possibly cause pathologic fracture.

- Soiled dressings should be handled carefully to prevent cross-contamination of the wound or spread of the infection to other patients. When the dressing is changed, sterile technique is essential.
- Good body alignment and frequent position changes prevent complications associated with immobility and promote comfort.

Foot drop can develop quickly in the lower extremity if the foot is not correctly supported. A splint is frequently applied to the involved extremity in an attempt to maintain immobilization, support, and comfort.

- The patient should be instructed to avoid any activities, such as exercise or heat application, that increase circulation and promote the spread of infection.
- Patients are frightened and discouraged because of the serious nature of the disease, pain, and the length and cost of treatment. Continued psychologic support is an integral part of nursing management.

▼ **Patient Teaching**

- If at home, the patient and family must be instructed on the proper care and management of the venous access device for delivering antibiotics. They must also be taught how to administer antibiotics.
- If there is an open wound, dressing changes may be necessary. The patient may require supplies and instruction on the technique.

OSTEOPOROSIS

Definition/Description

Osteoporosis, or porous bone, is a condition characterized by low bone mass and structural deterioration of bone tissue. This leads to increased bone fragility. Osteoporosis is the major cause of fractures in postmenopausal women and older adults in general. Osteoporosis is increasing in incidence because more people are surviving to an older age. At least 25 to 35 million persons in the United States have some degree of osteoporosis. Osteoporosis is eight times more common in women.

Risk factors for osteoporosis are female gender, increasing age, Caucasian or Asian race, oophorectomy, family history, small stature, anorexia, sedentary lifestyle, and insufficient dietary calcium. Increased risk is also associated with cigarette smoking and alcoholism.

Pathophysiology

Peak bone mass (maximum bone tissue) is achieved during adolescence. It is determined by a combination of four major factors: heredity, nutrition, exercise, and hormone function. Heredity may be responsible for up to 70% of peak bone mass.

- Bone loss from midlife (age 35 to 40 years) onward is inevitable, but the rate of loss varies. At menopause, with the loss of estrogen, women experience rapid bone loss with reduced rates after 8 to 10 years.

Bone is continually being deposited by osteoblasts and resorbed by osteoclasts, a process called *remodeling*. Normally the rates of bone deposition and resorption are equal to each other so that the total bone mass remains constant. In osteoporosis, bone resorption exceeds bone deposition.

- Although resorption affects the entire skeletal system, osteoporosis occurs most commonly in the bones of the spine, hips, and wrists. Over time, wedging and fractures of the vertebrae produce a gradual loss of height and a humped back known as *dowager's hump* or *kyphosis*.
- The usual first signs are back pain or spontaneous fractures. The loss of bone substance causes the bone to become mechanically weakened and prone to either spontaneous fractures or fractures from minimal trauma.
- Specific diseases associated with osteoporosis include intestinal malabsorption, kidney disease, rheumatoid arthritis, advanced alcoholism, cirrhosis of the liver, and diabetes mellitus (DM).
- Many medications are known to decrease calcium retention, including corticosteroids, antiseizure medications (phenytoin [Dilantin]), heparin, isoniazid (INH), aluminum-containing antacids, and tetracycline.
- A genetic marker, the vitamin D receptor gene, has been linked to bone density.

Clinical Manifestations

Osteoporosis is often called the "silent disease" because bone loss occurs without symptoms. People may not know they have osteoporosis until their bones become so weak that a sudden strain, bump, or fall causes a hip or vertebral fracture.

- Collapsed vertebrae may initially be manifested as back pain, loss of height, or spinal deformities such as kyphosis or severely stooped posture.

Diagnostic Studies

Osteoporosis often goes unnoticed because it cannot be detected by conventional x-ray until more than 25% to 40% of the calcium in the bone is lost.

- Serum calcium, phosphorus, and alkaline phosphatase levels remain normal, although alkaline phosphatase may be elevated after a fracture.
- Bone mineral density (BMD) measurements are used to measure bone density.

- One of the most common studies is the dual-energy x-ray absorptiometry (DEXA), which measures bone density in the spine, hips, and forearm (the most common sites of fractures due to osteoporosis).

Nursing and Collaborative Management

Care of the patient with osteoporosis focuses on proper nutrition, calcium and vitamin D supplementation, exercise, and medication. Prevention and treatment of osteoporosis focuses on adequate calcium intake (1000 mg/day in premenopausal women and postmenopausal women taking estrogen and 1500 mg/day in postmenopausal women who are not receiving supplemental estrogen).

- If the dietary intake of calcium is inadequate, supplemental calcium should be taken. The amount of elemental calcium varies in different calcium preparations (see Table 59-25, Lewis and others, *Medical-Surgical Nursing,* edition 5, p. 1814). Calcium supplementation inhibits age-related bone loss; however, no new bone is formed.
- Moderate amounts of exercise are important to build up and maintain bone mass. Exercise also increases muscle strength, coordination, and balance. Walking is preferred to high-impact aerobics or running, both of which may put too much stress on the bones of patients with osteoporosis.
- Patients should be instructed to quit smoking, cut down on alcohol intake, and decrease the intake of high-phosphate carbonated beverages to decrease the likelihood of losing bone mass.

Drug Therapy

Estrogen replacement therapy after menopause is used to prevent osteoporosis. Although the exact mechanism for the protective function of estrogen is not known, it is believed that estrogen inhibits osteoclast activity, leading to decreased bone resorption and preventing both cortical and trabecular bone loss.

- Estrogen replacement therapy is most effective when combined with calcium. The greatest benefit of estrogen is probably in the first 10 years after menopause. Transdermal estrogen treatment has been shown to be effective in the treatment of postmenopausal women with established osteoporosis.

Calcitonin is secreted by the thyroid gland and inhibits osteoclastic bone resorption by directly interacting with active osteoclasts. It is available in intramuscular (IM), subcutaneous (SC), and intranasal forms. When calcitonin is used, calcium supplementation is necessary to prevent secondary hyperparathyroidism.

Biphosphonates inhibit osteoclast-mediated bone resorption, thereby increasing BMD and total bone mass. This group of drugs includes etidronate (Didronel), alendronate (Fosamax), pamidronate (Aredia), and tiludronate (Skelid).

- Patients should be instructed on the proper administration of alendronate to aid in its absorption. It should be taken upon rising in the morning with a full glass of water. The patient should not eat or drink anything for 30 minutes after taking it. The patient should also be instructed not to lie down after taking this medication. These precautions have been proven to decrease GI side effects (especially esophageal irritation) and increase drug absorption.

Other drugs include selective estrogen receptor modulators, such as raloxifene (Evista). This drug mimics the effect of estrogen on bone by reducing bone resorption without stimulating breast or uterine tissues. Raloxifene in postmenopausal women significantly increases BMD and may also protect the heart. Unlike estrogen it does not relieve menopausal symptoms.

Efforts should be made to keep patients with osteoporosis ambulatory in order to prevent further loss of bone substance as a result of immobility. Treatment also involves protecting areas of potential pathologic fractures; for example, a corset can be used to prevent vertebral collapse.

OTITIS MEDIA

Definition/Description

Otitis media is usually an acute childhood disease associated with colds, sore throats, and blockage of the eustachian tube. It is the most common problem of the middle ear. Untreated or repeated attacks of acute otitis media may lead to chronic otitis media and hearing loss. Chronic infection of the middle ear is more common in the person who experienced episodes of acute otitis media in early childhood.

Pathophysiology

Although most patients have mixed infections, bacteria are the predominant etiologic agents. Because the mucous membrane is continuous, both the middle ear and the air cells of the mastoid can be involved in the chronic infectious process. Organisms involved in chronic otitis media include *Staphylococcus aureus, Streptococcus, Proteus mirabilis, Pseudomonas aeruginosa,* and *Escherichia coli.*

Untreated conditions can result in eardrum perforation and the formation of a *cholesteatoma,* a cystic mass composed of epithelial cells and cholesterol. Enzymes produced by it may destroy adjacent bones, including ossicles.

Clinical Manifestations

- *Acute otitis media:* pain, fever, malaise, headache, and reduced hearing.
- *Chronic otitis media:* purulent, foul-smelling discharge accompanied by hearing loss and occasionally by ear pain, nausea, and episodes of dizziness. Additional complaints may include hearing loss as a result of ossicle destruction, tympanic membrane perforation, or accumulation of fluid in the middle ear space. Chronic otitis media is usually painless. However, if pain is present, it indicates fluid under pressure.

Untreated otitis media can result in eardrum perforation, cholesteatoma (an accumulation of keratinizing squamous epithelium), sensorineural deafness, facial weakness, brain or subdural abscess, and meningitis.

Diagnostic Studies

- Otoscopic examination may reveal a perforated or convex eardrum.
- Culture and sensitivity tests if drainage is present to identify infectious agent.
- Sinus x-rays, MRI, or CT scan of temporal bone destruction.

Collaborative Care

The aim of treatment is to rid the middle ear of infection. Systemic antibiotic therapy based on sensitivity testing is usually initiated. In addition, the patient with chronic otitis media may need to undergo frequent evacuation of drainage and debris in an outpatient setting. Antibiotic eardrops and 2% acetic acid drops are used to reduce infection. If there is a recurrence, the patient may be treated with parenteral antibiotics.

Often, chronic tympanic membrane perforations will not heal in response to conservative treatment. A tympanoplasty is then indicated. In acute otitis media, a myringotomy (incision in the tympanum) may be needed to release increased ear pressure and exudate.

Since the advent of antibiotics, the incidence of severe and prolonged infections of the middle ear has been greatly reduced. Prompt treatment of an episode of acute otitis media generally prevents spontaneous perforation of the tympanic membrane.

Nursing Management
Goals
The patient with otitis media will verbalize satisfaction with pain relief, identify factors that increase risk injury, and have adequate postoperative knowledge to take care of himself or herself and identify the complications associated with untreated otitis media.

Nursing Diagnoses/Collaborative Problems
- Impaired verbal communication *related to* hearing loss
- Risk for injury *related to* decreased hearing acuity
- Pain *related to* surgical incision, infection, and pressure
- Potential complication: bleeding from the operative site

Nursing Interventions
Following a tympanoplasty, postoperative care includes:
- Assessing the degree of pain to plan appropriate intervention
- Assisting the patient when getting up for the first time because dizziness may occur.
- Instructing the patient to avoid blowing the nose because this causes increased pressure in the eustachian tube and middle ear and could dislodge graft to the tympanum. Coughing and sneezing can cause a similar disruption.
- Monitoring dressing tightness and the amount and type of drainage.

OVARIAN CANCER

Definition/Description
Ovarian cancer is the most deadly cancer of the female reproductive system because most patients with ovarian cancer have advanced disease at diagnosis. The median age of women with ovarian cancer is 60. Caucasian women of North American or European descent are at greater risk for ovarian cancer as compared to African-American women.

Cancer of the ovary seems to be linked to a family history of ovarian cancer, increasing age, and a high-fat diet. Women who have mutations of the BRCA 1 gene have an increased susceptibility (a 60% greater risk) for ovarian cancer. Breast feeding, oral contraceptives (taken for more than 5 years), and an early age upon first giving birth may reduce the risk.

Pathophysiology
Eighty to eighty-five percent of ovarian cancers are epithelial carcinomas. Germ cell tumors account for another 10%. Histologic grading is an important prognostic determinant (see Cancer, p. 97).

Ovarian cancer has two patterns of metastasis—lymphatic and direct spread. Primary lymphatic drainage of the ovary is through the retroperitoneal nodes surrounding the renal hilum; secondary drainage is through the iliac lymphatics; tertiary drainage is through the inguinal lymphatics. Ovarian cancer also metastasizes directly to the abdominal cavity, the diaphragm, and the omentum.

Clinical Manifestations

In its early stages, ovarian cancer is usually asymptomatic. As the malignancy grows, a variety of symptoms, such as an increase in abdominal girth, bowel and bladder dysfunction, pain, menstrual irregularities, and ascites can occur.

Diagnostic Studies

- Unlike the Pap test used to screen for cervical cancer, no screening test exists for ovarian cancer. For women with a high risk of ovarian cancer, a combination of serum CA-125 and ultrasound is recommended in addition to a yearly pelvic exam.
- CA-125 is positive in 80% of women with epithelial ovarian cancer and is used to monitor the disease course.
- Bimanual pelvic exam is used to identify the presence of a mass.
- Laparoscopy is performed to establish the diagnosis if a mass has been palpated.
- If the mass is malignant, staging is critical for guiding treatment decisions. Because of the numerous metastatic pathways for ovarian cancer, accurate staging usually involves multiple biopsies.

Collaborative Care

The usual treatment for stage I disease (limited to the ovaries) is a total abdominal hysterectomy and bilateral salpingo-oophorectomy with the removal of as much of the tumor as possible (i.e., tumor debulking). Ascitic fluid is submitted for cytologic study and appropriate biopsies are performed to determine the stage of the disease. The addition of chemotherapy or the instillation of intraperitoneal radioisotopes is usually done for stage I disease (see Chemotherapy, p. 643).

The patient with stage II disease (limited to the true pelvis) may receive external abdominal and pelvic radiation, intraperitoneal radiation, or systemic combined chemotherapy after tumor-reducing surgery. After the completion of systemic chemotherapy in patients who are clinically free of symptoms, a "second-look" surgical procedure is often performed to determine whether there is any evidence of disease. This option does not necessarily improve the outcome. If no disease is found, the chemotherapy is stopped and the patient is monitored for recurrent disease.

Chemotherapy (e.g., cisplatin [Platinol], carboplatin [Paraplatin]) is used for the treatment of stage III (limited to the abdominal cavity) and stage IV (distant metastases) diseases. Altretamine (Hexalen) is used for the palliative treatment of persistent, recurrent ovarian cancer. Pacletaxel (Taxol) and topotecan (Hycamtin) are used to treat metastatic ovarian cancer. Surgical debulking is often done in conjunction with chemotherapy for advanced disease. Intraperitoneal chemotherapy may be used for patients who have minimum residual disease after surgery.

- Radiation and chemotherapy may be used to shrink the size of the tumor, which relieves both pressure and pain.

Nursing Management: Cancers of the Female Reproductive Tract

See Cervical Cancer, p. 121.

PAGET'S DISEASE

Definition/Description

Paget's disease (osteitis deformans) is a skeletal bone disorder in which there is excessive bone resorption followed by the replacement of normal marrow by vascular, fibrous connective tissue and new bone that is larger, more disorganized, and weaker. It occurs most often after the fourth decade of life and most commonly in men. The cause of Paget's disease is unknown, although a viral etiology has been proposed.

Pathophysiology

The disease is characterized by deformities of the bone caused by unexplained abnormal remodeling and resorption of bone, fibrotic changes, and remodeling with structurally uneven bone. Regions of the skeleton commonly affected are the pelvis, long bones, spine, ribs, and cranium.

Clinical Manifestations

In milder forms of Paget's disease, patients may remain free of symptoms, and the disease may be discovered incidentally on x-ray or serum chemistry.

- Initial manifestations are usually an insidious development of skeletal pain (which may progress to severe intractable pain), complaints of fatigue, and the progressive development of a waddling gait.
- Pathologic fracture is the most common complication and may be the first indication of the disease. Other complications include malignant osteosarcoma, benign giant cell tumors, or fibrosarcoma.

Diagnostic Studies

- There are markedly elevated serum alkaline phosphatase levels in advanced forms of the disease.
- X-rays may reveal that the normal contour of the affected bone is curved and the bone cortex is thickened, especially in weight-bearing bones and the cranium.

Nursing and Collaborative Management

Management is usually limited to symptomatic and supportive care and correction of secondary deformities by either surgical implementation or braces. Bone resorption, relief of acute symptoms, and the lowering of the serum alkaline phosphatase levels may be significantly influenced by the administration of calcitonin, which inhibits osteoclastic activity. Response to calcitonin therapy is only partial and often stops when therapy is discontinued.

- Biphosphonates, such as alendronate (Fosamax), tiludronate (Skelid), and pamidronate (Aredia) are nonhormonal agents that are effective in reducing the bone resorption in Paget's disease.
- Radiation therapy and local surgical procedures such as periosteal stripping may be used for control of the patient's pain.

A firm mattress should be used to provide back support and to relieve pain. The patient may be required to wear a corset or light brace to relieve back pain and provide support when in the upright position. The patient should be proficient in the correct application of such devices and know how to regularly examine areas of the skin for friction damage.

- Activities such as lifting and twisting should be discouraged. Good body mechanics are essential.
- Analgesics and muscle relaxants may be administered to relieve pain.
- A properly balanced nutritional program, especially as it pertains to vitamin D, calcium, and protein (which are necessary to ensure the availability of the components for bone formation), is very important in the management of metabolic disorders of bone.

Because metabolic bone disorders increase the possibility of pathologic fractures, the nurse must use extreme caution when the patient is turned or moved. It is important to keep the patient as active as possible to retard demineralization of bone resulting from disuse or extended immobilization. A supervised exercise program is an essential part of the treatment program. If the patient's condition permits, ambulation without causing fatigue must be encouraged.

- Prevention measures such as patient education, the use of an assistive device, and environmental changes should be actively pursued to prevent falls and subsequent fractures.

PANCREATIC CANCER

Definition/Description
Carcinoma of the pancreas is the fifth leading cause of death from cancer. It is more common in men and in African-Americans. The risk increases with age, with the peak incidence occurring between 65 and 80 years of age.

The prognosis of a patient with cancer of the pancreas is poor. Most patients die within 5 to 12 months of the initial diagnosis, and the 5-year survival rate is only about 10%.

Pathophysiology

The cause of pancreatic cancer is unknown. There may be some relationship between cancer, diabetes mellitus (DM), and chronic pancreatitis. It is not clear whether the cancer follows these diseases or whether these diseases occur as a result of pancreatic cancer.

Major risk factors seem to be alcohol use, cigarette smoking, a high-fat high-meat diet, DM, and exposure to chemicals such as benzidine. Pancreatic cancer develops twice as frequently in persons with a history of heavy cigarette use (more than two packs a day) as in nonsmokers.

P

Clinical Manifestations

Manifestations include abdominal pain (dull or aching), anorexia, rapid and progressive weight loss, nausea, and jaundice.

- Pain is very common and is related to the location of the malignancy. Extreme, unrelenting pain is related to the extension of the cancer into the retroperitoneal tissues and nerve plexuses. The pain is frequently located in the upper abdomen or left hypochondrium and radiates to the back. It is commonly related to eating, and it also occurs at night.

Diagnostic Studies

Better diagnostic measures are needed for detection of pancreatic cancer, since current methods detect only advanced stages.

- Cytologic examination of pancreatic secretions may reveal malignant cells.
- A secretin test frequently indicates a decreased volume of pancreatic juice with normal bicarbonate and enzyme production.
- Carcinoembryonic antigen (CEA) is elevated with advanced disease. CA 19-9 is a more specific tumor marker.
- Endoscopic retrograde cholangiography (ERCP) shows obstruction or narrowing of the pancreatic ducts.
- A CT scan identifies a solid tumor mass.

Collaborative Care

Surgery provides the most effective treatment of cancer of the pancreas. The classic surgery is a radical pancreaticoduodenectomy or *Whipple's procedure.* This entails a resection of the proximal pancreas (proximal pancreatectomy), the adjoining duodenum (duodenectomy), the distal portion of the stomach (partial gastrectomy), and the distal segment of the common bile duct. An anastomosis of the pancreatic duct, common bile duct, and stomach to the jejunum is done.

Radiation therapy alters survival rates very little but is effective for pain relief. External radiation is usually used, but implantation of internal radiation seeds into the tumor has also been used. Chemotherapy has limited success.

- Adjuvant therapy, which uses surgical resection, radiation, and chemotherapy, is believed to be the most effective way to manage pancreatic cancer (see Radiation Therapy, p. 681, and Chemotherapy, p. 643).

Nursing Management

Because the patient with carcinoma of the pancreas has many of the same problems as the patient with pancreatitis, nursing care includes the same measures (see Pancreatitis, Acute, below).

- The nurse should provide symptomatic and supportive nursing care. Medications and comfort measures to relieve pain should be provided before the patient reaches the peak of pain.
- Psychologic support is essential, especially during times of anxiety or depression, which seem to occur frequently in these patients.
- Adequate nutrition is an important part of the care plan. Frequent and supplemental feedings may be necessary. Measures to stimulate the appetite as much as possible and to overcome anorexia, nausea, and vomiting should be included.
- Because bleeding can result from impaired vitamin K production, the nurse should assess for bleeding from body orifices and mucous membranes.
- A significant component of nursing care is helping the patient and the family or significant others through the grieving process.

PANCREATITIS, ACUTE

Definition/Description

Acute pancreatitis is an acute inflammatory process of the pancreas, with the degree of inflammation varying from mild edema to severe hemorrhagic necrosis. Some patients recover completely; others have recurring attacks; still others develop chronic pancreatitis. Acute pancreatitis can be life threatening.

Pathophysiology

Many factors can cause injury to the pancreas. The primary etiologic factors are biliary tract disease and alcoholism. In the United States the most common cause is alcoholism, followed by gall bladder disease. Other causes of acute pancreatitis include trauma (postsurgical or abdominal), viral infections (mumps), penetrating duodenal ulcer, cysts, abscesses, cystic fibrosis, certain drugs (corticosteroids, sulfonamides, nonsteroidal antiinflammatory drugs [NSAIDs]), and metabolic disorders such as hyperparathyroidism and renal failure. In some cases the cause is not known (idiopathic).

- The most common pathogenic mechanism is believed to be autodigestion of the pancreas. The etiologic factors cause injury to pancreatic cells or activation of the pancreatic enzymes in the pancreas rather than in the intestine.

The pathophysiologic involvement of acute pancreatitis ranges from *edematous pancreatitis* (which is mild and self-limiting) to *necrotizing pancreatitis* (in which the degree of necrosis correlates with the severity of the manifestations).

Clinical Manifestations

Abdominal pain is the predominant symptom of acute pancreatitis. The pain is usually located in the left upper quadrant but may be in the midepigastrium. It commonly radiates to the back because of the retroperitoneal location of the pancreas.

- The pain has a sudden onset and is described as severe, deep, piercing, and continuous or steady. It is aggravated by eating and frequently has its onset when the patient is recumbent; it is not relieved by vomiting. The pain may be accompanied by flushing, cyanosis, and dyspnea.

Other manifestations include nausea and vomiting, low grade fever, leukocytosis, hypotension, tachycardia, and jaundice. Abdominal tenderness with muscle guarding is common. Bowel sounds may be decreased or absent. The lungs are frequently involved, with crackles present.

Intravascular damage from circulating trypsin may cause areas of cyanosis or greenish to yellow-brown discoloration of the abdominal wall. Other areas of ecchymoses are the flanks (*Grey Turner's spots* or *sign,* a bluish flank discoloration) and the periumbilical area (*Cullen's sign,* a bluish periumbilical discoloration).

Complications

Local complications of acute pancreatitis are pseudocyst and abscess.

- A pancreatic *pseudocyst* is a cavity continuous with or surrounding the outside of the pancreas. Symptoms are abdominal pain, palpable epigastric mass, nausea, vomiting, and anorexia. The serum amylase level frequently remains elevated. These cysts usually resolve spontaneously within a few weeks, but may perforate, causing peritonitis, or rupture into the stomach or duodenum.
- A pancreatic *abscess* is a large fluid-containing cavity within the pancreas. It results from extensive necrosis in the pancreas. It may become infected or perforate into adjacent organs. Manifes-

tations include upper abdominal pain, abdominal mass, high fever, and leukocytosis. Pancreatic abscesses require prompt surgical drainage to prevent sepsis. Shock may occur because of hemorrhage into the pancreas or toxemia from the activated pancreatic enzymes.

Systemic complications of acute pancreatitis are pulmonary complications (pleural effusion, atelectasis, and pneumonia) and tetany due to hypocalcemia.

Diagnostic Studies

- Serum amylase (pancreatic isoamylase), serum lipase, and urinary amylase are elevated.
- Other laboratory abnormalities include hyperglycemia, hyperlipidemia, and hypocalcemia.
- Abdominal x-ray and ultrasound scan of the pancreas.

Collaborative Care

Objectives of management for acute pancreatitis include relief of pain, prevention or alleviation of shock, reduction of pancreatic secretions, control of fluid and electrolyte imbalance, prevention or treatment of infections, and removal of the precipitating cause, if possible.

- A primary consideration is the relief and control of pain. Meperidine (Demerol) is preferred because it causes less spasm of the smooth muscles of the ducts than morphine. It may be combined with an antispasmodic. If shock is present, blood volume replacements and expanders such as dextran or albumin may be given.

It is important to reduce or suppress pancreatic enzymes to decrease stimulation of the pancreas and allow it to rest. The patient is allowed to take nothing by mouth (NPO status). Nasogastric (NG) suction may be used to reduce vomiting and gastric distention and to prevent gastric digestive juices from entering the duodenum. Certain drugs may also be used for this purpose.

- Inflamed and necrotic pancreatic tissue is a good media source for bacterial growth. Antibiotic therapy should be instituted early if an infection occurs.
- When food is allowed, small, frequent feedings are given. The diet is usually high in carbohydrate content because it is the least stimulating to the exocrine portion of the pancreas. The diet combines high-carbohydrate intake with low-fat and high-protein intake.

Surgical intervention may be indicated when the diagnosis is uncertain and in patients who do not respond to conservative therapy. Surgery is necessary for an abscess, acute pseudocyst, and severe peritonitis. Percutaneous drainage of a pseudocyst can be performed, and a drainage tube is left in place. Surgical treatment of associated biliary tract disease may be necessary.

Several different drugs may be used in the treatment of both acute and chronic pancreatitis (see Table 41-21, Lewis and others, *Medical-Surgical Nursing*, edition 5, p. 1223).

Nursing Management

Goals

The patient with acute pancreatitis will have relief of pain, return of fluid and electrolyte balance, minimal to no complications, and no recurrent attacks.

See NCP 41-3 for the patient with acute pancreatitis, Lewis and others, *Medical-Surgical Nursing*, edition 5, p. 1225.

Nursing Diagnoses/Collaborative Problems

- Pain *related to* inflammation of the pancreas, peritoneal irritation, and ineffective pain and comfort measures
- Fluid volume deficit *related to* nausea, vomiting, NG suction, and restricted oral intake
- Altered nutrition: less than body requirements *related to* anorexia, dietary restrictions, nausea, loss of nutrients from vomiting, and impaired digestion
- Ineffective management of therapeutic regimen *related to* lack of knowledge of preventive measures, diet restrictions, and follow-up care
- Potential complication: hemorrhagic shock *related to* the destruction of blood vessel walls by proteolytic enzymes
- Potential complication: fluid and electrolyte imbalance *related to* loss of fluids into the peritoneal cavity

Nursing Interventions

The nurse should encourage the early diagnosis and treatment of alcohol abuse and biliary tract diseases such as cholelithiasis.

Because abdominal pain is a prominent symptom of pancreatitis, a major focus of nursing care is the relief of pain. Giving the prescribed medications before the pain becomes too severe makes the medication more effective. Measures such as comfortable positioning, frequent changes in position, and relief of nausea and vomiting assist in reducing the restlessness that usually accompanies the pain.

- Some patients experience reduced pain by assuming positions that flex the trunk and draw the knees up to the abdomen. A side-lying position with the head elevated 45 degrees decreases tension on the abdomen and may help ease the pain.

Nursing measures for the patient who is on NPO status or has an NG tube should be employed. Frequent oral and nasal care to relieve the dryness of the mouth and nose is comforting to the patient.

- Observation for electrolyte imbalances is important because frequent vomiting, along with gastric suction, may result in decreased chloride, sodium (Na^+), and potassium (K^+) levels. It is important to observe for symptoms of hypocalcemia such as tetany and numbness or tingling around the lips and in the fingers. The patient should be assessed for a positive Chvostek's or Trousseau's sign.
- Observation for fever and other manifestations of infection is important. Respiratory infections are common because the retroperitoneal fluid raises the diaphragm, which causes the patient to take shallow, guarded abdominal breaths. Prevention of respiratory infections includes turning, coughing, deep breathing, and assuming a semi-Fowler's position.

Most patients will need home care follow-up. The patient may have lost physical reserve and muscle strength. Physical therapy may be needed. Continued care to prevent infection and detect any complications is important.

▼ **Patient Teaching**

- The patient should be encouraged to eliminate alcohol intake, especially if there have been any previous episodes of pancreatitis. Attacks of pancreatitis become milder or disappear with the discontinuance of alcohol use.
- Beverages with caffeine should not be consumed. Because smoking and stressful situations can overstimulate the pancreas, they should also be avoided.
- Dietary teaching should include the restriction of fats because they stimulate the pancreas. Carbohydrates are less stimulating to the pancreas, so they should be encouraged. The patient should be instructed to avoid crash dieting and bingeing because these can precipitate attacks.
- The patient and the family should be given instructions regarding the recognition and reporting of symptoms of infection, diabetes mellitus (DM), or steatorrhea (foul-smelling, frothy stools). These changes indicate possible destruction of pancreatic tissue.
- The nurse should make sure the patient fully understands the prescribed regimen. Each aspect must be explained. The importance of taking required medications and following the recommended diet should be stressed.

PANCREATITIS, CHRONIC

Definition/Description
Chronic pancreatitis is the progressive destruction of the pancreas with fibrotic replacement of pancreatic tissue. Strictures and calcifications may also occur in the pancreas. Chronic pancreatitis may follow acute pancreatitis, but it may also occur in the absence of any history of an acute condition. In the United States chronic pancreatitis is found almost exclusively in alcoholics. Two major types are chronic obstructive pancreatitis and chronic calcifying pancreatitis.

Pathophysiology
Chronic obstructive pancreatitis is associated with biliary disease. The most common cause is inflammation of the sphincter of Oddi associated with cholelithiasis. Cancer of the ampulla of Vater, duodenum, or pancreas are additional causes.

Chronic calcifying pancreatitis is associated with inflammation and sclerosis that mainly occurs in the head of the pancreas and around the pancreatic duct. The ducts are obstructed with protein precipitates that block the pancreatic duct and eventually calcify. This is followed by fibrosis and glandular atrophy. Pseudocysts and abscesses commonly develop. This type of chronic pancreatitis is the most common form and is also called alcohol-induced pancreatitis.

Clinical Manifestations
As with acute pancreatitis, a major manifestation of chronic pancreatitis is abdominal pain. The patient may have episodes of acute pain, but it usually is chronic (recurrent attacks at intervals of months or years). The attacks may become more and more frequent until they are almost constant, or they may diminish as the pancreatic fibrosis develops. The pain is located in the same areas as in acute pancreatitis but is usually described as a heavy, gnawing feeling or sometimes as burning and cramplike. The pain is not relieved with food or antacids.

- Other manifestations include symptoms of pancreatic insufficiency, including malabsorption with weight loss, constipation, mild jaundice with dark urine, steatorrhea, and diabetes mellitus (DM). The steatorrhea may become quite severe with voluminous, foul, fatty stools. Urine and stool may be frothy. Some abdominal tenderness may be found.

Diagnostic Studies
- A secretin stimulation test is the most useful test in diagnosing chronic pancreatitis.

- Serum amylase, bilirubin, and alkaline phosphatase levels are elevated.
- Mild leukocytosis and elevated sedimentation rate.
- Hyperglycemia.
- Fatty stools *(steatorrhea)* are found in fecal fat determination with neutral fat indicative of maldigestion.
- Arteriography and x-rays may demonstrate fibrosis and calcification.

Nursing and Collaborative Management

When the patient with chronic pancreatitis is experiencing an acute attack, the therapy is identical to that for acute pancreatitis. At other times the focus is on the prevention of further attacks, the relief of pain, and the control of pancreatic exocrine and endocrine insufficiency. It sometimes takes large, frequent doses of analgesics to relieve the pain, and narcotic addiction may become a problem.

- The treatment of chronic pancreatitis sometimes requires surgery. When biliary disease is present or if obstruction or pseudocyst develops, surgery may be indicated. Other operations are performed to divert bile flow or relieve ductal obstruction.

▼ Patient Teaching

- The patient should be instructed to take measures to prevent further attacks. Dietary control, along with consistency of other treatment measures, such as taking pancreatic enzymes, is essential. Pancreatic extracts are usually given with meals or can be given with a snack. The patient's stools need to be observed for steatorrhea to help determine the effectiveness of the enzymes. The patient and the family need instructions regarding the observation of stools.
- Alcohol must be avoided, and the patient may need assistance with this problem. If the patient has developed a dependence on alcohol or narcotics, a referral to other agencies or resources may be necessary.
- If DM has developed, the patient will need instruction regarding testing of blood glucose levels and medications.
- The patient who is taking liquid antacids should be instructed to sip the medication slowly, and the nurse should make certain it is taken as ordered to help control gastric acidity. Antacids should be taken after meals. Both the antacid and the pancreatic enzymes may be left at the bedside to prepare the patient for self-management at home.

PARKINSON'S DISEASE

Definition/Description

Parkinsonism is a syndrome that consists of slowness in the initiation and execution of movement *(bradykinesia),* increased muscle tonus *(rigidity),* tremor, and impaired postural reflexes.

- Parkinson's disease is a form of parkinsonism. About 1.5% of the population in the United States over the age of 65 years of age is affected. The disease shows no gender, socioeconomic, or cultural preference. There is no apparent genetic cause and no known cure. The disease rarely occurs in African-Americans.

Pathophysiology

There are many causes of parkinsonism. Encephalitis lethargica, or type A encephalitis, has been associated with the onset of parkinsonism. Parkinson-like symptoms have also occurred after intoxication with a variety of chemicals, including carbon monoxide, manganese (among copper miners), and an analogue of meperidine (MPTP). Drug-induced parkinsonism can follow the use of reserpine (Serpasil), methyldopa (Aldomet), haloperidol (Haldol), and phenothiazine therapy. Most patients with parkinsonism have the degenerative or idiopathic form, for which the term *Parkinson's disease* is usually reserved.

- The pathology of Parkinson's disease is associated with degeneration of the dopamine-producing neurons in the substantia nigra of the midbrain. In Parkinson's disease the levels of dopamine-synthesizing enzymes and metabolites are reduced, and postmortem analysis shows a loss of the normal melanin pigment in the substantia nigra and a loss of neurons. In addition, deficient amounts of gamma-aminobutyric acid (GABA), serotonin, and norepinephrine have been found in the basal ganglia and substantia nigra.

Clinical Manifestations

The onset of Parkinson's disease is gradual and insidious, with a gradual progression and a prolonged course. The classic triad of symptoms is tremor, rigidity, and bradykinesia. In the beginning stages, only a mild tremor, slight limp, or a decreased arm swing may be evident. Later the patient may have a shuffling, propulsive gait with arms flexed and loss of postural reflexes. In some patients there may be a slight change in speech patterns.

- *Tremor,* often the first sign, may initially be minimal, so that the patient is the only one who notices it. Parkinsonian tremor is more prominent at rest and is aggravated by emotional stress or increased concentration. The hand tremor is described as "pill rolling" because the thumb and forefinger appear to move in a rotary fashion as if rolling a pill, coin, or other small object. Tremor can involve the diaphragm, tongue, lips, and jaw.

- *Rigidity* is increased resistance to passive motion when the limbs are moved through their range of motion. Parkinsonian rigidity is typified by a jerky quality, as if there were intermittent catches in the movement of a cogwheel, when the joint is moved. This is called *cogwheel rigidity.*

- *Bradykinesia* is particularly evident in the loss of automatic movements, which is secondary to the physical and chemical alteration of the basal ganglia. In the unaffected patient, automatic movements are involuntary and occur subconsciously; these include the blinking of the eyelids, swinging of the arms while walking, swallowing of saliva, self-expression with facial and hand movements, and minor movement of postural adjustment. The patient with Parkinson's disease does not execute these movements. This lack of spontaneous activity accounts for the stooped posture, masked facies ("deadpan" expression), drooling of saliva, and shuffling gait. There is difficulty in initiating movement.

Complications

Many of the complications are caused by the decomposition and loss of spontaneity of movement.

- Swallowing may become very difficult *(dysphagia)* in severe cases, leading to malnutrition or aspiration. General debilitation may lead to pneumonia, urinary tract infections, and skin breakdown.

- Mobility is greatly decreased. The gait slows and turning is especially difficult. The posture is that of the "old man" image, with the head and trunk bent forward and the legs constantly flexed. The lack of mobility may lead to constipation, ankle edema, and, more seriously, contractures.

- Orthostatic hypotension may occur and, along with the loss of postural reflexes, may result in falls or other injuries.

- Bothersome complications include seborrhea, excessive sweating, conjunctivitis, insomnia, incontinence, and depression.

- Many of the apparent complications of Parkinson's disease are due to the side effects of prolonged medication therapy, particularly levodopa.

- Dyskinesias (e.g., athetosis of the neck) and weakness and akinesia (total immobility) may cause problems.

- Dementia occurs in up to 40% of patients with Parkinson's disease.

Diagnostic Studies

Because there is no specific diagnostic test for Parkinson's disease, the diagnosis is based solely on the history and the clinical features.

- A firm diagnosis can be made only when there are at least two of the three characteristic signs of the classic triad: tremor, rigidity, and bradykinesia.
- The ultimate confirmation of Parkinson's disease is a positive response to antiparkinsonian medication.

Collaborative Care

Because there is no cure, management is aimed at relieving symptoms. Antiparkinson drugs either enhance dopamine release or supply (dopaminergic) or antagonize or block the effects of the overactive cholinergic neurons (anticholinergic).

Surgical therapy is aimed at relieving symptoms. Surgical procedures such as thalamotomy, thalamic stimulation, and pallidotomy are often reserved for patients who are unresponsive to drug therapy or who have developed severe motor complications. Stereotactic thalamotomy relieves tremor and (to a lesser extent) rigidity. Bilateral posteroventral pallidotomy relieves tremor rigidity and bradykinesia.

Chronic thalamic electrical stimulation has been used to reduce tremor and enhance motor function. Transplantation of fetal tissue into the caudate nucleus in an attempt to provide viable dopamine-producing cells to the brain has had variable results.

Drug Therapy

Drug therapy is aimed at correcting an imbalance of neurotransmitters within the central nervous system (CNS).

- Levodopa with carbidopa (Sinemet) is often the first drug to be used. Levodopa is a precursor of dopamine and is converted to dopamine in the basal ganglia. Sinemet is the preferred drug because it contains carbidopa, an enzyme which inhibits the breakdown of levodopa before it reaches the brain. This results in more levodopa reaching the brain.
- If symptoms are not severe, mild antiparkinsonian drugs, such as the dopamine agonists bromocriptine (Parlodel) and pergolide (Permax) can provide improvement in symptoms. Newer dopamine-receptor agonists such as ropinirole (Requip) and pramipexole (Mirapex) have also been shown to be effective in improving the symptoms of early Parkinson's disease. When more moderate to severe symptoms are present, carbidopa/dopa agents (e.g., Sinemet) are added to the drug regimen.
- Anticholinergic drugs are also used and act by decreasing the activity of acetylcholine. This provides a balance between cholinergic and dopaminergic actions. These drugs include trihexyphenidyl (Artane) and benztropine (Cogentin).

- Antihistamines (e.g., diphenhydramine [Benadryl]) with anticholinergic properties are sometimes used to manage tremors.
- The antiviral agent amantadine (Symmetrel) is also effective, although its exact mechanism of action is not known. Amantadine promotes the release of dopamine from the neurons.

Nutritional Therapy

Diet is of major importance because malnutrition and constipation can be serious consequences of inadequate nutrition. Patients who have dysphagia and bradykinesia need appetizing foods that are easily chewed and swallowed. The diet should contain adequate roughage and fruit to avoid constipation. Ample time should be planned for eating to avoid frustration and encourage independence.

Nursing Management

Goals

The patient with Parkinson's disease will maximize neurologic function, maintain independence in activities of daily living (ADLs) for as long as possible, and optimize psychosocial well-being.

See NCP 56-4 for the patient with Parkinson's disease, Lewis and others, *Medical-Surgical Nursing,* edition 5, p. 1699.

Nursing Diagnoses

- Impaired physical mobility *related to* rigidity, tremor, bradykinesia, and akinesia
- Altered nutrition: less than body requirements *related to* dysphagia
- Sleep pattern disturbance *related to* medication side effects (e.g., hallucinations), anxiety, rigidity, and muscle discomfort
- Impaired verbal communication *related to* dysarthria and tremor or bradykinesia
- Self-care deficits *related to* parkinsonian symptoms

Nursing Interventions

Promotion of physical exercise and a well-balanced diet are major concerns for nursing care. Exercise can limit the consequences of decreased mobility such as muscle atrophy, contractures, and constipation. Overall muscle toning as well as specific exercises to strengthen the muscles involved with speaking and swallowing should be included.

- Because Parkinson's disease is a chronic degenerative disorder with no acute exacerbations, nurses should note that health teaching and nursing care are directed toward the maintenance of good health, encouragement of independence, and avoidance of complications such as contractures.

▼ **Patient Teaching**

- Instructions for patients who tend to "freeze" while walking include (1) consciously thinking about stepping over imaginary lines on the floor, (2) dropping rice kernels and stepping

over them, (3) rocking from side to side, (4) lifting the toes when stepping and (5) taking one step backward and two steps forward.
- Getting out of a chair can be facilitated by using an upright chair with arms and placing the back legs on small (2-inch) blocks.
- Rugs and excess furniture can be removed to avoid stumbling.
- Clothing can be simplified by the use of slip-on shoes and velcro hook-and-loop fasteners or zippers on clothing instead of buttons and hooks.
- An elevated toilet seat can facilitate getting on and off the toilet.
- The nurse should work closely with the patient's family in exploring creative adaptations that allow the patient the greatest amount of independence and self-care.

PELVIC INFLAMMATORY DISEASE

Definition/Description
Pelvic inflammatory disease (PID) is an infectious condition of the pelvic cavity that may involve the fallopian tubes (salpingitis), ovaries (oophoritis), and pelvic peritoneum. PID remains a major cause of infertility and is often the result of untreated cervicitis.

Pathophysiology
The most frequent causative organisms of PID are *Neisseria gonorrhoeae* and *Chlamydia trachomatis.* These organisms, as well as mycoplasma, streptococci, and anaerobes, may gain entrance during sexual intercourse or after pregnancy termination, pelvic surgery, or childbirth.

Clinical Manifestations
The woman with PID usually goes to a health care provider because of lower abdominal pain.
- The pain starts gradually and is constant. The intensity may vary from mild to severe with movements such as walking increasing the pain.
- Spotting after intercourse and abnormal vaginal discharge are common.
- Fever and chills may also be present.
- Women with less acute symptoms notice increased cramping pain with menses, irregular bleeding, and some pain with intercourse. Women who have mild symptoms may go untreated either because they did not seek care or the health care provider misdiagnosed their complaints.

Complications

Septic shock can occur when PID spreads to the liver. The patient will have symptoms of right upper quadrant pain, but liver function tests will be normal. Pelvic and tubal ovarian abscesses may "leak" or rupture, resulting in pelvic or generalized peritonitis.

- Long-term complications include ectopic pregnancy, infertility, and chronic pelvic pain. PID can cause adhesions and strictures to develop in the fallopian tubes.

Diagnostic Studies

The diagnosis is based on data obtained during the bimanual portion of the pelvic exam. Women with PID have lower abdominal tenderness and bilateral adnexal tenderness when the cervix is moved.

- Diagnostic criteria also include fever and abnormal vaginal or cervical discharge.
- Cultures for gonorrhea and chlamydia should be obtained from the endocervix.
- A pregnancy test should always be done.
- When pain or obesity compromise the pelvic examination and an ovarian abscess may be present, a vaginal ultrasound is indicated.

Collaborative Care

Treatment of PID is usually on an outpatient basis. The patient is given a combination of antibiotics such as cefoxitin (Mefoxin) and doxycycline to provide broad coverage against the causative organisms. Instructions are given to avoid intercourse for 3 weeks, restrict general activities, get adequate rest and nutrition, and return to the clinic for reevaluation in 48 to 72 hours even if the symptoms are improving.

If outpatient treatment is not successful or if the patient is acutely ill or in severe pain, admission to the hospital is indicated. Maximum doses of parenteral antibiotics are given. In some situations corticosteroids are given to reduce inflammation and improve subsequent fertility. Analgesics to relieve pain and IV fluids to prevent dehydration are also prescribed.

Application of heat to the lower abdomen or sitz baths may be used to improve circulation and decrease pain. Bed rest in the semi-Fowler's position promotes drainage of the pelvic cavity by gravity and may prevent the development of abscesses high in the abdomen. Sexual partners of women with PID should also be examined and treated.

Indications for surgery include the presence of abscesses that fail to resolve with IV antibiotics. The abscesses may be drained by laparotomy or laparoscopy. Childbearing function in young women is preserved whenever possible.

Nursing Management

Goals

The patient with PID will experience a relief of symptoms, practice good perineal hygiene and safe sex, not become infertile as a result of the disease, and comply with the treatment regimen to prevent the disease from becoming chronic.

See NCP 51-1 for the patient with pelvic inflammatory disease, Lewis and others, *Medical-Surgical Nursing,* edition 5, p. 1536.

Nursing Diagnoses

- Pain *related to* infection process
- Anxiety *related to* imposed activity restrictions, perceived loss of control, and lack of knowledge of the outcome on reproductive status and the course of the disease

Nursing Interventions

Prevention, early recognition, and prompt treatment of vaginal and cervical infections can help prevent PID and its serious complications. Nurses can provide information regarding factors that place a woman at increased risk for PID, such as multiple sexual partners.

- The patient should be encouraged by the awareness that some discharges are not indicative of infection and that early diagnosis and treatment of an infection can prevent complications.
- Women should be informed of the methods of preventing infection as well as the signs of infection in their partners.

During hospitalization for PID, the nurse has an important role in implementing drug therapy, monitoring the patient's health status, and providing symptom relief and patient education. Vital signs and the character, amount, color, and odor of the vaginal discharge are recorded. Explanations about the need for limited activity (bed rest in a semi-Fowler's position) and increased fluid intake should increase patient cooperation. The nurse should assess the patient's pain level and plan appropriate interventions such as heat to the lower abdomen, sitz baths, and analgesics.

- The patient may have guilt feelings about the problem, especially if it was associated with a sexually transmitted disease. She may also be concerned about the complications associated with PID, such as adhesions and strictures of the fallopian tubes, sterility, and the increased incidence of ectopic pregnancy. Discussion with the patient and significant others regarding these feelings and concerns can assist her to cope more effectively with them.

PEPTIC ULCER DISEASE

Definition/Description
Peptic ulcer disease is an erosion of GI mucosa resulting from the digestive action of hydrochloric (HCl) acid and pepsin. Any portion of the GI tract that comes into contact with gastric secretions is susceptible to ulcer development, including the lower esophagus, stomach, duodenum, and at the margin of a gastrojejunal anastomosis site after surgical procedures.

Peptic ulcers can be classified as acute or chronic, depending on the degree of mucosal involvement, and gastric or duodenal, according to the location. Eighty percent of all peptic ulcers are duodenal.

- An *acute ulcer* is associated with superficial erosion and minimal inflammation. It is of short duration and resolves quickly when the cause is identified and removed.
- A *chronic ulcer* is of long duration, eroding through the muscular wall with the formation of fibrous tissue. It is continuously present for many months or intermittently throughout the person's lifetime. A chronic ulcer is at least four times as common as an acute ulcer.
- Gastric and duodenal ulcers, although defined as peptic ulcers, are distinctly different in etiology and incidence (Table 44).

Pathophysiology
Peptic ulcers develop only in the presence of an acid environment. Under specific circumstances the mucosal barrier can be impaired and back-diffusion of HCl acid and pepsin can occur. When the barrier is broken, HCl acid freely enters the mucosa and injury to the tissues occurs. This results in cellular destruction and inflammation. Histamine is released from the damaged mucosa, resulting in vasodilation and increased capillary permeability. A variety of agents are known to destroy the mucosal barrier (see Gastritis, p. 245). The critical pathologic process in gastric ulcer formation may not be the amount of acid that is secreted but the amount that is able to penetrate the mucosal barrier.

- Nonsteroidal antiinflammatory drug (NSAID) use is a risk factor for gastric ulcers.
- *Helicobacter pylori* is a dominant factor in the promotion of peptic ulcer formation. This organism promotes gastric mucosal destruction (see Gastritis, p. 245).

Clinical Manifestations
It is common with gastric or duodenal ulcers to have no pain or other symptoms (gastric and duodenal mucosa do not have pain sensory

Table 44 Comparison of Gastric and Duodenal Ulcers

Gastric	Duodenal
Superficial lesion; smooth margins; round/oval/cone-shaped	Penetrating lesion (associated with deformity of duodenal bulb from healing of recurrent ulcers)
Located predominantly in antrum; also in body and fundus of stomach	Located in first 1-2 cm of duodenum
Greater incidence in women; peak age fifth to sixth decade	Greater incidence in men, but increasing in women (especially postmenopausal); peak age 35-45 yr
More common in persons of low socioeconomic status and in unskilled laborers	Associated with psychologic stress and other diseases (e.g., chronic obstructive pulmonary disease, pancreatic disease, hyperparathyroidism, Zollinger-Ellison syndrome, chronic renal failure)
Increased with smoking; drug and alcohol use; incompetent pyloric sphincter; and stress ulcers after severe burns, head trauma, and major surgery	
Manifestations include burning or gaseous pressure in high left epigastrium and back and upper abdomen; pain 1-2 hr after meals; if penetrating ulcer, aggravation of discomfort with food; occasional nausea and vomiting; weight loss	Manifestations include burning, cramping, pressurelike pain across midepigastrium and upper abdomen; back pain with posterior ulcers; pain 2-4 hr after meals and in midmorning, midafternoon, middle of night; also periodic and episodic pain; pain relief with antacids and food; occasional nausea and vomiting

P

fibers). When pain does occur with a duodenal ulcer, it is described as "burning" or "cramplike" and is most often located in the midepigastrium region beneath the xyphoid process. Pain associated with gastric ulcer is located high in the epigastrium and occurs spontaneously about 1 to 2 hours after meals. The pain is described as "burning" or "gaseous." The pain can occur when the stomach is empty or when food has been ingested. Some persons do not experience any pain until a serious complication such as hemorrhage or perforation occurs.

Complications

Three major complications of chronic peptic ulcers are hemorrhage, perforation, and gastric outlet obstruction. All are considered emergency situations and are initially treated conservatively. However, surgery may become necessary at any time during the course of therapy.

Hemorrhage is the most common complication. It develops from the erosion of granulation tissue at the base of the ulcer during healing or from the erosion of an ulcer through a major blood vessel. Duodenal ulcers account for a greater percentage of upper GI bleeding than gastric ulcers.

Perforation, the most lethal complication, occurs when the ulcer penetrates the serosal surface with spillage of either gastric or duodenal contents into the peritoneal cavity. The size of the perforation is directly proportional to the length of time the patient has had the ulcer.

- Manifestations of perforation are sudden with a dramatic onset and include severe upper abdominal pain that quickly spreads throughout the abdomen. Shallow and rapid respirations and absent bowel sounds are also present.

Gastric outlet obstruction may occur over time due to edema, inflammation, fibrous scar tissue, and pylorospasm associated with active ulcer formation. Symptoms include upper abdomen discomfort and swelling, loud peristalsis, visible peristaltic waves, vomiting (often projectile), and constipation.

Diagnostic Studies

- Fiberoptic endoscopy is used to determine the characteristics and nature of the ulcer, obtain a tissue biopsy, obtain specimens to test for *H. pylori,* and assess the degree of ulcer healing following treatment.
- Barium studies for the diagnosis of pyloric obstruction by recurrent ulcers.
- Exfoliative cytology differentiates between benign and malignant tumors.
- A gastric analysis determines the amount and composition of gastric secretions.
- Complete blood count (CBC), urinalysis, liver enzyme studies, serum amylase determination, and stool examination may be performed for further diagnostic information.

Collaborative Care

The aim of treatment is to decrease gastric acidity, enhance mucosal defense mechanisms, and minimize the harmful effects on the mucosa.

Conservative Therapy

The prescribed regimen consists of adequate rest, dietary interventions, medications, elimination of smoking, and long-term follow-up care. Strict adherence to the prescribed regimen of drugs is mandatory because peptic ulcer recurrence is high without treatment. Drug therapy includes the use of antacids, histamine H_2-receptor antagonists (e.g., cimetidine [Tagamet], famotidine [Pepcid]), antisecretory agents (e.g., misoprostol [Cytotec]), proton pump inhibitor (e.g., omeprazole [Prilosec]) anticholinergics, and cytoprotective (e.g., sucralfate [Carafate]) agents. Aspirin and NSAIDs should be discontinued. The patient is placed on antibiotics to eradicate *H. pylori* infection.

Healing of a peptic ulcer requires many weeks of therapy. Pain disappears after 3 to 6 days, but ulcer healing is much slower. Complete healing may take 3 to 9 weeks, depending on the ulcer size and the treatment regimen employed.

Acute exacerbation of peptic ulcer can usually be treated with the same regimen used for conservative therapy. Blood products may be given for bleeding. However, the situation is considered more serious because of the chronicity of the ulcer and possible complications of perforation, hemorrhage, and obstruction.

- One method of symptom relief is to keep the stomach empty for 24 to 48 hours via nasogastric (NG) tube and intermittent suctioning, with IV fluid and electrolyte infusions given.
- In perforation, the focus of therapy is to stop the spillage of gastric contents by NG tube or surgery. Blood volume is replaced with antibiotics and pain medication is also given.
- In gastric outlet obstruction the aim of therapy is to decompress the stomach via NG tube.

Nutritional Therapy

Nutritional therapy is individualized with an avoidance of foods causing pain or discomfort. Protein is considered the best neutralizing food, but it also stimulates gastric secretions. Carbohydrates and fats are the least stimulating to HCl acid secretion, but they do not neutralize well. The patient must determine a suitable combination of these essential nutrients without causing undue distress to the ulcer. Small, frequent (six per day) meals may be recommended.

Surgical Therapy

Many physicians believe that surgery is necessary after therapy has been tried and proven unsuccessful. Types of surgery to treat ulcers include partial gastrectomy, vagotomy, or pyloroplasty. Postoperative complications from surgery are dumping syndrome, postprandial hypoglycemia, and bile reflux gastritis.

- *Dumping syndrome* is the direct result of the surgical removal of a large portion of the stomach and pyloric sphincter. These changes drastically reduce the reservoir capacity of the stomach. The onset of symptoms occurs at the end of a meal or within 15 to 30 minutes of eating. The patient usually describes feelings of generalized weakness, sweating, palpitations, and dizziness. Symptoms are self-limiting.
- *Postprandial hypoglycemia* is considered a variant of dumping syndrome, since it is the result of uncontrollable gastric emptying of a bolus of fluid high in carbohydrates, resulting in hyperglycemia into the small intestine. Symptoms are sweating, weakness, mental confusion, palpitations, and tachycardia. Treatment limits sugar intake, with small frequent meals recommended.
- The major symptom associated with *bile reflux gastritis* is continuous epigastric distress that increases after meals. Vomiting relieves distress but only temporarily. The administration of cholestyramine (Questran), either before or with meals, has met with considerable success.

Nursing Management
Goals
The patient with peptic ulcer disease will experience a reduction or absence of discomfort related to the disease, exhibit no signs of GI complications related to the ulcerative process, have complete healing of the peptic ulcer, make appropriate lifestyle changes to prevent recurrence, and comply with the prescribed therapeutic regimen.

See NCP 39-2 for the patient with a peptic ulcer, Lewis and others, *Medical-Surgical Nursing,* edition 5, p. 1120.

Nursing Diagnoses/Collaborative Problems
- Pain *related to* gastric secretions, decreased mucousal protection, and ingestion of gastric irritants
- Ineffective management of the therapeutic regimen *related to* lack of knowledge of long-term management of peptic ulcer disease and unwillingness to modify lifestyle
- Potential complication: perforation of GI mucosa secondary to impaired mucosal tissue integrity.

Nursing Interventions
Very often during the acute phase all that is necessary for the patient's immediate recovery is to maintain nothing by mouth (NPO) status for a few days, have an NG tube inserted and connected to intermittent suction, and replace fluids intravenously. The rationale for this therapy must be conveyed to the anxious patient and family. Vital signs are taken at least hourly with hematocrit (Hct) and hemoglobin (Hb) levels monitored so hemorrhage and perforation can be detected early.

Postoperative care of the patient after major abdominal surgery is similar to postoperative care after abdominal laparotomy (see Abdominal Pain, Acute, p. 3). Additional considerations include:

- Gastric aspirate from the NG tube must be carefully observed for color, amount, and odor during the immediate postoperative period.
- Observe the patient for signs of decreased peristalsis and lower abdominal discomfort that may indicate impending intestinal obstruction.
- Keep the patient comfortable and free of pain by the administration of prescribed medications and by frequent changes in position.
- Observe the dressing for signs of bleeding or odor and drainage indicative of an infection.
- Ambulation is encouraged and is increased daily.
- Because the patient is generally returning to the same home and work environment, there is always the danger of ulcer redevelopment, especially at the site of the anastomosis. Adequate rest, nutrition, and avoidance of known stressors are keys to complete recovery.

▼ **Patient Teaching**

General instructions for the newly diagnosed patient should cover aspects of the disease process itself, nutritional therapy, medication, possible changes in lifestyle, and regular follow-up care.

- Specifically, the patient must be well informed about each drug prescribed, why it is ordered, and the expected benefits.
- Stress reduction techniques should be taught to the patient as relaxation results in decreased acid production and reduction in pain.
- The need for long-term follow-up care must be stressed. Because successful treatment is frequently followed by a recurrence of ulcer disease, the patient should be encouraged to seek immediate intervention if symptoms such as pain and discomfort recur or if blood is noted in stools or vomitus.

PERICARDITIS, ACUTE

Definition/Description

Pericarditis is a syndrome caused by inflammation of the pericardial sac (the pericardium), which may occur on an acute basis. The pericardium provides lubrication to decrease friction during systolic and diastolic heart movements and assists in preventing excessive dilation of the heart during diastole.

Pathophysiology

Acute pericarditis is most often idiopathic with a variety of suspected viral causes. The coxsackievirus B group is the most commonly identified virus and tends to elicit pleuropericarditis in adults (Bornholm disease) and myopericarditis in children. In addition to idiopathic or viral pericarditis, other causes of this syndrome include uremia, bacterial infection, acute myocardial infarction (MI), tuberculosis (TB), neoplasm, and trauma.

Pericarditis in the acute MI patient may be described as two distinct syndromes. Acute pericarditis immediately follows myocardial damage within the initial 48 to 72 hour period. Dressler's syndrome (late pericarditis) appears 2 to 4 weeks after infarction.

An inflammatory response is the characteristic pathologic finding in acute pericarditis. There is an influx of neutrophils, increased periocardial vascularity, and eventual fibrin deposition on the visceral pericardium.

Clinical Manifestations

Characteristic manifestations found in acute pericarditis include chest pain, dyspnea, and a pericardial friction rub.

- Intense, pleuritic chest pain is generally sharpest over the left precordium or retrosternally but it may radiate to the trapezius ridge and neck (mimicking angina), or sometimes to the epigastrium or abdomen (mimicking abdominal or other noncardiac pathological conditions). The pain is aggravated by lying supine, deep breathing, coughing, swallowing, and moving the trunk and is eased by sitting up and leaning forward.
- Dyspnea is related to the patient's need to breathe in rapid, shallow breaths to avoid chest pain and may be aggravated by fever and anxiety.
- The hallmark finding is the *pericardial friction rub*. The rub is a scratching, grating, high-pitched sound believed to arise from friction between the roughened pericardial and epicardial surfaces. It is best heard with the stethoscope diaphragm firmly placed at the lower left sternal border of the chest. The pericardial friction rub does not radiate widely or vary in timing from the heartbeat, but may require frequent auscultation to identify because it may be elusive and transient. Timing the pericardial friction rub with the pulse (and not respirations) will help to distinguish it from pleural rub.

Complications

Complications that may result from acute pericarditis are pericardial effusion and cardiac tamponade.

Pericardial effusion is generally a rapid accumulation of excess pericardial fluid that occurs in chest trauma. However, a slowly developing effusion may result, as in TB pericarditis. Large effusions may compress adjoining structures. Pulmonary tissue compression can cause cough, dyspnea, and tachypnea. Phrenic nerve compression can induce hiccups, and compression of the recurrent laryngeal nerve may result in hoarseness. Heart sounds are generally distant and muffled. BP is usually maintained by compensatory changes.

Cardiac tamponade develops as the pericardial effusion increases in size. Compensatory mechanisms ultimately fail to adjust to the decreased cardiac output. The patient with pericardial tamponade is often confused, agitated, and restless and has tachycardia and tachypnea with a low-output state. The neck veins are usually markedly distended because of jugular venous pressure elevation, and a significant *pulsus paradoxus* is present. Pulsus paradoxus, an inspiratory drop in systolic BP >10 mm Hg, results because the normal inspiratory decline in systolic BP of <10 mm Hg is exaggerated in cardiac tamponade (see Table 35-1, Lewis and others, *Medical-Surgical Nursing,* edition 5, p. 948).

Diagnostic Studies
- Auscultation of chest for pericardial friction rub.
- ECG to detect arrhythmias.
- Echocardiography is used to determine the presence of pericardial effusion or cardiac tamponade.
- Pericardiocentesis and pericardial biopsy are done to determine the cause of pericarditis.
- CT scan and nuclear scan of heart.

Collaborative Care
The management of acute pericarditis is directed toward the identification and treatment of the underlying problem. Antibiotics should be used to treat bacterial pericarditis. Corticosteroids are generally reserved for patients with pericarditis secondary to systemic lupus erythematosus, patients already taking corticosteroids for a rheumatologic or other immune system condition, or patients who do not respond to nonsteroidal antiinflammatory drugs (NSAIDs). When necessary, prednisone is usually given in a tapering dosage schedule. Pain and inflammation are usually treated with nonsteroidal antiinflammatory agents. High-dose salicylates (300 to 900 mg orally four times a day) or indomethacin (Indocin) (25 to 50 mg orally four times a day) are commonly used.
- Pericardiocentesis is usually performed when acute cardiac tamponade has reduced the patient's systolic BP 30 mm Hg or more from baseline. Hemodynamic support as the patient is prepared for the pericardiocentesis may include the administration of volume expanders and inotropic agents.

Nursing Management

Management of the patient's pain and anxiety are primary nursing considerations. Assessment of the amount, quality, and location of the pain is important, particularly in distinguishing the pain of acute MI (or reinfarction) from the pain of pericarditis. Careful nursing observations should be made regarding ischemic chest pain, which is generally located retrosternal in the left shoulder and arm with a pressurelike, burning quality and is unaffected by posture. In contrast, pericarditic pain is usually located in the precordium, the left trapezius ridge, with a sharp, pleuritic quality that changes with respirations. Relief from this pain is often obtained by the patient leaning forward and is worsened by recumbency.

- Pain relief measures include maintaining the patient on bed rest with the head of the bed elevated to 45 degrees and providing a padded overbed table.
- Antiinflammatory medications help to alleviate the patient's pain. However, because of the potential for GI problems with the use of high doses of these medications, specific nursing interventions should include the administration of these drugs with food or milk, generally 30 minutes before or 2 hours after meals, and instructions to the patient to avoid alcoholic beverages while taking the medications.

Monitoring for the signs and symptoms of tamponade, along with preparations for possible pericardiocentesis, are important nursing responsibilities.

Anxiety-reducing measures for the patient include providing simple, complete explanations of all procedures performed. These explanations are particularly important for the patient during the time a diagnosis is being established and for the patient who has already experienced an acute MI and has pericarditis (Dressler's syndrome).

PERITONITIS

Definition/Description

Peritonitis is a localized or generalized inflammatory process of the peritoneum. It may appear in acute and chronic forms, and it may be caused by trauma or rupture of an organ containing chemical irritants or bacteria, which are released into the peritoneal cavity (Table 45).

Pathophysiology

The response of the peritoneum to the leakage of GI contents is localization of the offending agent by attempting to "wall it off." Adhesions may form. These adhesions may shrink and disappear

Table 45	Causes of Peritonitis
Primary	**Secondary**
Blood-borne organisms	Appendicitis with rupture
Genital tract organisms	Blunt or penetrating trauma to
Cirrhosis with ascites	abdominal organs
	Diverticulitis with rupture
	Ischemic bowel disorders
	Obstruction in the GI tract
	Pancreatitis
	Perforated peptic ulcer
	Peritoneal dialysis
	Postoperative (breakage of
	anastomosis)

P

when the infection is eliminated. Normally, peritoneal injuries heal without the formation of adhesions unless other factors, such as infection, ischemia, or foreign substances, are present.

Clinical Manifestations
- Abdominal pain is the most common symptom, followed by ascites.
- A universal sign is tenderness over the involved area. Rebound tenderness, muscular rigidity, and spasm are other major signs of irritation of the peritoneum.
- Abdominal distention (ascites), fever, tachycardia, tachypnea, nausea, vomiting, and altered bowel habits may also be present. Complications include hypovolemic shock, septicemia, intraabdominal abscess formation, paralytic ileus, and organ failure.

Diagnostic Studies
- Complete blood count (CBC) to determine hemoconcentration and leukocytosis.
- Peritoneal aspiration for analysis of blood, bile, pus, bacteria, fungi, and amylase content.
- Abdominal x-ray may show dilated loops of bowel consistent with paralytic ileus, free air if there is a perforation, or air and fluid levels if an obstruction is present.
- CT scan or ultrasound to identify ascites or abscesses.
- Peritoneoscopy is helpful in patients without ascites.

Collaborative Care
The goals of management are to identify and eliminate the cause, combat infection, and prevent complications. Patients with milder

cases of peritonitis or those who are poor surgical risks may be managed nonsurgically. Treatment consists of antibiotics, nasogastric (NG) suction, analgesics, and IV fluid administration. Patients who require surgery need preoperative preparation. These patients may be placed on total parenteral nutrition (TPN) (see Total Parenteral Nutrition, p. 684) because of increased nutritional requirements.

Nursing Management

Goals

The patient with peritonitis will have resolution of inflammation, relief of abdominal pain, freedom from complications (especially hypovolemic shock), and normal nutritional status.

Nursing Diagnoses/Collaborative Problems

- Pain *related to* inflammation of the peritoneum and abdominal distention
- Risk for fluid volume deficit *related to* collection of fluid in peritoneal cavity as a result of trauma, infection, or ischemia
- Altered nutrition: less than body requirements *related to* nausea, vomiting, and anorexia
- Anxiety *related to* uncertainty of cause or outcome of condition and pain
- Potential complication: hypovolemic shock *related to* loss of circulatory volume

Nursing Interventions

The patient with peritonitis is very ill and needs skilled supportive care. The patient is monitored for pain and the response to analgesic therapy. The patient may be positioned with knees flexed to increase comfort. The nurse should provide rest and a quiet environment. Sedatives may be given to allay anxiety.

- Accurate monitoring of fluid intake and output and electrolyte status is necessary to determine replacement therapy. Vital signs are monitored frequently.
- Antiemetics may be administered to decrease nausea and vomiting and further fluid losses. The patient is on nothing by mouth (NPO) status and may have an NG tube in place to decrease gastric distention.
- If the patient has an open-incision surgical procedure, drains are inserted to remove purulent drainage and excessive fluid. Postoperative care of the patient is similar to the care of the patient with an exploratory laparotomy (see Abdominal Pain, Acute, p. 3).

PHARYNGITIS, ACUTE

Acute pharyngitis is an acute inflammation of the pharynx caused by bacterial, viral, or fungal infection. Acute follicular pharyngitis ("strep throat") results from streptococcal bacterial invasion. *Neisseria gonorrhoeae* and *Corynebacterium diphtheriae* are other bacterial organisms that infect the pharynx. Fungal pharyngitis, especially candidiasis, can develop with prolonged use of antibiotics, inhaled corticosteroids, or in immunosuppressed patients, especially those with HIV infection.

Clinical manifestations of acute pharyngitis range in severity from complaints of a "scratchy throat" to pain so severe that swallowing is difficult.

- White, irregular patches suggest infection with *Candida albicans.*
- In viral infections the throat may appear mildly red with some congestion of the blood vessels.
- In strep throat the throat is typically an intense red-purple color with patchy yellow exudate and localized lymphadenopathy.
- In diphtheria a gray-white false membrane, termed a *pseudomembrane,* is seen covering the oropharynx, nasopharynx, and laryngopharynx and sometimes extending to the trachea.

Cultures are done to establish the cause and the appropriate management. Even with severe infection, cultures may be negative.

The goals of management are infection control, symptomatic relief, and the prevention of secondary complications. Because cultures can be negative even when infection is present, the patient suspected of having strep throat is often treated with antibiotics. *Candida* infections are treated with nystatin, an antifungal antibiotic. Treatment for pharyngitis should continue until symptoms are gone. The patient should be encouraged to increase fluid intake and to take cool, bland liquids and gelatin that will not irritate the pharynx. Citrus juices should be avoided because they irritate mucous membranes.

PHEOCHROMOCYTOMA

Pheochromocytoma is the most common disorder of the adrenal medulla. It is characterized by a neoplasm that produces excessive catecholamines. Most of these tumors (95%) are benign and encapsulated. Pheochromocytoma can occur at any age and in either gender, but it is found most commonly in patients between the ages of 30 and 50.

The most striking clinical features of pheochromocytoma are severe, episodic hypertension; severe, pounding headache; and profuse sweating. Attacks of episodic hypertension are due to sympathetic nervous system stimulation and are often accompanied by anxiety and profuse sweating.

- Attacks may be provoked by many medications including antihypertensives, opiates, and tricyclic antidepressants. The duration of the attacks may vary from a few minutes to several hours.

Measurement of urinary metanephrines (catecholamine metabolites) is the simplest and most reliable diagnostic test. Plasma catecholamines are also elevated. It is preferable to measure catecholamines during an "attack." CT and MRI scans are used for tumor localization.

Treatment consists of the surgical removal of the tumor. Before surgery the patient is hospitalized for treatment to correct hypovolemia and cardiovascular complications to decrease the risk of surgery.

- Sympathetic blocking agents (e.g., phenoxybenzamine [Dibenzyline], propranolol [Inderal]) are administered to reduce the BP and alleviate other symptoms of catecholamine excess.
- Preoperative and postoperative care is similar to that for any patient undergoing adrenalectomy except that blood pressure fluctuations from catecholamine imbalances tend to be severe and need to be carefully monitored.

Complete removal of the tumor cures the hypertension in the majority of patients. In the others, hypertension persists or returns but is usually well controlled by standard therapy (see Hypertension, p. 321).

PNEUMONIA

Definition/Description

Pneumonia is an acute inflammation of the lung parenchyma. It is the sixth leading cause of death in the United States. Pneumonia can be caused by bacteria, viruses, Mycoplasma, fungi, parasites, and chemicals.

- Although pneumonia can be classified according to the causative organism, a clinically more effective way is to classify pneumonia as community-acquired (CAP) or hospital-acquired (HAP) (Table 46). This classification helps in directing therapy.

Pathophysiology

Normally the airway distal to the larynx is sterile because of protective defense mechanisms. Pneumonia is more likely to result when defense mechanisms become incompetent or are overwhelmed by infectious agents. Risk factors for pneumonia are varied and include:

Table 46	Causes of Pneumonia

Community-acquired	Hospital-acquired
*Streptococcus pneumoniae**	*Pseudomonas aeruginosa*
Mycoplasma pneumoniae	*Enterobacter*
*Haemophilus influenzae***	*Escherichia coli*
Respiratory viruses	*Proteus*
Chlamydia pneumoniae	*Klebsiella*
Legionella pneumophila	*Staphylococcus aureus*
Oral anaerobes	*Streptococcus pneumoniae*
Moraxella catarrhalis	Oral anaerobes
Staphylococcus aureus	
Nocardia	
Enteric aerobic gram-negative bacteria (e.g., Klebsiella)	
Fungi	
Mycobacterium tuberculosis	

*Most common cause of community-acquired pneumonia (CAP)
**Second most common cause of CAP

- Decreased consciousness, which depresses the cough and epiglottal reflexes
- Tracheal intubation, which interferes with the normal cough reflex and the mucociliary mechanism
- Impaired mucociliary mechanism due to air pollution, cigarette smoking, viral upper respiratory tract infections, and normal aging changes
- Malnutrition, in which the formation and function of lymphocytes and polymorphonuclear leukocytes are altered
- Certain diseases such as leukemia, alcoholism, and diabetes mellitus (DM), which are associated with an increased frequency of gram-negative bacilli in the oropharynx
- Altered oropharyngeal flora, which can occur secondary to antibiotic therapy given for an infection elsewhere in the body

Clinical Manifestations and Complications

CAP has been thought to present as two syndromes: typical and atypical. *Typical* pneumonia syndrome is characterized by the sudden onset of fever, chills, cough productive of purulent sputum, and pleuritic chest pain.

- Signs of pulmonary consolidation, such as dullness to percussion, increased fremitus, bronchial breath sounds, and crackles, may be found.

- In the elderly or debilitated patient, confusion or stupor may be the predominant finding.

The *atypical* syndrome is characterized by a more gradual onset, a dry cough, and extrapulmonary manifestations such as headache, myalgias, fatigue, sore throat, nausea, vomiting, and diarrhea. Crackles are often heard.

Manifestations of viral pneumonia are highly variable. Viruses also cause pneumonia that is usually characterized by an atypical presentation with chills, fever, dry nonproductive cough, and extrapulmonary symptoms.

- Patients with hematogenous *Staphylococcus aureus* pneumonia may only present with dyspnea and fever. Necrotizing infection causes the destruction of lung tissue. These patients are usually very sick.

Most cases of pneumonia generally run an uncomplicated course. Complications can occur and develop more frequently in individuals with underlying chronic diseases and other risk factors.

Complications include pleurisy (inflammation of the pleura), pleural effusion, atelectasis (collapsed, airless alveoli), delayed resolution resulting from persistent infection, lung abscess, empyema (accumulation of purulent exudate in the pleural cavity), pericarditis, arthritis, meningitis, and endocarditis.

Diagnostic Studies

- Gram's stain of sputum and blood cultures to identify the causative organism.
- Sputum culture and sensitivity test using transtracheal aspiration or bronchoscopy with aspiration if patient is unable to voluntarily produce a sputum specimen.
- Chest x-ray often shows a typical pattern characteristic of infecting organism.
- Arterial blood gases (ABGs) usually reveal hypoxemia.
- Complete blood count (CBC) and white blood cell (WBC) count (leukocytosis usually found).

Collaborative Care

Prompt treatment with the appropriate antibiotic almost always cures bacterial and mycoplasma pneumonia. Currently, there is no definitive treatment for viral pneumonia. Tables 26-3 and 26-4, Lewis and others, *Medical-Surgical Nursing,* edition 5, pp. 613-614, outline the drug therapies used in the treatment of CAP and HAP.

In uncomplicated cases, the patient responds to drug therapy within 48 to 72 hours. Indications of improvement include decreased temperature, improved breathing, and reduced chest pain.

Supportive measures may be used, including oxygen (O_2) therapy, analgesics to relieve chest pain, and antipyretics such as aspirin or acetaminophen. During the acute febrile phase, the patient's activity should be restricted and rest should be encouraged and planned.

Pneumococcal vaccine is indicated primarily for the individual considered at increased risk who (1) has chronic illnesses such as lung and heart disease and DM, (2) is recovering from a severe illness, (3) is 65 years of age or older, or (4) is in a nursing home or other long-term care facility. The current recommendation is that the vaccine is good for the person's lifetime. In the immunosuppressed individual at increased risk for development of fatal pneumococcal infection, revaccination should be considered every 5 years.

Nursing Management

Goals
The patient with pneumonia will have clear breath sounds, normal breathing patterns, normal chest x-ray, and no complications related to pneumonia.

See NCP 26-1 for the patient with pneumonia, Lewis and others, *Medical-Surgical Nursing,* edition 5, p. 620.

Nursing Diagnoses/Collaborative Problems
- Ineffective breathing pattern *related to* pneumonia and pain
- Ineffective airway clearance *related to* pain, positioning, fatigue, and thick secretions
- Pain *related to* pleuritis and ineffective pain management or comfort measures
- Altered nutrition: less than body requirements *related to* increased metabolism, fatigue, anorexia, nausea, and vomiting
- Activity intolerance *related to* an interrupted sleep/wake cycle, hypoxia, and weakness
- Altered health maintenance *related to* a lack of knowledge regarding the treatment regimen after discharge
- Potential complication: hypoxemia *related to* impaired gas exchange in the lungs

Nursing Interventions
Interventions focus on preventing the occurrence of pneumonia. If possible, exposure to upper respiratory infections (URIs) should be avoided. If a URI occurs, it should be treated promptly with supportive measures (e.g., rest, fluids). If symptoms persist for more than 7 days, the person should obtain medical care. The individual at increased risk for pneumonia (e.g., the chronically ill patient and the older adult) should be encouraged to obtain both influenza and pneumococcal vaccines.

In the hospital, the nursing role involves identifying the patient at risk and taking measures to prevent the development of pneumonia.
- The patient with altered consciousness should be placed in positions (e.g., side-lying, upright) that will prevent or minimize aspiration. The patient should be turned and repositioned at

least every 2 hours to facilitate adequate lung expansion and to discourage the pooling of secretions.
- The patient who has a feeding tube generally requires attention to positioning of the tube to prevent aspiration.
- The patient who has difficulty swallowing (e.g., a stroke patient) needs assistance in eating, drinking, and taking medication to prevent aspiration.
- The gag reflex should be present in the individual who has had local anesthesia to the throat before the administration of fluids or food.
- The patient who has recently had surgery and others who are immobile need assistance with turning at frequent intervals.
- Overmedication with narcotics or sedatives, which can cause a depressed cough reflex, should be avoided.
- Strict medical asepsis and adherence to universal precautions should be practiced to reduce the incidence of nosocomial infections.

▼ **Patient Teaching**
- Instruct the patient to prevent the occurrence of pneumonia by practicing good health habits, such as proper diet and hygiene, adequate rest, and regular exercise.
- It is extremely important to emphasize to the patient the need to take all of the prescribed medication and to return for follow-up medical care and evaluation.
- Adequate rest is needed to maintain progress toward recovery and to prevent relapse. The patient needs to be told that it may be weeks before the usual vigor and sense of well-being are felt.
- The patient considered to be at increased risk for pneumonia should be told about available vaccines and should discuss them with the health care worker.
- Deep breathing exercises should be practiced for 6 to 8 weeks after the patient is discharged from the hospital.

PNEUMOTHORAX

Definition/Description
Pneumothorax is a complete or partial collapse of a lung as a result of an accumulation of air in the pleural space. This condition should be suspected after any blunt trauma to the chest wall. A pneumothorax may be closed or open.

Pathophysiology
Closed pneumothorax has no associated external wound; the most common form is *spontaneous pneumothorax,* which is caused by the

rupture of small blebs on the visceral pleural space. The cause of blebs is unknown; there is a tendency for this condition to recur. This condition occurs most commonly in male cigarette smokers between 20 and 40 years of age.

- Other causes of closed pneumothorax include injury to the lungs from mechanical ventilation, insertion of a subclavian catheter, perforation of the esophagus (see Flail Chest, p. 232, and Fracture, Rib, p. 243), and ruptured blebs or bullae in a patient with chronic obstructive pulmonary disease (COPD).

Open pneumothorax occurs when air enters the pleural space through an opening in the chest wall. Examples include stab or gunshot wounds and surgical thoracotomies. A penetrating chest wound is often referred to as a *sucking chest wound.*

Tension pneumothorax may result from an open or closed pneumothorax or when chest tubes are clamped or become blocked after insertion for a pneumothorax. In an open chest wound, a flap may act as a one-way valve; thus air can enter on inspiration but cannot escape. Intrathoracic pressure increases, the lung collapses, and the mediastinum shifts toward the unaffected side, which is subsequently compressed. As intrathoracic pressure increases, cardiac output (CO) is altered because there is decreased venous return and compression of the great vessels.

- Tension pneumothorax is a medical emergency because both the respiratory and circulatory systems are affected. It usually occurs with mechanical ventilation or resuscitative efforts.

Hemothorax is an accumulation of blood in the intrapleural space. It is frequently found in association with open pneumothorax and is then called a *hemopneumothorax.* The causes of hemothorax include chest trauma, lung malignancy, complication of anticoagulant therapy, and pulmonary embolus.

Clinical Manifestations

If the pneumothorax is small, only mild tachycardia and dyspnea may be present. If it is a large pneumothorax, shallow, rapid respirations, dyspnea, and air hunger may occur.

- Chest pain and a cough with or without hemoptysis may also be present.
- On auscultation there are no breath sounds over the affected area, and hyperresonance may be heard.

If a tension pneumothorax develops, severe respiratory distress, tachycardia, and hypotension occur. The trachea and point of maximal impulse (PMI) shift to the unaffected side.

Collaborative Care

If the amount of air or fluid accumulated in the intrapleural space is minimal, no treatment may be needed because the pneumothorax resolves spontaneously, or the pleural space can be aspirated with a large-bore needle. Needle aspiration is often a lifesaving measure.

- An open pneumothorax should be covered with a vented dressing. (A vented dressing is one secured on three sides with the fourth side left untaped.) This allows air to escape from the vent and decreases the likelihood of tension pneumothorax developing. If the object that caused the open chest wound is still in place, it should not be removed until the physician is present.

The most common treatment for a pneumothorax and hemothorax is to insert a chest tube and connect it to water-seal drainage (see Chest Tubes and Pleural Drainage, p. 649). Repeated spontaneous pneumothoraces may need to be treated surgically by a partial pleurectomy, stapling, or laser pleurodesis to promote the adherence of pleurae to one another.

POLYCYSTIC RENAL DISEASE

Polycystic renal disease is characterized by multiple renal cysts that enlarge and destroy surrounding tissue by compression. The cysts involve both kidneys and are filled with fluid, including blood or pus. The *childhood form* of polycystic disease is a rare autosomal recessive disorder that is often rapidly progressive. The *adult form* of polycystic disease is an autosomal dominant disorder which is latent for many years and usually manifests between 30 and 40 years old.

Symptoms appear when the cysts begin to enlarge. A common early symptom of adult cystic disease is abdominal or flank pain, which is either steady and dull or abrupt in onset, as well as episodic and colicky. On physical examination, palpable bilateral enlarged kidneys are often found.

- Other manifestations include hematuria, urinary tract infection (UTI), and hypertension.
- Usually the disease progresses to chronic renal failure.

The diagnosis is based on clinical manifestations, family history, intravenous pyelogram (IVP), ultrasound, or CT scan.

There is no specific treatment for polycystic kidney disease. A major aim of treatment is to prevent infections of the urinary tract or to treat them with appropriate antibiotics if they occur. Nephrectomy may be necessary if pain, bleeding, or infection becomes a chronic, serious problem. When the patient begins to experience progressive renal failure, therapeutic interventions are determined by the remaining renal function.

Nursing measures are those used for management of end-stage renal disease (see Renal Failure, Chronic, p. 496). They include diet modification, fluid restriction, medications (e.g., antihypertensives), helping the patient to accept the chronic disease process, and assisting the patient and the family to deal with the altered body image, financial concerns, and other issues related to the hereditary nature of the disease.

- The patient will need appropriate counseling regarding plans for having more children; each child of a parent with polycystic renal disease has a 50% chance of having the disease.

POLYCYTHEMIA

Definition/Description
Polycythemia is the production and presence of an increased number of red blood cells (RBCs). The increase in erythrocytes can be so great that blood circulation is impaired as a result of the increased blood viscosity (hyperviscosity) and volume (hypervolemia).

Pathophysiology
The two types of polycythemia are *primary polycythemia (polycythemia vera)* and *secondary polycythemia* (Figure 4). Their etiologies and pathogenesis differ, although their complications and clinical manifestations are similar.

Polycythemia vera is a myeloproliferative disorder arising from a chromosomal mutation in a single pluripotent stem cell. Therefore not

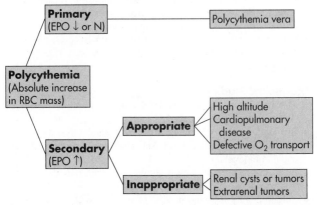

Fig. 4 Differentiating between primary and secondary polycythemia. *EPO,* Erythropoietin; *N,* normal; O_2, oxygen; *RBC,* red blood cell.

only are erythrocytes involved, but also granulocytes and platelets, leading to increased production of each of these blood cells. The disease develops insidiously and follows a chronic, vacillating course. It usually develops in patients over 50 years of age. Patients have enhanced blood viscosity and blood volume and congestion of organs and tissues with blood. Splenomegaly is common.

- The major cause of morbidity and mortality from polycythemia vera is thrombosis.

Secondary polycythemia is caused by hypoxia rather than a defect in RBC production. Hypoxia stimulates erythropoietin in the kidney, which stimulates erythrocyte production. The need for oxygen (O_2) may be due to high altitude, pulmonary and cardiovascular disease, defective O_2 transport, or tissue hypoxia.

Clinical Manifestations

Manifestations are due to hypertension caused by hypervolemia and hyperviscosity. These include subjective complaints of headache, vertigo, dizziness, tinnitus, and visual disturbances.

Manifestations caused by blood vessel distention, impaired blood flow, thrombosis, and tissue hypoxia include angina, congestive heart failure (CHF), intermittent claudication, and thrombophlebitis.

- Generalized pruritus may be a striking symptom and is related to histamine release from an increased number of basophils and mast cells.
- Hemorrhage can be acute or catastrophic and may result in petechiae, ecchymoses, epistaxis, or GI bleeding.
- Hepatomegaly and splenomegaly may contribute to patient complaints of satiety and fullness.
- Pain due to peptic ulcer may occur due to increased gastric secretions or liver and spleen engorgement.
- *Plethora* (ruddy complexion) may also be present.
- Hyperuricemia caused by the increase in RBC destruction that accompanies excessive RBC production may cause a secondary form of gout.

Diagnostic Studies

- Elevated hemoglobin (Hb), RBC count, and white blood cell (WBC) count with basophilia.
- Elevated platelets (thrombocytosis) and platelet dysfunction.
- Elevated leukocyte alkaline phosphatase, histamine, uric acid, and cobalamin levels.
- Bone marrow examination shows hypercellularity of RBCs, WBCs, and platelets.
- Splenomegaly is found in 90% of patients with primary polycythemia.

Collaborative Care

Treatment of polycythemia vera is directed toward reducing blood volume and viscosity and bone marrow activity. A phlebotomy may be done to diminish blood volume until the desired hematocrit (Hct) level is achieved. The aim of phlebotomy is to reduce and keep the Hct to less than 45% to 48%. An individual managed with repeated phlebotomies eventually becomes iron deficient, although this effect is rarely symptomatic. Iron supplementation should be avoided.

- Hydration therapy is used to reduce the blood's viscosity.
- Myelosuppressive agents such as busulfan (Myleran), hydroxyurea (Hydrea), melphalan (Alkeran), and radioactive phosphorus may be given to inhibit bone marrow activity.
- Allopurinol (Zyloprim) may reduce the number of acute gouty attacks.
- Antiplatelet agents, such as aspirin and dipyridamole (Persantine), used to prevent thrombotic complications are controversial because of the increased irritation of the gastric mucosa resulting in GI symptoms, including bleeding.

Nursing Management

Primary polycythemia vera is not preventable. However, because secondary polycythemia is generated by any source of hypoxia, problems may be prevented by maintaining adequate oxygenation. Therefore controlling chronic pulmonary disease and avoiding high altitudes may be important.

When acute exacerbations of polycythemia vera develop, the nurse has several responsibilities. Depending on the institution's policies, the nurse may either assist with or perform the phlebotomy.

- Fluid intake and output must be evaluated during hydration therapy to avoid fluid overload (which further complicates circulatory congestion) and underhydration (which can cause even greater blood viscosity).
- If myelosuppressive agents are used, the nurse must administer the drugs as ordered, observe the patient, and teach the patient about medication side effects.
- An assessment of the patient's nutritional status in collaboration with the dietitian may be necessary to offset the inadequate food intake that can result from GI symptoms of fullness, pain, and dyspepsia.
- Activities are needed to decrease thrombus formation. Active or passive leg exercises and ambulation when possible should be initiated.
- Because of its chronic nature, polycythemia vera requires ongoing evaluation. Phlebotomy may need to be done every 2 to 3 months. The nurse must evaluate the patient for the development of complications.

PRESSURE ULCER

Definition/Description

A pressure ulcer is a localized area of tissue necrosis caused by unrelieved pressure, tissue layers sliding over other tissue layers (shearing), and excessive moisture. The result is damage to the underlying tissues. Factors that may lead to the development of an ulcer include impaired circulation, obesity, anemia, contractures, immobility, incontinence, old age, and poor nutrition. More than 95% of all pressure ulcers occur over a bony prominence, primarily the pelvic girdle.

Clinical Manifestations

Pressure ulcers are staged according to the deepest level of tissue damage. Manifestations of pressure ulcers depend on the ulcer stage. Table 47 describes the four pressure ulcer stages.

When eschar is present, accurate staging is not possible until the eschar is removed by debridement. If the pressure ulcer becomes infected, signs of systemic infection such as leukocytosis and fever may occur.

Collaborative Care

Care of a patient with a pressure ulcer requires local wound care as well as support measures such as adequate nutrition and pressure relief. The current trend is to keep a pressure sore slightly moist, rather than dry, to enhance reepithelialization. Both conservative and surgical strategies are used in the treatment of pressure ulcers, depending on the ulcer's stage and condition.

Nursing Management

Goals

The patient with a pressure ulcer will have no deterioration of the ulcer stage, reduce or eliminate the factors that lead to pressure ulcers, not develop an infection in the pressure ulcer, and have no recurrence.

Nursing Diagnoses

- Impaired skin integrity *related to* pressure and inadequate circulation

Nursing Interventions

Patients should be assessed for pressure ulcer risk initially on admission and at periodic intervals. Risk assessment should be done using a validated assessment tool such as the Braden scale. Prevention remains the best treatment for pressure ulcers.

- Devices such as alternating pressure mattresses, foam mattresses with adequate stiffness and thickness, wheelchair cushions,

Table 47	Staging Pressure Ulcers
Stage I	A stage I pressure ulcer is an observable pressure-related alteration of intact skin whose indicators, as compared to an adjacent or opposite area on the body, may include changes in one or more of the following: skin temperature (warmth or coolness) tissue consistency (firm or boggy feel) sensation (pain or itching) The ulcer appears as a defined area of persistent redness in lightly pigmented skin, whereas in darker skin tones, the ulcer may appear with persistent red, blue, or purple hues.
Stage II	Partial-thickness skin loss involving epidermis, dermis, or both. The ulcer is superficial and presents clinically as an abrasion, blister, or shallow crater.
Stage III	Full-thickness skin loss involving damage to or necrosis of subcutaneous tissue that may extend down to, but not through, underlying fascia. The ulcer presents clinically as a deep crater with or without undermining of adjacent tissue.
Stage IV	Full-thickness skin loss with extensive destruction, tissue necrosis, or damage to muscle, bone, or supporting structures (e.g., tendon, joint capsule). Undermining and sinus tracts may also be associated with stage IV pressure ulcers.

Source: Fifth National NPUAP Conference: *Task Force on Darkly Pigmented Skin and Stage I Pressure Ulcers,* Approved Feb 1998 and Bergstrom N and others: *Treatment of pressure ulcers,* Clinical Practice Guideline, no. 15. Rockville, Md: U.S. Department of Health and Human Services, Public Health Service, Agency for Health Care Policy and Research, AHCPR Publication no. 95-0652, Dec. 1994.

padded commode seats, foam boots, and lift sheets are useful in reducing pressure and shearing force. However, they are not adequate substitutes for frequent repositioning.

- Once a person has been identified as being at risk for pressure ulcer development, prevention strategies should be implemented. Table 22-16 and NCP 22-2, Lewis and others, *Medical-Surgical Nursing,* edition 5, p. 519, list guidelines for preventing pressure ulcers.

Once a pressure ulcer has developed, the nurse should initiate interventions based on the ulcer's stage and the presence or absence of infection. Documentation should be made of the pressure ulcer size. Pressure ulcers should be reassessed at least weekly.

Local ulcer care may involve debridement, wound cleaning, and the application of a dressing.

- A pressure ulcer that has necrotic tissue or eschar (except for dry, stable necrotic heels) must have the tissue removed by either surgical/sharp, mechanical, enzymatic, or autolytic debridement methods. Once the pressure ulcer has been successfully debrided and has a clean granulating base, the goal is to provide an appropriate wound environment that supports moist wound healing and prevents the disruption of newly formed granulation tissue.
- Reconstruction of the pressure ulcer site by operative repair, including skin grafting, skin flaps, musculocutaneous flaps, or free flaps, may be necessary.
- Pressure ulcers that are not infected should be cleaned with noncytotoxic solutions (e.g., normal saline) that do not kill or damage cells such as fibroblasts.
- After the pressure ulcer has been cleansed, it needs to be covered with an appropriate dressing. (Dressings are discussed in Chapter 11 and Table 11-17, Lewis and others, *Medical-Surgical Nursing,* edition 5).

The maintenance of adequate nutrition is an important nursing responsibility for the patient with a pressure ulcer. Often the patient is debilitated and has a poor appetite secondary to the disease process or other reasons.

- Caloric intake may need to be as high as 4200 calories per day. Oral feedings should be high in calories and protein and should be supplemented with vitamins and minerals.
- Nasogastric (NG) feedings can be used to supplement oral feedings. If necessary, parenteral nutrition may be used.

▼ **Patient Teaching**

Since the recurrence of pressure ulcers is common, education of both the patient and the care provider in prevention techniques is extremely important.

- The care provider needs to know the etiology of pressure ulcers, prevention techniques, early signs, nutritional support, and care techniques for active pressure ulcers.
- Since the patient with a pressure ulcer often requires extensive care for other health problems, it is important that the nurse offer the care provider emotional and physical support.

PROSTATE CANCER

Definition/Description

Cancer of the prostate is the most common form of cancer in men. It is the second leading cause of cancer death in men after lung cancer. Because of new screening procedures (e.g., prostate specific antigen [PSA]) subclinical prostate cancer is being diagnosed with increasing frequency. Researchers are investigating high-fat diets and environmental factors for possible links to prostate cancer. A family history of prostate cancer is a major risk factor.

A higher incidence exists in men 60 years of age or older, in African-American men, and in married men.

Pathophysiology

Prostate cancer is an androgen-dependent adenocarcinoma. The tumor is slow growing and usually begins in the posterior or lateral portions of the prostate. Tumor spread is by three routes: direct extension, lymphatics, and bloodstream. Direct extension is by continuity to the seminal vesicles, urethral mucosa, bladder wall, and external sphincter. The cancer later spreads to the pelvic bones, head of the femur, lower lumbar spine, liver, and lungs.

Clinical Manifestations

Prostate cancer is asymptomatic in the early stages. Eventually the patient may have symptoms similar to those of benign prostatic hyperplasia (BPH), including dysuria, dribbling, frequency, hematuria, nocturia, and retention. The prostate feels hard, enlarged (unilateral), and fixed on rectal examination.

- Pain in the lumbosacral area that radiates down to the hips or legs, when coupled with urinary symptoms, may indicate metastasis. As the cancer spreads, the pain can become severe, especially in the back and legs because of spinal cord compression.

Diagnostic Studies

- Rectal examination with palpation of prostate gland.
- PSA level determination; elevated levels are indicative of prostatic pathology, not necessarily cancer.
- Elevated prostatic acid phosphatase (PAP) levels are specific for prostate cancer.
- Transrectal ultrasound scan allows visualization of prostate outer lobes.
- Biopsy of the prostate gland when suspicious lesion is noted.
- CT scan or MRI to assess cancer spread.
- Elevated serum alkaline phosphatase may indicate bone metastasis.

Collaborative Care

The management of prostate cancer depends upon the stage of the cancer. Prostate cancer is staged on the basis of tumor growth and spread (see Table 52-5, Lewis and others, *Medical-Surgical Nursing,* edition 5, p. 1564). The TNM system is also used to stage prostate cancer (see Table 11, p. 79). Surgery is the most accurate method of staging the extent of tumor growth and lymph node involvement.

- The decision of which treatment course to pursue is a joint decision between the patient and physician based on a careful analysis of the facts and the patient's unique situation.

Surgical therapy is often the first line of treatment, particularly in the earlier stages of the disease. In stages A or B a transurethral resection of the prostate (TURP) or total prostatectomy may be the treatment. If the patient is asymptomatic, he may be watched carefully with annual rectal exams and PSA testing.

- For patients with a stage C tumor, surgery is usually a radical prostatectomy involving the resection of the prostate gland, seminal vesicles, and part of the ampulla of the vas deferens.
- Surgery is usually not considered an option for stage D cancer, except to relieve obstruction, because metastasis outside the prostate has already occurred.

A nerve-sparing technique is sometimes used to prevent erectile dysfunction. This surgery is useful for patients who are younger and who have negative lymph nodes, no elevation of serum alkaline phosphatase levels, and no clinical evidence of extracapsular extension.

In advanced cases of prostate cancer, the surgical removal of the prostate followed by an orchiectomy (removal of the testes) removes the source of 90% of circulating androgens. Orchiectomy often provides rapid relief of bone pain and may induce sufficient shrinkage of the prostate to relieve urinary obstruction in the later stages of disease when surgery is not an option.

- Estrogen (e.g., diethylstilbestrol [DES]) treatment can be substituted for orchiectomy. It causes regression of the prostate size and metastatic bone lesions. Leuprolide (Lupron) and goserelin (Zoladex), agonists of luteinizing hormone releasing hormone (LHRH), block androgen secretion at the pituitary level.

External beam radiation therapy (especially for men over 70) and interstitial radioactive seed implants are also commonly used (see Radiation Therapy, p. 681). Prostatic cryosurgery is an experimental but promising approach to treating prostate cancer. The treatment takes about 2 hours under general or spinal anesthesia and does not involve a major abdominal incision.

Nursing Management

Goals

The patient with prostate cancer will be an active participant in the treatment plan, have satisfactory pain control, follow the therapeutic plan, accept the effect of the therapeutic plan on sexual function, and find a satisfactory way to manage bladder and bowel function.

Nursing Diagnoses

- Pain *related to* surgery, prostatic enlargement, bone metastasis, and bladder spasms
- Urinary retention *related to* the obstruction of the urethra or bladder neck by the prostate, blood clots, and loss of bladder tone
- Sexual dysfunction *related to* the effects of treatment
- Anxiety *related to* the uncertain outcome of the disease process on life and lifestyle and the effect of treatment on sexual functioning

Nursing Interventions

One of the most important roles for nurses in relation to prostate cancer is to encourage patients to have an annual prostate examination to increase early detection. Men should have an annual rectal examination starting at the age of 40.

- The nurse needs to provide psychologic support for the patient and his family to help them cope with the diagnosis of cancer.
- Preoperative and postoperative phases of therapy are the same as for BPH (see Benign Prostatic Hyperplasia, p. 72).
- Pain control is the primary nursing intervention for the terminally ill patient.
- Hospice care is often appropriate and most beneficial to the patient and family. (Hospice care is discussed in Chapter 2, Lewis and others, *Medical-Surgical Nursing,* edition 5.)

▼ Patient Teaching

If the patient is discharged with an indwelling catheter in place, the nurse must teach appropriate catheter care.

- The patient should be instructed to clean the urethral meatus with soap and water once a day; maintain a high fluid intake; keep the collecting bag lower than the bladder at all times; keep the catheter securely anchored to the inner thigh or abdomen; and report any signs of bladder infection, such as bladder spasms, fever, or hematuria.
- If urinary incontinence is a problem, the patient should be encouraged to practice pelvic floor muscle exercises (Kegel) at every urination and throughout the day. Continuous practice during the 4- to 6-week healing process improves the success rate.

PULMONARY EMBOLISM

Definition/Description

Pulmonary embolism is a thrombotic occlusion of the pulmonary arterial system. Pulmonary embolism is the most common complication in hospitalized patients. It is estimated to cause more than 50,000 deaths annually in the United States.

Pathophysiology

Most pulmonary emboli arise from thrombi in the deep leg veins. Other sites of origin include the right side of the heart (especially with atrial fibrillation), upper extremities (rare), and the pelvic veins (especially after surgery or childbirth). Lethal pulmonary emboli originate most commonly in the femoral or iliac veins. The lungs are an ideal location for emboli to lodge because of their extensive arterial and capillary network. The lower lobes are most frequently affected because they have a higher blood flow than other lobes.

- Thrombi in the deep veins can dislodge spontaneously. However, a more common mechanism is jarring of the thrombus by mechanical forces, such as sudden standing, and changes in the rate of blood flow, such as those that occur with the Valsalva maneuver.

Clinical Manifestations

The severity of manifestations depends on the size of the emboli and the size and number of blood vessels occluded. The most common manifestations are the sudden onset of unexplained dyspnea, tachypnea, and tachycardia.

- Other signs are cough, chest pain, hemoptysis, crackles, fever, accentuation of the pulmonic heart sound, and a sudden change in mental status due to hypoxemia.

Massive emboli may produce a sudden collapse of the patient with shock, pallor, severe dyspnea, and crushing chest pain. However, some people with massive emboli do not have pain. The pulse is rapid and weak, the BP is low, and an ECG indicates right ventricular strain. When rapid obstruction of 50% or more of the pulmonary vascular bed occurs, acute cor pulmonale may result because the right ventricle (RV) can no longer pump blood into the lungs.

Medium-sized emboli often cause pleuritic chest pain accompanied by dyspnea, slight fever, and a productive cough with blood-streaked sputum. A physical examination may indicate tachycardia and a pleural friction rub.

Small emboli frequently go undetected or produce vague, transient symptoms. The exception to this is the patient with underlying cardiopulmonary disease, in whom even small or medium-sized emboli may result in severe cardiopulmonary compromise.

Complications

Pulmonary infarction (death of lung tissue) occurs in less than 10% of patients with emboli. Infarction is more likely when (1) the occlusion is of a large or medium-sized pulmonary vessel (>2 mm in diameter), (2) insufficient collateral blood flows from the bronchial circulation, or (3) preexisting lung disease is present. Infarction results in alveolar necrosis and hemorrhage. Concomitant pleural effusion is frequently found.

Pulmonary hypertension occurs when more than 50% of the cross-sectional area of the normal pulmonary bed is compromised. Pulmonary hypertension also results from hypoxemia. As a single event an embolus does not cause pulmonary hypertension unless it is massive. However, recurrent small to medium-sized emboli may result in chronic pulmonary hypertension. Pulmonary hypertension eventually results in dilation and hypertrophy of the right ventricle (RV). Depending on the degree of pulmonary hypertension and its rate of development, death may result rapidly or only mild or transient alterations may be produced (see Pulmonary Hypertension, p. 485).

Diagnostic Studies

- Continuous ECG monitoring as arrhythmia is the most common finding with pulmonary emboli.
- Lung scan (perfusion and ventilation) screens for embolism.
- Chest x-ray is not useful unless an infarction has occurred.
- Arterial blood gases (ABGs) are abnormal with pulmonary occlusion.
- Complete blood count (CBC) count with differential.
- Pulmonary angiography is a definitive test for embolism.
- Venous studies may diagnose deep vein thrombosis as an embolism source.

Collaborative Care

The objectives of treatment are to (1) prevent further growth or multiplication of thrombi in the lower extremities, (2) prevent embolization from the upper or lower extremities to the pulmonary vascular system, and (3) provide cardiopulmonary support if indicated. Supportive therapy for the patient's cardiopulmonary status varies according to the severity of the pulmonary embolism.

- Administration of oxygen (O_2) by mask or cannula may be adequate for some patients. O_2 is given in a concentration determined by ABG analysis. In some situations, endotracheal intubation and mechanical ventilation may be needed to maintain adequate oxygenation.

- Respiratory measures such as turning, coughing, and deep breathing are important to prevent or treat atelectasis.
- If shock is present, vasopressor agents may be necessary to support systemic circulation. If heart failure is present, digitalis and diuretics are used.

Pain resulting from pleural irritation or reduced coronary blood flow is treated with narcotics, usually morphine. Properly managed anticoagulant therapy is effective for many patients. Heparin and warfarin (Coumadin) are the drugs of choice. Anticoagulant therapy may not be indicated in the presence of blood dyscrasias, hepatic dysfunction causing an alteration in the clotting mechanism, overt bleeding, a history of hemorrhagic cerebrovascular accident, or neurologic conditions. Thrombolytic agents, such as tissue plasminogen activator (tPA), dissolve pulmonary emboli as well as the thrombus source.

If the degree of pulmonary arterial obstruction is severe (usually >50%) and the patient does not respond to conservative therapy, an immediate embolectomy may be indicated.

- To prevent further pulmonary embolization, surgical procedures appropriate for thrombophlebitis may be used (see Thrombophlebitis, p. 573). These include the insertion of intracaval filter devices.

Nursing Management

Nursing measures aimed at prevention of pulmonary embolism parallel those for the prevention of thrombophlebitis (see Thrombophlebitis, p. 573).

The prognosis of a patient with pulmonary emboli is good if therapy is promptly instituted. The patient should be kept in bed in a semi-Fowler's position to facilitate breathing. An IV line should be maintained for medications and fluid therapy. O_2 therapy should be administered as ordered. Careful monitoring of vital signs, ECG, blood gases, and lung sounds is critical to assess the patient's status.

- The patient is usually anxious because of pain, an inability to breathe, and a fear of death. Carefully explain the situation and provide emotional support and reassurance to help relieve the patient's anxiety. During the acute phase someone should be with the patient as much as possible.

In addition to thromboembolic problems, the patient may have an underlying chronic illness requiring long-term treatment. To provide supportive therapy, the nurse must understand and differentiate between the various problems caused by the underlying disease and those related to thromboembolic disease.

▼ **Patient Teaching**
- Long-term management is similar to that for the patient with thrombophlebitis. (See NCP 36-3 for the patient with

thrombophlebitis, Lewis and others, *Medical-Surgical Nursing,* edition 5, p. 1001.)

- Discharge planning is aimed at limiting the progression of the condition and preventing complications. The nurse must reinforce the need for the patient to return to the health care facility for regular follow-up examinations.

PULMONARY HYPERTENSION

Definition/Description
Pulmonary hypertension is elevated pulmonary pressure due to an increase in pulmonary vascular resistance to blood flow through small arteries and arterioles. A 60% to 70% reduction in the pulmonary vascular bed is required before pulmonary hypertension develops.

Pathophysiology
The increase in pulmonary vascular resistance may be anatomic or vasomotor. Reasons for an anatomic increase in vascular resistance include the loss of capillaries as a result of alveolar wall damage (e.g., chronic obstructive pulmonary disease [COPD]), stiffening of the pulmonary vasculature (e.g., pulmonary fibrosis), and obstruction of the blood flow (e.g., pulmonary emboli).

A vasomotor increase in pulmonary vascular resistance is found in conditions characterized by alveolar hypoxia and hypercapnia. These conditions cause localized vasoconstriction and shunting of blood away from poorly ventilated alveoli.

- Alveolar hypoxia and hypercapnia can be caused by a wide variety of conditions, including Pickwickian syndrome, kyphoscoliosis, and neuromuscular disease.

Primary pulmonary hypertension is not associated with either pulmonary or cardiac disease. A person with this disorder is typically a woman between the ages of 20 and 40. The basic cause of the problem is unknown. No definitive therapy is available, and the course is often one of continual downhill progression within several years of onset of symptoms.

Clinical Manifestations
Common manifestations are dyspnea, fatigue, and chest pain. These symptoms initially occur only when there is an increased cardiac output (CO) (e.g., during exercise or with fever) or during hypoxia (e.g., with pulmonary infection). Eventually the condition occurs even during rest.

- Pulmonary hypertension increases the workload of the right ventricle (RV) and causes right ventricular hypertrophy *(cor pulmonale)* and eventual heart failure.

Collaborative Care

Treatment of pulmonary hypertension caused by pulmonary or cardiac disorders consists mainly of treating the underlying disorder.

In primary pulmonary hypertension, many patients can be effectively managed with calcium channel blocker therapy, such as nifedipine (Procardia), diltiazem (Cardizem), and epoprostenol (Flolan).

- IV adenosine (Adenocard) and inhaled nitric oxide have also been used to decrease pulmonary vascular resistance.
- Diuretic therapy relieves dyspnea and peripheral edema and may be useful in reducing right ventricular volume overload.
- Anticoagulant therapy has also been used based on evidence that thrombosis *in situ* is common.
- Lung transplantation is recommended for patients who do not respond to epoprostenol and progress to severe right-sided heart failure. Disease recurrence has not been reported in individuals who have undergone transplantation.

PYELONEPHRITIS

Definition/Description

Pyelonephritis is an acute or chronic inflammatory process of the renal pelvis and parenchyma of the kidney.

Pathophysiology

The inflammatory process is generally caused by bacterial invasion from normal inhabitants of the intestinal tract (e.g. *Escherichia coli*). Pyelonephritis can develop via the ascending route from cystitis, with the infection usually starting in the renal medulla and then spreading to the adjacent cortex. The infected portion then heals by fibrosis and scarring. Repeated attacks of acute pyelonephritis in conjunction with preexisting factors such as bladder tumors, prostatic hyperplasia, urinary stones, vesicoureteral reflux, and neurogenic bladder can result in chronic pyelonephritis.

Chronic pyelonephritis is usually the end result of long-standing urinary tract infection (UTI) with relapses and reinfections creating chronic inflammation and scarring.

Clinical Manifestations

Acute pyelonephritis manifestations vary from acute lassitude to the sudden onset of chills, fever, vomiting, malaise, flank pain, dysuria, costovertebral tenderness on the affected side, and frequent urination. Symptoms of cystitis may or may not be found (see Cystitis, p. 184). Acute manifestations generally subside within a few days even without specific therapy, although bacteriuria or pyuria may persist.

Bacteremia (the presence of bacteria in the blood) can occur secondary to a UTI ascending to the kidney and can result in sepsis. The patient will have a high fever and elevated white blood cell (WBC) count. Some patients develop septic shock syndrome as a result of endotoxins produced by gram-negative bacteria that are released in the blood (see Shock, p. 526).

Chronic pyelonephritis usually includes a history of recurrent acute infections that lead to the progressive destruction of functioning nephrons. Chronic pyelonephritis may progress to chronic renal failure (see Renal Failure, Chronic, p. 496).

Diagnostic Studies

- Urinalysis for culture, sensitivity, and Gram's stain
- Urinalysis for red blood cells (RBCs), WBCs, WBC casts, pyuria, and antibody-coated bacteria
- Palpation for flank pain
- Blood culture if bacteremia suspected
- Intravenous pyelogram (IVP), ultrasound, or CT scan to reveal structural abnormalities

Collaborative Care

An essential principle of management is to consider factors that may be contributing to infection. The acute management of mild symptoms includes bed rest, outpatient management or short hospital stay for IV antibiotics, administration of oral antibiotics (e.g., trimethoprim-sulfamethoxazole [Bactrim, Septra], ciprofloxacin [Cipro]) for 14 days, a high fluid intake, and follow-up urine cultures. For more severe symptoms management includes hospitalization, parenteral antibiotics such as gentamicin, a high fluid intake, and follow-up urine culture.

Nursing Management

Goals

The patient with pyelonephritis will have relief of pain, normal body temperature, no complications, and no recurrence of symptoms.

See NCP 43-1 for the patient with a UTI, Lewis and others, *Medical-Surgical Nursing,* edition 5, p. 1265.

Nursing Diagnoses

- Pain *related to* dysuria, urgency, frequency, and bladder spasms secondary to inflammation or tissue trauma

- Altered urinary elimination *related to* UTI
- Risk for reinfection *related to* lack of knowledge regarding the prevention of recurrence and the signs and symptoms of recurrence

Nursing Interventions

Measures for acute pyelonephritis are similar to those with cystitis (see Cystitis, p. 184). Because the patient with structural abnormalities of the urinary tract is at increased risk for infection, the need for regular medical care should be stressed. Interventions vary depending on the severity of the symptoms. Bed rest is often indicated to increase patient comfort.

▼ **Patient Teaching**

- Instruct the patient regarding the (1) need to continue medications as prescribed, (2) need for a follow-up urine culture to ensure proper management, and (3) identification of recurrence of infection or relapse.
- In addition to antibiotic therapy, the patient should be encouraged to drink at least eight glasses of fluid every day. Increased fluid intake should be continued, even after the infection has been treated.
- The patient with frequent relapses or reinfections may be treated with long-term, low-dose antibiotics.
- Understanding the rationale for therapy is important to enhance patient compliance.

RAYNAUD'S PHENOMENON (ARTERIOSPASTIC DISEASE)

Definition/Description

Raynaud's phenomenon (arteriospastic disease) is an episodic vasospastic disorder of the small cutaneous arteries, most frequently involving the fingers and toes. The condition occurs primarily in young women, with the exact etiology unknown. It may occur secondary to an exaggerated reflex to sympathetic vasoconstriction. It is seen frequently in association with collagen diseases such as rheumatoid arthritis, scleroderma, and systemic lupus erythematosus. Other contributing factors include occupationally related trauma and pressure to fingertips as noted in typists, pianists, and those who use handheld vibrating equipment. Exposure to heavy metals may also be a contributing etiologic factor. Symptoms are usually precipitated by exposure to cold, emotional upsets, caffeine, and tobacco use.

Clinical Manifestations

- The disorder is characterized by three color changes (white, red, and blue). Initially, a vasoconstrictive effect produces pallor (white), followed by cyanosis (bluish-purple). These changes are subsequently followed by rubor or hyperemia. Because Raynaud's phenomenon is a vasospastic disorder of the small blood vessels, the radial and ulnar pulses are never lost.
- The patient usually describes cold and numbness in the vasoconstrictive phase with throbbing, aching pain; tingling; and swelling in the hyperemic phase. This type of episode usually lasts only minutes but in severe cases may persist for several hours.
- Complications include punctate (small hole) lesions of the fingertips and superficial gangrenous ulcers in advanced stages.

Nursing and Collaborative Management

There are no specific diagnostic tests for Raynaud's phenomenon. If symptoms persist for several years in the absence of an associated underlying disorder, the diagnosis of primary Raynaud's disease may be made. It is of diagnostic importance to search for an underlying disease so that appropriate treatment can be instituted. Otherwise, treatment is generally not required because the symptoms are self-limiting.

Treatment of symptoms with calcium channel blockers has been encouraging. Adrenergic blocking agents have been used with variable success. Sympathectomy is considered only in advanced cases.

▼ **Patient Teaching**

Patient education should be directed toward the reassurance that no serious underlying disorder is present and that prevention of recurrent episodes is possible.

- Loose, warm clothing should be worn as protection from cold, including gloves when a refrigerator or freezer is used or when cold objects are being handled.
- Temperature extremes should be avoided. Moving to a warmer climate is not necessarily beneficial because symptoms may still occur during cooler weather and in an air-conditioned environment.
- Patients should stop smoking, avoid caffeine, and develop techniques to cope with anxiety-producing situations. The immersion of the hands in warm water often decreases the spasm.

REFRACTIVE ERRORS

Refractive errors are the most common visual problem. This defect in vision prevents light rays from converging into a single focus on the retina. Defects are due to corneal curvature irregularities, lens-focusing power, or eye length.

Types of refractive errors include the following:

- *Myopia* (nearsightedness), the most common refractive error, is caused by light rays focusing in front of the retina.
- *Hyperopia* (farsightedness) is caused by light rays focusing behind the retina.
- *Presbyopia* is a loss of accommodation due to age, with the crystalline lens becoming larger, firmer, and less elastic.
- *Astigmatism* is associated with unequal corneal curvature so that incoming light rays are bent unequally.
- *Aphakia* is the absence of the crystalline lens due to a congenital defect or cataract extraction surgery.
- The major symptom of refractive errors is blurred vision. Additional complaints may include ocular discomfort, eye strain, or headaches.
- Management of refractive errors is correction, which may include eyeglasses, contact lenses, or keratorefractive surgery.

REITER'S SYNDROME

Reiter's syndrome is a self-limiting disease associated with arthritis, urethritis, conjunctivitis, and mucocutaneous lesions. Although the exact etiology is unknown, Reiter's syndrome appears to be a reactive arthritis after certain enteric (e.g., *Shigella*) or venereal (e.g., *Chlamydia trachomatis*) infections. The prognosis is favorable, with most patients recovering after 2 to 16 weeks.

- The disease usually affects men, and 85% of patient's with Reiter's are positive for HLA-B27, which provides evidence for a genetic predisposition.

The arthritis of Reiter's syndrome tends to be asymmetric, frequently involving the weight-bearing joints of the lower extremities and sometimes the lower part of the back. Arthralgias usually begin 1 to 3 weeks after the appearance of the initial infection.

- The full attack may be accompanied by fever and other constitutional complaints, including anorexia with considerable weight loss, and may prove highly debilitating. Soft-tissue manifestations include Achilles tendinitis.

Many patients have a complete remission with full joint function. About one half of the patients have recurring acute attacks; others follow a chronic course, having continued synovitis and progression of x-ray changes closely resembling those of ankylosing spondylitis (AS). Progressive disease may result in major disability.

- Treatment is symptomatic. Joint inflammation is treated with nonsteroidal antiinflammatory drugs (NSAIDs).

RENAL CELL CARCINOMA

Renal cell carcinoma (adenocarcinoma) is the most common type of malignant kidney tumor. Renal adenocarcinoma is twice as frequent in men as in women and is typically discovered when the person is 50 to 70 years old. The most significant risk factor is cigarette smoking. Other risk factors include exposure to cadmium, asbestos, and gasoline.

There are no characteristic early symptoms. Generalized symptoms of weight loss, weakness, and anemia are the earliest manifestations. The classic manifestations of gross hematuria, flank pain, and a palpable mass are those of advanced disease. Local extension of renal cancer into the renal vein and vena cava is common. The most common sites of metastases include the lungs, liver, and long bones.

Diagnostic studies include the following:
- Intravenous pyelogram (IVP) with nephrotomography detects most masses.
- Ultrasound helps differentiate between a tumor and a cyst.
- Angiography, percutaneous needle aspiration, CT scan, and MRI are also used for diagnosis.

The TNM classification is used for renal cancer staging (see Table 11, p. 79). Robson's system for staging renal carcinoma is also used, as determined by limitation to the renal capsule (stage I) through the presence of distant metastases (stage IV).

The treatment of choice is a radical nephrectomy, which is the removal of the kidney, adrenal gland, surrounding fascia, part of the ureter, and the draining lymph nodes. Radiation therapy is used palliatively in inoperable cases and when there are metastases to the bone or lungs (see Radiation Therapy, p. 681). No effective chemotherapy is available for metastatic disease. Biologic therapies, including α-interferon and interleukin-2, are the most promising in the treatment of metastatic disease.

RENAL FAILURE, ACUTE

Definition/Description

Renal failure is a severe impairment or total lack of kidney function. Renal failure is classified as *acute* or *chronic*. Acute renal failure most commonly has a rapid onset. In contrast, chronic renal failure usually develops insidiously over time.

- Acute renal failure is characterized by a rapid decline in renal function with progressive *azotemia* (an accumulation of nitrogenous waste products such as blood urea nitrogen [BUN]) and increasing levels of serum creatinine. *Uremia* is the condition in which azotemia progresses to a symptomatic state.
- Acute renal failure is usually associated with a decrease in urinary output to less than 400 ml/day, although it is possible to have normal or increased urinary output.
- Acute renal failure usually develops over hours or days. It most commonly follows severe, prolonged hypotension, hypovolemia, or contact with a nephrotoxic agent.

Pathophysiology

Acute renal failure is categorized according to pathogenesis into prerenal, intrarenal (or renal parenchyma), and postrenal causes.

- *Prerenal* causes consist of factors outside the kidneys that impair renal blood flow and lead to decreased glomerular perfusion and filtration. Prerenal causes are the most common, accounting for 70% of all cases of acute renal failure. Examples include hypovolemia, decreased cardiac output (CO), and decreased peripheral vascular resistance. Prerenal disease can lead to intrarenal disease (acute tubular necrosis) if renal ischemia is prolonged.

- *Intrarenal* causes include conditions that cause direct damage to the renal tissue (parenchyma) resulting in malfunctioning nephrons. Primary renal diseases such as acute glomerulonephritis and acute pyelonephritis may lead to acute renal failure. More commonly, the predisposing insult is acute tubular necrosis (ATN), which may be caused by ischemia, nephrotoxins (e.g., antibiotics), or myoglobin from necrotic muscle cells.
- *Postrenal* causes involve a mechanical obstruction of urinary outflow. As the flow of urine is blocked, urine backs up into the renal pelvis, ultimately resulting in renal failure. The most common causes are prostate cancer, benign prostatic hyperplasia (BPN), calculi, trauma, and tumors. These causes are almost always treatable if identified before permanent damage occurs.

Clinical Manifestations

Acute renal failure may progress through the phases of oliguria, diuresis, and recovery. In some situations the patient does not recover from acute renal failure, and chronic renal failure results.

The *oliguric phase* is commonly manifested by oliguria, which is caused by a reduction in the glomerular filtration rate (GFR). Oliguria usually occurs within 1 to 7 days of the causative event. Additional urinary changes include bloody urine with casts, red blood cells (RBCs), white blood cells (WBCs), a specific gravity fixed at around 1.010, and urine osmolality at about 300 mOsm/L. This is the same specific gravity and osmolality as plasma. The average duration of this phase is 10 to 14 days. The longer the oliguric phase lasts, the poorer the prognosis.

- Fluid volume excess occurs, neck veins become distended, the pulse becomes more bounding, and edema and hypertension may develop. Fluid overload can lead to congestive heart failure (CHF), pulmonary edema, and pericardial and pleural effusions.
- Metabolic acidosis results when the kidneys cannot synthesize ammonia, which is needed for excretion of hydrogen (H^+). The patient may develop Kussmaul's (rapid, deep) respirations to increase the excretion of carbon dioxide (CO_2).
- Serum potassium (K^+) levels increase and may exceed 6 mEq/L (6 mmol/L). Treatment must be initiated immediately to prevent cardiac arrhythmias.

- Azotemia occurs with oliguria as BUN and creatinine levels are elevated.

The *diuretic phase* begins with a gradual increase in urine output of 1 to 3 L/day but may reach 3 to 5 L/day or more. In this phase the kidneys have recovered their ability to excrete wastes but not to concentrate urine. Uremia may still be severe.

- The diuretic phase may last 1 to 3 weeks with the patient's acid-base, electrolyte, and waste product parameters beginning to normalize near the end of this phase. Because of large losses of fluid and electrolytes, the patient must be monitored for hyponatremia, hypokalemia, and dehydration.

The *recovery phase* begins when GFR increases so that BUN and serum creatinine levels start to stabilize and then decrease. Although major improvements occur in the first 1 to 2 weeks of this phase, renal function can continue to improve for up to 12 months after acute renal failure.

- The outcome is influenced by the patient's overall health, the severity of renal failure, and the number and type of complications. Mortality rates from acute renal failure vary from 30% to 60% depending on the cause. The most common cause of death is infection, with the incidence of infection highest in patients where surgery or traumatic injury contributed to renal failure.

Diagnostic Studies
- History is the most important tool for identification of a possible cause.
- Serum creatinine and BUN levels are elevated initially.
- Serum electrolytes, especially K^+, are altered.
- Urinalysis is done to assess sediment, casts, hematuria, pyuria, and crystals.
- Retrograde pyelogram, renal scan, and ultrasound.
- CT scan or MRI.

Collaborative Care
Because acute renal failure is potentially reversible, the primary goal of treatment is to maintain the patient in as normal a state as possible while the kidneys are repairing themselves. The precipitating cause is determined and corrected if possible. Management is focused on controlling patient symptoms and preventing complications. This includes (1) correcting hypovolemia and maintaining CO for adequate kidney perfusion, with a trend to initiate early and frequent dialysis (see Dialysis, p. 654), (2) monitoring fluid intake during the oliguric phase, (3) decreasing K^+ levels, and (4) initiating nutritional therapy to decrease the body's catabolism of protein by providing carbohydrate and fat sources.

Nursing Management

Goals

The patient with acute renal failure will completely recover with no residual loss of kidney function, be maintained in normal fluid and electrolyte balance, have decreased anxiety, and comply with and understand the need for careful follow-up care.

Nursing Diagnoses/Collaborative Problems

- Fluid volume excess *related to* renal failure and fluid retention
- Risk for infection *related to* invasive lines, uremic toxins, and altered immune responses secondary to renal failure
- Altered nutrition: less than body requirements *related to* altered metabolic state and dietary restrictions
- Fatigue *related to* anemia and uremic toxins
- Anxiety *related to* the disease process, therapeutic interventions, and the uncertainty of the prognosis
- Potential complication: hyperkalemia *related to* decreased renal excretion of K^+
- Potential complication: arrhythmias *related to* electrolyte imbalances

Nursing Interventions

Prevention of acute renal failure is essential because of the high mortality rate and is primarily directed toward (1) identifying and monitoring high-risk populations, (2) controlling industrial chemicals and nephrotoxic drugs, and (3) preventing prolonged episodes of hypotension and hypovolemia. In the hospital the patient at greatest risk for developing acute renal failure is the person who has experienced massive trauma, extensive burns, cardiac failure, obstetric complications, or the individual who has a baseline renal insufficiency as a result of another chronic disease.

- These patients must be monitored carefully for intake and output, fluid and electrolyte balance, and possible blood transfusion reactions. Extrarenal losses of fluid from vomitus, diarrhea, and hemorrhage must be assessed and recorded.
- Prompt replacement of lost extracellular fluids will help prevent ischemic tubular damage associated with trauma, burns, and extensive surgery. Intake and output records and the patient's weight provide valuable indicators of fluid volume status.
- Aggressive diuretic therapy for the patient with fluid overload as a result of any cause can lead to inadequate renal vascular perfusion.

Acute intervention involves managing the fluid and electrolyte balance during the oliguric and diuretic phases, including the observation and recording of accurate intake and output of fluids and daily weights.

- The nurse must be knowledgeable about common signs and symptoms that result from hypervolemia (in the oliguric phase) or hypovolemia (in the diuretic phase), hypernatremia or hyponatremia, hyperkalemia or hypokalemia, and other electrolyte imbalances that may occur in acute renal failure.

- Because infection is the leading cause of death in acute renal failure, meticulous aseptic technique is critical.
- Respiratory complications, especially pneumonitis, can be prevented. Humidified oxygen (O_2), intermittent positive-pressure breathing, turning, coughing, deep breathing, and ambulation are measures the nurse can use to help the patient maintain adequate respiratory ventilation.
- Skin care and measures to prevent pressure ulcers should be performed because the patient usually develops edema as well as a loss of muscle tone. Mouth care is important to prevent stomatitis.

▼ **Patient Teaching**

Once kidney function has returned, follow-up care and regular evaluation of renal function should be emphasized.

- The patient should be taught the signs and symptoms of recurrent renal disease, especially the manifestations of fluid and electrolyte imbalances. Measures to prevent the recurrence of acute renal failure must be addressed.
- The long-term convalescence of 3 to 12 months may cause social and financial hardships for the family; appropriate counseling and referrals should be made.

RENAL FAILURE, CHRONIC

Definition/Description

Chronic renal failure is the progressive, irreversible destruction of both kidneys. The disease progresses until many nephrons are destroyed and replaced by nonfunctional scar tissue. Although there are many different causes of chronic renal failure, the end result is a systemic disease involving every body organ.

- In the United States the leading causes of chronic renal failure are diabetes mellitus (DM) and hypertension.

Pathophysiology

In the vast majority of cases the individual passes through the early stages of chronic renal failure without recognizing the disease state because the remaining nephrons hypertrophy to compensate. The prognosis and course of chronic renal failure are highly variable.

Although there are no distinct stages in chronic renal failure, the disease progression may be divided into three stages:

1. *Diminished renal reserve.* This stage is characterized by normal blood urea nitrogen (BUN) and serum creatinine levels and an absence of symptoms.
2. *Renal insufficiency.* This stage occurs when the glomerular filtration rate (GFR) is about 25% of normal. BUN and serum creatinine levels are increased. Easy fatigue and weakness are common symptoms. As renal failure progresses, nocturia, polyuria, headaches, nausea, and pruritus may occur.
3. *End-stage renal disease* (ESRD) or *uremia.* The last stage occurs when the GFR is less than 5% to 10% of normal or when creatinine clearances are less than 5 to 10 ml/min. It is at this stage that most patients are no longer able to carry out basic activities of daily living (ADLs) because of the extent of the symptoms.

Clinical Manifestations

As renal function progressively deteriorates, every body system becomes involved. Manifestations are a result of retained substances including urea, creatinine, hormones, and abnormal electrolyte concentrations. Manifestations of uremia vary among patients, according to the etiology of renal failure, comorbid conditions, age, and the degree of compliance with the prescribed medical regimen.

Specific manifestations include:

- *Urinary system.* Polyuria, nocturia, a fixed specific gravity at 1.010 with renal insufficiency followed by oliguria and anuria as renal failure progresses.
- *Metabolic disturbances.* Increased BUN and creatinine levels; insulin resistance causes moderate hyperglycemia and hyperlipidemia.
- *Electrolyte and acid-base imbalances.* Hyperkalemia, sodium (Na^+) retention, and metabolic acidosis.
- *Hematologic system.* Anemia, bleeding tendencies, and infection.

Additional systemic signs include hypertension, peripheral edema, pulmonary edema, diarrhea, nausea and vomiting, constipation, peripheral neuropathy, osteomalacia, yellowish discoloration of skin, hypothyroidism, and personality changes.

Diagnostic Studies

- Identification of reversible renal disease by renal scan, CT scan, and renal ultrasound.
- Hematocrit (Hct) and hemoglobin (Hb) levels are decreased.
- BUN and serum creatinine are elevated.
- Serum electrolytes are abnormal.
- Urinalysis and urine culture are used.

Collaborative Care

When a patient is diagnosed as having chronic renal insufficiency, conservative therapy is attempted before maintenance dialysis begins (see Dialysis, p. 654). Every effort is made to detect and treat potentially reversible causes of renal failure (e.g., cardiac failure, dehydration, pyelonephritis, nephrotoxins, lower urinary tract obstruction). Conservative therapy is directed toward preserving existing renal function, treating symptoms, preventing complications, and providing for patient comfort. This primarily consists of drug and nutritional therapy and supportive care.

Drug therapy includes administration of erythropoietin, calcium supplements, antihypertensive medication, and measures to lower potassium (K^+). Drug dosages are adjusted for decreased renal function.

Nutritional therapy includes the restriction of protein, water, Na^+, and K^+.

Nursing Management

Goals

The patient with chronic renal failure will demonstrate the knowledge and ability to comply with the therapeutic regimen, participate in decision making for the plan of care and future treatment modality, demonstrate effective coping strategies, and continue with ADLs within physiologic limitations.

See NCP 44-1 for the patient with chronic renal failure, Lewis and others, *Medical-Surgical Nursing,* edition 5, p. 1316.

Nursing Diagnoses

- Fluid volume excess *related to* an inability of the kidney to excrete fluid, excessive fluid intake, and elevated plasma Na^+ levels
- Anticipatory grieving *related to* the loss of kidney function
- Risk for injury: fracture *related to* alterations in the absorption of calcium and excretion of phosphate and altered vitamin D metabolism
- Impaired skin integrity *related to* a decrease in oil and sweat gland activity, deposition of calcium-phosphate precipitates, capillary fragility, excess fluid, and neuropathy
- Sexual dysfunction *related to* the effects of uremia on the reproductive and endocrine systems and the psychosocial impact of renal failure and its treatment

Nursing Interventions

If a patient has a history of renal disease, hypertension, DM, or a family history of renal disease, regular check-ups, including serum creatinine, BUN, and urinalysis, are essential.

- When a patient is prescribed potentially nephrotoxic drugs, it is important to monitor renal function with serum creatinine and BUN determinations.

- Individuals need to be instructed on maintaining an adequate fluid intake each day (at least 2 L). Any changes in urine appearance (color), odor, frequency, or volume need to be reported to the health care provider. Routine urinalysis should be part of a physical examination.
- While the patient is being maintained on conservative therapy, the decision regarding future therapies, if any, should be made. This should be done before complications such as mental status changes, bleeding, progressive neuropathies, and persistent congestive heart failure (CHF) occur.
- The patient and family need a clear explanation of what is involved in dialysis and transplantation.

▼ **Patient Teaching**

It is important to educate the patient and family because the patient is responsible for diet, medications, and follow-up care.

- The patient should weigh daily, learn to take daily BP, and learn to identify the signs and symptoms of edema, hyperkalemia, and other electrolyte imbalances.
- The patient and family need to understand the importance of strict dietary adherence. The dietitian and nurse need to meet with the patient and family on a continuing basis to assist in diet planning. A diet history and a consideration of cultural variations make diet planning and adherence more easily achieved goals.
- The patient needs a complete understanding of the drugs, dosages, and common side effects. It may be helpful to make a list of medications and the times of administration that can be posted in the home in convenient locations. The patient needs to be instructed to avoid certain over-the-counter drugs such as laxatives and antacids that contain magnesium.

It is important that the patient be motivated to assume the primary role in management of the disease.

RESPIRATORY FAILURE, ACUTE

Definition/Description

The major function of the respiratory system is gas exchange, which involves the transfer of oxygen (O_2) and carbon dioxide (CO_2) between the atmosphere and the blood. *Respiratory failure* results when one or both of these gas exchanging functions is inadequate. Respiratory failure is not a disease; it is a condition that occurs as a result of one or more diseases involving the lungs or other body system. Respiratory failure can be classified as hypoxemic or hypercapnic (Table 48).

| Table 48 | Types of Respiratory Failure and Common Causes |

Hypoxemic respiratory failure*	Hypercapnic respiratory failure*
Respiratory System ARDS Respiratory distress syndrome of the newborn Pneumonia	**Respiratory System** Asthma COPD Cystic fibrosis
Cardiac System Cardiogenic pulmonary edema	**Central Nervous System** Brainstem infarction Sedative and narcotic overdose Severe head injury
Pulmonary Vascular System Massive pulmonary embolism (e.g., thrombus emboli or fat emboli)	**Chest Wall** Flail chest Kyphoscoliosis Massive obesity
	Neuromuscular System ALS Phrenic nerve injury Cervical cord injury Guillain-Barré syndrome Poliomyelitis Muscular dystrophy MS

ALS, Amyotrophic lateral sclerosis; *ARDS,* acute respiratory distress syndrome; *COPD,* chronic obstructive pulmonary disease; *MS,* multiple sclerosis.
*This list is not all inclusive.

- *Hypoxemic respiratory failure* is also referred to as *oxygenation failure* because the primary problem is inadequate O_2 transfer. Although no universal definition exists, hypoxemic respiratory failure is commonly defined as a partial pressure of oxygen in arterial blood (PaO_2) ≤60 mm Hg when the patient is receiving an inspired O_2 concentration ≥60%.
- *Hypercapnic respiratory failure* is also referred to as *ventilatory failure* because the primary problem is insufficient CO_2 removal. Hypercapnic respiratory failure is commonly defined as a partial pressure of carbon dioxide in arterial blood ($PaCO_2$) above normal (>45 mm Hg) in combination with acidemia (pH <7.35).

Many patients experience both hypoxemic and hypercapnic respiratory failure.

Pathophysiology

Hypoxemic respiratory failure. Common diseases and conditions that cause hypoxemic respiratory failure are listed in Table 49. There are four physiologic mechanisms that may cause hypoxemia and subsequent hypoxemic respiratory failure: (1) mismatch between ventilation (V) and perfusion (Q), commonly referred to as $\dot{V}/\dot{Q}$ mismatch; (2) shunt; (3) diffusion limitation; and (4) hypoventilation. The most common causes are $\dot{V}/\dot{Q}$ mismatch and shunt.

- Many diseases and conditions cause *$\dot{V}/\dot{Q}$ mismatch*. The most common are those in which increased secretions are present in the airways (e.g., chronic obstructive pulmonary disease [COPD]) or alveoli (e.g., pneumonia) or when bronchospasm is present (e.g., asthma). $\dot{V}/\dot{Q}$ mismatch may also result when alveoli collapse (atelectasis).

- *Shunt* occurs when blood exits the heart without being exposed to O_2. A shunt can be viewed as an extreme $\dot{V}/\dot{Q}$ mismatch. There are two types of shunt: anatomic and intrapulmonary. O_2 therapy may be ineffective in increasing the PaO_2 if hypoxemia is due to shunt because (1) blood passes from the right to the left side of the heart without passing through the lungs (anatomic shunt); or (2) the alveoli are filled with fluid, which prevents gas exchange (intrapulmonary shunt).

- *Diffusion limitation* occurs when the gas exchange across the alveolar-capillary membrane is compromised by a process that thickens or destroys the membrane. Pulmonary capillary blood flow may be reduced as a result of obstruction or destruction of vessels, as in severe emphysema or recurrent pulmonary emboli. Some diseases cause the alveolar-capillary membrane to become thicker (fibrotic), which slows gas transport. These diseases include pulmonary fibrosis, interstitial lung disease, and acute respiratory distress syndrome. The classic sign of diffusion limitation is hypoxemia, which is present during exercise but not at rest.

- *Alveolar hypoventilation* is a generalized decrease in ventilation that results in an increase in the $PaCO_2$ and a consequent decrease in PaO_2. Hypoventilation may be the result of lung disease, central nervous system (CNS) disease, chest wall dysfunction, or neuromuscular disease.

- Frequently, hypoxemic respiratory failure is caused by a combination of $\dot{V}/\dot{Q}$ mismatch, shunting, diffusion limitation, or hypoventilation.

Table 49 Predisposing Factors for Acute Respiratory Failure*

Predisposing factors	Mechanisms of respiratory failure
Respiratory System	
Acute respiratory distress syndrome (ARDS)	Direct lung injury from aspiration of gastric contents, diffuse infection, near-drowning, toxic gas inhalation, or airway contusion. Indirect lung injury from sepsis syndrome, severe nonthoracic trauma, or cardiopulmonary bypass. Fluid enters the interstitial space and, ultimately, the alveoli, markedly impairing gas exchange. The result is an initial ↓ in PaO_2 and later ↑ in $PaCO_2$.
Asthma	Bronchospasm escalates in severity rather than responding to therapy. Bronchospasm, edema of the bronchial mucosa, and plugging of small airways with secretions greatly reduce airflow. Work of breathing increases, causing respiratory muscle fatigue. ↓ PaO_2 and ↑ $PaCO_2$.
Chronic obstructive pulmonary disease (COPD)	Alveoli are destroyed by protease-antiprotease imbalance or respiratory infection or an exacerbation of COPD escalates in severity rather than responding to therapy. Secretions obstruct airflow. Work of breathing increases and causes respiratory muscle fatigue. ↓ PaO_2 and ↑ $PaCO_2$.
Cystic fibrosis	Abnormal Na^+ and Cl^- transport produces secretions that are viscous, poorly cleared, and therefore a foci for infection. Over time the airways become clogged with viscous, purulent, often greenish-colored sputum. Secretions obstruct airflow. Repeated infections destroy alveoli. Work of breathing increases, causing respiratory muscle

Central Nervous System

Narcotic or other drug overdose	Respirations slowed by drug effect. Insufficient CO_2 is excreted, resulting in an increase in $PaCO_2$.
Brainstem infarction, head injury	Medulla cannot alter respiratory rate in response to change in $PaCO_2$ caused by brainstem injury.

Chest Wall

Flail chest	Fractures prevent normal rib cage expansion, resulting in inadequate gas exchange.
Kyphoscoliosis	Change in spinal configuration compresses the lungs and prevents normal expansion of the chest wall.
Massive obesity	Weight of the chest and abdominal contents prevents normal rib cage movement.

Neuromuscular Conditions

Cervical cord injury, phrenic nerve injury	Neural control is lost, preventing use of the diaphragm, the major muscle of respiration. As a consequence, the patient inspires a smaller tidal volume, which predisposes to ↑ $PaCO_2$.
Amyotrophic lateral sclerosis (ALS), Guillain-Barré, muscular dystrophy, multiple sclerosis (MS), poliomyelitis	Respiratory muscle weakness or paralysis occurs, preventing normal CO_2 excretion. Dysfunction may be slowly progressive (muscular dystrophy, MS), progressive with no potential of recovery (ALS), rapid with good expectation of recovery (Guillain-Barré), or stable for extended periods of time (poliomyelitis).

R

CO_2, Carbon dioxide; Na^+, sodium; $PaCO_2$, partial pressure of carbon dioxide in arterial blood; PaO_2, partial pressure of oxygen in arterial blood.
*This list is not all inclusive.

Hypercapnic respiratory failure. This condition results from an imbalance between ventilatory supply and ventilatory demand. Normally, ventilatory supply far exceeds ventilatory demand. Patients with lung diseases do not have this advantage. Hypercapnic respiratory failure is sometimes called pump failure because the primary problem is the inability of the respiratory system to expel (pump out) sufficient CO_2 to maintain a normal $PaCO_2$.

- Many diseases can cause a limitation in ventilatory supply (see Table 49). They can be grouped into four categories: (1) abnormalities of the respiratory system; (2) abnormalities of the CNS; (3) abnormalities of the chest wall; and (4) neuromuscular conditions.

Clinical Manifestations

Respiratory failure may develop suddenly (in minutes or hours) or gradually (taking several days or longer). A sudden decrease in PaO_2 or a rapid rise in $PaCO_2$ implies a serious condition that can rapidly become a life-threatening emergency.

- Manifestations are related to the extent of the change in PaO_2 and $PaCO_2$, the rapidity of change (acute versus chronic), and the ability to compensate to overcome this change. When the patient's compensatory mechanisms fail, respiratory failure occurs. Because manifestations are variable, it is important to monitor arterial blood gas (ABG) values or use pulse oximetry to evaluate the extent of change.
- Restlessness, confusion, and combative behavior suggest inadequate delivery of O_2 to the brain.
- Tachycardia and mild hypertension are also early signs. A severe morning headache suggests hypercapnia may have occurred during the night. Rapid shallow breaths suggest that the tidal volume may be inadequate to remove CO_2 from the lungs.
- As the PaO_2 decreases and acidosis increases, the heart may be unable to function and arrhythmias may occur. Permanent brain damage may occur because of O_2 deprivation. Renal function may be impaired, and sodium (Na^+) retention, edema formation, acute tubular necrosis, and uremia may result.
- The patient may have a rapid, shallow breathing pattern or a respiratory rate which is slower than normal. A change from a rapid to a slower rate in a patient in acute respiratory distress suggests tiring and the possibility of respiratory arrest.
- There may be a change in the inspiratory (I) to expiratory (E) (I:E) ratio. Normally the I:E ratio is 1:2. In patients in respiratory distress, the ratio may increase to 1:3 or 1:4. This change signifies airflow obstruction.

- The nurse may observe *retraction* (inward movement) of the intercostal spaces or the supraclavicular area and the use of accessory muscles during inspiration or expiration. Use of the accessory muscles signifies moderate distress. Paradoxical breathing indicates severe distress.
- Any deterioration in mental status, such as combative behavior, confusion, or a decreased level of consciousness (LOC), should be reported immediately, as this change may indicate the onset of rapid deterioration and the need for mechanical ventilation.

Diagnostic Studies

- Arterial blood gas (ABG) analysis is used to determine $PaCO_2$, PaO_2, and blood pH.
- An indwelling catheter may be inserted into an artery for monitoring pressures.
- Pulse oximetry is used for the monitoring of oxygenation status, but in respiratory failure, ABGs are necessary to obtain both oxygenation (PaO_2) and ventilation ($PaCO_2$) status.
- Other studies may include a chest x-ray, complete blood count (CBC), serum electrolytes, urinalysis, pulmonary function tests, and ECG.
- Cultures of sputum and blood are obtained as necessary to determine sources of possible infection.
- If pulmonary embolus is suspected, a ventilation-perfusion lung scan or pulmonary angiography may be done.
- In severe respiratory failure, the measurement of cardiac output (CO) and mixed venous blood gases by pulmonary artery catheter may be performed. Pulmonary artery, pulmonary artery wedge, and left atrial pressures are monitored.

Nursing and Collaborative Management

Because there are many different problems that cause respiratory failure, specific care of the patient varies.

Goals

The patient in acute respiratory failure will have ABG values within the patient's baseline, baseline breath sounds, no dyspnea or dyspnea at the patient's baseline, and an effective cough and the ability to clear secretions.

See the NCP 62-1 for the patient with acute respiratory failure, Lewis and others, *Medical-Surgical Nursing,* edition 5, p. 1902.

Nursing Diagnoses

Nursing diagnoses for the patient with acute respiratory failure include, but are not limited to, those presented under Acute Respiratory Distress Syndrome, p. 7.

Nursing Interventions
Respiratory Therapy

The goals of respiratory care include maintaining adequate oxygenation and ventilation. This includes O_2 therapy, mobilization of secretions, and positive pressure ventilation (PPV).

O_2 therapy. The primary goal of O_2 therapy is to correct hypoxemia (see Oxygen Therapy, p. 676). If hypoxemia is secondary to $\dot{V}/\dot{Q}$ mismatch, supplemental O_2 administered at 1 to 3 L/min by nasal cannula or 24% to 32% by simple face mask should improve the PaO_2 and SpO_2. Hypoxemia secondary to an intrapulmonary shunt is usually not responsive to high O_2 concentrations and the patient will usually require PPV (see Mechanical Ventilation, p. 668).

- Patients with chronic hypercapnia should receive O_2 through a low-flow device such as a nasal cannula at 1 to 2 L/min or a Venturi mask at 24% to 28%. They should be closely monitored for changes in mental status, respiratory rate, and ABG results until their PaO_2 level has reached their normal value.

Mobilization of secretions. Retained pulmonary secretions may cause or exacerbate acute respiratory failure by blocking O_2 movement into the alveoli. Secretions can be mobilized through effective coughing, adequate hydration and humidification, chest physical therapy, and suctioning.

Effective coughing and positioning. If secretions are obstructing the airway, the patient should be encouraged to cough. The patient with a neuromuscular weakness due to the disease or exhaustion may not be able to generate sufficient airway pressures to produce an effective cough. *Augmented coughing (quad coughing)* may be helpful. It is performed by placing the palm of the hand or hands on the abdomen below the xiphoid process. As the patient ends a deep inspiration and begins the expiration, the hands should be moved forcefully downward, increasing abdominal pressure and facilitating the cough.

- Positioning the patient by elevating the head of the bed to at least 45 degrees or by using a reclining chair bed may assist to maximize thoracic expansion.
- The patient should be side-lying if there is a possibility that the tongue will obstruct the airway or that aspiration may occur. An oral or nasal airway should be kept at the bedside for use if necessary.

Hydration and humidification. Thick and viscous secretions are difficult to raise and should be thinned. Adequate fluid intake (2 to 3 L per day) is necessary to keep secretions thin and easy to expel. If the patient is unable to take sufficient fluids orally, IV hydration will be used.

Drug Therapy

The goals of drug therapy for patients in acute respiratory failure include relief of bronchospasm, reduction of airway inflammation and pulmonary congestion, treatment of pulmonary infection, and reduction of severe anxiety and restlessness.

Relief of bronchospasm. Alveolar ventilation will be increased with the relief of bronchospasm. Short-acting bronchodilators such as metaproterenol (Alupent) and albuterol (Venolin) are frequently administered to reverse bronchospasm, using either a hand-held nebulizer or a metered-dose inhaler with a spacer. If severe bronchospasm continues, IV aminophylline may be administered.

Reduction of airway inflammation. Corticosteroids may be used in conjunction with bronchodilating agents when bronchospasms and inflammation are present. Inhaled corticosteroids are not used for acute respiratory failure, as they require 4 to 5 days before optimum effects are seen. However, IV corticosteroids (e.g., methylprednisolone) have an immediate onset.

Reduction of pulmonary congestion. IV diuretics (e.g., furosemide [Lasix]) are used to decrease the pulmonary congestion caused by heart failure. Digitalis may also be used if left ventricular failure or atrial fibrillation is present.

Treatment of pulmonary infections. Pulmonary infections can either cause or exacerbate acute respiratory failure. IV antibiotics are frequently administered to inhibit bacterial growth.

Reduction of severe anxiety and restlessness. Anxiety, restlessness, and agitation result from cerebral hypoxia. In addition, fear due to the inability to breathe and a sense of loss of control may exacerbate anxiety.

- Low-dose sedation (e.g., lorazepam [Ativan]) may be used to decrease anxiety. Patients receiving any sedative medication must be monitored for respiratory depression. In the critical care setting, sedation and neuromuscular paralysis are commonly used for severely restless and agitated patients in acute respiratory failure who breathe asynchronously with mechanical ventilation.

Nutritional Therapy

The maintenance of protein and energy stores is especially important because nutritional depletion causes a loss of muscle mass, including the respiratory muscles, and may prolong recovery. During the acute manifestations of respiratory failure, the risk of aspiration typically prevents oral nutritional intake. Enteral or parenteral nutrition may therefore be administered.

RETINAL DETACHMENT

Definition/Description

Retinal detachment is a separation of the sensory retina and underlying pigment epithelium with fluid accumulation between the two
layers. Risk factors include high myopia, aphakia, proliferative
diabetic retinopathy, retinal lattice degeneration, and ocular trauma.

Pathophysiology

The most common cause is a retinal break, which is an interruption in
the full thickness of the retinal tissue. Additional causes for detachment include retinal holes with spontaneous atrophic breaks and retinal tears where the vitreous shrinks with aging and pulls on the retina.

Once there is a retinal break, liquid vitreous enters between the sensory and retinal pigment epithelium layers causing detachment. Untreated retinal detachment will lead to blindness in the involved eye.

Clinical Manifestations

The symptoms of a detached retina include photopsia ("light
flashes"), floaters, and a "cobweb" or ring in the vision field. Once
the retina is detached, complaints of a painless loss of peripheral or
central vision are described.

Diagnostic Studies

- Visual acuity measurements
- Direct visualization of the retina using direct and indirect oph-
  thalmoscopy or slit-lamp microscopy
- Ultrasound to help identify a detachment

Collaborative Care

Retinal breaks are evaluated to determine if prophylactic laser photocoagulation or cryopexy is necessary to avoid retinal detachment.
Some breaks will not progress to detachment, so the patient may be
observed and given precise information about the warning signs of
impending detachment and instructions to seek immediate evaluation if these signs occur. The general ophthalmologist will usually
refer the patient with a retinal detachment to a retinal specialist.

Retinal detachment treatment has two objectives: (1) to seal any
retinal breaks, and (2) to relieve inward retinal traction. Surgical
treatment to seal breaks may include laser photocoagulation and
cryopexy. Management of inward retina traction involves scleral
buckling, pneumatic retinopexy, and vitrectomy.

- Reattachment is successful in 90% of all cases with the visual
  prognosis dependent on the extent, length, and area of detachment.

Nursing Management
Goals
The patient with a retinal detachment will experience minimal anxiety throughout the event and maintain an acceptable level of comfort postoperatively.

Nursing Diagnoses
- Pain *related to* surgical correction and unusual positioning
- Fear *related to* the possibility of permanent vision loss in the affected eye
- Self-care deficits *related to* imposed activity restrictions and visual deficits

Nursing Interventions
Retinal detachment is a situation with an urgent need for surgery. The patient needs emotional support, especially during the immediate preoperative period.

- With postoperative pain the nurse should administer prescribed pain medications and teach the patient to take medication as necessary when discharged.
- Discharge planning is important and the nurse should begin this process as early as possible because the patient may not be hospitalized long.
- See NCP 20-1 for the patient following eye surgery, Lewis and others, *Medical-Surgical Nursing,* edition 5, p. 457.

▼ Patient Teaching
- Instruct the patient with an increased risk of retinal detachment about the signs of detachment.
- Promote the use of proper protective eyewear to help avoid retinal detachments related to trauma.
- Verify the prescribed level of activity with the patient's surgeon and help the patient plan for any necessary assistance related to activity restrictions.
- Teach the postoperative patient the signs of retinal detachment because the risk of detachment in other eye is approximately 2% to 25%.

RHEUMATIC FEVER AND HEART DISEASE

Definition/Description
Rheumatic fever is an inflammatory disease of the heart, potentially involving all layers (endocardium, myocardium, and pericardium). The resulting damage to the heart from rheumatic fever is called rheumatic heart disease, a chronic condition characterized by scarring and deformity of the heart valves.

Pathophysiology

Rheumatic fever almost always occurs as a delayed sequela (usually 2 to 3 weeks) following a group A β-hemolytic streptococcal infection of the upper respiratory system, usually a pharyngeal infection. Acute rheumatic fever (ARF) affects the heart, joints, central nervous system (CNS), and skin because of an abnormal humoral and cell-mediated immune response to group A hemolytic streptococcal antigens. It is possible that these antigens cross-react with other tissues and bind to receptors on heart, muscle, joint, and brain cells, triggering immune and inflammatory responses.

About 40% of ARF episodes are marked by carditis, and all layers of the heart (endocardium, myocardium, and pericardium) may be involved.

- Rheumatic endocarditis is found primarily in the valves, with swelling and erosion of the valve leaflets. Vegetations form and create a fibrous thickening of the valve leaflets, fusion of commissures and chordae tendineae, and fibrosis of the papillary muscle. Stenosis and regurgitation may occur in valve leaflets.
- Myocardial involvement is characterized by *Aschoff's bodies,* which are nodules formed by a reaction to inflammation with accompanying swelling and fragmentation of collagen fibers.
- Rheumatic pericarditis affects the pericardium, which becomes thickened and covered with a fibrinous exudate.

The lesions of rheumatic fever are systemic, especially involving the connective tissue. The joints (polyarthritis), skin (subcutaneous [SC] nodules), CNS (chorea), and lungs (fibrinous pleurisy and rheumatic pneumonitis) can be involved in rheumatic fever.

Clinical Manifestations

The presence of two major criteria or one major and two minor criteria indicates a high probability of ARF (Table 50). Either combination must have evidence of an existing streptococcal infection.

Major Criteria

- *Carditis* is the most important manifestation of ARF, with three signs including (1) an organic heart murmur or murmurs of mitral or aortic regurgitation, or mitral stenosis; (2) cardiac enlargement and congestive heart failure (CHF) occurring secondary to myocarditis; and (3) pericarditis resulting in distant heart sounds, chest pain, a pericardial friction rub, or signs of effusion.
- *Polyarthritis,* the most common finding in rheumatic fever, involves swelling, heat, redness, tenderness, and limitation of motion. The arthritis is migratory, affecting one joint and then moving to another.
- *Chorea (Sydenham's chorea)* is the major CNS manifestation. It is characterized by weakness, ataxia, and choreic movement

| Table 50 | Modified Jones Criteria for Acute Rheumatic Fever |

Major criteria	Minor criteria
Carditis	Fever
Polyarthritis	Previous occurrence of rheumatic fever
Chorea	or rheumatic heart disease
Erythema	Arthralgia
marginatum	Prolonged PR interval on ECG
SC nodules	Laboratory findings*

Source: American Heart Association.
SC, Subcutaneous.
*See Table 35-13 (Lewis and others, *Medical-Surgical Nursing,* edition 5, p. 961).

R

that is spontaneous, rapid, purposeless, and tends to intensify with voluntary activity.
- *Erythema marginatum* lesions are a less common feature. The bright pink, maplike macular lesions occur mainly on the trunk or inner aspects of the upper arm and thigh; they never appear on the face. The rash is nonpruritic and nonpainful and is neither indurated nor raised. It is usually transitory (lasting for a few hours), may recur intermittently for months, and is exacerbated by heat (e.g., a warm bath).
- *Subcutaneous nodules* are firm, small, hard, painless swellings found most commonly over bony prominences (e.g., knees, elbows, spine, scapulae).

Minor Criteria
Minor clinical manifestations are frequently present and are helpful in recognizing the disease. These include fever, arthralgia, a prolonged PR interval, and a previous occurrence of rheumatic fever or rheumatic heart disease.

Diagnostic Studies
- Antistreptolysin O (ASO) titer is the most specific test to confirm group A streptococcal infection.
- A throat culture is usually negative at the onset of the disease.
- Erythrocyte sedimentation rate is elevated; C-reactive protein is positive.
- White blood cell (WBC) count is elevated.
- Chest x-ray may show an enlarged heart, possibly due to CHF.

- Echocardiography may show valvular insufficiency and pericardial fluid or thickening.
- ECG reveals a prolonged PR interval with delayed atrioventricular (AV) conduction.

Collaborative Care

No specific treatment will cure rheumatic fever. Treatment consists of drug therapy and supportive measures. Antibiotic therapy does not modify the course of the acute disease or the development of carditis. Penicillin eliminates residual group A β-hemolytic streptococci remaining in the tonsils and pharynx and prevents the spread of organisms to close contacts. Salicylates and corticosteroids are effective in controlling the fever and joint manifestations. Corticosteroids are also used if severe carditis is present.

- The patient without carditis may be ambulatory as soon as the acute symptoms have subsided and may return to normal activity when antiinflammatory therapy has been discontinued.
- When carditis is present, ambulation is postponed until CHF has been controlled with treatment. Full activities should not be resumed until antiinflammatory therapy has been discontinued.

Nursing Management

Goals

The patient with rheumatic fever will have no residual cardiac disease, resume daily activities without joint pain, and verbalize the ability to manage the disease.

See NCP 35-2 for the patient with rheumatic fever and heart disease, Lewis and others, *Medical-Surgical Nursing,* edition 5, p. 964.

Nursing Diagnoses

- Activity intolerance *related to* arthralgia
- Ineffective management of therapeutic regimen *related to* a lack of knowledge concerning the need for long-term prophylactic antibiotic therapy and possible disease sequelae, lack of compliance, and a lack of resources

Nursing Interventions

Rheumatic fever is one of the few cardiovascular diseases that is preventable. Prevention is frequently classified as primary and secondary.

Primary prevention involves the early detection and immediate treatment of group A β-hemolytic streptococcal pharyngitis. Adequate treatment of streptococcal pharyngitis prevents initial attacks of rheumatic fever. The nurse's role is to educate people in the community to seek medical attention for symptoms of streptococcal pharyngitis and emphasize the need for adequate treatment of a streptococcal sore throat.

Secondary prevention focuses on the use of prophylactic antibiotics to prevent recurrent rheumatic fever. A person who has had rheumatic fever is more susceptible to a second attack after a streptococcal infection. The best prevention is monthly injections of penicillin G benzathine.

- Prophylactic treatment should continue for life in individuals who had rheumatic carditis as children. Rheumatic fever without carditis after the age of 18 may need only 5 years of prophylactic antibiotic therapy, or may continue indefinitely in patients with frequent exposure to group A streptococcus.

The primary goals of acute intervention are to control and eradicate the infecting organism; prevent cardiac complications; relieve joint pain, fever, and other symptoms; and support the patient psychologically and emotionally.

- The nurse should administer antibiotics as ordered and teach the patient that oral antibiotics require adherence to the full 10-day course of therapy. Precautions with respiratory secretions should be maintained for 24 hours after the initiation of antibiotic therapy.
- Antipyretics should be administered as prescribed. Oral fluids should be encouraged if the patient is able to swallow; IV fluids should be administered as prescribed.
- The promotion of optimal rest is essential to reduce the cardiac workload and diminish the metabolic needs of the body. After acute symptoms have subsided, the patient without carditis should ambulate.
- Relief of joint pain is important. Painful joints should be positioned for comfort and proper alignment. The removal of covers from painful joints can be done with a bed cradle. Heat may be applied, and salicylates administered to relieve joint pain.
- Psychologic and emotional care can be more important than physical care. Any alteration in cardiac function may be perceived as a threat to the person's body image.

▼ **Patient Teaching**
- The patient with a previous history of rheumatic fever should be taught about the disease process, possible sequelae, and the continual need for prophylactic antibiotics.
- The patient must be made aware of the increased risk of recurrence if a streptococcal infection develops and should be informed about the risk of exposure to streptococcal infections from contact with school-age children, individuals in the military services, and people in health care positions.
- Ongoing patient education and reinforcement should encourage good nutrition and hygienic practices as well as the importance of adequate rest.

- The patient should be instructed in the use of prophylactic antibiotic therapy. The dosage of antibiotics used in maintenance prophylaxis is not adequate to prevent infective endocarditis when invasive procedures are performed. Additional prophylaxis is necessary if a patient with known rheumatic heart disease has dental or surgical procedures involving the upper respiratory, GI, or genitourinary (GU) tract.
- The patient should be cautioned about the possibility of development of valvular heart disease. The nurse should teach the patient to seek medical attention if symptoms such as excessive fatigue, dizziness, palpitations, or dyspnea on exertion develop.

RHEUMATOID ARTHRITIS

Definition/Description

Rheumatoid arthritis (RA) is a chronic, systemic disease characterized by recurrent inflammation of the diarthrodial joints and related structures. It is frequently accompanied by a variety of extraarticular manifestations, such as rheumatoid nodules, arteritis, neuropathy, scleritis, pericarditis, lymphadenopathy, and splenomegaly.

Rheumatoid arthritis is characterized by periods of remission and exacerbation. The course of the illness varies, ranging from episodes of illness separated by periods of remission to a more continuous, progressive disease.

Of the approximately 6 million Americans who have RA, 75% are women. There are no geographic or racial predispositions. Although RA can occur at any age, it most often occurs in women of childbearing age.

Pathophysiology

The cause of RA remains unknown. Several etiologies are possible including infection (e.g., Epstein-Barr virus, paroviruses, mycobacteria) and autoimmunity. RA is characterized by the presence of autoantibodies against altered immunoglobulin G (IgG). The autoantibodies to altered IgG are known as *rheumatoid factor*. These autoantibodies combine with altered IgG to form immune complexes that deposit in the joints, blood vessels, and pleura.

Certain familial factors may influence the development of RA. An increased prevalence of human leukocyte antigen (HLA) HLA-DR4 occurs in 65% of persons with RA.

The pathogenesis of RA is more clearly understood than its etiology. If unarrested, the disease progresses through four stages:

- *First stage.* An unknown etiologic factor initiates joint inflammation, or synovitis, with swelling of the synovial lining membrane and production of excess synovial fluid.
- *Second stage. Pannus* (granulation inflammatory tissue) is formed at the juncture of synovium and cartilage. This extends over the surface of the articular cartilage and eventually invades the joint capsule and subchondral bone.
- *Third stage.* Tough fibrous connective tissue replaces pannus, occluding the joint space. Fibrous ankylosis results in decreased joint motion, malalignment, and deformity.
- *Fourth stage.* As fibrous tissue calcifies, bony ankylosis may result in total joint immobilization.

Clinical Manifestations

RA typically develops insidiously. Nonspecific manifestations such as fatigue, anorexia, weight loss, and generalized stiffness may precede the onset of arthritic complaints. The stiffness becomes more localized after weeks to months. Some patients report a history of a precipitating stressful event such as infection, childbirth, surgery, or emotional upset.

Articular involvement is manifested by pain, stiffness, limitation of motion, and signs of inflammation (heat, swelling, and tenderness). Joint symptoms are bilaterally symmetric and frequently affect the small joints of the hands and feet as well as the larger peripheral joints, including wrists, knees, and hips.

- The patient characteristically has joint stiffness on arising in the morning and after periods of inactivity. (See Table 43, p. 422, for a comparison of the manifestations of RA and osteoarthritis [OA].)
- As RA progresses, inflammation and fibrosis of the joint capsule and supporting structures may lead to deformity and disability. Atrophy of muscles and destruction of tendons around the joint cause one articular surface to slip past the other (subluxation). Typical hand deformities include "ulnar drift," "swan neck," and boutonniere deformities.

Rheumatoid nodules are present in 25% to 50% of all people with RA and are the most common extraarticular finding. They appear subcutaneously as firm, nontender masses and are usually found on the olecranon bursae or along the extensor surface of the forearm. Nodules develop insidiously and can persist or regress spontaneously. They are usually not removed unless they are significantly disabling because of the high probability of recurrence. Nodules may also appear on the eye or lungs; these indicate active disease and a poor prognosis.

Vasculitis (inflammation of blood vessels) may be responsible for peripheral neuropathy, myopathy, cardiopulmonary involvement, and ischemic ulcerations of the skin. (For the extraarticular manifestations of RA, see Fig. 60-5, Lewis and others, *Medical-Surgical Nursing,* edition 5, p. 1829.)

Diagnostic Studies

Although no single laboratory test is conclusive, several findings are helpful in diagnosing RA in conjunction with the history and physical examination.

- Moderate anemia is common.
- Erythrocyte sedimentation rate (ESR) is elevated in 85% of patients and is useful in monitoring the response to therapy
- Serum rheumatoid factor is present in titers greater than 1:160 in nearly 80% of cases.
- Antinuclear antibody and lupus cell tests may be positive.
- Synovial fluid analysis may show increased volume and turbidity but decreased viscosity. The white blood cell (WBC) count is elevated (often as high as $30,000/\mu L$ [$30 \times 10^9/L$]) and consists predominantly of polymorphonuclear leukocytes.
- Inflammatory changes in the synovium can be confirmed by tissue biopsy.
- X-ray findings (not specifically diagnostic) may reveal bone demineralization and soft tissue swelling during the early months of the disease. Later, narrowing of the joint space, destruction of articular cartilage, erosion, subluxation, and deformity are present. Malalignment and ankylosis occur in advanced disease.

Collaborative Care

Management of RA begins with a comprehensive program of drug therapy and education. Physical comfort is promoted by nonsteroidal antiinflammatory drugs (NSAIDs) and rest. The patient and family are educated about the disease process and home management strategies. Responsible compliance with medications includes correct administration, reporting of side effects, and frequent medical and laboratory follow-up visits. Physical therapy maintains joint motion and muscle strength. Occupational therapy develops upper extremity function and encourages joint protection through the use of splinting, pacing techniques, and assistive devices.

Drug Therapy

In the past, aspirin and NSAIDS were commonly used. A more aggressive approach is now more common as recent research has shown that the destructive process starts within the first 2 years of the disease.

- Many patients are now receiving a disease-modifying agent (such as methotrexate) early in the disease course. A disease-modifying agent is a drug that has the potential to lessen the permanent effects of RA, such as joint deformity. The damaging effects of RA may be prevented or postponed by this plan.

For patients with mild disease, hydroxychloroquine (Plaquenil) is often prescribed. A low dose of prednisone may be given with or instead of hydroxychloroquine. Intraarticular corticosteroid injections are administered for a flare in one or two joints. *Bridge therapy* (5 mg orally of the prescribed corticosteroid for 4 to 6 weeks) is used until one of the longer-acting drugs, such as hydroxychloroquine (Plaquenil), gold, or D-penicillamine (Cuprimine), has been taken long enough to suppress disease activity. *Burst corticosteroid therapy* consists of a high-dose (e.g., 60 mg) corticosteroid used for a severe articular flare, which is then quickly tapered in 10 to 14 days. *Pulse therapy* (Solu-Medrol at dosages of no more than 1 g/day intravenously for 3 days) is used to achieve fast control of inflammation and results in fewer side effects over the long term as a result of taking a smaller daily dose.

For patients with moderate to severe disease with symmetric joint involvement and a positive rheumatoid factor assay, a more aggressive drug regimen may be initiated. Methotrexate, usually the first drug of choice, has a rapid antiinflammatory effect and reduces clinical symptoms in days to weeks. Methotrexate therapy requires frequent laboratory follow-up. Gold therapy may be considered for patients who do not respond to methotrexate. Azathioprine (Imuran) or penicillamine may be used if the patient does not respond to either methotrexate or gold therapy. Aspirin and NSAIDS are still commonly used.

Nutritional Therapy

There is no special diet; however, balanced nutrition is important. A sensible weight-loss program consisting of balanced nutrition and exercise will reduce stress on arthritic joints. Limited sodium (Na⁺) intake may help minimize weight gain caused by Na^+ retention. The patient must be encouraged to continue a balanced diet and not to alter the corticosteroid dose or stop therapy abruptly. Weight slowly adjusts to normal several months after the cessation of therapy.

Nursing Management

Goals

The patient with RA will have satisfactory pain relief, have minimal loss of functional ability of the affected joints, participate in the planning and carrying out of the therapeutic regimen, maintain a positive self-image, and perform self-care to the maximum amount possible.

Nursing Diagnoses

- Fatigue *related to* exacerbation of disease activity, anemia, drug side effects, sleep disturbance, or depression
- Pain *related to* joint inflammation, overuse of joint, and ineffective pain and comfort measures

- Impaired physical mobility *related to* joint pain, stiffness, and deformity
- Altered family processes *related to* the patient's inability to function secondary to chronic illness and the complexity of the treatment regimen
- Self-care deficits *related to* the disease progression, weakness, and contractures
- Ineffective management of therapeutic regimen *related to* the complexity of the chronic health problem, pain, and fatigue
- Body image disturbance *related to* chronic disease activity, long-term treatment program, deformities, stiffness, and an inability to perform usual activities

Nursing Interventions

Prevention of RA is not possible at this time. However, community education programs should include information concerning the symptoms of RA to promote early diagnosis and treatment. The primary objectives in management may be approached by a comprehensive program of daily antiinflammatory medications, rest, joint protection, therapeutic heat, exercise, and patient and family education.

Nursing interventions begin with a careful assessment of physical needs (joint pain, swelling, range of motion, and general health status), psychosocial needs (family support, sexual satisfaction, emotional stress, financial constraints, vocation and career limitations), and environmental needs (transportation, home and work modifications).

- The suppression of inflammation is most effectively achieved through the administration of antiinflammatory or disease-modifying agents. Education centers around the action and side effects of each drug and the importance of laboratory monitoring. The nurse must make the drug regimen as clear and simple as possible. High-dose IV corticosteroid therapy requires careful observation for changes in BP, peripheral edema, and signs of congestive heart failure (CHF).
- Nonpharmacologic relief of pain includes the use of therapeutic heat and cold, rest, relaxation techniques, biofeedback, transcutaneous electrical nerve stimulation (TENS), and hypnosis.
- Lightweight splints are sometimes used to rest an inflamed joint and prevent deformity from muscle spasms and contractures. These splints should be removed, skin care given, range-of-motion (ROM) exercises performed, and splints reapplied as prescribed.
- Morning care and procedures should be planned around the patient's morning stiffness. Sitting or standing in a warm shower, sitting in a tub with warm towels around the shoulders, or soaking the hands in a basin of warm water may help to relieve joint stiffness and allow the patient to comfortably perform activities of daily living.

- Regularly scheduled rest periods alternated with activity throughout the day help relieve fatigue and pain and minimize excessive weight-bearing. The nurse should assist the patient to pace activities and set priorities on the basis of realistic goals.
- Good body alignment while resting is important. A firm mattress or bedboard should be used. Positions of extension should be encouraged, and positions of flexion should be avoided. Pillows should never be placed under the knees. A small, flat pillow may be used under the head and shoulders. Splints and casts may be helpful in maintaining proper alignment and promoting rest, especially when joint inflammation is present.

Protecting the joints from stress is very important. Nursing interventions include helping the patient identify ways to modify tasks. Sample activities that protect small joints are listed in Table 60-8, Lewis and others, *Medical-Surgical Nursing,* edition 5, p. 1835.

- Patient independence may be increased by occupational therapy training with assistive devices that help simplify tasks, such as built-up utensils, buttonhooks, and raised toilet seats. A cane or a walker offers support and relief of pain when walking.
- Heat and cold therapy help to relieve stiffness, pain, and muscle spasm. Application of ice may be beneficial in an acute episode, and moist heat appears to offer better relief of chronic stiffness.
- The nurse should reinforce compliance with an individualized exercise program and evaluate that the exercises are being done correctly. Gentle ROM exercises are usually done daily to keep the joints functional.

▼ **Patient Teaching**

Self-management and adherence to an individualized home program are contingent on a thorough understanding of RA, the nature and course of the disease, and the treatment objectives. In addition, the patient's perception of the disease and value system must be considered.

- The nurse can help the patient recognize common fears and concerns faced by all people living with a chronic illness. Evaluation of the family support system is important. The patient is constantly threatened by problems of limited function and fatigue, loss of self-esteem, and fear of disability and deformity.
- Alterations in sexuality should be discussed. Financial planning may be necessary. Community resources such as a home care nurse, homemaker services, and vocational rehabilitation may be considered. Self-help groups are beneficial for some patients.

SEIZURE DISORDERS

Definition/Description
A seizure is the paroxysmal, uncontrolled electrical discharge of neurons in the brain that interrupts normal function. Seizures may accompany a variety of disorders, or they may occur spontaneously without any apparent cause.

- In the adult, metabolic disturbances that cause seizures include acidosis, electrolyte imbalances, hypoglycemia, hypoxia, alcohol and barbiturate withdrawal, and dehydration.
- Extracranial disorders that can cause seizures include heart, lung, liver, and kidney disease; systemic lupus erythematosus; diabetes mellitus (DM); hypertension; and septicemia.

Epilepsy is a condition in which a person has spontaneously recurring seizures. Two million persons have epilepsy in the United States. Incidence rates are very high during the first year of life, decline through childhood and adolescence, plateau in middle age, and rise sharply again among the elderly.

Pathophysiology
The most common causes of epilepsy during the first 6 months of life are severe birth injury, congenital defects involving the central nervous system (CNS), infections, and inborn errors of metabolism. In individuals between 20 and 30 years of age, epilepsy usually occurs as a result of structural lesions, such as trauma, brain tumors, or vascular disease. After the age of 50, primary causes of epilepsy are cerebrovascular lesions and metastatic brain tumors. Three fourths of all cases cannot be attributed to a specific cause.

In recurring seizures (epilepsy), a group of abnormal neurons *(seizure focus)* seem to undergo spontaneous firing. This firing spreads by physiologic pathways to involve adjacent or distant areas of the brain. Often the brain area from which epileptic activity arises is found to have scar tissue *(gliosis).* Scarring is thought to interfere with the normal chemical and structural environment of brain neurons, making them more likely to fire abnormally.

Clinical Manifestations
The preferred method of classifying epileptic seizures is the International Classification System (see Table 56-6, Lewis and others, *Medical-Surgical Nursing,* edition 5, p. 1679). This system is based on the clinical and electroencephalograph (EEG) manifestations of seizures.

Seizures are divided into two major classes, *generalized* and *partial.* Depending on the type, a seizure may progress through several phases, which include (1) *prodromal* phase with signs or activity that precede a seizure, (2) *aural* phase with a sensory warning, (3) *ictal* phase with full seizure, and (4) *postictal* phase, which is the period of recovery after the seizure.

Generalized Seizures

Generalized seizures are characterized by bilateral synchronous epileptic discharge in the brain. Because the entire brain is affected at the onset of the seizures, there is no warning or aura. In most cases the patient loses consciousness for a few seconds to several minutes.

- *Tonic-clonic (grand mal) seizures* are the most common generalized seizures. This type of seizure is characterized by a loss of consciousness and falling to the ground if the patient is upright, followed by stiffening of the body (tonic phase) for 10 to 20 seconds and subsequent jerking of the extremities (clonic phase) for another 30 to 40 seconds. Cyanosis, excessive salivation, tongue or cheek biting, and incontinence may accompany the seizure. In the postictal phase the patient usually has muscle soreness, is very tired, and may sleep for several hours. The patient has no memory of the seizure activity.

- *Typical absence (petit mal) seizures* usually occur in children and rarely continue beyond adolescence. The typical clinical manifestation is a brief staring spell that lasts only a few seconds. There may be an extremely brief loss of consciousness. When untreated, the seizures may occur up to 100 times a day. Typical absence seizures are often precipitated by hyperventilation and flashing lights.

- *Atypical absence seizures* are another type of generalized seizure characterized by a staring spell. A brief warning, peculiar behavior during the seizure, and confusion after the seizure are also common.

Partial Seizures

Partial (focal) seizures begin in a specific region of the cortex, as indicated by the EEG and the clinical manifestations. Partial seizures may be confined to one side of the brain and remain partial or focal in nature, or they may spread to involve the entire brain, culminating in a generalized tonic-clonic seizure. Any tonic-clonic seizure preceded by an aura or warning is a partial seizure that generalizes secondarily.

- Partial seizures are further divided into those with simple motor or sensory phenomena and those with complex symptoms (also called *psychomotor seizures*). The terms *focal motor, focal sensory,* and *Jacksonian* have been used to describe seizures of the simple partial type.

Complications

Status epilepticus is the most serious complication and a neurologic emergency. This is a state in which seizures recur in rapid succession and the patient does not regain consciousness or normal function between seizures.

- Status epilepticus can involve any type of seizure. During repeated seizures the brain uses more energy than can be supplied. Neurons become exhausted and cease to function. Permanent brain damage may result.
- Tonic-clonic status epilepticus is the most dangerous because it can cause ventilatory insufficiency, hypoxemia, cardiac arrhythmias, and systemic acidosis, all of which can be fatal.

Diagnostic Studies

- Complete history and physical examination to include birth and development history, significant illnesses and injuries, family history, history of febrile seizures, and comprehensive neurologic assessment
- Seizure history to include precipitating factors, antecedent events, and a seizure description (including onset, duration, frequency, postictal state)
- Complete blood count (CBC), urinalysis, electrolytes, blood urea nitrogen (BUN), and fasting blood glucose to rule out metabolic disorders
- Lumbar puncture and EEG
- CT scan and MRI to rule out a structural lesion

Collaborative Care

Most seizures do not require professional emergency medical care because they are self-limiting and rarely cause bodily injury. However, if status epilepticus occurs, if significant bodily harm occurs, or if the event is a first-time seizure, medical care should be sought immediately. Table 56-8, Lewis and others, *Medical-Surgical Nursing,* edition 5, p. 1682, summarizes the emergency care of the patient with a generalized tonic-clonic seizure.

Epilepsy is treated primarily with antiseizure medication. Therapy is aimed at preventing seizures, because cure is not possible. Medications generally act by stabilizing the nerve cell membranes and preventing the spread of the epileptic discharge. Alternative therapies such as vagal nerve stimulation and biofeedback may also be used.

Surgery may be considered to control intractable seizures, prevent cerebral degeneration from repeated seizures, and improve the quality of life.

Drug Therapy

The primary goal of antiseizure drug therapy is to obtain maximum seizure control with a minimum of toxic side effects. The principle of drug therapy is to begin with a single drug and increase the dosage until the seizures are controlled or toxic side effects occur.

- The primary drugs for the treatment of generalized tonic-clonic and partial seizures may include phenytoin (Dilantin), carbamazepine (Tegretol), phenobarbital, primidone (Mysoline), and divalproex (Depakote). The primary drugs for the treatment of absence, akinetic, and myoclonic seizures may include ethosuximide (Zarontin), divalproex (Depakote), and clonazepam (Klonopin). New antiseizure drugs are gabapentin (Neurontin), lamotrigine (Lamictal), and topiramate (Topamax).

Nursing Management
Goals
The patient with seizures will be free from injury during a seizure, have optimal mental and physical functioning while taking antiseizure medication, and have satisfactory psychosocial functioning.

Nursing Diagnoses
- Ineffective airway clearance *related to* tracheobronchial obstruction
- Ineffective individual coping *related to* a perceived loss of control and a denial of the diagnosis
- Ineffective breathing pattern *related to* neuromuscular impairment secondary to the prolonged tonic phase of seizure or during postictal period
- Self-esteem disturbance *related to* the diagnosis of epilepsy
- Ineffective management of therapeutic regimen *related to* a lack of knowledge about the management of epilepsy
- Risk for injury *related to* seizure activity and subsequent impaired physical mobility secondary to postictal weakness or paralysis

Nursing Interventions
The patient with epilepsy should practice good general health habits (e.g., maintaining a proper diet, getting adequate rest, and exercising). The patient should be helped to identify events or situations that precipitate their seizures and given suggestions for avoiding them or handling them better.

The nurse caring for a hospitalized epileptic patient or a patient who has had seizures as a result of metabolic factors should focus on observation and treatment of the seizure, education, and psychosocial intervention.

- When a seizure occurs, the nurse should carefully observe and record details of the event because the diagnosis and subsequent treatment depend on the seizure description.
- Assessment of the postictal period should include a detailed description of the level of consciousness (LOC), vital signs,

memory loss, muscle soreness, speech disorders (aphasia, dysarthria), weakness or paralysis, sleep period, and the duration of each sign or symptom.
- During the seizure it is important to maintain a patent airway. This may involve supporting and protecting the head, turning the patient to the side, loosening constrictive clothing, or easing the patient to the floor if sitting in a chair. After the seizure the patient may require suctioning and oxygen.
- A seizure can be a frightening experience for the patient and for others who may witness it. The nurse should assess the level of their understanding and provide information about how and why the event occurred.

▼ **Patient Teaching**

The prevention of recurring seizures is the major goal in the treatment of epilepsy. Because epilepsy cannot be cured, medication must be taken regularly and continuously, often for a lifetime. Table 51 lists patient and family teaching guidelines.

Table 51	Patient and Family Teaching Guide: Seizures

The patient with a seizure disorder should be taught the following:
1. Medications need to be taken as prescribed. Any and all side effects of medications should be reported to the health care provider. When necessary, blood drawings are done to ensure that therapeutic levels are maintained.
2. Use of nondrug techniques, such as relaxation therapy and biofeedback training to potentially reduce the number of seizures.
3. Availability of resources in the community.
4. Need to wear a medical-alert bracelet, necklace, and identification card.
5. Avoidance of excessive alcohol intake, fatigue, and loss of sleep.
6. Eat regular meals and snack in between if feeling shaky, faint, or hungry.

Family members should be taught the following:
1. First aid treatment of tonic-clonic seizure. It is not necessary to call an ambulance or send the patient to the hospital after a single seizure unless the seizure is prolonged, another seizure immediately follows, or extensive injury has occurred.
2. During an acute seizure, it is important to protect the patient from injury. This may involve supporting and protecting the head, turning the patient to the side, loosening constrictive clothing, and easing the patient to the floor, if seated.

- The nurse should ensure that the patient knows the specifics of the medication regimen and what to do if a dose is missed.
- The patient should be cautioned not to adjust medications without professional guidance because this can increase seizure frequency and even cause status epilepticus.
- The patient should be encouraged to report any medication side effects and to keep regular appointments with the health care provider.
- The nurse should teach family members and significant others the first-aid treatment of tonic-clonic seizures.
- The nurse should provide psychosocial support for the patient by providing education and helping to identify coping mechanisms.

SEXUALLY TRANSMITTED DISEASES

Sexually transmitted diseases (STDs) are infectious diseases usually associated with intimate sexual contact. Historically, they have been referred to as *venereal diseases*. There are many diseases that can be sexually transmitted (Table 52).

Some STDs, such as chancroid and granuloma inguinale, are more common in tropical and semitropical areas. However, with the mobility of modern society, their occurrence in other areas of the world is increasing.

- Diseases that are associated with sexual transmission can also be contracted by other routes, such as through blood, blood products, and accidental inoculation. (See the more detailed listings for Gonorrhea, p. 260, Syphilis, p. 553, Genital Herpes, p. 303, and Chlamydial Infection, p. 127.)

There are contributing factors to the increased incidence of STDs. Earlier reproductive maturity and increased longevity have resulted in a longer sexual life span. The increase in the total population has resulted in an increase in the number of susceptible hosts.

- Other factors include greater sexual freedom, changing roles of women, changes in the institutions of marriage and the family, decreased social control by religious institutions, and an increased emphasis on sexuality on the part of the media.
- In many studies, the incidence of drug abuse is closely correlated with the increasing number of STDs.

Table 52	Microorganisms Responsible for Diseases Transmitted by Sexual Activity

Organism	Disease
Chlamydia trachomatis	Nongonococcal urethritis (NGU), cervicitis, lymphogranuloma venereum
Cytomegalovirus (CMV)	Multiple diseases
Hepatitis B virus (HBV)	Hepatitis B
Herpes simplex virus (HSV)	Genital herpes
Human immunodeficiency virus (HIV)	HIV infection, acquired immunodeficiency syndrome (AIDS)
Human papillomavirus	Genital and anal warts
Molluscum contagiosum virus	Molluscum contagiosum
Neisseria gonorrhoeae	Gonorrhea
Treponema pallidum	Syphilis

SHOCK

Definition/Description

Shock is a clinical syndrome characterized by an inadequate supply of oxygen (O_2) and nutrients to the cells due to impaired tissue perfusion.

- Shock presents with many signs and symptoms and may be precipitated by a variety of etiologic factors. Although the cause and initial presentation of various types of shock differ, the physiologic responses to cellular hypoxia are the same, leading to the same sequence of events if shock is not recognized and treated early.

Pathophysiology

Shock is a dynamic event in which several different processes may be occurring at the same time. A patient may progress toward death or toward recovery over widely varying time periods. Shock may develop rapidly or gradually, depending on the severity of the initial insult and the adequacy of compensatory mechanisms. If these mechanisms can maintain adequate arterial pressure and cardiac output (CO), a compensatory stage is reached. If compensatory mechanisms are insufficient to restore effective perfusion to vital organs, clinical evidence of reduced organ perfusion and progression through the stages of shock will occur. The shock syndrome can be divided into the following 3 stages:

1. The *compensated stage* is a potentially reversible stage in which a variety of compensatory mechanisms maintain adequate perfusion to vital organs.
2. In the *progressive stage,* compensatory mechanisms are ineffective and fail to maintain vital organ perfusion. Aggressive management is necessary to reverse the shock state.
3. In the *irreversible* or *refractory stage,* compensatory mechanisms are nonfunctioning or totally ineffective. Cellular necrosis and multiple organ dysfunction syndrome (MODS) may occur. Death becomes imminent with attempts to restore the BP having failed.

Classification of Shock

Table 53 presents one classification system that lists the common types of shock and their precipitation factors. This classification of shock is based upon the three primary mechanisms responsible for adequate circulation: (1) vascular tone *(distributive shock),* (2) the ability of the heart to pump *(cardiogenic shock),* and (3) intravascular volume *(hypovolemic shock).* Patients may have more than one form of shock simultaneously.

- *Distributive shock* includes neurogenic, septic, and anaphylactic shock. In distributive shock, relative hypovolemia occurs when vasodilation increases the size of the vascular space. This results in a decrease in the vascular tone with no change in blood volume.
- *Neurogenic shock,* an uncommon and often transitory disorder, is caused by massive vasodilation without compensation. It is caused by a loss of sympathetic vasoconstrictor tone in the vascular smooth muscles. This massive vasodilation causes pooling of the blood in the venous vasculature, decreased venous return to the heart, decreased CO, and (eventually) inadequate tissue perfusion. Typically, the patient with neurogenic shock will develop hypotension and bradycardia.
- *Septic shock* is sepsis with hypotension in spite of adequate fluid resuscitation. Sepsis is a systemic inflammatory response syndrome (SIRS) due to infection. The causes of septic shock are listed in Table 53. Cardiovascular parameters that are associated with high mortality include a persistent elevation in both heart rate (HR) and CO with low systemic vascular resistance (SVR) and refractory hypotension for more than 24 hours.

Table 53	Classification and Precipitating Factors of Shock

Distributive Shock
Neurogenic shock
- Injury and disease to the spinal cord at or above T6
- Spinal anesthesia, deep general anesthesia, or epidural block
- Vasomotor center depression (severe pain, drugs, hypoglycemia)

Septic shock
- Infection (urinary tract, respiratory tract, septic abortion, postpartum, invasive procedures [especially urological procedures], and indwelling lines and catheters)
- High-risk patients: older adults, patients with chronic diseases (diabetes, cancer, HIV/AIDS), patients receiving immuno-suppressive therapy, malnourished and debilitated patients

Anaphylactic shock
- Contrast media
- Drugs (especially antimicrobials)
- Insect bites/stings
- Anesthetic agents
- Foods/food additives
- Vaccines
- Environmental agents (pet dander, molds, pollens)

Hypovolemic Shock
Absolute hypovolemia
- Loss of whole blood (hemorrhage from trauma or surgery, GI bleeding)

AIDS, acquired immunodeficiency syndrome; *GI,* gastrointestinal; *HIV,* human immunodeficiency virus.

- *Anaphylactic shock* is an acute and life-threatening allergic reaction. It is an immediate hypersensitivity reaction that causes massive vasodilation and increased capillary perme-ability, causing microvascular leakage throughout the body. Anaphylactic shock can lead to respiratory failure as a result of laryngeal edema or severe bronchospasm and circulatory failure as a result of massive vasodilation. Generally, the severity of an anaphylactic shock reaction is directly related to how rapid the onset of symptoms occurs.
- *Hypovolemic shock* occurs when there is a loss of intravascular fluid volume. In hypovolemic shock the volume is inadequate to fill the vascular space. External loss of fluid from the body is de-

Table 53	Classification and Precipitating Factors of Shock—cont'd

Hypovolemic Shock—cont'd
Absolute hypovolemia—cont'd
- Loss of plasma (burn injuries)
- Loss of other body fluids (vomiting, diarrhea, excessive use of diuretics and laxatives, diaphoresis, diabetes insipidus (DI), diabetes ketoacidosis)

Relative hypovolemia
- Pooling of blood (ascites, peritonitis, bowel obstruction)
- Internal bleeding (fracture of long bones, ruptured spleen, hemothorax, severe pancreatitis, femoral arterial punctures, or catheters in patients on anticoagulant therapy)
- Massive vasodilation (as can occur in conditions that cause distributive shock)

Cardiogenic Shock
- Primary ventricular dysfunction (acute myocardial infarction [MI], cardiac surgery)
- Arrhythmias
- Structural problems (septal rupture, papillary muscle rupture, ventricular aneurysm, cardiomyopathy)
- Obstructive causes (pericardial tamponade, pericardial diseases, tension pneumothorax, acute valvular damage, pulmonary embolism)

S

fined as *absolute hypovolemia,* while internal fluid shifting from the intravascular to the extravascular space (either interstitial or intracellular space) is defined as *relative hypovolemia* (see Table 53). The vascular compartment has not changed, but the volume of blood or plasma has decreased. The loss of fluid results in decreased venous return to the heart, decreased stroke volume, decreased CO, circulatory insufficiency, and eventual inadequate tissue perfusion.

- *Cardiogenic shock,* often referred to as *pump failure,* occurs when the heart can no longer pump blood efficiently to all parts of the body and CO is decreased. There is no decreased intravascular volume or vasodilation of the vascular space. Cardiogenic shock is usually the result of left ventricular dysfunction. The most common cause of cardiogenic shock is an acute myocardial infarction (MI). Other causes of cardiogenic shock are listed in Table 53. Regardless of the cause, the extent of pump failure depends on the degree of heart muscle impairment and the adequacy of compensatory mechanisms.

Clinical Manifestations

According to the three stages of shock (Table 54):

1. *Compensated stage.* Subtle symptoms that are often overlooked include sensorium changes (restlessness, irritability), slight HR increase and increased respirations, pupil dilation, decreased urine output, thirst, and cool, pale extremities (except in septic shock, in which the extremities are warm and dry).

2. *Progressive stage.* Symptoms for this stage include listlessness; confusion; falling BP and narrowed pulse pressure; tachycardia; shallow increased respirations; a further decrease in urine output; hypothermia; cold, pale, and clammy skin; and thirst with dry lips and mucosa.

3. *Irreversible or refractory stage.* In this stage, all body systems are affected, with decompensation evident; symptoms include unconscious and unresponsiveness to all stimuli, systolic BP falling with diastolic BP towards zero, cardiac arrhythmias, weak pulse and slow HR, Cheyne-Stokes respirations, renal ischemia with minimal urine output, hypothermia, and cyanosis.

Diagnostic Studies

- History and physical examination provide initial clues for the diagnosis of shock.
- Blood studies, which may include complete blood count (CBC), disseminated intravascular coagulation (DIC) screen, erythrocyte sedimentation rate (ESR), blood urea nitrogen (BUN), glucose, electrolytes, arterial blood gases (ABGs), lactate, blood cultures, and liver enzymes.
- Urine specific gravity and urine output.
- Placement of central venous pressure (CVP) or pulmonary artery catheter as indicated.
- Chest x-ray may reveal changes consistent with shock or acute respiratory distress syndrome (ARDS).
- Twelve-lead ECG and cardiac monitor.

See Table 61-6, Lewis and others, *Medical-Surgical Nursing,* edition 5, p. 1877, for further information. See Table 61-2 for the hemodynamic effects of shock, *Medical-Surgical Nursing,* p. 1867.

Collaborative Care

The critical factor in management is early recognition and treatment. Prompt intervention can alter the shock process and prevent

Table 54	Clinical Manifestations Correlated with Stage of Shock		
Clinical manifestations	Compensated stage	Progressive stage	Irreversible or refractory stage
Neurologic Status			
Level of consciousness	Restlessness, irritability, and apprehension	Listlessness or agitation, apathy, confusion, alteration or decrease in response to painful stimuli	Unconsciousness, absent reflexes likely
Orientation	Oriented, verbal	Orientation possible, slowed speech	Confusion and disorientation with slurred, incoherent speech
Cardiovascular Status			
HR	Increased (20 beats/min above patient's normal)	Tachycardia (rate of 100-150 beats/min), often irregular	Slow and irregular
Peripheral pulses	Bounding (septic shock) or thready	Weak, thready, may be absent	Absent
BP			
Systolic	Normal or slight decrease	Hypotension <90 mm Hg with decrease in pulse pressure	Falling to unobtainable
Diastolic	Normal or slight increase	Falling	Approaching zero

Continued

BP, blood pressure; *HR,* heart rate.

S

Table 54   Clinical Manifestations Correlated with Stage of Shock—cont'd

Clinical manifestations	Compensated stage	Progressive stage	Irreversible or refractory stage
Respiratory Status			
Rate	> patient's normal rate	Rapid (>20/min)	Slow
Depth	Deeper than normal	Shallow	Shallow with irregular rhythm such as Cheyne-Stokes or Biot's respirations
Renal Status			
Urine output	Slight decrease but within normal limits	Oliguria (<.5 ml/kg/hr) with increase in specific gravity	≤18 ml/hr, progressing to anuria with proteinuria
General Status			
Appearance of skin	Pale and cool (warm and flushed in septic shock)	Cold and clammy, cyanosis possible	Cold, clammy, cyanotic, and mottled
Body temperature	Decreased, normal, or increased	Usually subnormal (subnormal or elevated in sepsis)	Significant decrease
Degree of thirst	Normal or slight increase	Marked increase	Severe increase if patient conscious
Bowel sounds	Normal or hypoactive	Hypoactive or absent	Absent

the development of the irreversible refractory stage and death. Successful management depends on the ability to (1) identify patients at increased risk for shock, (2) diagnose shock syndrome swiftly and accurately, (3) eliminate or treat the primary cause, (4) implement appropriate therapeutic measures to correct pathologic changes and enhance tissue perfusion, (5) protect target organs from dysfunction, and (6) provide supportive care. The emergency care of the patient in shock is presented in Table 61-8, Lewis and others, *Medical-Surgical Nursing,* edition 5, p. 1879.

Whenever possible, the patient in shock should be treated in an intensive care unit and receive continuous ECG monitoring. A general goal is to keep the mean arterial BP >60 mm Hg. Overall areas of focus include:

- O_2 and ventilatory assistance (Artificial Airways: Endotracheal Tubes, p. 626, Oxygen Therapy, p. 676, and Mechanical Ventilation, p. 668).
- Supine positioning with legs elevated at angle of 45 degrees (after neck and spine injuries have been ruled out)
- Fluid replacement
- Maintenance of fluid and electrolyte balance and acid-base balance
- Monitoring and treatment of cardiac arrhythmias (see Arrhythmias, p. 54).

In addition to general management of shock, there are specific interventions for different types of shock (Table 55). Drugs used in the treatment of shock are presented in Table 61-10, Lewis and others, *Medical-Surgical Nursing,* edition 5, p. 1882.

During the acute phase of shock, maintenance of nutrition is vital to decreasing patient morbidity. Some type of nutrition should be implemented within the first 24 hours of therapy for shock. Generally, parenteral feeding is used if enteral feedings have failed, are contraindicated, or fail to meet the patient's caloric requirements (see Total Parenteral Nutrition, p. 684, and Tube Feedings, p. 689).

- A patient in shock should be weighed daily (on the same scale at the same time of day) to determine whether caloric needs are being met.
- The measurement of BUN levels provides pertinent data because falling levels may indicate overhydration or malnutrition (although renal failure may mask this decrease).

Nursing Management
Goals
The patient with shock will have adequate tissue perfusion, normal BP, a return of organ function, and no complications related to shock.

See NCP 61-1 for the patient with hypovolemic shock, Lewis and others, *Medical-Surgical Nursing,* edition 5, p. 1886.

Table 55	Collaborative Care: Shock

Hypovolemic Shock
- Control of bleeding (surgery if indicated)
- Reduction of fluid loss from vomiting, diarrhea, and diuresis
- Volume replacement and blood/blood products (if necessary)
- Discontinue thrombolytics and anticoagulants (as indicated)

Cardiogenic Shock
- Correction of arrhythmias
- Cardiac catheterization with coronary angioplasty and/or stenting
- Administration of inotropic agents (e.g., dopamine [Intropin]) to increase cardiac contractility
- Careful fluid administration if patient volume depleted (monitor PAWP)
- Reduction of workload of the heart by decreasing afterload with vasodilator drugs (e.g., nitroglycerin)
- IABP to increase coronary perfusion and decrease afterload (if indicated)
- Use of ventricular assist device
- Emergency cardiac surgery or cardiac transplantation

Distributive Shock
Neurogenic shock
- Treatment according to cause (e.g., pain relief, management of hypoxemia)
- Correction of underlying cause (if possible)
- Careful administration of fluid

BP, Blood pressure; *IABP,* intraaortic balloon pump; *PAWP,* pulmonary artery wedge pressure; *SVR,* systemic vascular resistance.

Nursing Diagnoses/Collaborative Problems
- Decreased CO *related to* shock state
- Fear and anxiety *related to* the severity of the condition
- Potential complication: organ ischemia or dysfunction *related to* decreased neurologic, renal, GI, respiratory, and/or peripheral vascular tissue perfusion

Nursing Interventions

To prevent shock, the nurse must first identify persons who are at risk. In general, the very old, the very young, and persons with chronic, debilitating diseases are at increased risk. More specifically,

Table 55	Collaborative Care: Shock—cont'd

Distributive Shock—cont'd
Neurogenic shock—cont'd
- Administration of dopamine for hypotension and bradycardia (as indicated)
- Administration of phenylephrine (Neo-Synephrine) or norepinephrine (Levophed) to increase SVR

Anaphylactic shock
- Maintenance of patent airway
- Administration of epinephrine for vasoconstriction and bronchodilation
- Administration of fluid
- Administration of inhaled albuterol (Proventil) for bronchodilation (aminophylline if ineffective)
- Administration of aerosolized epinephrine for laryngeal edema
- Administration of diphenhydramine (Benadryl) to counteract effects of histamine
- Administration of vasopressors (e.g., norepinephrine [Levophed]) as indicated

Septic shock
- Administration of fluid
- Collection of cultures to identify organism
- Use of vasopressors (e.g., norepinephrine [Levophed]) to support BP as indicated
- Administration of appropriate antibiotics
- Control of temperature

S

any person who sustains surgical or accidental trauma is at risk of shock resulting from hemorrhage, spinal cord injury, and burn injuries.

The prevention of shock can include interventions such as early mobilization of spinal cord injuries to prevent neurogenic shock, careful monitoring of fluid balance to prevent hypovolemic shock, and monitoring the patient at risk for sepsis for signs of infection. Aseptic technique must be used with all invasive procedures. Frequent handwashing is essential.

When shock develops, it is important to monitor the patient's ongoing physical and emotional status to detect subtle changes in condition, plan and implement nursing interventions and therapy, evaluate the patient's response to therapy, and provide emotional support to the patient and significant others. Nursing responsibilities also include judging when it is necessary to alert other health team members to changes in patient status that may require a reevaluation of treatment. Detailed information regarding specific nursing interventions during the acute stages of shock is presented on p. 1884, Lewis and others, *Medical-Surgical Nursing,* edition 5. Ongoing reassessment of the patient's condition is important.

Communication with the patient is important. It includes:

- Talking to the patient, even if the patient is intubated or appears comatose.
- Simple explanations of procedures for the patient before they are carried out, as well as information regarding the current plan of care and rationale.
- Simple and honest answers if the patient asks questions about his or her progress and prognosis.
- Avoiding conversations about the patient where the patient can overhear them. Hearing is often the last sense to go, and even if the patient cannot respond, he or she may still be able to hear.
- The patient's family and significant others need support and comfort. The family needs to be kept informed of the patient's condition.
- Rehabilitation necessitates the prevention or early treatment of complications and the correction of the precipitating cause of shock. The nurse should continue to assess the patient for indications of complications throughout the recovery period. These complications include chronic renal failure after acute tubular necrosis or the development of fibrotic lung disease as a result of ARDS.

SJÖGREN'S SYNDROME

Sjögren's syndrome is an immunologic disorder characterized by deficient moisture production of the lacrimal, salivary, and other glands, resulting in abnormal dryness of the mouth, eyes, and other mucous membranes. Sjögren's syndrome is characterized by autoantibodies to two ribonucleic acid (RNA) complexes termed SS-A/Ro and SS-B/La. Manifestations are caused by inflammation and dysfunction of the exocrine glands, particularly the salivary and lacrimal glands. More than 90% of the patients are women, and one half have rheumatoid arthritis (RA) or another connective tissue disease.

Decreased tearing leads to a "gritty" sensation in the eyes, burning, and photosensitivity.

- Dry mouth produces buccal membrane fissures, dysphagia, and frequent dental caries.
- Dry nasal and respiratory passages are common and can result in a cough. The parotid glands are often enlarged.
- Other exocrine glands may also be affected; for example, vaginal dryness may lead to dyspareunia.
- Histologic study reveals lymphocyte infiltration of the salivary and lacrimal glands, but the disease may become more generalized and involve the lymph nodes, bone marrow, and visceral organs (pseudolymphoma). Extraglandular proliferation may become malignant (e.g., lymphoma).
- Rheumatoid and antinuclear factors are present in the majority of patients.
- Anemia, leukopenia, hypergammaglobulinemia, and elevated erythrocyte sedimentation rate (ESR) are usually found.
- Ophthalmologic examination (Schirmer's test), salivary flow rates, and lower lip biopsy of the minor salivary glands confirm the diagnosis.

Treatment is symptomatic, including (1) artificial tears instillation as often as necessary to maintain adequate hydration and lubrication, (2) surgical punctal occlusion, and (3) increased fluids with meals. Dental hygiene is important.

- Increased humidity at home may reduce respiratory infections. Vaginal lubrication with a water-soluble product such as K-Y jelly may increase comfort during intercourse.
- Corticosteroids and immunosuppressive drugs are indicated for the treatment of pseudolymphoma.

SPINAL CORD INJURY

Definition/Description

Spinal cord injuries are classified by the mechanism of injury, level of injury, or degree of injury. The major mechanisms of injury are flexion, hyperextension, flexion-rotation, extension-rotation, and compression. The level of injury may be cervical, thoracic, or lumbar. Cervical and lumbar injuries are the most common because these levels are associated with the greatest flexibility and movement.

The degree of spinal cord involvement may be either complete or incomplete (partial).

- *Complete cord involvement* results in flaccid paralysis and total loss of sensory and motor function below the level of the lesion (injury). If the cervical cord is involved, paralysis of all four extremities (particularly the hands and forearms) occurs, resulting in quadriplegia. If the thoracic or lumbar cord is damaged, the result is paraplegia.

- *Incomplete cord lesion involvement* (partial transection) results in a mixed loss of voluntary motor activity and sensation and leaves some tracts intact. The degree of sensory and motor loss varies depending on the level of the lesion and reflects the specific nerve tracts damaged and those spared.

The risk population for spinal cord injury is primarily young adult men between the ages of 15 and 30 and those who are impulsive or risk takers in daily living. A history of numerous injuries before the cord injury is common. The causes of spinal cord injury frequently include motor vehicle accidents, falls, acts of violence, and sports injuries. The resulting spinal cord injury can be due to cord compression by bone displacement, interruption of blood supply to the cord, or traction resulting from pulling on the cord.

Pathophysiology

Penetrating trauma, such as gunshot and stab wounds, can result in tearing and transection of the spinal cord. Complete cord dissolution in severe trauma is related to autodestruction of the cord.

Shortly after the injury, petechial hemorrhages are noted in the center gray matter of the cord. Within 4 hours there may be infarction in the gray matter. Hemorrhage, edema, and metabolites act together to produce ischemia, which progresses to necrotic destruction of the cord. By 24 hours permanent damage has occurred because of the development of edema.

Hemorrhagic necrosis causes the lesion to be complete after 48 hours, and any function of the nerves that arise in and pass through this level is lost. Because additional edema extends the level of the injury beyond the immediate level of destruction for 72 hours to 1 week, the exact extent of injury cannot be determined before that time.

In addition to discrete damage at the trauma site, the entire cord below the level of the lesion fails to function, resulting in *spinal shock* characterized by hypotension, bradycardia, and warm, dry extremities. The loss of sympathetic innervation causes peripheral vasodilation, venous pooling, and a decreased cardiac output (CO). These effects are generally associated with a cervical or high thoracic injury. With spinal shock there is also flaccid paralysis below the level of injury. This affects musculoskeletal, bowel, and bladder function.

- Spinal shock generally lasts for 7 to 10 days after onset but can last from weeks to months. Indications that spinal shock has ended include spasticity, reflex emptying of the bladder, and hyperreflexia.

Clinical Manifestations

The manifestations of spinal cord injury are related to the level and degree of injury. The patient with an incomplete lesion may demonstrate a mixture of symptoms. The higher the injury, the more serious the sequelae because of the proximity of the cervical cord to the medulla and brainstem. Movement and rehabilitation potential related to specific locations of the spinal cord injury are described in Table 57-3, Lewis and others, *Medical-Surgical Nursing,* edition 5, p. 1725. In general, sensory function closely parallels motor function at all levels.

- Accidents that cause spinal cord trauma can also result in head injury. The patient should be assessed for signs of concussion and increased intracranial pressure (ICP) (see Increased Intracranial Pressure, p. 343). In addition, a careful assessment for musculoskeletal injuries and trauma to internal organs should be performed. Urinary output is examined for hematuria, which is also indicative of internal injuries.

Complications

Respiratory system. Cervical injury or fracture above the level of C4 presents with a total loss of respiratory muscle function. Mechanical ventilation is required to keep the patient alive.

Cardiovascular system. Any cord transection above the level of T5 markedly decreases the influence of the sympathetic nervous system. Bradycardia occurs as a result of the unopposed effect of the parasympathetic nervous system on the heart, and peripheral vasodilation results in hypotension. Close cardiac monitoring is necessary.

Urinary system. Retention is common in acute spinal cord injuries and spinal shock. While the patient is in spinal shock, the bladder is atonic and will become overdistended. An indwelling catheter is inserted to drain the bladder.

GI system. If the cord transection has occurred above the level of T5, the primary problems are related to hypomotility. Decreased GI activity will contribute to the development of a paralytic ileus and gastric distention. A nasogastric (NG) tube for intermittent suctioning may relieve the gastric distention.

Integumentary system. A major consequence of the lack of movement is tissue breakdown in the area of denervation, which can occur quickly and lead to major infection or sepsis. A certain degree of muscle atrophy occurs during the flaccid paralysis state, whereas contractures tend to occur during the spastic state.

Peripheral vascular problems. Deep vein thrombosis (DVT) is a common problem accompanying spinal cord injury. Pulmonary embolism is one of the leading causes of death in patients with spinal cord injury. Techniques for the assessment of DVT include Doppler exam, impedance plethysmography, and the measuring of leg and thigh girth.

Autonomic dysreflexia (hyperreflexia) is a massive uncompensated cardiovascular reaction mediated by the sympathetic nervous system. It occurs in response to visceral stimulation once spinal shock is resolved in patients with spinal cord lesions above T7.

- The condition is a life-threatening situation that requires immediate resolution. If resolution does not occur, this condition can lead to status epilepticus, stroke, and even death.
- The most common precipitating cause is a distended bladder or rectum (from hard stool), although any sensory stimulation may cause autonomic dysreflexia.
- Manifestations include hypertension (up to 300 mm Hg systolic), blurred vision, throbbing headache, marked diaphoresis above the level of the lesion, bradycardia (30 to 40 beats/minute), piloerection (erection of body hair), nasal congestion, and nausea. It is important that BP be measured when a patient with a spinal cord injury complains of a headache.
- The patient and family must be taught the causes and symptoms of autonomic dysreflexia (see Table 57-7, Lewis and others, *Medical-Surgical Nursing,* edition 5, p. 1736). They must understand the life-threatening nature of this dysfunction and must know how to relieve the cause.

Diagnostic Studies
- Complete neurologic examination to evaluate the degree of deficit and establish the level and degree of injury
- Arterial blood gases (ABGs), electrolytes, glucose, hemoglobin (Hb), and hematocrit (Hct) levels
- Urinalysis
- Anteroposterior, lateral, and odontoid spinal x-ray studies to document injury
- CT scan and MRI of spinal cord
- Myelography and electromyogram (EMG)

Collaborative Care
After stabilization at the accident scene, the person is transferred to a medical facility. Respiratory, cardiac, urinary, and GI functions are monitored closely. The patient may go directly to surgery following initial immobilization and stabilization or to the intensive care unit (ICU) for monitoring and management.

Surgical Therapy
When cord compression is certain or the neurologic disorder progresses, benefits are noted with immediate surgery. Surgery stabilizes the spinal column. Other criteria for early surgery include (1) evidence

of cord compression, (2) progressive neurologic deficit, (3) compound fracture of the vertebrae, (4) bony fragments (may dislodge and penetrate the cord), and (5) penetrating wounds of the spinal cord or surrounding structures.

- More common surgical procedures include decompression laminectomy by anterior cervical and thoracic approaches with fusion, posterior laminectomy with the use of acrylic wire mesh and fusion, and the insertion of stabilizing rods (e.g., Harrington rods for the correction and stabilization of thoracic deformities). (Specific surgical and nursing interventions for these techniques are discussed in Chapter 59, Lewis and others, *Medical-Surgical Nursing,* edition 5, p. 1809.)

Drug Therapy

Vasopressor agents such as dopamine (Intropin) are employed in the acute phase and are adjuvants to treatment. Methylprednisolone (MP), when administered early, results in an increased recovery of neurologic function. MP has become a standard of care and is administered IV. MP, a blocker of lipid peroxidation byproducts, has been found to improve blood flow and reduce edema in the spinal cord. MP produces a number of effects that may account for the overall improvement noted in the patient with a spinal cord injury. These effects include reduction of posttraumatic spinal cord ischemia, improvement of energy balance, restoration of extracellular calcium, improvement of nerve impulse conduction, and repression of the release of free fatty acids from spinal cord tissues.

- Drug therapy is used to treat specific autonomic dysfunctions such as GI hyperactivity, bleeding, bradycardia, orthostatic hypotension, inadequate emptying of the bladder, and autonomic dysreflexia.

Nursing Management
Goals

The patient with a spinal cord injury will maintain an optimal level of neurologic functioning, have minimal or no complications of immobility, and return to his or her home and the community at an optimal level of functioning.

See NCP 57-1 for the patient with a spinal cord injury, Lewis and others, *Medical-Surgical Nursing,* edition 5, p. 1729.

Nursing Diagnoses

- Impaired physical mobility *related to* spinal cord injury, vertebral column instability, or forced immobilization by traction
- Impaired skin integrity *related to* immobility and poor tissue perfusion
- Constipation *related to* the injury, inadequate fluid intake, a diet low in roughage, and immobility

- Altered urinary elimination *related to* injury and limited fluid intake
- Sexual dysfunction *related to* inability to achieve erection or perceive pelvic sensations and a lack of knowledge of alternate means of achieving sexual satisfaction
- Risk for injury *related to* sensory deficit and the lack of self-protective abilities
- Altered family processes *related to* a change in function of the ill family member
- Inability to sustain spontaneous ventilation *related to* diaphragmatic fatigue or paralysis

Nursing Interventions

High cervical injury due to flexion-rotation is the most complex spinal cord injury and will be discussed in this section. Interventions for this type of injury can be modified for patients with less severe problems.

Immobilization. Proper immobilization of the neck involves the maintenance of a neutral or extension position. The body should always be correctly aligned and turning should be performed so that the patient is moved as a unit to prevent lateral rotation movement of the cervical spine. For cervical injuries, skeletal traction is usually provided by Crutchfield, Vinke, Gardner-Wells, or another type of skull tongs.

- Infection at the sites of tong insertion is a potential problem. Preventive care includes cleansing the sites twice a day with normal saline solution and applying an antibiotic ointment that acts as a mechanical barrier to the bacteria.
- Meticulous skin care is critical because decreased sensation and circulation make the patient particularly susceptible to skin breakdown.
- Patients should be removed from backboards as soon as possible and have cervical collars properly fitted or replaced with other forms of immobilization to prevent coccygeal and occipital area skin breakdown.

Respiratory problems. If the patient is exhausted from labored breathing or ABGs deteriorate (indicating inadequate oxygenation), endotracheal intubation or tracheostomy and mechanical ventilation should be initiated. (See Artificial Airways: Endotracheal Tubes, p. 626, Tracheostomy, p. 686, and Mechanical Ventilation, p. 668.) Respiratory arrest is a possibility that requires careful monitoring and prompt action should it occur. Pneumonia and atelectasis are potential problems because of the loss of vital capacity.

- The nurse should regularly assess breath sounds, ABGs, tidal volume, vital capacity, skin color, breathing patterns (especially the use of accessory muscles), subjective comments about the ability to breathe, and the amount and color of sputum.

- In addition to monitoring activities, the nurse can intervene in maintaining ventilation by the administration of oxygen (O_2) until ABGs stabilize, chest physiotherapy and quad-assist coughing, incentive spirometry, and tracheal suctioning.

Cardiovascular problems. If bradycardia is symptomatic, an anticholinergic medication such as atropine is administered. A temporary pacemaker may be inserted in some instances (see Pacemakers, p. 677). Hypotension is managed with a vasopressor agent, such as dopamine, and fluid replacement.

- Compression gradient stockings can be used to prevent thromboemboli and to promote venous return.
- The nurse should perform range-of-motion (ROM) exercises and heel-cord stretching regularly. The thighs and calves of the legs should be assessed every shift for the signs of DVT.
- The nurse should also monitor the patient for indications of hypovolemic shock secondary to hemorrhage.

Fluid and nutritional maintenance. During the first 48 to 72 hours after the injury the GI tract may stop functioning (paralytic ileus) and a NG tube must be inserted.

- Once bowel sounds are present or flatus is passed, oral food and fluids can gradually be introduced. Because of severe catabolism, a high protein, high caloric diet is necessary for energy and tissue repair.
- In patients with high cervical cord injuries, swallowing must be evaluated before starting oral feedings. If the patient is unable to resume eating, total parenteral nutrition (TPN) may be started to provide nutritional support.

Bowel and bladder management. An indwelling catheter is usually inserted as soon as possible after injury. Its patency must be ensured by irrigation and frequent inspection. Strict aseptic technique for catheter care is essential to avoid introducing infection.

Urinary tract infections (UTIs) are a common problem. A large fluid intake and the liberal use of juices such as cranberry, grape, and apple help prevent infections.

Suppositories are used in combination with a laxative to assist in bowel evacuation. Enemas are used only if absolutely necessary because they can overdistend the rectum.

Temperature control. Because there is no vasoconstriction, piloerection, or heat loss through perspiration below the level of injury, temperature control is largely external to the patient. The nurse needs to monitor the environment closely to maintain an appropriate temperature for the patient.

Sensory deprivation. The nurse must compensate for the patient's absent sensations to prevent sensory deprivation. This is done by stimulating the patient above the level of injury. Conversation, music, strong aromas, and interesting flavors should be a part of nursing care. Prism glasses are provided so that the patient can read and watch television. Every effort should be made to prevent the patient from withdrawing from the environment.

Reflexes. Erections can occur from a variety of stimuli, causing embarrassment and discomfort. Spasms ranging from mild twitches to convulsive movements below the level of the lesion may also occur. Spasms may be relieved with the use of warm baths, whirlpool treatments, antispasmodics, and muscle relaxants. Peak spasticity occurs after 2 years, and if it is severe, destruction of the reflexes (cordotomy) may be necessary. This procedure compromises retraining and should only be done as a last resort.

Rehabilitation. Physiologic and psychologic rehabilitation is complex and involved. Many of the problems identified in the acute period become chronic and continue throughout life. Rehabilitation focuses on refined retraining of physiologic processes.

- Braces, electronic wheelchairs, and mechanical devices are used to maximize the patient's remaining function.
- The patient with a high cervical spinal cord injury has greatly increased mobility with phrenic nerve stimulators or electronic diaphragmatic pacemakers.

If the patient can be successfully brought through the acute period, the patient's life can be fuller and richer than previously believed possible. Unfortunately, other patients may not have such a positive future outlook. The nurse has a pivotal role in the coordinated efforts of the health team to influence a positive outcome.

SPINAL CORD TUMORS

Definition/Description

Tumors that affect the spinal cord account for 0.5% to 1% of all neoplasms. These tumors are classified as primary (arising from some component of cord, dura, nerves, or vessels), and secondary (from primary growths in the breast, prostate, lung, kidney, and other sites).

- Spinal cord tumors are further classified as extradural, intradural-extramedullary, and intradural-intramedullary tumors (see Table 57-15, Lewis and others, *Medical-Surgical Nursing,* edition 5, p. 1742).
- Neurofibromas, meningiomas, gliomas, and hemangiomas are the most frequently occurring neoplasms.

Because many of these tumors are slow growing, their symptoms stem from the mechanical effects of slow compression and irritation of nerve roots, displacement of the cord, or gradual obstruction of the vascular supply. The slowness of growth does not cause autodestruction as in traumatic lesions. Therefore complete functional restoration is possible when the tumor is removed, except with the intradural-intramedullary tumors.

Clinical Manifestations

The most common early symptom of a spinal cord tumor outside the cord is pain in the back with a radiation of pain simulating intercostal neuralgia, angina, or herpes zoster. The location of the pain depends on the level of compression. The pain worsens with activity, coughing, straining, and lying down.

- Sensory disruption is manifested by coldness, numbness, and tingling in an extremity or in several extremities, slowly progressing upward until it reaches the level of the lesion.
- Impaired sensation of pain, temperature, and light touch precedes a deficit in vibration and position sense that may progress to complete anesthesia.
- Motor weakness accompanies sensory disturbances and consists of slowly increasing clumsiness, weakness, and spasticity.
- Bladder disturbances are marked by urgency with difficulty in starting the flow and progressing to retention with overflow incontinence.

Manifestations of intradural spinal tumor develop as progressive damage to the long spinal tracts, producing paralysis, sensory loss, and bladder dysfunction. Pain can be severe as a result of the compression of spinal roots or vertebrae.

Diagnostic Studies

Extradural tumors are seen early on routine spinal x-rays, whereas intradural and intramedullary tumors require MRI or CT scans for detection. Cerebrospinal fluid (CSF) analysis may reveal tumor cells.

Nursing and Collaborative Management

Compression of the spinal cord is an emergency. Relief of the ischemia related to the compression is the goal of therapy. Corticosteroids are generally prescribed immediately to relieve tumor-related edema. Dexamethasone is usually used, often in large doses (up to 100 mg initially).

Treatment for nearly all spinal cord tumors is surgical removal. The exception is the metastatic tumor that is sensitive to radiation and that has caused only minimal neurologic deficits in the patient. In general, tumors of the extradural or intradural-extramedullary group can be completely removed surgically.

- Radiation therapy after surgery is fairly effective. Chemotherapy has also been used in conjunction with radiation therapy (see Radiation Therapy, p. 681, and Chemotherapy, p. 643).

The relief of pain and the return of function are the ultimate goals of treatment.

- Nurses need to be aware of the neurologic status of the patient before and after treatment. Ensuring that the patient receives pain medication as needed is an important nursing responsibility. Depending on the amount of neurologic dysfunction exhibited, the patient may need to be cared for as though recovering from a spinal cord injury (see Spinal Cord Injury, p. 537).

SPLEEN DISORDERS

The spleen performs many functions and is affected by many illnesses. There are many different causes of splenomegaly, including sickle cell anemia, infection, cirrhosis, congestive heart failure (CHF), and polycythemia vera. The term *hypersplenism* refers to the occurrence of splenomegaly and peripheral cytopenias (anemia, leukopenia, and thrombocytopenia).

- The degree of splenic enlargement varies with the disease. For example, massive splenic enlargement occurs with chronic myelocytic leukemia and thalassemia major, while mild splenic enlargement occurs with CHF and systemic lupus erythematosus. When the spleen enlarges, its normal filtering and sequestering capacity increases. Consequently, there is often a reduction in the number of circulating blood cells.

A slight to moderate enlargement of the spleen is usually asymptomatic and found during a routine examination of the abdomen. Massive splenomegaly can be tolerated but patients may complain of abdominal discomfort and early satiety. Other techniques to assess spleen size include Tc-colloid liver-spleen scan, CT scan, and ultrasound scan.

Management of an enlarged spleen may involve a *splenectomy*. Spleen removal can have a dramatic effect in increasing peripheral red blood cell (RBC), white blood cell (WBC), and platelet counts. Another indication for splenectomy is splenic rupture. The spleen may rupture from trauma, inadvertent tearing during other surgical procedures, and diseases such as mononucleosis.

Nursing responsibilities for patients with spleen disorders vary depending on the nature of the problem.

- Splenomegaly may be painful and require analgesic administration; care in moving, turning, and positioning; and evaluation of lung expansion, since spleen enlargement may impair diaphragmatic excursion.

- If anemia, thrombocytopenia, or leukopenia develops from splenic enlargement, nursing measures must be instituted to support the patient and prevent life-threatening complications.
- Postsplenectomy patients are vulnerable to infection. A younger patient is at significantly greater risk than an older patient, but the risk is present for all ages. These patients are highly susceptible to infection from encapsulated organisms such as pneumococcus. This complication is prevented by immunization with polyvalent pneumococcal vaccine (Pneumovax).

SPRUE

Two closely related malabsorption conditions are *nontropical sprue* and *tropical sprue*. Tropical and nontropical sprue are found in adults. Nontropical sprue is most commonly referred to as *celiac sprue* (especially in children) but is also called *adult celiac disease* and *gluten-induced enteropathy*.

In celiac disease there is marked atrophy and flattening of the villi. As a result, absorption within the small intestine is reduced. The proposed reason for the injury to the villi is a hypersensitivity response initiated by gluten and gliadin (a breakdown product of gluten). Gluten is a protein found in wheat, rye, barley, and oats. The hypersensitivity leads to an inflammatory response of the mucosa.

Tropical sprue is a chronic disorder acquired in endemic tropical areas. The exact cause is unknown, but the disorder has been linked to an infectious agent. Folate deficiency is also believed to play a role in the development of this disease. Clinically, it resembles nontropical sprue.

Patients may become symptomatic at any age with celiac sprue, but the incidence peaks in childhood when gluten is first introduced and then during the fourth and fifth decades.

- Clinical manifestations include steatorrhea (bulky, foul-smelling, yellow-gray, greasy stools with puttylike consistency), diarrhea, weight loss, abdominal distention, and excessive flatulence. There may also be signs of multiple vitamin deficiencies (e.g., glossitis, cheilosis).

The diagnosis of sprue may be made by stool content analyses or intestinal biopsy. A barium enema may demonstrate abnormalities, including the obliteration of intestinal folds.

Treatment of sprue syndrome is based on the underlying cause.

- In *nontropical sprue,* a gluten-free diet usually leads to clinical recovery. Wheat, barley, oats, and rye products should be avoided. Soybean flours may be used. For those patients who are unresponsive to dietary exclusion therapy (gluten-free diet), corticosteroids may be used to treat nontropical sprue.

- *Tropical sprue* is treated with broad-spectrum antibiotics (e.g., tetracycline) in conjunction with folic acid therapy. The patient who responds to this therapy and achieves a remission is usually maintained on folic acid.

STOMACH (GASTRIC) CANCER

Definition/Description

The rate of stomach (gastric) cancer has been steadily declining in the United States since the 1930s. It is the sixth leading cause of cancer mortality in the United States. Worldwide, gastric adenocarcinoma is the second most common malignant growth. Stomach cancer is typically at an advanced stage when diagnosed and is not amenable to surgical resection.

Pathophysiology

Many factors have been implicated in gastric cancer. It is believed that a diet of smoked, highly salted, or spiced foods may have a carcinogenic effect. A genetic etiology has also been postulated. In addition, persons with blood group A have a greater incidence of gastric cancer than the general population. Other predisposing factors are atrophic gastritis, pernicious anemia, benign gastric polyps, and achlorhydia.

Tumors located at the cardia and fundus are associated with a poor prognosis. These tumors typically infiltrate rapidly to the surrounding tissue, regional lymph nodes, and liver. Patients with tumor growth along the lesser curvature have a better survival rate.

- Tumor growth is insidious and follows a pattern of continuous infiltration.
- Cancer of the stomach may spread by direct extension along the mucosal surface and infiltrate through the gastric wall.
- Evidence of spread to the peritoneal cavity is manifested by ascites and by spread to the ovaries.

Clinical Manifestations

Manifestations can be categorized by signs and symptoms of anemia, peptic ulcer disease, or indigestion.

- Anemia occurs with chronic blood loss as the lesion erodes the stomach mucosa. The patient appears pale and weak with fatigue, weakness, and positive occult stools.
- Symptoms associated with peptic ulcer disease (pain and discomfort) also occur.

- Indigestion signs include vague epigastric fullness with early satiety after meals.
- Weight loss, dysphagia, and constipation may also occur.

Diagnostic Studies
- Complete blood cell (CBC) count determines anemia and its severity.
- Stool examination for occult or gross bleeding.
- Exfoliative cytologic examination from washings obtained with gastric analysis demonstrate malignancy.
- Carcinoembryonic antigen (CEA) may be used to detect and monitor the progression of malignancy.
- Further studies may include upper GI barium tests, fiberoptic endoscopy, and biopsy.

Collaborative Care
The treatment of choice is a surgical removal of the tumor. Surgical procedures used are similar to those used for peptic ulcer disease (see Peptic Ulcer, p. 454).

- Preoperative management focuses on the correction of nutritional deficits, special bowel preparation, packed red blood cell (RBC) transfusions for the treatment of anemia, and the replacement of blood volume.
- Chemotherapy and radiation may be used if a surgical cure is not feasible (see Chemotherapy, p. 643, and Radiation Therapy, p. 681).
- Single-agent chemotherapy is of little value. Combination chemotherapy including 5-fluorouracil (5-FU), doxorubicin (Adriamycin), and methotrexate (MTX) has shown a better response rate.
- Gastric tumor sensitivity to radiation therapy is low; it is of little value except for obstructions.

Nursing Management
Goals
The patient with gastric cancer will experience minimal discomfort, achieve optimal nutritional status, and maintain a degree of spiritual and psychologic well-being appropriate to the disease stage.

Nursing Diagnoses
- Altered nutrition: less than body requirements *related to* the inability to ingest, digest, or absorb nutrients
- Anxiety *related to* a lack of knowledge of diagnostic tests, an unknown diagnostic outcome, the disease process, and the therapeutic regimen
- Pain *related to* the underlying disease process and side effects of surgery, chemotherapy, or radiation therapy

- Anticipatory grieving *related to* perceived unfavorable diagnosis and impending death

Nursing Interventions

The nursing role in the early detection of stomach cancer is focused primarily on the identification of the patient at risk (e.g., one with pernicious anemia).

When diagnostic tests confirm the presence of malignancy, the nurse must give emotional and physical support, provide information, clarify test results, and maintain a positive attitude with respect to the patient's immediate recovery and long-term survival.

The preoperative teaching plan is very similar to that for peptic ulcer disease surgery (see Peptic Ulcer, p. 454).

Postoperative care generally includes close observation for signs of fluids leaking at the site of anastomosis, as evidenced by an elevation in temperature and increasing dyspnea.

Because most radiation therapy and chemotherapy are completed on an outpatient basis, the nurse should assess the patient's knowledge of radiation, skin care, need for good nutrition and fluid intake during therapy, and appropriate use of antiemetic drugs (see Radiation Therapy, p. 681, and Chemotherapy, p. 643).

▼ **Patient Teaching**

Before discharge, instruction should be given for the relief of pain, including comfort measures and the judicious use of analgesics; additional considerations include the following:

- Wound care, if needed, must be taught to the primary caregiver in the home situation. Dressings, special equipment, or special services may be required for the patient's continued care at home.
- A list of community agencies that are available for assistance should be provided.
- Long-term follow-up must be stressed to the patient. The patient must be encouraged to comply with the prescribed dietary and medication regimens, keep appointments for chemotherapy or radiation treatments, and keep the physician informed of changes in physical condition.

SYNDROME OF INAPPROPRIATE ANTIDIURETIC HORMONE

Definition/Description

The syndrome of inappropriate antidiuretic hormone (SIADH) occurs when antidiuretic hormone (ADH) is released in amounts far in excess of those indicated by the plasma osmotic pressure. It is more common in the elderly.

Pathophysiology

SIADH has various causes. Ectopic ADH production by carcinomas is not a primary pituitary disorder but has similar manifestations. Bronchogenic carcinoma is a common ADH-secreting tumor.

- Pulmonary conditions, such as pneumonia, tuberculosis (TB), lung abscess, and positive pressure breathing, have been associated with SIADH.
- The syndrome is also associated with such diverse conditions as trauma (most frequently head trauma), meningitis, subarachnoid hemorrhage, peripheral neuropathy, delirium tremens, Addison's disease, psychoses, vomiting, stress, and many medications.

The excess ADH increases renal tubular permeability and reabsorption of water into the circulation. Consequently, extracellular fluid volume expands, plasma osmolality declines, glomerular filtration rate (GFR) rises, and sodium (Na^+) levels decline.

Clinical Manifestations

- SIADH is characterized by fluid retention, serum hypoosmolality, dilutional hyponatremia, hypochloremia, concentrated urine in the presence of intravascular volume depletion, and normal renal function.
- Problems related to SIADH include low urinary output and weight gain without edema.
- Initially, thirst, dyspnea on exertion, fatigue, and dulled sensorium may be evident.
- As plasma osmolality and serum Na^+ levels continue to decline, cerebral edema may occur, leading to lethargy, anorexia, confusion, headache, convulsions, and coma.
- Other effects of hyponatremia include muscle cramps and weakness.

Diagnostic Studies

- Simultaneous measurements of urine and serum osmolality. A serum osmolality much lower than the urine osmolality indicates the inappropriate excretion of concentrated urine in the presence of very dilute serum.
- Other laboratory findings are decreased blood urea nitrogen (BUN), creatinine clearance, hemoglobin (Hb), and hematocrit (Hct).

Collaborative Care

The treatment goal is to restore normal fluid volume and osmolality. Fluids may be restricted to 800 to 1000 ml per day. If fluid restriction alone does not improve symptoms, an IV of 3% to 5% (hypertonic) saline solution may be administered. A diuretic such as furosemide (Lasix) may be used to promote diuresis if cardiac symptoms develop. Because furosemide increases potassium (K^+) excretion, K^+ supplements may be needed.

- SIADH tends to be self-limiting when caused by head trauma or drugs, but chronic in nature when associated with tumors or metabolic diseases. Treatment of the underlying cause, or discontinuing the causal medication, is indicated to improve the clinical course.
- In chronic symptomatic SIADH, demeclocycline (Declomycin), a tetracycline that causes nephrogenic diabetes insipidus (DI), is useful. This drug blocks the action of ADH at the level of the distal and collecting tubules, regardless of the ADH source.

Nursing Management

Careful nursing assessment of patients who have had brain surgery or those susceptible to the syndrome can help in the early detection of SIADH. The nurse should be alert for low urinary output with a high specific gravity, a sudden weight gain, or a serum Na^+ decline. If a patient has SIADH, nursing measures include:

- Restriction of total fluid intake to no more than 1000 ml/day and restriction of oral intake until normalization of serum Na^+ (if appropriate)
- Positioning the head of the bed flat or with no more than 10 degrees of elevation to enhance venous return to the heart and increase left atrial filling pressure, reducing ADH release
- Positioning siderails up because of potential alterations in mental status. Turning of patient every 2 hours, proper positioning, range-of-motion (ROM) exercise, and massage (if patient bedridden)
- Use of seizure precautions such as padded siderails and dim lighting
- Assistance with ambulation and provision of frequent oral hygiene

When SIADH is chronic, patients must learn to self-manage their treatment regimens.

- Fluids are restricted to 800 to 1000 ml/day. Sucking on hard candy or ice chips can help decrease thirst. The patient may be treated with a diuretic to remove excess fluid volume.
- The diet should be supplemented with Na^+ and K^+, especially if diuretics are prescribed. Salts of these electrolytes must be well diluted to prevent GI irritation or damage.
- The patient should be taught the symptoms of fluid and electrolyte imbalances, especially those involving Na^+ and K^+, so that they can monitor their responses to treatment.
- If a patient is to be treated with demeclocycline, the need for close follow-up care should be stressed because of the nephrotoxic side effects and the potential for fungal infections associated with this drug.

SYPHILIS

Definition/Description
Syphilis is a disease of the blood vessels characterized by dilation and swelling of the capillaries and a proliferation of the endothelium. The causative organism of syphilis is *Treponema pallidum,* a spirochete.

- Syphilis is an ulcerative disease, and as such, facilitates the transmission of HIV infection during sexual contact. If untreated in early pregnancy, syphilis can lead to fetal infection and/or perinatal death.

Pathophysiology
The organism, *T. pallidum,* is thought to enter the body through very small breaks in the skin or mucous membranes. Its entry is facilitated by the minor abrasion that often occurs during intercourse. It is extremely fragile and is easily destroyed by drying, heating, or washing.

- Not all people who are exposed to syphilis acquire the disease; about one third become infected after intercourse with an infected person.
- In addition to sexual contact, syphilis may be spread through contact with infectious lesions and through the sharing of needles among drug addicts.
- Congenital syphilis is transmitted from an infected mother to the fetus in utero.
- The incubation period for syphilis ranges from 10 to 90 days but is usually considered to be 3 weeks.
- Scar tissue formation is the method of healing for syphilis. The severity and extent of the damage varies.

There is an association between syphilis and HIV infection. Persons at increased risk for acquiring syphilis are also at increased risk for acquiring HIV. Often, both infections are present in the same person. Therefore the evaluation of all patients with syphilis should include serologic testing for HIV with the patient's consent.

Clinical Manifestations
Syphilis presents with a variety of signs and symptoms that can mimic a number of less serious diseases. Consequently, it is more difficult to recognize syphilis than other venereal diseases. If it is not treated, specific clinical stages are characteristic of the disease progression.

- In the *primary stage,* chancres (painless indurated lesions found on the penis, vulva, and lips and in the mouth, vagina, and rectum) are seen at the site of bacterial invasion. *T. pallidum* multiplies in the epithelium, producing a granulomatous tissue reaction (chancre).

- In the *secondary stage,* syphilis is systemic. During this stage blood-borne bacteria spread to all major organ systems. Manifestations characteristic of the secondary stage include cutaneous eruptions, *alopecia* (hair loss), and generalized adenopathy. Cutaneous eruptions include a bilateral, symmetric rash usually involving the palms and soles; mucous patches in the mouth, tongue, or cervix; and *condylomata* (moist papules) in the anal and genital area.

- *Latent syphilis* follows the secondary stage and is a period during which the immune system is able to suppress the infection. There are no signs or symptoms of syphilis during this time.

- *Late syphilis* (also called *tertiary syphilis*) is the most severe stage of the disease. Because antibiotics can cure syphilis, manifestations of late syphilis are rare. However, when it does occur, it is responsible for significant morbidity and mortality. *Gummas* (destructive skin, bone, and soft tissue lesions associated with late syphilis) are probably caused by a severe hypersensitivity reaction to the microorganism. Within the cardiovascular system late syphilis may cause aneurysms, heart valve insufficiency, and heart failure. Within the central nervous system (CNS), the presence of *T. pallidum* in the cerebrospinal fluid (CSF) may cause manifestations of neurosyphilis.

Complications

Complications occur in late syphilis. The gummas of benign late syphilis may produce irreparable damage to bone, liver, or skin but seldom result in death.

- In cardiovascular syphilis, the resulting aneurysm may press on structures such as the intercostal nerves, resulting in pain. Scarring of the aortic valve results in aortic valve insufficiency and eventual heart failure.

- *Neurosyphilis* (general paresis) is responsible for degeneration of the brain with mental deterioration. Problems related to sensory nerve involvement are a result of *tabes dorsalis* (progressive locomotor ataxia). There may be sudden attacks of pain anywhere in the body; loss of vision and position sense in the feet and legs can also occur. Walking may become even more difficult as joint stability is lost.

Diagnostic Studies

- Dark-field microscopy confirms the diagnosis with the presence of spirochetes from tissue scrapings of primary or secondary lesions.

- Venereal Disease Research Laboratory (VDRL) and rapid plasma reagin (RPR) testing for screening of nonspecific antitreponemal antibodies is usually positive 10 to 14 days after chancre appearance.
- Fluorescent treponemal antibody absorption (FTA-ABS) test and the microhemagglutination (MHA) test detect specific antitreponemal antibodies and are used to confirm the diagnosis.

Collaborative Care

Management is aimed at the eradication of all syphilitic organisms. However, treatment cannot reverse damage that is already present in the late stage of the disease.

- Parenteral penicillin remains the treatment of choice for all stages of syphilis. To date, there is no evidence to suggest a decrease in the effectiveness of penicillin against *T. pallidum*. Table 50-5, Lewis and others, *Medical-Surgical Nursing,* edition 5, p. 1501 describes therapy for the various stages of syphilis and is in accordance with United States Public Health Service recommendations. All stages of syphilis should be treated.
- Appropriate antibiotic treatment of maternal syphilis before the eighteenth week of pregnancy prevents infection of the fetus. Appropriate treatment after 18 weeks of pregnancy cures both mother and fetus because the antibiotics can cross the placental barrier. Treatment administered in the second half of pregnancy may pose a risk of premature labor.
- All patients with neurosyphilis must be carefully followed with periodic serologic testing, clinical evaluation at 6-month intervals, and repeat CSF examinations for at least 3 years.

Nursing Management

For the nursing management of sexually transmitted diseases, see Chlamydial Infection, p. 127.

SYSTEMIC LUPUS ERYTHEMATOSUS

Definition/Description

Systemic lupus erythematosus (SLE) is a chronic multisystem inflammatory disease of connective tissue that often involves the skin, joints, serous membranes (pleura, pericardium), kidney, hematologic system, and central nervous system (CNS). SLE is characterized by its variability within and among persons, with a chronic unpredictable course of exacerbations alternating with periods of remission. Women have a higher incidence of SLE than men. The disease is observed three times more often in African-American women than in Caucasian women.

Pathophysiology

The exact etiology of SLE is unknown. However, factors implicated in the etiology of SLE include genetic predisposition, sex hormones, race, environmental factors (e.g., ultraviolet [UV] radiation, drugs, chemicals), viruses and infections, stress, and immunologic abnormalities. SLE is a disorder of immune regulation.

- Hormones are known to play a role in the etiology of SLE. The disease often worsens during pregnancy and the immediate postpartum period. Healthy women are more immunologically reactive than healthy men because estrogens enhance immune reactivity. The onset or exacerbation of disease symptoms sometimes occurs after the onset of menarche, with the use of oral contraceptives, and during and after pregnancy.

The pathologic features relate to autoimmune reactions directed against constituents of the cell nucleus, particularly deoxyribonucleic acid (DNA). In SLE, autoantibodies are produced against nuclear antigens (DNA, histones, ribonucleoproteins, and nucleolar factors), cytoplasmic antigens (ribosomal and cardiolipin), and blood cell surface antigens (white blood cells [WBCs], red blood cells [RBCs], platelets, and granulocytes).

- Accumulation of antigen-antibody (immune) complexes within the blood vessel walls and subsequent complement activation leads to a condition called lupus vasculitis. The ensuing ischemia within the blood vessel walls gradually leads to thickening of the internal cell lining, fibrinoid degeneration, and thrombus formation.

Clinical Manifestations and Complications

There is no characteristic pattern of progressive organ involvement, nor is it predictable which systems may become affected. General constitutional complaints, including fever, weight loss, arthralgia, and excessive fatigue, may precede an exacerbation of disease activity.

Dermatologic manifestations. The most common feature is an erythematous rash that can occur on the face, neck, and extremities. The classic butterfly rash, which is distributed across the bridge of the nose and cheeks, may appear as discoid (coinlike) lesions or as a diffuse maculopapular rash; it may occur anywhere on the body but is most frequently seen on the face and chest.

- Exposure to sunlight and to other sources of UV radiation can cause a severe skin reaction and may precipitate a flare-up of disease activity in persons who are photosensitive. Ulcers of the oral or nasopharyngeal membranes may occur. Transient diffuse or patchy hair loss (alopecia) is common, with or without underlying scalp lesions.

Musculoskeletal problems. Polyarthralgia with morning stiffness is often the patient's first complaint and may precede the onset of multisystem disease by many years. Arthritis occurs in 95% of all patients with SLE at some time in the disease course. Joint symptoms are typically migratory, producing pain without objective signs of inflammation.

- Lupus-related arthritis is generally nonerosive, but it may cause deformities such as swan neck, ulnar deviation, and subluxation with hyperlaxity of the joints.

Cardiopulmonary problems. Pericarditis may be present and is usually associated with myocardial disease. Patients treated with corticosteroids have a higher incidence of atherosclerosis. Pleurisy with or without effusion is seen in many patients at some time during the illness, and pulmonary function studies are generally abnormal. Raynaud's phenomenon may occur. Cardiovascular involvement is an ominous sign of advanced disease and contributes significantly to morbidity and mortality.

Renal problems. Renal involvement is present in nearly one half of all patients and includes microscopic hematuria, excessive cellular casts in the urine sediment, proteinuria, and elevation of the serum creatinine level. Kidney involvement varies in degree but may eventually end in renal failure. Nearly all patients with SLE show histologic abnormalities in renal biopsy studies or autopsy results. Nephritis is the leading cause of death in SLE.

Infection. Patients appear to have increased susceptibility to infections, possibly related to defects in their ability to phagocytize invading bacteria, deficiencies in the production of antibodies, and the immunosuppressive effect of many antiinflammatory drugs. Pneumonia is the most common infection.

Central nervous system problems. CNS involvement ranks close behind kidney disease and infection as a leading cause of death in SLE. Seizures are the most common neurologic manifestation and they may be of the grand mal, petit mal, or psychomotor type; they are generally controlled by corticosteroids or antiseizure therapy.

- Organic brain syndrome may result from the deposition of immune complexes within the brain tissue. It is characterized by disordered thought processes, disorientation, memory deficits, and psychiatric symptoms such as severe depression and psychosis. Recovery is expected, although some residual impairment may result. Occasionally a cerebrovascular accident (stroke) or aseptic meningitis may be attributable to SLE.

Hematologic problems. The formation of antibodies against blood cells such as erythrocytes, leukocytes, thrombocytes, and coagulation factors is a common feature. Anemia, mild leukopenia, and thrombocytopenia are often present. Some patients show a tendency to bleed while others show a tendency toward blood clots.

Diagnostic Studies

The diagnosis is based on the history, physical examination, and laboratory findings.

- Elevated erythrocyte sedimentation rate (ESR), increased gamma globulin levels, anemia, decreased WBC and platelet counts.
- ECG or chest x-ray may show pericarditis or pleural effusions.
- Urine sediment abnormalities (cellular casts, proteinuria), reduced serum complement, and tissue specimens demonstrate changes compatible with SLE.

Autoantibodies directed against nuclear antigens (ANA) have been detected in 99% of persons with SLE. Although extremely sensitive, ANA is not specific for SLE because it is present in 5% of normal persons and 38% of all persons more than 60 years of age.

- Anti-DNA is found most commonly in SLE and rarely seen in other rheumatic diseases.
- Anti–Smith antigen (Sm) antibody, an antibody to the Smith nuclear antigen, is a definitive serologic marker for SLE.

Collaborative Care

Corticosteroids remain the mainstay for treatment of severe illness. Their use should be reserved for acute generalized exacerbation or serious organ involvement, although a reduced maintenance dosage is sometimes used. Immunosuppressive drugs may be used for symptoms which are resistant to corticosteroid therapy. The efficacy of treatment is most appropriately monitored by serial serum complement levels and anti-DNA titers. Survival is influenced by several factors, including age, race, gender, socioeconomic status, accompanying morbid conditions, and the severity of the disease.

Drug Therapy

Aspirin or other nonsteroidal antiinflammatory drugs (NSAIDs) may reduce mild symptoms such as fever and arthritic complaints. Antimalarial drugs such as hydroxychloroquine sulfate (Plaquenil) may be used to improve skin and musculoskeletal problems. Topical corticosteroid preparations and intralesional corticosteroid injections are effective treatments for skin lesions.

- Corticosteroids are used for acute generalized exacerbations and for treatment of serious organ involvement, including hematologic abnormalities. As clinical and laboratory values improve, dosages are gradually tapered.

- Immunosuppressive drug therapy, such as azathioprine (Imuran) and cyclophosphamide (Cytoxan), is often used in life-threatening situations for symptoms unresponsive to more conservative treatment.

Nursing Management
Goals
The patient with SLE will have satisfactory pain relief, comply with the therapeutic regimen to achieve maximum symptom management, avoid activities which induce disease exacerbation, and maintain a positive self-image.

See NCP 60-2 for the patient with systemic lupus erythematosus, Lewis and others, *Medical-Surgical Nursing,* edition 5, p. 1846.

Nursing Diagnoses
- Pain *related to* the disease process and inadequate comfort measures
- Impaired skin integrity *related to* photosensitivity, skin rash, and alopecia
- Body image disturbance *related to* changes in physical appearance
- Fatigue *related to* the disease process
- Activity intolerance *related to* arthralgia, weakness, and fatigue
- Altered nutrition: less than body requirements *related to* anorexia, fatigue, oral ulcerations, and immunosuppressive therapy
- Ineffective management of therapeutic regimen *related to* a lack of knowledge of the long-term management of the disease

Nursing Interventions
Prevention of SLE is not possible at this time. The education of health professionals and the community may promote a clearer understanding of the disease and earlier diagnosis and treatment.

During an exacerbation, patients may become abruptly and dramatically ill. Nursing interventions include accurately recording the severity of symptoms and documenting the response to therapy. Fever pattern, joint inflammation, limitation of motion, location and degree of discomfort, and fatigability should be specifically assessed.

- The patient's weight and fluid intake and output should be monitored because of the fluid retention effect of corticosteroids and the possibility of renal failure. Careful collection of 24-hour urine for protein may be required.
- The nurse should observe for signs of bleeding that result from drug therapy, such as pallor, skin bruising, petechiae, or tarry stools.
- A careful assessment of neurologic status includes observation for visual disturbances, headaches, personality changes, and forgetfulness. Psychosis may indicate CNS disease or may be

the effect of corticosteroid therapy. Irritation of the nerves of the extremities (peripheral neuropathy) may produce numbness, tingling, and weakness of the hands and feet. Less frequently, a stroke may result.

- The nurse must explain the nature of the disease and the modes of therapy and prepare the patient for numerous diagnostic procedures. Emotional support for the patient and family is essential.

▼ **Patient Teaching**

The patient must understand that adherence to the treatment plan is not a guarantee against exacerbation because the disease course is unpredictable. Patient and family education should include the following:

- Education on the disease process
- The names, actions, side effects, dosage, and administration of medications
- Energy conservation and pacing techniques
- Daily heat and exercise program (for arthralgia)
- Avoidance of physical and emotional stress, overexposure to UV light, and unnecessary exposure to infection
- Regular medical and laboratory follow-up
- Referral resources to community and health care agencies.

The nurse should counsel the patient and family that SLE has a good prognosis for the majority of persons. Many young couples require pregnancy and sexual counseling. Pacing techniques and relaxation therapy can help keep the patient actively involved. Daily planning should include recreational as well as occupational activities.

SYSTEMIC SCLEROSIS (SCLERODERMA)

Definition/Description

Systemic sclerosis, or scleroderma, is a disorder of the connective tissue characterized by fibrotic, degenerative, and occasionally inflammatory changes in the skin, blood vessels, synovium, skeletal muscle, and internal organs. Skin thickening and tightening are the cardinal features.

- The disease may range from a diffuse cutaneous thickening with rapidly progressive and fatal visceral involvement to a more benign variant called *CREST syndrome* (*c*alcinosis, *R*aynaud's phenomenon, *e*sophageal hypomotility, *s*clerodactyly [skin change of the fingers] and telangiectasia (macule-like angioma on the skin).

Systemic sclerosis (SS) affects women three times more frequently than men, with the female/male ratio increasing to 15:1 during the childbearing years. Although symptoms may begin at any time, the usual age at onset is between 30 and 50 years.

Pathophysiology

The exact cause of SS remains unclear. Collagen is overproduced and disrupts the normal functioning of internal organs, such as the lungs, kidney, heart, and GI tract. Widespread systemic disease may be the result of primary vessel injury or immune dysregulation. Disruption of the cell is followed by platelet aggregation, myointimal cell proliferation, and fibrosis.

Clinical Manifestations

Raynaud's phenomenon (paroxysmal vasospasm of the digits) occurs in most patients with SS and is the most common initial complaint in CREST syndrome. Raynaud's phenomenon may precede the onset of systemic disease by months, years, or even decades (see Raynaud's Phenomenon, p. 489).

- Symmetric painless swelling or thickening of the skin of the fingers and hands may progress to diffuse scleroderma of the trunk. In CREST syndrome, skin thickening is generally limited to the fingers and face. The skin loses elasticity and becomes taut and shiny, producing the typical expressionless facies with tightly pursed lips.
- Flexion contractures and atrophy of soft tissue may give the hands a clawlike appearance. Polyarthralgias and morning stiffness may be early symptoms.

Esophageal hypomotility causes the frequent reflux of gastric acid, causing heartburn, and substernal dysphagia for solid foods. If swallowing becomes difficult, the patient often decreases food intake and loses weight. GI complaints also include abdominal distention, diarrhea, malodorous floating stools (malabsorption syndrome) as a result of small bowel disease, and constipation.

Lung involvement includes pleural thickening and pulmonary fibrosis as well as pulmonary function abnormalities. Pulmonary hypertension is seen almost exclusively in CREST syndrome.

Primary heart disease consists of pericarditis, pericardial effusion, and cardiac arrhythmias. Myocardial fibrosis resulting in congestive failure occurs most frequently in those persons with diffuse SS.

- Renal disease is a major cause of death. Arterial hypertension associated with rapidly progressive and irreversible renal insufficiency is often present.

Diagnostic Studies

- Erythrocyte sedimentation rate (ESR) may be mildly elevated with hypergammaglobinemia.
- Antinuclear antibody (ANA) titers are elevated with autoantibody Scl-70 seen in diffuse SS.
- Nail-bed capillary microscopy shows capillary loop dilation with limited disease and dilation with avascular areas in patients with diffuse disease.
- If renal involvement is present, urinalysis may show proteinuria, microscopic hematuria, and casts.
- X-ray evidence of subcutaneous (SC) calcification, digital tuft resorption, distal esophageal hypomotility, and/or bilateral pulmonary fibrosis.
- Pulmonary function studies reveal a decreased vital capacity.
- Skin biopsy shows dermal collagen thickening, condensation, or homogenization.

Collaborative Care

The management of SS offers no specific treatment with long-term effects. Therapy is directed toward attempts to prevent or treat the secondary complications of involved organs. Various drugs, such as antiinflammatory agents, D-penicillamine, and colchicine have been used with varying degrees of success.

Physical therapy helps maintain joint mobility and preserve muscle strength. Occupational therapy assists the patient in maintaining functional abilities. Gastroesophageal reflux may be treated by antacids and periodic dilation of the esophagus. Raynaud's phenomenon may be temporarily relieved by thoracic sympathectomy.

Drug Therapy

No specific drugs or combinations of drugs have been proven effective. Corticosteroids are generally reserved for patients with myositis or overlap syndromes (e.g., mixed connective tissue disease). Penicillamine (Cuprimine) increases the solubility of dermal collagen and may cause thinning of the skin, but it has many side effects. Colchicine is being used to inhibit the accumulation of collagen, but evidence is still insufficient to prove its therapeutic worth. The use of immunosuppressive agents is under investigation.

Supportive measures include oral or topical vasodilating drugs and intraarterial injections of reserpine. Calcium channel blockers (nifedipine [Procardia], diltiazem [Cardizem]) are the treatment of choice for Raynaud's phenomenon. Infected ulcers of the fingertips may be treated by soaking with hyaluronidase and using a bacterial antibiotic ointment. Joint symptoms may be relieved by aspirin and other nonsteroidal antiinflammatory drugs (NSAIDs). Antacids may be useful for heartburn. Combinations of antihypertensive medications, including hydralazine (Apresoline), minoxidil (Loniten), captopril (Capoten), propranolol (Inderal), and methyldopa (Aldomet), have been used in the treatment of hypertension and renal failure.

Nursing Management

Because prevention is not possible, nursing interventions often begin during hospitalization for diagnostic purposes. Emotional stress and a cold environment may aggravate Raynaud's phenomenon. Patients with SS should not have fingerstick blood testing done because of compromised circulation and poor digital healing. The nurse may help the patient to resolve feelings of helplessness by providing information about the illness and encouraging active participation in planning care.

- Hands and feet should be protected from cold exposure and possible burns or cuts that might heal slowly. Smoking should be avoided because of its vasoconstricting effect. Lotions may help to alleviate skin dryness and cracking but must be rubbed in for an unusually long time because of skin thickness. Signs of infection should be reported.
- Dysphagia may be reduced by eating small, frequent meals, chewing carefully and slowly, and drinking fluids. Heartburn may be minimized by using antacids 45 to 60 minutes after each meal and by sitting upright for 30 to 45 minutes after eating. Using additional pillows or raising the head of the bed may help reduce nocturnal gastroesophageal reflux.
- Job modifications are often necessary as stair climbing, typing, writing, and cold exposure may pose particular problems.
- Some people need to wear gloves to protect fingertip ulcers and to provide extra warmth. Sensitive areas on the fingertips resulting from ulcers may require padded utensils or special assistive devices to reduce discomfort.
- Daily oral hygiene must be emphasized, or neglect may lead to increased tooth and gingival problems.
- Psychologic support reduces stress and may positively influence peripheral motor response.
- Biofeedback training and relaxation techniques may be used to reduce tension, improve sleeping habits, and raise digital temperature.

The patient must actively carry out therapeutic exercises at home. The nurse should reinforce heat therapy, the use of assistive devices, and the organization of activities to preserve strength and reduce disability. Sexual dysfunction resulting from body changes, pain, muscular weakness, limited mobility, decreased self-esteem, and decreased vaginal secretions may require sensitive counseling by the nurse.

TESTICULAR CANCER

Definition/Description

Testicular tumors occur primarily in men between 20 and 40 years of age. Testicular tumors are more common in men who have had undescended testicles (cryptorchidism) or a family history of testicular cancer or anomalies.

- Other predisposing factors include a history of mumps, orchitis, inguinal hernia in childhood, maternal exposure to diethylstilbestrol (DES), and testicular cancer in the contralateral testis.
- The etiology of testicular neoplasms is unknown. Testicular tumors may develop from the cellular components of the testis or from the embryonal precursors (germ cell tumors). Testicular germ cell tumors are almost always malignant. Non-germ cell tumors are rare, usually benign, and can occur at any age.

Clinical Manifestations

Germ cell tumors may have a slow or rapid onset depending on the type.

- The patient may notice a lump in his scrotum, as well as scrotal swelling and a feeling of heaviness. The scrotal mass is usually nontender, very firm, and cannot be transilluminated.
- Manifestations associated with metastasis include abdominal masses, back pain, cough, dyspnea, hemoptysis, dysphagia, alterations in vision or mental status, and seizures.

Diagnostic Studies

Palpation of the scrotal contents is the first step in diagnosing testicular cancer. Additional tests that aid in diagnosis include a testicular sonogram and MRI.

- If a testicular neoplasm is suspected, blood may be drawn to look for certain glycoprotein tumor markers including α-fetoprotein (AFP) and human chorionic gonadotropin (hCG). After diagnosis and staging, AFP and hCG will continue to be monitored, if appropriate, to detect metastases and assess the therapy response.
- Following orchiectomy, tumor staging is done on the biopsy specimen. Testicular cancer is histologically classified as germ cell tumors (seminomas and nonseminomas) or non-germ cell tumors.

Nursing and Collaborative Management

As with many forms of cancer, the survival of the patient is closely associated with early tumor recognition. The scrotum is easily examined, and beginning tumors are usually palpable. Every male between the ages of 20 to 40 years should be taught and encouraged to perform a monthly testicular self-exam for the purpose of detecting testicular tumors or other scrotal abnormalities such as varicoceles. (See Table 52-8 and Fig. 52-5 for scrotum self-examination guidelines, Lewis and others, *Medical-Surgical Nursing,* edition 5, p. 1570.)

- The patient may indicate some reluctance to examine his own genitals. With encouragement the patient can learn this simple procedure. He should be encouraged to do self-examinations frequently until he is comfortable with the procedure. The scrotum should be examined once a month.

Collaborative management generally involves a radical orchiectomy, spermatic cord removal, and resection of the regional and paraaortic lymph nodes.

- Radiation of the remaining lymph nodes may be used if the tumor is radiosensitive. Single or multiple chemotherapeutic agent regimens such as bleomycin (Blenoxane), vincristine (Oncovin), cisplatin (Platinol), etoposide (VePesid), and vinblastine (Velban) are also used before and after surgery depending on the histologic findings and disease stage.

The prognosis for patients with testicular cancer has improved and 75% of all patients obtain complete remission if the disease is detected in the early stages.

- All patients with testicular cancer, regardless of pathology or stage, require meticulous follow-up and monthly physical examinations, chest x-ray, CT scan, and assessment of hCG and AFP (if appropriate). The goal is to detect relapse when the tumor burden is minimal.
- The man with testicular cancer should have the opportunity to discuss fertility and sperm banking prior to any treatment.
- The nurse should be sensitive to any psychosocial problems this type of cancer can have on a man's feelings of maleness or self-worth. Treatment has the potential to interfere with both erections and fertility.

TETANUS

Definition/Description

Tetanus (lockjaw) is an extremely severe polyradiculitis and polyneuritis affecting spinal and cranial nerves. It results from the effects of a potent neurotoxin released by the anaerobic bacillus *Clostridium tetani.* The toxin interferes with the function of the reflex arc by blocking inhibitory transmitters at the presynaptic sites in the spinal cord and brainstem. The spores of the bacillus are present in soil, garden mold, and manure. Worldwide, the number of cases per year is estimated to be 1 million. Overall, mortality rates range from 45% to 55%.

Pathophysiology

Clostridium tetani enters the body through a traumatic or suppurative wound, which provides an appropriate low-oxygen environment for the organisms to mature and produce toxin. Other possible sources include dental infection, injections of heroin, human and animal bites, frostbite, compound fractures, and gunshot wounds.

- The incubation period is usually 7 days but can range from 3 to 21 days, with symptoms frequently appearing after the original wound is healed. In general, the longer the incubation period, the milder the illness and the better the prognosis.

Clinical Manifestations

The manifestations of generalized tetanus include a feeling of stiffness in the jaw *(trismus)* or neck, a slight fever, and other symptoms of general infection. Generalized tonic spasms occur because of the lack of reciprocal innervation.

- As the disease progresses, the neck muscles, back, abdomen, and extremities become progressively rigid. In severe forms, continuous tonic convulsions may occur with *opisthotonos* (extreme arching of the back and retraction of the head). Laryngeal and respiratory spasms cause apnea and anoxia.
- Additional effects are manifested by overstimulation of the sympathetic nervous system; these include profuse diaphoresis, labile hypertension, episodic tachycardia, hyperthermia, and arrhythmias. The slightest noise, jarring motion, or bright light can set off a seizure. These seizures are agonizingly painful.
- Death is usually attributable to asphyxia or heart failure, the result of constantly recurring spasms.
- Residual injury, such as vertebral fracture, muscular contraction, and brain damage secondary to hypoxia, may remain.

Diagnostic Studies

- Serum electrolytes, complete blood count (CBC), albumin, clotting factors, glucose, and arterial blood gases (ABGs) are monitored.
- ECG with monitoring of cardiac function.

Collaborative Care

Management includes the administration of tetanus toxoid booster (Td) and tetanus immune globulin (TIG) before the onset of symptoms to neutralize circulating toxins. Because of laryngospasm, a tracheostomy (see Tracheostomy, p. 686) is usually performed early and the patient is maintained on mechanical ventilation. Any recognized wound should be debrided; any abscesses should be drained.

- Control of spasms is essential and is managed by deep sedation, usually with diazepam (Valium), barbiturates, or chlorpromazine (Thorazine). A 10-day course of penicillin is recommended to inhibit further growth of the organism.
- If sedation does not control seizures, skeletal muscle paralyzing drugs such as D-tubocurarine (curare) are used.
- Pain is relieved by means of codeine or meperidine, often with the addition of promethazine (Phenergan).

Nutrition is maintained through parenteral or tube feeding. Those who recover have a long convalescence that includes extensive physiotherapy.

Nursing Management

Health teaching is aimed at ensuring tetanus prophylaxis, which is the most important factor influencing the incidence of this disease.

- The patient should be taught that immediate, thorough cleansing of all wounds with soap and water is important in prevention.
- If an open wound occurs and the patient has not been immunized within the past 10 years, the primary care provider should be contacted so that a tetanus booster can be given.

Acute intervention is aimed at supportive care based on the treatment of the clinical manifestations. The patient should be placed in a quiet, darkened room insulated against noise. Judicious sedation should be given.

- Nursing care should be administered with the utmost caution to avoid triggering spasms. For example, the nurse should avoid unnecessary touching, use firm touching when necessary, avoid the use of linens to cover the patient, and maintain a slightly higher than normal ambient temperature.
- Nursing care related to tracheostomy and mechanical ventilation is given as appropriate.
- An indwelling bladder catheter may be used to prevent bladder distention and urinary reflux in the presence of spasms in the muscles of the pelvic floor.
- The patient needs emotional support during the acute phase because the fear of death is real. The family also needs support and education.

THALASSEMIA

Definition/Description

Thalassemia is a disease of decreased erythrocyte (red blood cell [RBC]) production due to an inadequate production of normal hemoglobin (Hb). Hemolysis also occurs in thalassemia.

- In contrast to iron deficiency anemia, in which heme synthesis is the problem, thalassemia involves a problem with the globin protein. Therefore the basic defect of thalassemia is abnormal Hb synthesis.

Pathophysiology

Thalassemias are a group of autosomal recessive genetic disorders commonly found in members of ethnic groups whose origins are near the Mediterranean Sea. An individual with thalassemia may have a heterozygous or homozygous form of the disease.

- A person who is heterozygous has one thalassemic gene and one normal gene. They are said to have *thalassemia minor* or *thalassemic trait,* which is a mild form of the disease.
- A homozygous person has two thalassemic genes, causing a severe condition known as *thalassemia major.*

Clinical Manifestations

- The patient with thalassemia minor is frequently asymptomatic because of adjustment to the gradually acquired chronic state of anemia. Occasionally, splenomegaly may develop, and mild jaundice may occur if malformed erythrocytes are rapidly hemolyzed.
- The patient who has thalassemia major is pale and displays other general symptoms of anemia (see Anemia, p. 22). In addition, the person has marked splenomegaly, hepatomegaly, and jaundice from RBC hemolysis. Chronic bone marrow hyperplasia leads to expansion of the marrow space. This may cause thickening of the cranium and maxillary cavity, leading to an appearance resembling Down syndrome.
- Thalassemia major is a life-threatening disease in which growth, both physical and mental, is often retarded.

Collaborative Care

The laboratory findings in thalassemia major are summarized in Table 7, p. 28.

- Thalassemia minor requires no treatment because the body adapts to the reduction of normal Hb.
- Thalassemia major is usually treated with blood transfusions and chelation therapy (therapy to reduce iron overloading that

can occur with chronic transfusion therapy). Drug and nutritional therapy are not effective in treating thalassemia. Transfusions are administered to keep the Hb level at about 10 g/dl (100 g/L). This level is low enough to foster the patient's own erythropoiesis without enlarging the spleen.

- Because RBCs are sequestered in the enlarged spleen, thalassemia may be treated by splenectomy. However, even with collaborative therapy, the person with thalassemia major will experience retarded growth, hemochromatosis, and cardiac failure.

THROMBOANGIITIS OBLITERANS (BUERGER'S DISEASE)

Thromboangiitis obliterans (Buerger's disease) is an inflammatory, thrombotic disorder of the medium-sized arteries and veins of the upper or lower extremities. Occlusion of the vessels occurs with the development of collateral circulation around the areas of obstruction. The disorder, generally asymmetric, occurs predominantly in men between 25 and 40 years of age who smoke. A familial tendency has been observed.

- The basic cause is not known. There is a direct relationship to cigarette smoking; the disease occurs only in smokers, and when smoking is stopped, the disease improves. Unlike atherosclerosis, lipid accumulation does not occur in the vessel media.

The symptom complex of Buerger's disease is often confused with that of atherosclerotic occlusive disease.

- The patient may have intermittent claudication. The development of pain at rest is a premonitory sign of gangrene and may develop in the advanced stages of the disease.
- Other signs and symptoms may include color and temperature changes in the affected limb or limbs, paresthesia, thrombophlebitis, and cold sensitivity. Painful ulceration and gangrene may necessitate toe amputations.

The treatment includes the avoidance of trauma to the extremity and a complete cessation of smoking. Supportive psychotherapy and drug therapy of underlying anxiety disorders are sometimes helpful in assisting the patient to stop smoking.

- The disorder is difficult to treat; anticoagulants and vasodilator therapy have met with little success. Amputation, generally below the knee, may be necessary in advanced cases.

THROMBOCYTOPENIC PURPURA

Definition/Description

Immune thrombocytopenic purpura (ITP), the most common acquired thrombocytopenia, is a syndrome of abnormal destruction of circulating platelets. It was originally termed *idiopathic thrombocytopenic purpura* because its cause was unknown; however, it is now believed that ITP is an autoimmune disease.

- In ITP, platelets are coated with antibodies. Although these platelets function normally, when they reach the spleen the antibody-coated platelets are recognized as foreign and destroyed by macrophages. Platelets normally survive 8 to 10 days, but in ITP, survival is only 1 to 3 days.
- Acute ITP is seen predominantly in children following a viral illness. Chronic ITP occurs most commonly in women between 20 and 40 years of age. Chronic ITP has a gradual onset and transient remissions occur.

Thrombotic thrombocytopenia purpura (TTP) is an uncommon syndrome characterized by microangiopathic hemolytic anemia, thrombocytopenia, neurologic abnormalities, fever (in the absence of infection), and renal abnormalities.

- The disease is associated with enhanced agglutination of platelets, which form microthrombi that deposit in arterioles and capillaries. The cause of the platelet agglutination is unknown.
- TTP is seen primarily in adults between the ages of 20 and 50 with a slight female predominance.
- The syndrome is occasionally precipitated by the use of estrogen or by pregnancy.
- TTP is a medical emergency because bleeding and clotting occur simultaneously.

Clinical Manifestations

Despite different etiologies, the clinical manifestations of ITP and TTP are similar.

- Thrombocytopenia is most commonly manifested by the appearance of small, flat, pinpoint, red or reddish brown microhemorrhages known as *petechiae*. When the platelet count is low, red blood cells (RBCs) may leak out of the blood vessels and into the skin to cause petechiae.
- When petechiae are numerous, the resulting reddish skin bruise is known as *purpura*.

- Larger purplish lesions caused by hemorrhage are called *ecchymoses*. Ecchymoses may be flat or raised; on occasion pain and tenderness are present.
- Prolonged bleeding after routine procedures, such as venipuncture or intramuscular (IM) injection, may indicate thrombocytopenia. Because bleeding may be internal, the nurse must be aware of manifestations that reflect this type of blood loss including weakness, fainting, dizziness, tachycardia, abdominal pain, and hypotension.

The major complication of thrombocytopenia is hemorrhage, which may be insidious or acute and internal or external. It may occur in any area of the body, including the joints, retina, and brain. Cerebral hemorrhage may be fatal. Insidious hemorrhage may first be detected by discovering the anemia that accompanies blood loss.

Diagnostic Studies

- Platelet count is decreased; spontaneous life-threatening hemorrhages (e.g., intracranial bleeding) may occur with counts below 20,000/μl (20 × 10⁹/L).
- Bleeding time is prolonged.
- Bone marrow analysis may show normal or increased megakaryocytes; it is done to rule out leukemia, aplastic anemia, and other myeloproliferative disorders.
- Flow cytometry may detect antiplatelet antibodies.
- Hematocrit (Hct) and hemoglobin (Hb) levels reflect anemia.

Collaborative Care

Immune thrombocytopenic purpura. Multiple therapies are used to manage the patient with ITP.

- Corticosteroids are used to suppress the phagocytic response of splenic macrophages. This alters the spleen's recognition of platelets and increases platelet life span. In addition, corticosteroids depress autoimmune antibody formation. Corticosteroids also reduce capillary fragility and bleeding time.
- Treatment may also include high doses of IV immunoglobulin in the patient who is unresponsive to corticosteroids or splenectomy. The immunoglobulin works by competing with the antiplatelet antibodies for macrophage receptors. IV immunoglobulin raises the platelet count, but the beneficial effects are temporary.
- Danazol, an attenuated androgen, has been used with success in some patients. Immunosuppressive therapy used in refractory cases includes vincristine (Oncovin), vinblastine (Velban), azathioprine (Imuran), and cyclophosphamide (Cytoxan).
- Splenectomy is indicated if the patient does not respond to prednisone initially or requires unacceptably high doses to maintain an adequate platelet count. Approximately 80% of

- patients benefit from splenectomy, which results in a complete or partial remission.
- Platelet transfusions may be used to increase platelet counts in cases of life-threatening hemorrhage. Platelets should not be administered prophylactically because of the possibility of antibody formation.
- Aspirin and aspirin-containing compounds should be avoided.

Thrombotic thrombocytopenic purpura. TTP is treated with emergency plasma infusion or plasmapheresis. Treatment should be continued daily until the patient is in complete remission. Splenectomy, corticosteroids, dextran (an antiplatelet agent), and vinca alkaloids have also been used with success.

Nursing Management

Goals
The patient with thrombocytopenia will have no gross or occult bleeding, maintain vascular integrity, and manage home care to prevent any complications related to an increased risk for bleeding.

See NCP 29-2 for the patient with thrombocytopenia, Lewis and others, *Medical-Surgical Nursing,* edition 5, p. 759.

Nursing Diagnoses
- Fluid volume deficit *related to* acute blood loss
- Altered oral mucous membrane *related to* the treatment, the disease, or blood-filled bullae
- Risk for injury *related to* interventions and tissue sensitivity to trauma
- Ineffective management of therapeutic regimen *related to* a lack of knowledge of disease process, activity, nutrition, and medication

Nursing Interventions
It is important for the nurse to discourage excessive use of over-the-counter (OTC) medications known to be possible causes of acquired thrombocytopenia. Many medications contain aspirin as an ingredient. Aspirin reduces platelet adhesiveness, thus potentially contributing to thrombocytopenia.

The nurse should encourage persons to have a complete medical evaluation if manifestations of bleeding tendencies (e.g., prolonged epistaxis, petechiae) develop. In addition, the nurse must be observant for early signs of thrombocytopenia in patients receiving cancer chemotherapy drugs.

The goal during acute episodes of thrombocytopenia is to prevent or control hemorrhage. In the patient with thrombocytopenia, bleeding is usually from superficial sites; deep bleeding (into the muscles, joints, and abdomen) usually occurs only when clotting factors are diminished. It is important to emphasize that a seemingly minor nosebleed may lead to hemorrhage in a patient with severe thrombocytopenia.

- In a woman with thrombocytopenia, menstrual blood loss may exceed the usual amount and duration. Counting sanitary napkins or tampons used during menses is an important intervention to detect excess blood loss.
- The proper administration of platelet transfusions is an important nursing responsibility. Platelet concentrates, derived from fresh whole blood, can effectively increase the platelet level.
- Patients with ITP who are receiving corticosteroids should be monitored for a response to therapy.

▼ **Patient Teaching**

- Teach the patient about the disease process, medication, and activity and dietary recommendations to decrease anxiety and prevent complications.
- Teach the patient to avoid the Valsalva maneuver and suppositories, and to cough, sneeze, or blow the nose gently to decrease the risk of hemorrhage.
- Discuss complications and signs that should be reported, trauma prevention, the need for a high fluid intake, medication management, and the need for periods of rest and exercise so the patient will be knowledgeable and able to manage his or her own care or direct others in providing care.
- Provide opportunities for the patient to verbalize concerns to decrease his or her anxiety.
- Foster care decisions and planning by the patient to increase the sense of control and self-esteem.

THROMBOPHLEBITIS

Definition/Description

Thrombophlebitis is the formation of a thrombus (clot) in association with inflammation of the vein. The terms *phlebothrombosis* and *phlebitis* have been used to indicate whether the predominant process is thrombus formation or inflammation. In general, the preferred term is *thrombophlebitis* because both clots and inflammation are usually present. The initiating event is usually thrombus formation. Thrombophlebitis is classified as either *superficial* or *deep* (Table 56).

- Deep vein thrombophlebitis (DVT) is of greater significance and can result in embolization of thrombi from deep veins to the lungs. This can result in prolonged hospitalization and is potentially fatal.

Table 56 Clinical Manifestations of Thrombophlebitis

	Superficial	Deep	
		Small veins	Major venous trunks
Usual causes	Varicose veins; direct trauma; IV catheters; thromboangiitis obliterans; caustic IV medications such as chemotherapy, radiopaque contrast material; IV drug use	Postoperatively, before and after childbirth, direct or distant trauma, CHF, prolonged bed rest, acute febrile disease, sepsis, debilitating disease, malignant disease, blood dyscrasias	Systemic lupus erythematosus, pressure of tumors on veins, estrogen therapy, malignant disease, blood dyscrasias, idiopathic cause
Usual location	Saphenous veins and their tributaries; forearm	Soleal; posterior tibial, other deep calf veins; popliteal; pelvis	Femoral; iliac; inferior or superior vena cava; axillary; subclavian
Clinical findings	Tender, red, inflamed induration along course of SC vein (visible and palpable)	Possible tenderness to deep pressure induration of overlying muscle, minimal or no venous distention	Swelling, cyanosis, venous distention, mild to moderate pain, tenderness over involved vein (groin or axilla)
Edema of extremities	Almost never	Occasionally	Frequently
Embolization	Almost never	Always a threat	Always a threat
Chronic venous insufficiency	Almost never	Usually not	Frequently

CHF, Congestive heart failure; *IV*, intravenous; *SC*, subcutaneous.

Pathophysiology

The three important factors in the etiology of thrombophlebitis are (1) stasis of venous flow, (2) damage of the endothelium (inner lining of the vein), and (3) hypercoagulability of the blood. The patient who is at risk for thrombophlebitis usually has predisposing conditions related to these three disorders.

Venous stasis occurs if venous valves are dysfunctional or if the muscles of the extremities are inactive.

- Venous stasis occurs in people who are obese, have congestive heart failure (CHF), have been on long trips without regular exercise, or are immobile for long periods (e.g., with spinal cord injuries or fractured hips). Also at risk are pregnant women and women in the postpartum period, patients with atrial fibrillation, and patients who are on corticosteroid medication, which promotes venous stasis and clot formation.

Damage of the endothelium is caused by trauma or external pressure. This occurs any time a venipuncture is performed. Damaged endothelium has decreased fibrinolytic properties, which facilitates thrombus development.

- Endothelial damage occurs when patients on IV therapy are receiving high-dose antibiotics, potassium (K^+), chemotherapeutic agents, or hypertonic solutions such as contrast media.
- Other factors predisposing to endothelial inflammation and damage include the presence of an IV catheter in the same site (for >48 hours), the use of contaminated IV equipment, a fracture that causes damage to the blood vessels, diabetes mellitus (DM), blood pooling, burns, and any unusual physical exertion that results in muscular strain.

Hypercoagulability of the blood occurs in many hematologic disorders, particularly polycythemia, severe anemias, and various malignancies. A patient with systemic infections in which endotoxins are released also has hypercoagulability.

- The patient who takes estrogen-based oral contraceptives is at increased risk for thromboembolic disease. Women who take contraceptives and who smoke double their risk because of the constricting effect of nicotine on the blood vessel wall.

Thrombus formation results from the adherence of red blood cells (RBCs), white blood cells (WBCs), platelets, and fibrin. Frequent site of thrombus formation are the valve cusps of veins, where venous stasis allows the accumulation of blood products.

- As the thrombus enlarges, increased amounts of blood cells and fibrin collect behind it, producing a larger clot with a "tail" that eventually occludes the lumen of the vein.
- If a thrombus only partially occludes the vein, the thrombus becomes covered by endothelial cells and the thrombotic process stops.

- If the thrombus does not become detached, it undergoes lysis or becomes firmly organized and adherent within 5 to 7 days. The organized thrombi may detach and then give rise to emboli. These emboli generally flow through the venous circulation, back to the heart, and into the pulmonary circulation.
- Turbulence of the blood flow is a major factor contributing to the thrombus' detachment from the vein wall.

Clinical Manifestations

Manifestations vary according to the size and location of the thrombus and the adequacy of collateral circulation.

- The patient with *superficial thrombophlebitis* may have a palpable, firm, subcutaneous (SC) cordlike vein with the surrounding area tender to the touch, reddened, and warm. A mild systemic temperature elevation and leukocytosis may be present. Edema of the extremity may or may not occur. The most common cause of superficial thrombophlebitis in the lower extremities is related to varicose veins.
- The patient with *deep thrombophlebitis* may have no symptoms or may have unilateral leg edema, pain, warm skin, and a temperature $>100.4°$ F ($>38°$ C). If the calf is involved, tenderness may be present on palpation. *Homans' sign,* pain on dorsiflexion of the foot when the leg is raised, is a classic but unreliable sign because it is not specific for DVT.

Complications

The most serious complications of thrombophlebitis are pulmonary embolism, chronic venous insufficiency, and phlegmasia cerulea dolens. Pulmonary embolism is the most feared complication of thrombophlebitis because of its lethal potential (see Pulmonary Embolism, p. 482).

- Chronic venous insufficiency, a common complication resulting from recurrent thrombophlebitis, results in valvular destruction, allowing retrograde flow of blood. Persistent edema, increased pigmentation, secondary varicosities, ulceration, and cyanosis of the limb when it is placed in a dependent position may develop in a person with this complication. Signs and symptoms of chronic venous insufficiency often do not develop for many years following deep thrombophlebitis.
- *Phlegmasia cerulea dolens* (swollen, blue, painful leg) may develop with severe thrombophlebitis of the lower extremities. It presents as sudden, massive swelling and intense bluish discoloration of the extremity. Gangrene may occur as a result of arterial occlusion resulting from the obstruction of venous outflow.

Diagnostic Studies

- Coagulation studies (platelet count, bleeding time, prothrombin time [PT], partial thromboplastin time [PTT]) may be elevated with blood dyscrasias and decreased with polycythemia.
- Duplex scanning and venous Doppler evaluation determine venous flow.
- Plethysmography records abnormal findings with slow venous outflow.
- Venogram (phlebogram) can determine clot location.

Collaborative Care

Management of the patient with superficial thrombophlebitis includes elevation of the affected extremity until the tenderness has subsided. Warm, moist heat may be used to relieve pain and treat inflammation. Mild oral analgesics (e.g., aspirin, codeine) are used to relieve pain. Nonsteroidal antiinflammatory agents (e.g., ibuprofen) are used to treat the inflammatory process and accompanying pain.

- Anticoagulant therapy is usually not indicated for superficial thrombophlebitis but is routinely used for DVT. The goals of anticoagulation therapy are to prevent propagation of the clot, development of a new thrombus, and embolization. Anticoagulation therapy does not dissolve the clot. Lysis of the clot begins spontaneously through the body's intrinsic fibrinolytic system.
- Bed rest with elevation of the affected extremity above the level of heart is indicated until the therapeutic levels of anticoagulation are achieved and the edema subsides.
- If edema still persists when the patient is ambulatory, elastic compression stockings are recommended. Elastic gradient stockings are recommended for several months to support the vein walls and valves and decrease pain and swelling on ambulation.

Most patients are treated conservatively, but a small percentage require surgical intervention. The primary indication for surgery is to prevent pulmonary emboli. Surgical procedures include venous thrombectomy (rarely performed) and inferior vena cava interruption. Venous thrombectomy involves the removal of an occluding clot through an incision in the vein. This procedure is done to prevent pulmonary embolism and chronic venous insufficiency.

Nursing Management

Goals

The patient with thrombophlebitis will have relief of pain, decreased edema, no skin ulceration, and no evidence of pulmonary emboli.

See NCP 36-3 for the patient with thrombophlebitis, Lewis and others, *Medical-Surgical Nursing,* edition 5, p. 1001.

Nursing Diagnoses/Collaborative Problems

- Pain *related to* edema from impaired circulation in the extremities
- Altered health maintenance *related to* a lack of knowledge about the disorder and its treatment
- Risk for impaired skin integrity *related to* an alteration in peripheral tissue perfusion and possible valvular destruction
- Potential complication: anticoagulant therapy adverse effects
- Potential complication: pulmonary embolism *related to* dehydration, immobility, and embolization of thrombus

Nursing Interventions

Prophylactic measures in surgical patients to prevent thrombus formation include early ambulation and postoperative leg exercises, the use of compression stockings, adequate hydration, and low-dose anticoagulant therapy. Heparin, low molecular weight heparin, or oral anticoagulants are often recommended for the high-risk patient who is predisposed to thrombus formation.

- Another preventive measure is to avoid prolonged standing or sitting in a motionless, leg-dependent position. Frequent knee flexion, ankle rotation, and active walking should be done during long periods of sitting or standing, especially on long trips.
- The patient should be encouraged to stop smoking and to perform deep breathing and range-of-motion (ROM) exercises. In addition, identify patients at increased risk for DVT and institute appropriate preventive measures.

Acute care is directed toward the reduction of inflammation and the prevention of emboli formation.

- Intervention for superficial thrombophlebitis involves the use of warm moist packs or soaks, elevation of the affected extremity, removal of an IV catheter if present, and analgesia to minimize pain and inflammation.
- Intervention for DVT involves IV and oral anticoagulation, 3 to 6 days of bed rest with elevation of the affected extremity, and the use of elastic support (elastic bandages or compression stockings) to promote venous return.

While the patient is receiving anticoagulation therapy, closely observe for any indications of bleeding, including epistaxis and bleeding gingiva.

- Urine should be assessed for gross or microscopic hematuria. A smoky appearance to the urine is sometimes noted if blood is present.
- Particular attention should be paid to the protection of skin areas that may be traumatized. Surgical incisions should be closely observed for bleeding.

- Stools should be tested to determine the presence of occult blood from the GI tract.
- Mental status changes, especially in the older patient, should be assessed as a possible indication of cerebral bleeding.
- PTT, international normalized ratio (INR) for PT, hemoglobin (Hb), hematocrit (Hct), and platelet levels should be monitored when the patient is receiving anticoagulant drugs. The nurse should first check the results of clotting studies prior to administering either heparin or Coumadin. The antidote for heparin is protamine sulfate, and vitamin K is used as the antidote for Coumadin. These drugs must be immediately available if hemorrhage occurs.

▼ Patient Teaching

Discharge teaching should stress the avoidance of contraceptives for the patient with recurrent thrombophlebitis, the hazards of smoking, the importance of elastic compression stockings, and the need to avoid constrictive girdles or garters.

- Exercise programs should be developed with an emphasis on swimming and wading, which are particularly beneficial because of the gentle, even pressure of the water. A balanced program of rest and exercise, along with proper posture and the avoidance of long periods of sitting, improves arterial filling and venous return.
- The older patient should be taught safety precautions to prevent injury, such as from falls.
- Dietary considerations for the overweight patient are aimed at limiting caloric intake to maintain desired weight. Fat intake should be reduced if lipid or triglyceride levels are above normal. Sodium (Na^+) may be limited if edema is present. Fluid deficits should be avoided to prevent hypercoagulability of the blood. A well-balanced diet is important because calcium, vitamin E, and vitamin K all play active roles in clotting.
- Review with the patient any medications currently being taken that may interfere with anticoagulant therapy.
- If the patient is discharged while receiving anticoagulant medication, both the patient and family need careful explanations of its dosage, actions, and side effects, as well as the importance of routine blood tests and the need to report symptoms to the health care provider.

TRIGEMINAL NEURALGIA

Definition/Description

Trigeminal neuralgia (tic douloureux) is a relatively uncommon cranial nerve disorder. It is more commonly seen in women and usually begins in the fifth or sixth decade of life. Although this condition is considered benign, the severity of the pain and the disruption of lifestyle can result in almost total physical and psychologic dysfunction or even suicide.

Pathophysiology

The trigeminal nerve is the fifth cranial nerve (CN V) and has both motor and sensory branches. The sensory branches, primarily the maxillary and mandibular branches, are involved in trigeminal neuralgia.

- Although no specific cause has been identified, nerve compression by tortuous arteries of the posterior fossa blood vessels, demyelinating plaques, herpes virus infection, infection of the teeth and jaw, and a brainstem infarct have been suggested as initiating pathologic events.
- The effectiveness of antiseizure drug therapy may be related to the ability of these drugs to stabilize the neuronal membrane.

Clinical Manifestations

The classic feature of trigeminal neuralgia is an abrupt onset of paroxysms of excruciating pain described as burning or knifelike, or a lightning-like shock in the lips, upper or lower gums, cheek, forehead, or side of the nose.

- Intense pain, twitching, grimacing, and frequent blinking and tearing of the eye occur during the acute attack (giving rise to the term *tic*).
- The attacks are usually brief, lasting seconds to 2 or 3 minutes, and are generally unilateral.
- Recurrences are unpredictable; they may occur several times a day or weeks or months apart.
- After the refractory (pain-free) period, a phenomenon known as *clustering* can occur; it is characterized by a cycle of pain and refractoriness that continues for hours.

The painful episodes are usually initiated by a triggering mechanism of light cutaneous stimulation at specific points *(trigger zones)* along the distribution of the nerve branches.

- Precipitating stimuli include chewing, teeth brushing, a hot or cold blast of air on the face, washing the face, yawning, or even talking. Touch and tickle seem to predominate as causative triggers rather than pain or changes in temperature.

- As a result, the patient may not eat properly, neglect hygienic practices, wear a cloth over the face, and withdraw from interaction with other individuals. The patient may sleep excessively as a means of coping with the pain.

Diagnostic Studies
- Brain scan or CT scan; MRI
- Audiologic evaluation
- Electromyography
- Cerebrospinal fluid (CSF) analysis
- Arteriography and posterior myelography

Collaborative Care
The goal of treatment is the relief of pain, either medically or surgically.

- The majority of patients obtain adequate relief through antiseizure drugs such as phenytoin (Dilantin) and carbamazepine (Tegretol). These drugs may prevent an acute attack or promote a remission of symptoms, although the mechanism by which they work is not known. These drugs may not provide permanent pain relief.
- Nerve blocking with local anesthetics is another treatment possibility. Local nerve blocking results in complete anesthesia of the area supplied by the injected branches. The relief of pain is temporary, lasting from 6 to 18 months.
- Biofeedback is another strategy for pain management. In addition to controlling the pain, the patient may experience a strong sense of personal control by mastering the technique and altering certain body functions.

Surgical Therapy
If a conservative approach is not effective, surgical therapy is available. Percutaneous radiofrequency rhizotomy (electrocoagulation) and microvascular decompression afford the greatest relief of pain.

- *Percutaneous radiofrequency rhizotomy* consists of placing a needle into the trigeminal rootlets that are adjacent to the pons and destroying the area by means of a radiofrequency current. This can result in anesthesia of the face (although some degree of sensation may be retained) or trigeminal motor weakness. This procedure is easily performed with minimal risk to the patient.
- *Microvascular decompression* of the trigeminal nerve is accomplished by displacing and repositioning blood vessels that appear to be compressing the nerve at the root-entry zone where it exits the pons. This procedure relieves pain without residual sensory loss but is potentially dangerous, as is any

surgery near the brainstem. This procedure has a long-term success rate equal to or superior to percutaneous procedures without the higher rate of permanent neurologic sequelae.

- *Glycerol rhizotomy* has become more popular in the last 10 years and is preferred over percutaneous radiofrequency rhizotomy. Glycerol rhizotomy consists of an injection of glycerol through the foramen ovale into the trigeminal cistern. Glycerol rhizotomy is a more benign procedure with less sensory loss and fewer sensory aberrations than radiofrequency rhizotomy and with comparable or better pain relief.

- *Gamma knife radiosurgery* is another surgical treatment now available. Radiosurgery using the gamma unit provides precise radiation of the proximal trigeminal nerve identified on high-resolution imaging.

Nursing Management
Goals
The patient with trigeminal neuralgia will be free of pain, maintain adequate nutritional and oral hygiene status, have minimal to no anxiety, and return to normal or previous socialization and occupational activities.

Nursing Diagnoses
- Pain *related to* inflammation or compression of the trigeminal nerve
- Altered nutrition: less than body requirements *related to* a fear of triggering pain by eating or chewing
- Anxiety *related to* the uncertainty of the timing and initiating event of pain and an uncertainty regarding the effectiveness of pain-relieving treatments
- Altered oral mucous membrane *related to* an unwillingness to practice oral hygiene measures secondary to the potential for initiating pain
- Social isolation *related to* anxiety over pain attacks and a desire to maintain a nonstimulating environment

Nursing Interventions
Pain relief is primarily obtained by the administration of the recommended drug therapy.

- The nurse should monitor the patient's response to therapy and note any side effects. Strong narcotics such as morphine should be used cautiously because of the potential for addiction over time.
- Alternative pain relief measures, such as biofeedback, should be explored for the patient who is not a surgical candidate and whose pain is not controlled by other therapeutic measures.
- Careful assessment of pain, including history, pain relief, and drug dependency, can assist in selecting appropriate interventions.

Environmental management is essential during an acute period to lessen triggering stimuli. The room should be kept at an even, moderate temperature and free of drafts. A private room is preferred during an acute period.

- The nurse must use care to avoid touching the patient's face or jarring the bed. Many patients prefer to carry out their own care, fearing that they will be inadvertently injured by someone else.

The nurse should instruct the patient about the importance of nutrition, hygiene, and oral care, conveying understanding if previous neglect is apparent.

- The nurse should provide lukewarm water and soft cloths or cotton saturated with solutions not requiring rinsing for cleansing the face. A small, very soft bristled toothbrush or a warm mouthwash assist in promoting oral care.
- Hygiene activities are best carried out when analgesia is at its peak.

The patient will probably not engage in extensive conversation during the acute period. Alternative communication methods such as paper and pencil should be provided.

Food should be high in protein and calories and easy to chew. It should be served lukewarm and offered frequently. When oral intake is markedly reduced and the patient's nutritional status is compromised, a nasogastric (NG) tube is inserted on the unaffected side for NG feedings.

For the patient who has had surgery, the patient's postoperative pain should be compared with the preoperative level. The corneal reflex, extraocular muscles, hearing, sensation, and facial nerve function are evaluated frequently. General postoperative nursing care after a craniotomy is appropriate if intracranial surgery is performed.

- After a radiofrequency percutaneous electrocoagulation procedure, an ice pack is applied to the jaw on the operative side for 3 to 5 hours. To avoid injuring the mouth, the patient should not chew on the operative side until sensation has returned.

▼ **Patient Teaching**

Regular follow-up care should be planned.

- The patient needs instruction regarding the dosage and side effects of medications.
- The patient should be encouraged to keep environmental stimuli to a moderate level and to use stress reduction methods.

Long-term management after surgical intervention depends on the residual effects of the procedure used.

- If anesthesia is present or the corneal reflex is altered, the patient should be taught to (1) chew on the unaffected side, (2) avoid hot foods or beverages that can burn the mucous membranes, (3) check the oral cavity after meals to remove food

particles, (4) practice meticulous oral hygiene and continue with semiannual dental visits, (5) protect the face against extremes of temperature, (6) use an electric razor, and (7) wear a protective eye shield.
- The patient may have developed protective practices to prevent pain and may need counseling or psychiatric assistance in the readjustment, especially in reestablishing personal relationships.

TUBERCULOSIS

Definition/Description

Tuberculosis (TB) is an infectious disease caused by *Mycobacterium tuberculosis.* It usually involves the lungs, but can also occur in the kidneys, bones, lymph nodes, meninges, and adrenal glands. TB can be disseminated throughout the body.

With the introduction of antibiotic therapy in the late 1940s and early 1950s, there was a dramatic decrease in the prevalence of TB. Today 10 to 15 million people are infected with or harbor the tubercle bacillus; the majority of these individuals have healed or dormant TB. There have been approximately 29,000 cases a year of new active TB, with approximately 10% of these cases representing relapses. These statistics indicate that TB, in spite of being potentially curable and preventable, is still a major public health problem in the United States.
- The major factors that have contributed to the resurgence of TB are (1) the emergence of multidrug-resistant strains of *M. tuberculosis* and (2) the epidemic proportions of TB among patients with HIV infections.

Pathophysiology

M. tuberculosis, a gram-positive, acid-fast bacillus, is usually spread via airborne droplet nuclei, which are produced when the infected individual coughs, sneezes, or speaks.
- Once released into a room, organisms are dispersed and can be inhaled. Brief exposure to a few tubercle bacilli rarely causes infection.
- TB is not highly infectious, and transmission usually requires close, frequent, or prolonged exposure. The disease cannot be spread by hands, books, glasses, dishes, or other fomites.

When bacilli are inhaled, they pass down the bronchial system and implant themselves on respiratory bronchioles or alveoli. Lower parts of the lungs are usually the site of the initial bacterial implantation.

- After implantation, bacilli multiply with no initial resistance from the host.
- While a cellular immune response is being activated, bacilli can be spread through lymphatic channels to regional lymph nodes and via the thoracic duct to the circulating blood.

A characteristic tissue reaction called an *epithelioid cell granuloma* results after the cellular immune system is activated. This granuloma (also called an *epithelioid cell tubercle*) is a result of fusion of infiltrating macrophages. This reaction usually takes 10 to 20 days.

Healing of the primary lesion takes place by resolution, fibrosis, and calcification.

- When a tuberculous lesion regresses and heals, the infection enters a *latent period* in which it may persist without producing clinical illness. The infection may remain dormant or it may develop into clinical disease if persisting organisms begin to multiply rapidly.
- If the initial immune response is not adequate, control of the organisms is not maintained and clinical disease results. Certain individuals at increased risk for clinical disease include those who are immunosuppressed or have diabetes mellitus (DM).
- Dormant but viable organisms persist for years. TB reactivation can occur if the host's defense mechanisms become impaired.

The classification of TB according to the American Thoracic Society is presented in Table 57.

Clinical Manifestations

In the early stages the patient is usually free of symptoms. Many cases are found incidentally when routine chest x-rays are taken, especially in older adults.

- Systemic manifestations may initially consist of fatigue, malaise, anorexia, weight loss, low grade fevers (especially in the late afternoon), and night sweats. Weight loss may not be excessive until late in the disease. Irregular menses may be present in premenopausal women.

A characteristic pulmonary manifestation is a cough that becomes frequent and produces mucoid or mucopurulent sputum. Chest pain characterized as dull or tight may also be present. Hemoptysis is not a common finding and is associated with more advanced cases.

- Sometimes TB has more acute, sudden manifestations; the patient has a high fever, chills, generalized flulike symptoms, pleuritic pain, and a productive cough.
- The HIV-infected patient with TB often has atypical physical examinations and chest x-ray findings. Classical signs such as fever, cough, and weight loss may be attributed to *Pneumocystis carinii* pneumonia or other HIV-associated opportunistic diseases.

Table 57	Classification of Tuberculosis

Class 0
No tuberculosis (TB) exposure, not infected (no history of exposure, negative tuberculin skin test)

Class 1
TB exposure, no evidence of infection (history of exposure, negative tuberculin skin test)

Class 2
TB infection without disease (significant reaction to tuberculin skin test, negative bacteriologic studies, no x-ray findings compatible with TB, no clinical evidence of TB)

Class 3
TB infection with clinically active disease (positive bacteriologic studies or both a significant reaction to tuberculin skin test and clinical or x-ray evidence of current disease)

Class 4
No current disease (history of previous episode of TB or abnormal, stable roentgenographic findings in a person with a significant reaction to tuberculin skin test; negative bacteriologic studies if done; no clinical or x-ray evidence of current disease)

Class 5
TB suspected (diagnosis pending); person should not be in this classification for more than 3 months

Source: American Thoracic Society

Complications

If a necrotic lesion erodes through a blood vessel, large numbers of organisms invade the bloodstream and spread to all body organs. This is called *miliary* or *hematogenous TB.*

- The patient may be either acutely ill with fever, dyspnea, and cyanosis or chronically ill with systemic manifestations of weight loss, fever, and GI disturbance.
- Hepatomegaly, splenomegaly, and generalized lymphadenopathy may also be present.

Pleural effusion may occur and is caused by the release of caseous material into the pleural space. Manifestations include localized pleuritic pain on deep inspiration.

Acute pneumonia may result when large amounts of tubercle bacilli are discharged from the liquefied necrotic lesion into the lungs or lymph nodes.

- Manifestations are similar to those of bacterial pneumonia, including chills, fever, productive cough, pleuritic pain, and leukocytosis.

Diagnostic Studies

- Tuberculin skin test; a positive reaction indicates an active or post-TB infection.
- Chest x-ray; a diagnosis cannot be based solely on x-ray because other diseases may mimic TB.
- Bacteriologic studies.
- A sputum smear positive for acid-fast bacillus (AFB).
- Sputum culture, which detects mycobacterium.

Collaborative Care

Most patients with TB are treated on an outpatient basis and many can continue to work and maintain their lifestyles with few changes. Hospitalization may be used for diagnostic evaluation, for the severely ill or debilitated, and for those who experience adverse drug reactions or treatment failures.

Drug Therapy

The mainstay of TB treatment is drug therapy. Drug therapy is used to treat an individual with clinical disease as well as to prevent disease in an infected person. In view of the growing prevalence of multidrug-resistant TB, the patient with active TB should be managed aggressively. The treatment of TB usually consists of a combination of at least four drugs. The reason for combination therapy is to increase therapeutic effectiveness and decrease the development of *M. tuberculosis*-resistant strains.

- The five primary drugs used are isoniazid (INH), rifampin, pyrazinamide, streptomycin, and ethambutol (Myambutol). Combinations of isoniazid and rifampin and of isoniazid, rifampin, and pyrazinamide are available.
- Other drugs are primarily used for the treatment of resistant strains or if the patient develops toxicity to the primary drugs.
- Newer drugs include the quinolones, especially ciprofloxacin (Cipro) and ofloxacin (Floxin).
- An important reason for follow-up care in the patient with TB is to ensure adherence to the treatment regimen. Noncompliance is a major factor in the emergence of multidrug resistance and treatment failures.

Drug therapy can be used to prevent TB infection from developing into clinical disease. Isoniazid prophylaxis is generally recommended for adult tuberculin reactors who have additional risk factors for active TB such as immunosuppression or DM.

Nursing Management

Goals

The patient with tuberculosis will comply with the therapeutic regimen, have no recurrence of disease, have normal pulmonary function, and take appropriate measures to prevent the spread of the disease.

Nursing Diagnoses

- Ineffective breathing pattern *related to* decreased lung capacity
- Altered nutrition: less than body requirements *related to* anorexia, fatigue, and productive cough
- Noncompliance *related to* a lack of knowledge of the disease process, a lack of motivation, and long-term treatment
- Altered health maintenance *related to* a lack of knowledge about the disease process and the therapeutic regimen
- Activity intolerance *related to* fatigue, decreased nutritional status, and chronic febrile episodes

Nursing Interventions

The public health nurse and clinical nurse have especially important responsibilities; these include the following:

- Selective screening programs in known high-risk groups are of value in detecting persons with TB
- Encouraging chest x-rays to assess for the presence of TB in persons with a positive tuberculin skin test
- Identification of contacts of the individual who has TB. These contacts should be assessed for the possibility of infection and the need for prophylactic drug treatment.
- When an individual has respiratory symptoms such as cough, dyspnea, or productive sputum, especially if accompanied by night sweats and unexplained weight loss, the nurse should assess for the presence of TB.

If acute in-hospital care is needed:

- Respiratory isolation is indicated until the patient has been on adequate drug therapy for at least 2 weeks and has shown a clinical response to the therapy.
- Masks are of limited value unless they are made of fabric designed to filter out droplet nuclei. Any mask used needs to be molded to fit tightly around the nose and mouth.

Follow-up care may be indicated during the subsequent 12 months after the medication regimen is completed; this includes bacteriologic studies and chest x-rays.

▼ Patient Teaching

- In the hospital the patient should be taught to cover the nose and mouth with paper tissue every time he or she coughs, sneezes, or produces sputum. Masks are necessary only during face-to-face contacts; it is preferable that the patient wears the mask.

- The patient should be educated so that the need for dedication to the prescribed medication regimen is fully understood. The patient should be reassured that TB can be cured if the regimen is followed.
- Because approximately 5% of individuals experience relapses, the patient should be taught to recognize symptoms that indicate the recurrence of TB. If these symptoms occur, immediate medical attention should be sought.
- The patient also needs to be instructed about factors that could reactivate TB, such as immunosuppression and malignancy.

T

ULCERATIVE COLITIS

Definition/Description

Ulcerative colitis is characterized by inflammation and ulceration of the colon and rectum. It may occur at any age but peaks between the ages of 15 and 25 years. Ulcerative colitis affects both sexes but has a higher incidence in women. It is more common in Jewish and upper middle-class urban populations.

Pathophysiology

The inflammation of ulcerative colitis is diffuse and involves the mucosa and submucosa with alternate periods of exacerbations and remissions (see Table 26, p. 174). The disease usually begins in the rectum and sigmoid colon and spreads up the colon in a continuous pattern.

- The mucosa of the colon is hyperemic and edematous in the affected area. Multiple abscesses develop in the intestinal glands. As the disease advances, the abscesses break through the crypts into the submucosa, leaving ulcerations. These ulcerations also destroy mucosal epithelium, causing bleeding and diarrhea.

Losses of fluid and electrolytes occur because of decreased mucosal surface area for absorption. The breakdown of cells results in protein loss through the stool. Areas of inflamed, undermined mucosa form *pseudopolyps.* Granulation tissue develops and the mucosa musculature becomes thickened, shortening the colon.

Clinical Manifestations

Ulcerative colitis may appear as an acute fulminating crisis or, more commonly, as a chronic disorder with mild to severe acute exacerbations that occur at unpredictable intervals over many years.

- The major symptoms are bloody diarrhea and abdominal pain. Pain may vary from the mild, lower abdominal cramping associated with diarrhea to the severe, constant abdominal pain associated with acute perforations.
- With *mild disease,* diarrhea may consist of semiformed stools containing little blood.
- The patient may have no other systemic manifestations.
- In *moderate disease* there is increased stool output (4 to 5 stools per day), increased bleeding, and systemic symptoms including fever, malaise, and anorexia.
- In *severe disease,* diarrhea is bloody, contains mucus, and occurs 10 to 20 times a day. In addition, fever, weight loss (10% of total body weight), anemia, tachycardia, and dehydration are present.

Complications

Complications may be classified into those that are intestinal and those that are extraintestinal. Intestinal complications include hemorrhage, strictures, perforation, toxic megacolon (dilation and paralysis of the colon), and colonic dilation. Extraintestinal complications may be directly related to the colitis and small intestine pathology (malabsorption). Colitis-related complications are associated with active inflammation and can involve the joints, skin, mouth, and eyes. Skin lesions such as erythema nodosum and pyoderma gangrenosum are among the most frequently seen extraintestinal manifestations. Uveitis is the most common eye problem.

- A patient who has had ulcerative colitis for more than 10 years is at greater risk for colon cancer.

Diagnostic Studies

- Complete blood count (CBC) shows anemia from blood loss.
- An elevated white blood cell (WBC) count may indicate toxic megacolon or perforation.
- Serum electrolyte decreases from diarrhea and vomiting include sodium (Na^+), potassium (K^+), chloride, bicarbonate, and magnesium.
- Stool is examined for blood; culture and sensitivity are done.
- Hypoalbuminemia with severe disease is due to protein loss from the bowel.
- Flexible sigmoidoscope to view the rectum and sigmoid colon and colonoscope to view all of the large intestine.
- Barium enema (double-contrast) may show areas of granular inflammation with ulcerations.

Collaborative Care

The goals of treatment are to rest the bowel, control inflammation and infection, correct malnutrition, alleviate stress, and provide symptomatic relief using drug therapy. Hospitalization is indicated if the patient does not respond to corticosteroid therapy or if complications are suspected.

Drug therapy is an extremely important aspect of treatment. Sulfasalazine (Azulfidine) is the principal drug used. It is effective in the maintenance of remission and in the treatment of mild to moderate attacks.

Corticosteroids are of benefit for active ulcerative colitis. Oral prednisone or prednisolone or corticosteroid enemas are effective in the treatment of mild to moderate disease. If remission is not achieved, the patient requires hospitalization and IV corticosteroid therapy.

- The patient is placed on a regimen of bowel rest. Fluids and electrolytes are administered IV. Hydrocortisone enemas and

foams are effective in the treatment of colitis limited to the rectosigmoid area.

- The patient on corticosteroids needs to be monitored for signs of Cushing's syndrome, hypertension, hirsutism, and mood swings. In some cases, psychosis may develop.
- Immunosuppressive drugs (e.g., 6-mercaptopurine [6-MP]) are used in severe cases of ulcerative colitis when a patient has failed to respond to the usual medications and before surgery is considered.

Surgical Therapy

Surgery is indicated if the patient fails to respond to treatment; exacerbations are frequent and debilitating; massive bleeding, per-foration, strictures, obstruction, or changes that suggest dysplasia occur; or carcinoma develops.

- Surgical procedures include (1) total proctocolectomy with permanent ileostomy, (2) total proctocolectomy with continent ileostomy (Kock pouch), and (3) total colectomy with rectal mucosal stripping and ileoanal reservoir.

For descriptions of these procedures, see Lewis and others, *Medical-Surgical Nursing,* edition 5, p. 1156, and NCP 40-4 for the patient with a colostomy or ileostomy, *Medical-Surgical Nursing,* p. 1175.

Nutritional Therapy

An important component in the treatment of ulcerative colitis is diet. The dietitian is an important member of the team and should be consulted regarding dietary recommendations.

- The goals of diet management are to provide adequate nutrition without exacerbating symptoms, to correct and prevent malnutrition, to replace fluid and electrolyte losses, and to prevent weight loss. The diet for each patient must be individualized.

Nursing Management

Goals

The patient with ulcerative colitis will experience a decrease in the number and severity of acute exacerbations, maintain normal fluid and electrolyte balance, be free from pain or discomfort, comply with medical regimens, maintain nutritional balance, and have regular follow-ups.

See NCP 40-3 for the patient with ulcerative colitis, Lewis and others, *Medical-Surgical Nursing,* edition 5, p. 1160.

Nursing Diagnoses/Collaborative Problems

- Diarrhea *related to* irritated bowel and intestinal hyperactivity
- Sleep pattern disturbance *related to* frequent stools

- Impaired skin integrity *related to* excoriation and/or irritation of perianal area due to diarrhea, immobility, and altered nutritional status
- Ineffective individual coping *related to* chronic disease, lifestyle changes, stress, and pain
- Anxiety *related to* possible social embarrassment, unfamiliar environment, diagnostic tests, and treatment
- Altered nutrition: less than body requirements *related to* decreased nutrient intake, increased nutrient loss through diarrhea, and decreased absorption in the intestine
- Potential complication: hypovolemia and electrolyte imbalances

Nursing Interventions

During the acute phase, attention is focused on hemodynamic stability, pain control, fluid and electrolyte balance, and nutritional support. Accurate intake and output records need to be maintained, with the number and appearance of stools also noted. Nursing care is directed toward an intensive therapeutic and supportive program.

- Emotional support is important because the patient may feel insecure, dependent, and sensitive. It is important that the nurse establish a good working relationship and encourage the patient to talk about himself or herself and his or her daily activities. An explanation of all procedures and treatments is necessary and may allay some apprehension.
- Bed rest may be ordered if the patient has a severe exacerbation. Interventions to prevent complications of immobility should be instituted. A sedative or tranquilizer may be prescribed to ensure rest. Rest is important because patients may lose sleep due to frequent episodes of diarrhea and abdominal pain. Activities should be scheduled around rest periods.
- Nutritional deficiencies and anemia leave the patient feeling weak and listless.
- Until diarrhea is controlled, the patient must be kept clean, dry, and free of odor. A bedpan and wipes should be kept within reach of the patient. The bedpan should be emptied as soon as possible. A deodorizer should be placed in the room. Antidiarrheal agents should be administered as ordered. If the patient has continuous diarrhea, the enterostomal therapy nurse or therapist may give helpful suggestions.
- Meticulous perianal skin care using plain water (no harsh soap) is necessary to treat and prevent skin breakdown. Dibucaine (Nupercainal), witch hazel, or other soothing compresses and/or prescribed ointment and sitz baths may reduce irritation and relieve discomfort of the anus.

U

URETHRITIS

Urethritis is an inflammation of the urethra that is often difficult to diagnose. Causes of urethritis include a bacterial or viral infection, *Trichomonas* and monilial infection (especially in women), chlamydia, and gonorrhea (especially in men).

Clinical manifestations of urethritis are the same as those of cystitis (see Cystitis, p. 184).

- The female urethra may be extremely tender, or there may be a discharge, especially in men.
- Inflammatory changes may make the recovery of bacteria difficult because they become entrapped in urethral tissue and do not appear in the urine.
- Urethritis may coexist with cystitis. Cultures on split urine collections or any urethral discharge may confirm a diagnosis of urethral infection.

Treatment is based on identifying and treating the cause and providing symptomatic relief.

- Sulfamethoxazole with trimethoprim (Bactrim, Septra) or nitrofurantoin (Furadantin) are examples of medications used for bacterial infections. Metronidazol (Flagyl) and clotrimazole (Lotrimin) may be used for *Trichomonas*. Medications such as nystatin (Mycostatin) may be prescribed for monilial infections. In chlamydial infections, doxycycline may be used.
- Women with negative urine cultures and no pyuria do not usually respond to antibiotics. Hot sitz baths without perfumed bath oil or bath salts may relieve the symptoms.

Patient teaching should include avoiding the use of vaginal deodorant sprays, properly cleansing the perineal area after bowel movements and urination, and avoiding intercourse until the symptoms subside.

See Cystitis, p. 184, for further information on the management of a urinary tract infection (UTI).

URINARY INCONTINENCE AND RETENTION

Definition/Description

Urinary incontinence, or the involuntary loss of urine, affects an estimated 13 million people (11 million are women) in the United States. Incontinence involves physical (infection, pressure sores, perineal rashes), psychosocial (embarrassment, isolation, depression), and economic costs. However minor the problem, incontinence can cause severe psychologic distress.

- Incontinence is not a natural consequence of aging; in most cases among older adults it can be significantly improved.

Retention is the inability to urinate in spite of the presence of urine in the bladder. Both incontinence and retention may occur in the same person.

Pathophysiology

Urinary incontinence can result from anything that interferes with bladder or urethral sphincter control.

- Causes may be transient; these include confusion or depression, infection, medications, and restricted mobility.
- Congenital disorders that produce incontinence include exstrophy of the bladder, epispadias, spina bifida with myelomeningocele, and ectopic ureteral orifice.
- Acquired disorders include stress, overflow, urge, and reflex incontinence. (For a complete description of urinary incontinence, see Table 43-16, Lewis and others, *Medical-Surgical Nursing*, edition 5, p. 1286.)

Retention can be found in association with incontinence but can also be independent of incontinence. Drugs that may cause retention include (1) antihypertensives (methyldopa [Aldomet], hydralazine [Apresoline]), (2) antiparkinsonian drugs (levodopa), (3) antihistamines, (4) anticholinergics (atropine), (5) antispasmodics (belladonna), (6) sedatives, and (7) anesthesia (especially spinal anesthesia).

- Postoperative urinary retention is not uncommon and is related to preoperative medication, anesthesia, supine position after surgery, and a low fluid intake. Postoperative retention may also be related to the effects of surgical manipulation of the sacral nerves.
- Another cause of retention is urethral obstruction, which may be caused by congenital urethral stenosis, benign prostatic hyperplasia (BPH), fecal impaction, or tumors (involving the bladder outlet).
- Psychologic problems may also contribute to urinary retention. Psychogenic urinary retention is found more commonly in women than in men.

Diagnostic Studies

- Intravenous pyelogram (IVP) and cystoscopy (including urethroscopy)
- Urodynamic studies to assess sphincter, perineal, and muscle activity
- Catheterization or ultrasound for residual urine

Collaborative Care

Treatment should correct the factors responsible for incontinence or retention if possible. Treatment includes behavioral techniques, medications, electrostimulation, and surgery.

Surgical approaches vary, depending on the underlying problem.

- A transurethral resection of the prostate is used to treat BPH.
- Urethral strictures are dilated.
- Several surgical procedures help correct anatomic malpositions of the bladder neck and urethra that cause female stress incontinence, including the Marshall-Marchetti procedure and the Pereyra procedure.
- The injection of urethral bulking agents, such as teflon or collagen, and the implantation of a prosthetic urethral sphincter, are also done for stress incontinence in selected cases.

Drug Therapy

- Vaginal or oral estrogen replacement is often prescribed for postmenopausal women to restore urethral suppleness.
- Muscarinic receptor antagonists, such as oxybutynin (Ditropan) and dicyclomine hydrochloride (Bentyl), are used to treat hyperreflexic bladders by suppressing the unwanted contractions that occur when the bladder has only a small volume of urine. These drugs have significant anticholinergic effects, such as drying of the mouth and eyes.
- α-Adrenergic blockers such as prazosin (Minipress) can be used to relax spastic bladder necks.
- Imipramine (Tofranil) and calcium channel blockers (nifedipine [Procardia]) reduce detrusor contractions and improve continence. Side effects from these drugs are common, especially in older patients.

Nursing Management

The nurse must recognize both the physical and the emotional problems that accompany incontinence. The patient's dignity, privacy, and feelings of self-worth must be maintained or enhanced. Most persons suffering from incontinence can be helped with proper diagnosis and modern therapeutic approaches.

- A patient with stress incontinence can be taught to do pelvic floor (perineal) muscle exercises (Kegel exercises). Consistency and persistence are necessary for success, and exercise regimens have to be individualized.
- Vaginal weights or biofeedback may help patients to gain awareness and control of their pelvic muscles.

The nurse has a major responsibility to help patients with incontinence problems in a variety of settings.

- In the hospital, nursing measures aimed at maintaining urinary continence include identifying transient causes and assessing the patient for signs of bladder infection, fecal impaction, or bladder distention. The nurse should offer the urinal or bedpan or help the patient to the bathroom every 2 hours or at scheduled times.

- Assuming the usual position for urination (standing for the man and sitting and leaning forward for the woman) or using relaxation techniques often help a patient to urinate successfully, particularly in unfamiliar settings.
- Applying pressure over the bladder area (Credé's maneuver) may be helpful when bladder outlet obstruction is not a problem.
- The nurse should be sure the patient has privacy and is not rushed when trying to urinate.
- Techniques to stimulate urination include running water in the sink, placing the hands in water, and pouring warm water over the perineum.

Fluid restriction, incontinence pads, and keeping a urinal in place at all times are only temporary measures to reduce the occurrence or effects of incontinence. Long-term use of these measures discourages continence and can lead to dehydration and skin problems.

- The patient should be taught that incontinence is not a normal part of aging and that it can be eliminated or controlled in most cases.
- If bladder retraining cannot be achieved, external appliances or intermittent self-catheterization may be indicated.

URINARY TRACT CALCULI

U

Definition/Description
Each year an estimated 500,000 people in the United States have *nephrolithiasis* (kidney stone disease). Except for *struvite* (an infected stone), which is more common in women, stone disorders are more common in men. The majority of patients are between 20 and 55 years of age.

- The incidence is also higher in persons with a family history of stone formation. Recurrence of stones can occur in up to 80% of patients.
- The term *calculus* refers to the stone and *lithiasis* refers to stone formation.

Pathophysiology
Many factors are involved in the incidence and type of stone formation, including metabolic, dietary, genetic, climatic, lifestyle, and occupational influences. Many theories have been proposed to explain the formation of stones in the urinary tract.

- Crystals, when in a supersaturated concentration, can precipitate and unite to form a stone. Keeping urine dilute and free-flowing reduces the risk of recurrent stone formation in many individuals.
- Urinary pH, solute load, and inhibitors in the urine affect the formation of stones. The higher the pH, the less soluble are calcium and phosphate. The lower the pH, the less soluble are uric acid and cystine.

Other important factors in the development of stones include obstruction with urinary stasis and urinary infection with urea-splitting bacteria (e.g., *Proteus, Klebsiella, Pseudomonas,* and some species of staphylococci). These bacteria cause the urine to become alkaline and contribute to the formation of calcium-magnesium-ammonium phosphate stones (struvite or triple phosphate stones).

- Infected stones, when entrapped in the kidney, may assume a staghorn configuration as they enlarge. Infected stones are frequent with an external urinary diversion, long-term indwelling catheter, neurogenic bladder, or urinary retention.
- There are five major categories of stones: calcium phosphate, calcium oxalate, uric acid, cystine, and struvite (magnesium ammonium phosphate). Stone composition may be mixed, although calcium stones are the most common.

Clinical Manifestations

Urinary stones cause manifestations when they obstruct the urinary flow; manifestations include hematuria, abdominal or flank pain, and renal colic.

- The type of pain is determined by the location of the stone. If the stone is nonobstructing, pain may be absent. If it produces obstruction in a calyx or at the ureteropelvic junction (UPJ), the patient may experience dull costovertebral flank pain or even colic. Pain resulting from the passage of a calculus down the ureter is intense and colicky. The patient may be in mild shock with cool, moist skin. As a stone nears the ureterovesical junction (UVJ), pain will be felt in the lateral flank and sometimes down into the scrotum, labia, or groin.
- Other manifestations include the presence of urinary infection accompanied by fever, vomiting, nausea, and chills.

Diagnostic Studies

- Blood urea nitrogen (BUN) and serum creatinine to assess renal function
- CT scan to differentiate a nonopaque stone from a tumor
- Urine and serum levels of substances involved in stone formation (e.g., calcium, phosphate, oxalate, and uric acid)

- Urine pH for struvite stones (tendency for acidic pH) and renal tubular necrosis (tendency for alkaline pH)
- X-rays of kidneys, ureters, and bladder (KUB) with tomograms to determine the location, size, and number of radiopaque stones
- Intravenous pyelogram (IVP) or retrograde pyelogram to further localize the degree and site of obstruction and confirm the presence of nonradiopaque stones (uric acid, cystine).

Collaborative Care

Evaluation and management of the patient consists of two concurrent approaches.

The *first approach* is directed toward management of the acute attack. This involves treating the symptoms of pain, infection, or obstruction. At frequent intervals, narcotics are typically required for relief of renal colic pain. Many stones pass spontaneously. However, stones >4 mm in size are unlikely to pass through the ureter.

The *second approach* is directed toward evaluation of the etiology of the stone formation and the prevention of further development of stones. Information to be obtained from the patient includes family history of stone formation, geographical residence, nutritional assessment (including the intake of vitamins A and D), activity pattern (active or sedentary), history of periods of prolonged illness with immobilization or dehydration, and any history of disease or surgery involving the GI or genitourinary (GU) tract.

Indications for surgical, endoscopic, or lithotripsy stone removal include:

- Stones too large for spontaneous passage, associated with bacteriuria or symptomatic infection, causing impaired renal function, persistent pain, nausea, or ileus
- An inability of the patient to be treated medically
- A patient with one kidney

If the stone is located in the bladder, a *cystoscopy* is done to remove small stones. For large stones, a *cystolithoplaxy* is done. A *cystoscopic lithotripsy* is used to pulverize stones. Complications with these cystoscopic procedures include hemorrhage, retained stone fragments, and infection.

Lithotripsy techniques include percutaneous ultrasonic lithotripsy, electrohydraulic lithotripsy, laser lithotripsy, and extracorporeal shock wave lithotripsy. Laser lithotripsy and extracorporeal shock wave lithotripsy are the most common.

- In *laser lithotripsy* probes are used to fragment lower ureteral and large bladder stones.
- In *extracorporeal shock wave lithotripsy,* a noninvasive procedure, the patient is anesthetized (spinal or general) and placed

in a water bath. Fluoroscopy or ultrasound is then used to focus the lithotripter on the affected kidney, and a high-voltage spark generator produces high-energy acoustic shock waves that shatter the stone without damaging the surrounding tissues. The stone is broken down into fine sand, which is excreted into the patient's urine within a few days of the procedure.

Hematuria is common after lithotripsy procedures. A self-retaining ureteral stent is often placed after the procedure to promote passage of this sand and to prevent obstruction caused by *steinstrasse* (a buildup of sand in the ureter). The stent is removed 1 to 2 weeks after lithotripsy. A primary advantage of these techniques compared with open surgery is the decrease in the length of hospitalization and the patient's earlier return to normal activities.

There is a small group of select patients who need open surgical procedures, such as very obese patients or those with complex abnormalities in the calyces or at the UPJ. The type of open surgery needed depends on the location of the stone.

- A *nephrolithotomy* is an incision into the kidney to remove a stone. A *pyelolithotomy* is an incision into the renal pelvis to remove a stone. If the stone is located in the ureter, a *ureterolithotomy* is performed. A *cystotomy* may be indicated for bladder calculi. For open surgery on the kidney or ureter, a flank incision directly below the diaphragm and across the side is usually the preferred surgical approach.

Nutritional Therapy

A high fluid intake (at least 3000 ml/day) is recommended after an episode of urolithiasis to produce a urine output of at least 2 L/day.

- A high urine output prevents the supersaturation of minerals (i.e., dilutes the concentration) and flushes them out before they have a chance to precipitate.
- Increasing the fluid intake is especially important for those who live in a dry climate, perform physical exercise, have a family history of stone formation, or work in an occupation that requires outdoor work that can lead to dehydration.

Dietary intervention may be important in the management of urolithiasis.

- Recent research suggests that a high level of calcium in the diet, which was previously thought to contribute to kidney stones, may actually lower the risk by reducing the urinary excretion of oxalate, a common factor in many stones.
- Initial nutritional therapy should include limiting oxalate-rich foods, thereby reducing oxalate excretion. Foods high in calcium, oxalate, and purines are presented in Table 43-11, Lewis and others, *Medical-Surgical Nursing,* edition 5, p. 1276.

Nursing Management

Goals

The patient with urinary tract calculi will have relief of pain, no urinary tract obstruction, and an understanding of measures to prevent further recurrence of stones.

See NCP 43-2 for the patient with acute renal lithiasis, Lewis and others, *Medical-Surgical Nursing,* edition 5, p. 1278.

Nursing Diagnoses/Collaborative Problems

- Pain *related to* irritation from stone obstruction of urine flow and inadequate pain control or comfort measures
- Ineffective management of therapeutic regimen *related to* a lack of knowledge about prevention of recurrence, diet, fluid requirements, and symptoms of recurrence
- Anxiety *related to* the uncertain outcome and lack of knowledge regarding possible surgery
- Potential complication: urinary obstruction *related to* the presence of a stone in the path of urine flow

Nursing Interventions

Preventive measures relate to the person who is on bed rest or is relatively immobile for a prolonged time.

- It is important to maintain a high fluid intake as well as prevent urinary stasis by turning the patient every 2 hours and helping the patient to sit or stand if possible.
- In the acute phase it is important to retrieve the stone if passed. All urine voided by the patient should be strained through gauze or a special urine strainer in an effort to detect the stone. Encouraging fluids and ambulation help the stone pass down the urinary tract.
- Narcotics will be required for renal colic because the pain is excruciating. Pain management and patient comfort are primary nursing responsibilities.

▼ Patient Teaching

Stone formation can be prevented and the recurrence rate can be greatly reduced. After the acute phase, it is important for the nurse to teach the patient ways to prevent its recurrence.

- Dietary restriction of oxalate is important for patients who have calcium oxalate stones. Diets that restrict purines may be helpful to patients at risk of developing uric acid stones.
- Follow-up care includes monitoring the patient's compliance with fluid and dietary recommendations.
- Periodic urine cultures may be indicated. Testing the pH of the urine is important, especially to assess the effectiveness of acidifying or alkalinizing agents.
- It is important to emphasize the need to avoid inadvertent dehydration from excessive exercise and to increase fluid consumption during illness.

URINARY TRACT INFECTION

Definition/Description

Urinary tract infections (UTIs) are a common bacterial disease. The most common cause is a microbial invasion of the tissues of the urinary tract, most often by *Escherichia coli*.

- Bacterial counts in the urine of 10^5 organisms or more generally indicate a UTI. However, bacterial counts as low as 10^2 to 10^3 in a person with symptoms are also indicative of UTI.
- Viral, fungal, and parasitic UTIs are not as common, but are seen most frequently in the patient who is immunosuppressed, has diabetes mellitus (DM), or has taken multiple courses of antibiotics.

Classification

Infections may be broadly classified as upper and lower UTIs based on the patient's symptoms. Terminology may specifically delineate the site of inflammation or infection. Examples of terms are *pyelonephritis* (involvement of the kidney and kidney pelvis) or *cystitis* (involvement of the bladder).

- It may be difficult to determine the specific location of a UTI. A patient may have a simultaneous infection in both the upper and lower urinary tract, an infection of adjacent organs causing urinary infection–like symptoms, or no symptoms at all.

Determining whether a UTI is uncomplicated or complicated is a significant factor in determining the treatment plan.

- *Uncomplicated infections* are those that occur in an otherwise normal urinary tract.
- *Complicated infections* include the coexisting presence of obstruction, stones, or catheters; the existence of diabetes or neurologic diseases; or when an infection is a recurrent one. The individual with a complicated infection is at an increased risk of renal damage.

Only about 25% of individuals who develop an acute infection develop recurrent UTIs. Recurrent UTIs can be classified as *relapses* (recurrences with the same strain of bacteria from within the urinary tract that occur within 1 to 2 weeks of stopping antibiotic therapy) or *reinfections* (recurrences with a new organism following successful treatment).

Pathophysiology

The organisms that usually cause UTIs are introduced via the ascending route from the urethra. Other less common routes are via the blood stream or lymphatic system. Most infections are due to gram-negative aerobic bacilli normally found in the GI tract.

- A common factor contributing to ascending infection is urologic instrumentation (e.g., catheterization, cystoscopic examinations). Instrumentation allows bacteria that are normally present at the opening of the urethra to enter the urethra or bladder.
- Sexual intercourse promotes the milking of bacteria from the vagina and perineum and may cause minor urethral trauma that predisposes women to UTIs.
- Rarely do UTIs result from a hematogenous route, where blood-borne bacteria secondarily invade the kidneys, ureters, or bladder from elsewhere in the body.

The following risk factors may predispose a patient to infection:

- Renal scarring from previous UTI
- Diminished ureteral peristalsis (e.g., in pregnancy)
- Urinary retention for any reason
- Presence of a foreign body (e.g., a urinary catheter)
- Vesicoureteral reflux of urine in a retrograde direction from the bladder toward the kidney
- Humoral or cellular immune deficiency in an otherwise normal urinary tract
- Shorter urethra in females
- Presence of urinary calculi
- Clinical disorders (e.g., neurogenic bladder, spinal cord injury, DM)

An important source of UTIs is hospital-acquired, or *nosocomial,* infection. The cause is often *Escherichia coli* and (less frequently) *Pseudomonas* organisms.

- The occurrence of UTIs is often related to the presence of abnormalities of the urinary tract, such as strictures and obstructions. An untreated UTI can lead to chronic pyelonephritis and a progressive decrease in renal function. If no abnormality exists, uncomplicated pyelonephritis rarely leads to progressive renal damage and renal failure.

For further information on UTIs, including manifestations, diagnostic studies, and management, see Cystitis, p. 184, Pyelonephritis, p. 486, and Urethritis, p. 594.

VAGINAL, CERVICAL, AND VULVAR INFECTIONS

Definition/Description

Infection and inflammation of the vagina, cervix, and vulva tend to occur when the natural defenses of the acid vaginal secretions (maintained by sufficient estrogen levels) and the presence of *Lactobacillus* are disrupted. A woman's resistance may also be decreased as a result of aging, poor nutrition, and the use of drugs that alter the mucosa.

Pathophysiology

Organisms gain entrance to these areas through contaminated hands, clothing, douche nozzles, and during intercourse, surgery, and childbirth. Table 58 presents the etiology, clinical manifestations, diagnostic methods, and collaborative care of common infections of the lower genital tract.

- Most lower genital tract infections are related to sexual intercourse. Vulvar infections, such as herpes and genital warts, can be sexually transmitted when no lesions are present.
- Drugs such as oral contraceptives, antibiotics, and corticosteroids may produce changes in the vagina and trigger an overgrowth of the organisms present. For example, *Candida albicans* may be present in small numbers in the vagina. An overgrowth of this organism causes yeast vaginitis.

Clinical Manifestations

- Abnormal vaginal discharge and vulvar lesions are common. Cervicitis and vaginal problems may be accompanied by an abnormal vaginal discharge.
- In addition to a thick white curdy discharge, women with monilial vaginitis often experience intense itching and dysuria.
- The hallmark of bacterial vaginosis is the fishy odor of the discharge.
- Women with cervicitis may notice spotting after intercourse.
- Common vulvar lesions include herpes infection and genital warts. Initial or primary herpes infections may be extremely painful, tender, or even go unnoticed. Herpes begins as a small vesicle followed by superficial red ulcers. Dysuria is common when urine touches the lesion.
- Genital warts, caused by the human papillomavirus (HPV), vary in appearance. Irregularly shaped "cauliflower"-type lesions are common. Genital warts are painless unless traumatized.

Table 58 Infections of the Lower Genital Tract

Infection/etiology	Clinical manifestations and diagnostic methods	Drug management
■ Monilial vaginitis Candida albicans (fungus)	Commonly found in mouth, GI tract, and vagina; pruritus, thick white curdy discharge; KOH microscopic examination—pseudohyphae; pH 4.0-4.7	Antifungal agents (e.g., Monistat, Gyne-Lotrimin, Mycelex [available over the counter]) available in cream or suppository.
■ Trichomoniasis Trichomonas vaginalis (protozoa)	Sexually transmitted; pruritus, frothy greenish or gray discharge; hemorrhagic spots on cervix or vaginal walls; saline microscopic examination—swimming trichomonads; pH 5.0-7.0.	Metronidazole (Flagyl) po in single dose for patient and partner.
■ Bacterial vaginosis Gardnerella vaginalis Corynebacterium vaginale	Watery discharge with fishy odor; may or may not have other symptoms; saline microscopic examination—epithelial cells; pH 5.0-5.5.	Sexually transmitted; metronidazole (Flagyl) 500 mg po or clindamycin (Cleocin) 300 mg po bid for 7 days; examine and treat partner.
■ Cervicitis Chlamydia trachomatis Neisseria gonorrhoeae Staphylococcus aureus	Sexually transmitted; mucopurulent discharge with postcoital spotting from cervical inflammation; culture for chlamydia and gonorrhea.	Azithromycin (Zithromax) po single dose or doxycycline po bid for 7 days and ciprofloxacin (Cipro) po single dose or ceftriaxone (Rocephin) IM in single dose. Treat partners with same drugs.
■ Severe recurrent vaginitis Candida albicans (most often)	May be indication of HIV infection; all women who are unresponsive to first-line treatment should be counseled and offered HIV testing.	Drug appropriate to opportunistic organism.

bid, Twice a day; *GI,* gastrointestinal; *HIV,* human immunodeficiency virus; *IM,* intramuscular; *po,* orally; *WBCs,* white blood cells.

V

- Older women may develop vulvar dystrophies, including lichen sclerosis and squamous cell hyperplasia. These conditions are associated with intense itching. The lesions are white initially, although scratching in response to itching produces changes in the appearance.

Diagnostic Studies
Genital problems
- History, physical exam, and sexual history need to be obtained.
- Ulcerative lesions need to be cultured.
- Blood test for syphilis when ulcerative lesions are present.
- Vulva dystrophies are examined by colposcope, and biopsies are taken for diagnosis.

Vaginal discharge problems
- Microscopy and culture of vaginal discharge.
- Most common vaginal conditions (bacterial vaginosis, monilial vaginitis, and trichomoniasis) are diagnosed by a wet mount.
- For cervicitis, endocervical cultures are obtained for chlamydia and gonorrhea. If purulent discharge is observed coming from the cervix, endocervical cells may be taken to conduct a Gram's stain.

Collaborative Care
Antibiotics taken as directed will cure bacterial infections. Antifungal preparations, usually creams, are indicated for monilial vaginitis. Women with vaginal conditions or cervical infection should abstain from intercourse for at least 1 week. Douching should be avoided as it disrupts the normal protective mechanisms within the vagina. Sexual partners must be evaluated and treated if the patient is diagnosed with trichomoniasis or cervicitis.

Viral infections such as herpes and genital warts cannot be cured. Systemic antiviral drugs may reduce the duration and severity of recurrent herpes outbreaks (see Herpes, Genital, p. 303). Non-drug measures such as wearing loose fitting clothes and sitz baths may decrease discomfort. Many women with visible genital warts want them removed for cosmetic reasons. Application of liquid nitrogen is a common treatment. Women with genital warts or those who have partners with genital warts are advised to get annual Pap tests.

Drug therapy for dystrophies is symptomatic because a cure is not available. Treatment involves controlling the itching and hence the scratching. Interrupting the "itch-scratch cycle" prevents further secondary damage to the skin. Women should be monitored annually for squamous cell cancer because it also presents as a vulvar lesion with intense itching.

Nursing Management
Nurses have the opportunity to educate women about common genital conditions and how women can reduce their risks. Understanding

the symptoms that may indicate a problem will help women seek care in a timely manner. Matters involving genitals or sexual intercourse are frequently difficult for people to discuss. The nurse's nonjudgmental attitude in providing information will allow women to feel more comfortable and ask the questions that may be especially worrisome.

- When a woman is diagnosed with cervicitis or a vaginal or vulvar condition, the nurse should ensure that she fully understands the directions for treatment. Taking the full course of medication is especially important to decrease the chance of relapse. Because genitals are such a private area, the use of graphs and models is especially helpful for patient teaching.
- When a woman will be using a vaginal medication, such as an antifungal cream, for the first time, showing her the applicator and how to fill it is important. The woman should be taught where and how the applicator should be inserted by using visual aids or models.

VALVULAR HEART DISEASE

Definition/Description

The types of valvular heart disease are defined according to the valve(s) affected and the two types of functional alterations, *stenosis* and *regurgitation*.

- The pressure on either side of an open valve is normally equal. However, in a stenotic valve the valve orifice is restricted, impeding the forward flow of blood and creating a pressure gradient difference across an open valve. The degree of stenosis is reflected in the pressure gradient differences (i.e., the higher the gradient, the greater the stenosis).
- In regurgitation (also called *valvular incompetence* or *insufficiency*) incomplete closure of valve leaflets results in a backward flow of blood.

Valvular disorders occur in children and adolescents primarily from congenital conditions such as tricuspid atresia, pulmonary stenosis, and aortic stenosis. Rheumatic heart disease is a common cause of adult valvular disease.

Mitral Stenosis

Pathophysiology. The majority of adult cases of mitral stenosis result from rheumatic heart disease. Less common causes include congenital mitral stenosis, rheumatoid arthritis, and systemic lupus erythematous (SLE).

V

- Rheumatic endocarditis causes scarring of valve leaflets and chordae tendineae. Contractures develop with adhesions between the commissures (junctional areas) of the two leaflets.
- The stenotic mitral valve assumes a funnel shape because of the thickening and shortening of the structures composing the mitral valve. Flow obstruction increases left atrial pressure and volume, resulting in increased pressure in the pulmonary vasculature.

Clinical manifestations. Dyspnea, sometimes accompanied by hemoptysis, is the primary symptom of mitral stenosis because of reduced lung compliance (Table 59).

- Palpitations from atrial fibrillation and fatigue may be present. Auscultatory findings generally include a loud or accentuated first heart sound, an opening snap (best heard at apex with stethoscope diaphragm), and a low-pitched, rumbling diastolic murmur (best heard at apex with stethoscope bell).
- Less frequently, patients with mitral stenosis may have hoarseness, chest pain, seizures, or a cerebrovascular accident (CVA).

Mitral Regurgitation

Pathophysiology. Mitral valve patency depends on the integrity of mitral leaflets, chordae tendineae, papillary muscles, left atrium (LA), and left ventricle (LV). An anatomic or functional abnormality of any of these structures can result in regurgitation.

- Causes of chronic and acute mitral regurgitation are numerous and may be inflammatory, degenerative, infective, structural, or congenital. The majority of cases may be attributed to chronic rheumatic heart disease, mitral valve prolapse, and infectious endocarditis.
- In chronic mitral regurgitation, volume overload on the LV, LA, and pulmonary bed is created by the backward flow of blood from the LV into the LA during ventricular systole, resulting in varying degrees of left atrial enlargement and left ventricular dilation.
- Acute mitral regurgitation does not result in dilation of the LA or LV. Without dilation to accommodate regurgitant volume, pulmonary vascular pressures rise, ultimately causing pulmonary edema.

Clinical manifestations

- The clinical picture in acute mitral regurgitation is that of pulmonary edema and shock (see Table 59). Patients will have thready, peripheral pulses and cool, clammy extremities.
- Auscultatory findings of a new systolic murmur may be obscured by a low cardiac output (CO) state.
- Patients with chronic mitral regurgitation may remain asymptomatic for many years until the development of some degree of left ventricular failure.

Table 59   Clinical Manifestations and Diagnostic Findings of Valvular Heart Diseases

	Clinical manifestations	Electrocardiogram
Mitral valve stenosis	Dyspnea, hemoptysis; fatigue; palpitations; loud, accentuated S_1; opening snap; low-pitched, rumbling diastolic murmur	Right axis deviation, left atrial enlargement, right ventricular hypertrophy, P "mitrale," P "mitrale" (wide, M-shaped P wave), atrial flutter or fibrillation
Mitral valve regurgitation	Acute—generally poorly tolerated with fulminating pulmonary edema and shock developing rapidly; systolic murmur	Left atrial enlargment, atrial fibrillation
	Chronic—weakness, fatigue, exertional dyspnea, palpitations; an S_3 gallop, holosystolic or pansystolic murmur	P mitrale, left ventricular hypertrophy, atrial flutter or fibrillation
Mitral valve prolapse	Palpitations, dyspnea, chest pain, activity intolerance, syncope; mobile midsystolic nonejection click and a late or holosystolic murmur	Usually normal; occasionally T wave inversion or biplasticity in leads II, III, and aVF are noted; complications of PVCs and tachyarrhythmias reported

Continued

V

Table 59 Clinical Manifestations and Diagnostic Findings of Valvular Heart Diseases—cont'd

	Clinical manifestations	Electrocardiogram
Aortic valve stenosis	Angina pectoris, syncope, heart failure, normal or soft S_1, prominent S_4, crescendo-decrescendo murmur	Left ventricular hypertrophy, left bundle branch block, complete atrioventricular heart block
Aortic valve regurgitation	*Acute*—abrupt onset of profound dyspnea, transient chest pain, progression to shock *Chronic*—fatigue, exertional dyspnea; Corrigan's pulse; heaving precordial impulse; diastolic high-pitched soft decrescendo diastolic murmur, characteristic Austin-Flint murmur at diastolic rumble, systolic ejection click	Left ventricular strain Left ventricular hypertrophy
Tricuspid stenosis and regurgitation	Peripheral edema, ascites, hepatomegaly; diastolic low-pitched, decrescendo murmur with increased intensity during inspiration (stenosis), pansystolic murmur with increased intensity at inspiration (regurgitation)	Tall, peaked P waves; atrial fibrillation

- Initial symptoms include weakness, fatigue, and dyspnea that gradually progress to orthopnea, paroxysmal nocturnal dyspnea, and peripheral edema.
- Patients with chronic mitral regurgitation have brisk carotid pulses.
- Auscultatory findings reflect accentuated left ventricular filling leading to an audible third heart sound (S_3), even in the absence of left ventricular dysfunction.

Mitral Valve Prolapse

Pathophysiology. Mitral valve prolapse (MVP) is a failure of one or both leaflets to fit together, resulting in displacement of an involved leaflet edge toward the atrium during systole.

- The etiology of MVP is unknown but is related to diverse pathogenic mechanisms. MVP can occur in the presence of redundant mitral valve leaflets, enlarged mitral annulus, and abnormally contracting left ventricular wall segments.
- MVP is the most common form of valvular heart disease in the United States. MVP is eight times as common among women as men.
- It is usually benign, but serious complications can occur, including mitral regurgitation, infective endocarditis, sudden death, and cerebral ischemia.
- There is an increased familial incidence in some patients resulting from a connective tissue defect affecting only the valve or arising as part of Marfan syndrome or other hereditary conditions that influence the structure of collagen in the body.

Clinical manifestations. MVP encompasses a broad spectrum of severity. Most patients are asymptomatic and remain so for their entire lives.

- A characteristic of MVP is a murmur from insufficiency that gets more intense through systole (see Table 59). This could be a late or holosystolic murmur.
- Another major sign is one or more clicks usually heard in mid- to late systole (between first heart sound [S_1] and second heart sound [S_2]) and less frequently in early systole. MVP does not alter S_1 or S_2 heart sounds.
- Arrhythmias, premature ventricular contractions (PVCs), paroxysmal supraventricular tachycardia, and ventricular tachycardia may cause palpitations, lightheadedness, and dizziness.
- Patients may or may not have chest pain. If episodes of chest pain occur, the episodes tend to occur in clusters, especially during periods of emotional stress. The chest pain may occasionally be accompanied by dyspnea, palpitations, and syncope.

Aortic Stenosis

Pathophysiology. Congenitally abnormal stenotic aortic valves are generally discovered in childhood, adolescence, or young adulthood.

V

A patient seen later in life usually has aortic stenosis from traumatic heart disease, calcific degeneration of a bicuspid valve, or senile calcific degeneration of a normal valve.

- Aortic stenosis results in an obstruction to flow from the LV to the aorta during systole. The effect is concentric left ventricular hypertrophy and increased myocardial oxygen consumption because of increased myocardial mass.
- As the disease course progresses and compensatory mechanisms fail, reduced CO leads to pulmonary hypertension.

Clinical manifestations. Symptoms of aortic stenosis (see Table 59) develop when the valve orifice becomes approximately one third its normal size and classically include angina pectoris, syncope, and heart failure.

- The prognosis is poor for a patient with symptoms and whose valve obstruction is not relieved.
- Auscultatory findings of aortic stenosis typically reveal a normal or soft first heart sound (S_1), a diminished or absent second heart sound (S_2), a systolic, crescendo-decrescendo murmur that ends before the second heart sound (S_2), and a prominent fourth heart sound (S_4).

Aortic Regurgitation

Pathophysiology. Aortic regurgitation may be the result of a primary disease of the aortic valve leaflets, the aortic root, or both.

- Acute aortic regurgitation is caused by bacterial endocarditis, trauma, or aortic dissection. It constitutes a life threatening emergency.
- Chronic aortic regurgitation is generally the result of rheumatic heart disease, a congenital bicuspid aortic valve, syphilis, or chronic arthritic conditions such as ankylosing spondylitis (AS) or Reiter's syndrome.
- The basic physiologic consequence of aortic regurgitation is retrograde blood flow from the ascending aorta into the LV, resulting in volume overload.
- Myocardial contractility eventually declines and blood volumes increase in the LA and pulmonary vasculature. Ultimately, pulmonary hypertension and right ventricular failure develop.

Clinical manifestations. Patients with acute aortic regurgitation have sudden clinical manifestations of cardiovascular collapse (see Table 59).

- The LV is exposed to aortic pressure during diastole and the patient develops weakness, severe dyspnea, and hypotension that generally constitutes a medical emergency.
- Patients with chronic, severe aortic regurgitation have pulses that are of the water-hammer or collapsing type with abrupt distention during systole and quick collapse during diastole *(Corrigan's pulse).*

- Auscultatory findings may include a soft or absent S_1, presence of a S_3 or S_4, and a soft, decrescendo high-pitched diastolic murmur. A systolic ejection murmur may also be heard, and the *Austin-Flint murmur*, a low frequency diastolic rumble similar to that of mitral stenosis, may be auscultated.
- The patient with chronic aortic regurgitation generally remains asymptomatic for years and is seen with exertional dyspnea, orthopnea, and paroxysmal nocturnal dyspnea only after considerable myocardial dysfunction has occurred.
- A nocturnal angina accompanied by diaphoresis and abdominal discomfort may be present.

Diagnostic Studies

- Chest x-ray reveals heart size, alterations in pulmonary circulation, and valve calcification.
- ECG shows variations in heart rate (HR), rhythm, and possible ischemia or chamber enlargement.
- Echocardiography provides information on valve structure and function and on chamber enlargement.
- Cardiac catheterization detects chamber pressure changes and pressure gradients across the valves.

Collaborative Care

An important aspect of conservative therapy is the prevention of recurrent rheumatic fever and infective endocarditis. Treatment of valvular heart disease depends on the valve involved and the severity of the disease. It focuses on preventing exacerbations of heart failure, acute pulmonary edema, thromboembolism, and recurrent endocarditis. If manifestations of congestive heart failure (CHF) develop, digitalis, diuretics, and a low-sodium (Na^+) diet are recommended.

- Anticoagulant therapy is used to prevent and treat systemic or pulmonary embolization, and it is also used as a prophylactic measure in patients with atrial fibrillation.
- Arrhythmias, especially atrial arrhythmias, are common with valvular heart disease and are treated with digitalis, antiarrhythmic drugs, or electrical cardioversion. β-Adrenergic blocking drugs may be used to slow the ventricular rate in patients with atrial fibrillation.
- Oral nitrates may be prescribed for patients with aortic valvular disease because the resulting peripheral vasodilation reduces the blood volume returning to the heart and subsequently decreases the pressure gradient between the aorta and LV, allowing the ventricle to pump more effectively. In addition, nitrates improve coronary artery perfusion and reduce myocardial oxygen consumption.

An alternative treatment for some patients with valvular heart disease is the *percutaneous transluminal balloon valvuloplasty* (PTBV) procedure. Balloon valvuloplasty has been used for pulmonic, aortic, and mitral stenosis. The procedure, performed in the cardiac catheterization laboratory, involves threading a balloon-tipped catheter from the femoral artery to the stenotic valve so that the balloon may be inflated in an attempt to separate valve leaflets.

- The PTBV procedure is generally indicated for older adult patients and patients who are poor surgical candidates.
- Complications are fewer for those undergoing PTBV versus valve replacement. The long-term results of PTBV seem promising.

Surgical Therapy

The type of surgery used for a particular patient depends on the valves involved, valvular pathology, the severity of the disease, and the patient's clinical condition. All types of valve surgery are palliative, and patients will require lifelong health care.

- Valve repair is becoming the surgical procedure of choice. Reparative or reconstructive procedures are often used in mitral or tricuspid valvular heart disease. Repair of these valves has a lower operative mortality than does replacement.
- *Mitral commissurotomy* (valvulotomy) is the procedure of choice for patients with pure mitral stenosis. The less precise *closed* (without cardiopulmonary bypass) *method* of commissurotomy has generally been replaced by the open method in the United States, Canada, and Western Europe. The closed mitral commissurotomy is generally performed in developing nations. Cost considerations are a major factor.
- Further repair or reconstruction of the valve may be necessary and can be achieved by *annuloplasty,* a procedure also used in cases of mitral or tricuspid regurgitation. Annuloplasty entails reconstruction of valve leaflets and the annulus, with or without aid of prosthetic rings (e.g., Carpentier ring).
- Open surgical *valvuloplasty* involves repairing the valve or suturing the torn leaflets. It is primarily performed to treat mitral regurgitation or tricuspid regurgitation. The main advantage of a reparative procedure is that it avoids the risks associated with valve replacement. The disadvantage is that it may not be possible to establish total valve competence.

Prosthetic valves. Valvular replacement may be required for mitral, aortic, tricuspid, and occasionally, pulmonic valvular disease. The surgical treatment of choice for combined aortic stenosis and aortic regurgitation is valvular replacement.

- The two categories of prosthetic valves are *mechanical* and *biologic (tissue) valves.* Mechanical valves are made of combinations of metal alloys, pyrolite carbon, and Dacron. Biologic valves are constructed from bovine, porcine, and human cardiac tissue. Mechanical prosthetic valves are more durable and last longer than biologic tissue valves but have an increased risk of thromboembolism, which necessitates the use of long-term anticoagulant therapy. Biologic valves offer the patient freedom from anticoagulant therapy as a result of their low thrombogenicity. However, their durability is limited by the tendency for early calcification, tissue degeneration, and stiffening of leaflets.

- Long-term anticoagulation is recommended for all patients with mechanical prostheses and for patients with biologic tissue valves who are in atrial fibrillation. Some patients with biologic tissue valves or annuloplasty with prosthetic rings may require anticoagulation during the first few months after surgery.
- The choice of a valvular prosthesis depends on many factors. For example, if a patient cannot take anticoagulant therapy (e.g., women of childbearing age), a biologic valve may be considered. A mechanical valve may be considered for a younger patient because it is more durable and lasts longer. For patients over the age of 65 the importance of durability is less of an issue, but the risks of noncompliance or hemorrhage from anticoagulants may be greater.

Nursing Management

Goals

The patient with valvular heart disease will have normal cardiac function, improved activity tolerance, and an understanding of the disease process and preventive measures.

See NCP 35-3 for the patient with valvular heart disease, Lewis and others, *Medical-Surgical Nursing,* edition 5, p. 974.

Nursing Diagnoses/Collaborative Problems

- Activity intolerance *related to* insufficient oxygenation secondary to decreased CO
- Ineffective management of therapeutic regimen *related to* a lack of knowledge about the disease process and prevention and treatment strategies
- Sleep pattern disturbance *related to* pulmonary congestion
- Potential complication: decreased CO
- Potential complication: hypervolemia
- Potential complication: systemic and pulmonary emboli

Nursing Interventions

Prevention of acquired rheumatic valvular disease is achieved by diagnosing and treating streptococcal infection and providing prophylactic antibiotics for patients with a history of rheumatic fever. Patients at risk for endocarditis and any patient with valvular heart disease must also be treated with prophylactic antibiotics.

- The patient must adhere to the recommended therapies. The individual with a history of rheumatic fever, endocarditis, and congenital heart disease should know the symptoms suggestive of valvular heart disease so that early medical treatment may be obtained.

A patient with progressive valvular heart disease may require hospitalization or outpatient care for the management of CHF, endocarditis, embolic disease, or arrhythmias. CHF is the most common reason for ongoing medical care.

The role of the nurse is to implement and evaluate the effectiveness of therapeutic management.

- Activities should be designed after considering the patient's limitations. An appropriate exercise plan can increase cardiac tolerance. However, activities that regularly produce fatigue and dyspnea should be restricted and an explanation should be provided to the patient.
- The patient should be assisted in planning activities of daily living (ADLs), with an emphasis on conserving energy, setting priorities, and taking planned rest periods.
- Referral to a vocational counselor may be necessary if the patient has a physically or emotionally demanding job.
- Auscultatory assessment of the heart should be performed to monitor the effectiveness of digitalis, β-adrenergic blocking agents, and antiarrhythmic drugs.
- The patient who is on anticoagulation therapy after surgery for valve replacement needs to have their prothrombin time (PT) checked regularly (usually monthly) to assess the adequacy of therapy and to prevent side effects.

▼ **Patient Teaching**

- Explain the nature and cause of the disease process to ensure patient has adequate knowledge base on which to make decisions.
- Teach the signs and symptoms of heart failure and infective endocarditis to ensure early reporting and treatment of complications.
- Explain the need to avoid all invasive surgical or diagnostic procedures that may predispose the patient to bacteremia until prophylactic antibiotics are given. Emphasize the importance of notifying the dentist, urologist, and gynecologist of valvular disease so prophylactic antibiotic treatment can be initiated prior to procedures.
- Explain the need for good oral hygiene and the avoidance of fatigue to decrease the opportunity for infection.
- Instruct patient to wear a medical alert bracelet.
- Discourage smoking to prevent an increased cardiac workload.
- Discuss prescribed medications, including dosage, purpose, and side effects, to promote safe and accurate self-medication.

- Teach the patient to monitor urinary output and daily weight when diuretics are prescribed. The patient's diet should be well balanced nutritionally, with Na^+ restriction to prevent fluid retention.

The patient needs to realize that valve surgery is not a cure and that regular follow-up examinations by the health care provider will be required.

- The nurse also needs to teach the patient about when to seek medical care. Any manifestations of infection, CHF, signs of bleeding, and any planned invasive or dental procedures require the patient to notify the health care provider.

VARICOSE VEINS

Definition/Description

Varicose veins (varicosities) are dilated, tortuous subcutaneous (SC) veins most frequently found in the saphenous system. They may be small and innocuous or large and bulging.

- *Primary* varicosities are those in which the superficial veins are dilated and the valves may or may not be rendered incompetent. The condition tends to be familial, is usually found bilaterally, and is probably caused by congenital weakness of the veins.
- *Secondary* varicosities result from previous thrombophlebitis of deep femoral veins with subsequent valvular incompetence. Secondary varicose veins may also occur in the esophagus as varices, in the anorectal area as hemorrhoids, and as abnormal arteriovenous connections (fistulas and malformations).

Pathophysiology

The etiology of varicose veins is unknown. Increased venous pressure may be due to congenital weakness of the vein structure, obesity, pregnancy, venous obstruction resulting from thrombosis or extrinsic pressure by tumors, or occupations that require prolonged standing.

- As the veins enlarge, valves are stretched and become incompetent, allowing blood flow to be reversed. As back pressure increases and the calf muscle pump (muscle movement that squeezes venous blood back toward the heart) fails, further venous distention results.
- Increased venous pressure is transmitted to the capillary bed, and edema develops.

Clinical Manifestations

Discomfort from varicose veins varies dramatically among people and tends to be worsened by superficial thrombophlebitis. The most common symptom is an ache or pain after prolonged standing, which is relieved by walking or by elevating the limb. Some patients feel pressure or a cramplike sensation. Swelling may accompany the discomfort. Nocturnal leg cramps, especially in the calf area, may occur.

Superficial thrombophlebitis is a serious consequence of varicose veins and may occur either spontaneously or after trauma, surgical procedures, or pregnancy. Uncommonly, rupture of varicose veins may occur because of weakening of the vessel wall. Ulceration as a result of skin infections or trauma may develop.

Diagnostic Studies

- Duplex ultrasound can detect obstruction and reflux in the venous system.

Collaborative Care

Treatment is usually not indicated if varicose veins are only a cosmetic problem. If incompetency of the venous system develops, management involves rest with the affected limb elevated, compression stockings, and walking exercise.

Sclerotherapy is used in the treatment of unsightly superficial varicosities. Direct IV injection of a sclerosing agent such as sodium tetradecyl (Sotradecol) induces inflammation and results in eventual thrombosis of the vein. This procedure can be performed safely in an office setting and causes minimal discomfort. After injection the leg is wrapped with an elastic bandage for 24 to 72 hours to maintain pressure over the vein. Local tenderness subsides within 2 to 3 weeks, and eventually the thrombosed vein disappears. After injection the patient should be advised to wear compression stockings to help prevent the development of further varicosities.

Surgical intervention for varicose veins involves ligation of the entire vein (usually saphenous) and the dissection and removal of its incompetent tributaries. Surgical intervention is indicated when chronic venous insufficiency cannot be controlled with conservative therapy. Recurrent thrombophlebitis in varicose veins is another indication for surgery.

Nursing Management

The patient should be instructed to avoid sitting or standing for long periods of time, maintain ideal body weight, take precautions against injury to extremities, and avoid wearing constrictive clothing.

After a patient has vein ligation surgery, encourage deep breathing, which helps promote venous return to the right side of the heart.

Extremities should be checked regularly for color, movement, sensation, temperature, presence of edema, and pedal pulses. Bruising and discoloration are considered normal.

- Postoperatively, the extremities are elevated at a 15-degree angle to prevent the development of venous stasis and edema. Compression stockings are applied, removed every 8 hours for short periods, and reapplied.

Long-term management of varicose veins is directed toward improving circulation, relieving discomfort, improving cosmetic appearance, and avoiding complications, such as superficial thrombophlebitis and ulceration. Varicose veins can recur in other veins after surgery.

▼ **Patient Teaching**

- The patient should be taught proper care of the lower extremities, including cleanliness and the use of individually fitted compression stockings. Instruct the patient to put on the stockings while still lying down, just before rising in the morning.
- The importance of periodic positioning of the legs above the heart should be stressed.
- The overweight patient may need assistance with weight reduction.
- The patient whose occupation requires prolonged periods of standing or sitting should be encouraged to change position as frequently as possible.

PART TWO

TREATMENTS AND PROCEDURES

AMPUTATION

Description

The clinical features that indicate the need for an amputation depend on the underlying diseases or traumas. Common indications for amputation include circulatory impairment resulting from a peripheral vascular disorder, traumatic and thermal injuries, malignant tumors, uncontrolled or widespread infection of the extremity, and congenital disorders.

These conditions may manifest as a loss of sensation, inadequate circulation, pallor, sweating, and local or systemic infection. Although pain is often present, it is not usually the primary reason for an amputation. The underlying problem dictates whether the amputation is performed as elective or emergency surgery.

- The goal of amputation surgery is to preserve extremity length and function, while removing all infected or ischemic tissue. This improves the possibility of good prosthetic, cosmetic, and functional satisfaction. (See Fig. 59-18 for the levels of amputation of the upper and lower extremities, Lewis and others, *Medical-Surgical Nursing,* edition 5, p. 1779).

Types of Amputation

The type of amputation depends on the reason for the surgery.

- A *closed amputation* is performed to create a weight-bearing residual limb (stump); an anterior skin flap with dissected soft-tissue padding covers the bony part of the residual limb. Special care is necessary to prevent the accumulation of drainage, which can produce pressure and harbor infection.
- *Disarticulation* is an amputation performed through a joint. A Symes amputation is a form of disarticulation at the ankle.
- An *open amputation* leaves a surface on the residual limb that is not covered with skin. This type of surgery is generally indicated for control of actual or potential infection. The wound is usually closed later by a second surgical procedure or by skin traction surrounding the residual limb. This type of amputation is often referred to as a *guillotine amputation.*

Nursing Management

Most lower limb amputations are needed because of peripheral vascular disease, and most upper limb amputations result from severe trauma. Control of causative illnesses such as peripheral vascular disease, diabetes mellitus (DM), chronic osteomyelitis, and skin ulcers can eliminate or delay the need for amputation.

- Patients with these problems must be taught to carefully examine the lower extremities daily for signs of potential problems. If the patient cannot assume this responsibility, a family member should be instructed on the procedure. The patient and family should be instructed to report problems such as changes in skin color or temperature, a decrease in or absence of sensation, tingling, pain, or the presence of a lesion to the health care provider.

The nurse must recognize the tremendous psychologic and social implications of a lower limb amputation for the patient.

- The disruption in body image caused by an amputation often causes a patient to go through psychologic stages similar to the grieving process of death. Allowing the patient to go through a period of depression and recognizing it as a normal consequence of the amputation may do much to aid the patient's acceptance of the amputation. The patient's family must also be helped to work through the process to arrive at a realistic and positive attitude about the future.

Preoperative Care

Before surgery, the nurse should reinforce information that the patient and family have received about the reasons for the amputation, the proposed prosthesis, and the mobility training program. In addition to the usual preoperative instructions, the patient undergoing an amputation has special education needs.

- To meet these needs, the nurse must know the level of amputation, the type of postsurgical dressing to be applied, and the type of prosthesis planned.
- The patient should receive instruction in the performance of upper extremity exercises such as push-ups in bed or the wheelchair to promote arm strength.

Patients should be warned that they may feel as though their amputated limbs are still present after surgery. This *phantom sensation* (a sensation of aching, tingling, or itching of the amputated limb) usually disappears but may cause patients grave concern unless they are forewarned. If pain was present in the affected limb preoperatively, the patient may experience *phantom limb pain* postoperatively. The patient may have feelings of coldness and heaviness or cramping, shooting, burning, or crushing pain.

- Often, the patient may be extremely anxious about this pain because the patient knows the limb is gone but still feels pain in it. Usually, phantom limb pain goes away in time, although it can become chronic.

Postoperative Care

The prevention and detection of complications are important nursing responsibilities during the postoperative period. Careful monitoring of the patient's vital signs and dressing can alert the nurse to hemorrhage in the operative area. Careful attention to sterile technique during dressing changes reduces the potential for wound infection and subsequent interruption of rehabilitation.

- If an immediate postoperative prosthesis has been applied, the nurse must monitor vital signs carefully, since the surgical site is heavily covered and may not be visible.
- A surgical tourniquet must always be available for emergency use. If hemorrhage occurs, the surgeon should be notified immediately and efforts to control the hemorrhage should begin at once.

The surgeon must decide the type of prosthetic fitting that will be used after surgery.

- An *immediate prosthetic fitting*, often called the *immediate post-surgical fitting* or the *immediate postoperative fitting*, is done in the operating room after the amputation. The main advantages of this device are reduction of edema and the psychologic benefit of early ambulation. A disadvantage is the inability to directly visualize the surgical site.
- The *delayed prosthetic fitting* may be the best choice for certain patients. Patients who have had amputations above the knee or below the elbow, older adults, debilitated individuals, and those with infection usually have delayed prosthetic fittings. A temporary prosthesis may be used for partial weight-bearing once the sutures are removed.

Not all patients are candidates for a prosthesis. It is important that the surgeon discuss ambulation possibilities frankly with the patient and family. The seriously ill or debilitated patient may not have the energy required to use a prosthesis. Mobility with a wheelchair may be the most realistic goal for this type of patient.

Flexion contractures may delay the rehabilitation process. The most common and debilitating contracture is hip flexion. To prevent flexion contractures, patients should avoid sitting with hips flexed in a chair or having pillows under the surgical extremity for long intervals.

▼ Patient Teaching

As the patient's overall condition improves, the nurse begins instruction in the principles and techniques of transferring from bed to chair and back.

- Active exercise and conditioning are essential in developing ambulation skills. Active range-of-motion exercises of all joints should be started as soon after surgery as the patient's pain level and medical status permit.
- Crutch walking is started as soon as the patient is physically able. If a patient has immediate postsurgical fitting, orders related to weight-bearing must be carefully followed to avoid disruption of the skin flap and delay of the training process.

Table 60	Patient and Family Teaching Guide: Following an Amputation

1. Inspect the residual limb daily for signs of skin irritation, especially redness and abrasion. Pay particular attention to areas prone to pressure.
2. Discontinue use of the prosthesis if irritation develops. Have the area checked before resuming use of the prosthesis.
3. Wash residual limb thoroughly each night with warm water and a bacteriostatic soap. Rinse thoroughly and dry gently. Expose the residual limb to air for 20 minutes.
4. Do not use any substance such as lotions, alcohol, powders, or oil unless prescribed by the physician.
5. Wear only a residual limb sock that is in good condition and supplied by the prosthetist.
6. Change residual limb sock daily. Launder in a mild soap, squeeze, and lay flat to dry.
7. Utilize prescribed pain management techniques.
8. Perform ROM to all joints daily. Perform general strengthening exercises, including on the upper extremities, daily.
9. Do not elevate residual limb on a pillow.
10. Lay prone with hip extension for 30 minutes three to four times daily.

ROM, range of motion.

Before discharge, the patient and family need careful instruction related to residual limb care, ambulation, prevention of contractures, recognition of complications, exercise, and follow-up care. Table 60 outlines patient and family teaching following an amputation.

ARTIFICIAL AIRWAYS: ENDOTRACHEAL TUBES

Description

An artificial airway is created by inserting a tube into the trachea, bypassing upper airway and laryngeal structures. A tube is placed into the trachea via the mouth or nose past the larynx *(endotracheal [ET] intubation).* ET intubation is more common in intensive care unit (ICU) patients. It can be performed quickly without taking the patient to surgery. ET tubes are illustrated in Fig. 5.

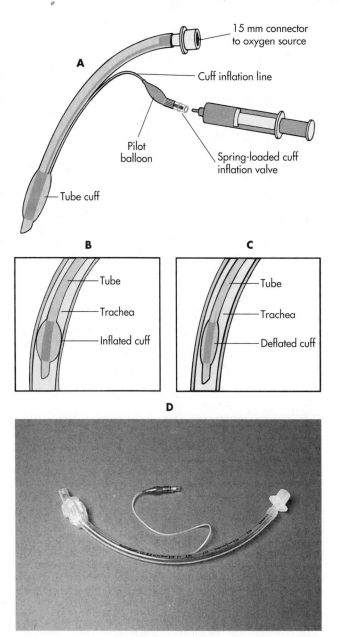

Fig. 5 A, Parts of a cuffed endotracheal tube. **B,** Tube in place with the cuff inflated. **C,** Tube in place with the cuff deflated. **D,** Endotracheal tube.

- Indications for an artificial airway are to (1) prevent or relieve upper airway obstruction, (2) decrease aspiration, (3) facilitate secretion removal, and (4) provide a closed system for positive pressure mechanical ventilation.

If *oral intubation* is selected, the endotracheal tube is passed through the mouth and vocal cords and into the trachea with the aid of a laryngoscope or bronchoscope.

- Oral ET intubation is the procedure of choice for most emergencies because the airway can be secured rapidly. It is easier to remove secretions and perform fiberoptic bronchoscopy if needed.
- There are disadvantages of oral ET intubation. It is difficult to place an oral tube if head and neck mobility are limited. Salivation is increased and swallowing is difficult. Mouth care is a challenge.

If *nasal intubation* is selected, insertion is performed by manipulating the tube through the nose, nasopharynx, and vocal cords.

- Nasal ET intubation is sometimes preferred because the tube is more stable than the oral tube and more difficult to dislodge. It can be placed "blindly" without visualizing the larynx; thus it is indicated when head and neck manipulation is risky.
- The nasal tube may be uncomfortable for some because it presses on the septum, while others may prefer it because there is no need for a bite-block and mouth care is more easily accomplished.

Before intubation, the nurse should ensure that the patient is properly oxygenated.

- The nurse should explain why endotracheal intubation is necessary, the procedure involved, and the sensations (gagging and a feeling of suffocation) that may be experienced during the procedure.
- The nurse should explain that because of the inflated cuff, it will not be possible to talk when the tube is in place, but speech will be possible after the tube is removed.

Nursing responsibilities for the patient with an artificial airway include (1) maintaining correct tube placement, (2) maintaining proper cuff inflation, (3) maintaining and monitoring ventilation status, including oxygenation and acid-base status, (4) maintaining tube patency, (5) providing mouth care and rotating the tube placement, (6) and fostering communication and comfort and assessing for complications. See NCP 63-1 for the patient with an artificial airway, Lewis and others, *Medical-Surgical Nursing,* edition 5, p. 1932.

The nurse monitors tube position by confirming that the exit mark on the tube remains at the point of exit from the body . The nurse observes for the symmetrical rise and fall of both sides of the chest and auscultates to confirm bilateral breath sounds.

Table 61 Complications of Endotracheal Tubes and Nursing Management

Complications	Causes	Prevention/treatment
■ Tube obstruction	Patient biting tube Tube kinking during repositioning Cuff herniation Dried secretions, blood, or lubricant Tissue from tumor Trauma Foreign body	*Prevention:* Place bite block. Sedate patient prn. Suction prn. Humidify inspired gases. *Treatment:* Replace tube.
■ Tube displacement	Movement of patient's head Movement of tube by patient's tongue Traction on tube from ventilator tubing Self-extubation	*Prevention:* Secure tube to upper lip. Restrain patient's hands. Sedate patient prn. Ensure that only 2 in of tube extend beyond lip. Support ventilator tubing. *Treatment:* Replace tube.

Continued

Source: Thelan LA and others, editors: *Critical care nursing: diagnosis and management,* ed 3, St Louis, 1998, Mosby. *NG,* Nasogastric; *prn,* as needed; *q8hr,* every 8 hours.

Table 61   Complications of Endotracheal Tubes and Nursing Management—cont'd

Complications	Causes	Prevention/treatment
■ Sinusitis and nasal injury	Obstruction of paranasal sinus drainage Pressure necrosis of nares	*Prevention:* Avoid nasal intubations. Cushion nares from tube and tape/ties. Position and stabilize tube properly. *Treatment:* Remove all tubes from nasal passages. Stabilize airway Administer antibiotics.
■ Tracheoesophageal fistula	Pressure necrosis of posterior tracheal wall resulting from overinflated cuff and rigid NG tube	*Prevention:* Inflate cuff with minimal amount of air necessary. Monitor cuff pressures q8hr. Use small bore feeding tube for enteral feeding. *Treatment:* Position cuff of tube distal to fistula. Place gastrostomy tube for enteral feedings. Place esophageal tube for secretion clearance

■ Mucosal lesions	Pressure at tube and mucosal interface	*Prevention:* Inflate cuff with minimal amount of air necessary. Monitor cuff pressures q8hr. Use appropriate size tube. *Treatment:* May resolve spontaneously. Perform surgical intervention.
■ Laryngeal or tracheal stenosis	Injury to area from end of tube or cuff, resulting in scar tissue formation and narrowing of airway	*Prevention:* Inflate cuff with minimal amount of air necessary. Monitor cuff pressures q8hr. Suction area above cuff frequently. *Treatment:* Perform tracheostomy. Place laryngeal stent. Perform surgical repair.
■ Cricoid abscess	Mucosal injury with bacterial invasion	*Prevention:* Inflate cuff with minimal amount of air necessary. Monitor cuff pressures q8hr. Suction area above cuff frequently. *Treatment:* Perform incision and drainage of area. Administer antibiotics.

- If the ET tube is not positioned properly, this is an emergency. The nurse stays with the patient, maintains the airway, supports ventilation, and secures the appropriate assistance to immediately reposition the tube.

See Table 63-11 for suctioning the patient with an artificial airway, *Medical-Surgical Nursing,* p. 1935.

The cuff is an inflatable, pliable sleeve encircling the outer wall of the ET tube. The inflated cuff stabilizes and seals the ET tube within the trachea. It prevents the escape of ventilating gases.

- The nurse should measure and record cuff pressure after intubation and once every 8 hours to confirm that the cuff is properly inflated. (For the nursing management of ET tubes, see Table 63-10, *Medical-Surgical Nursing,* p. 1935).

Meticulous care is required to prevent skin excoriation or pressure sores as a result of pressure from the tube, bite-block, or tube-holder.

- For the orally intubated patient, the outer layer of adhesive tape is removed every shift and the tube is moved to the other side of the mouth.

Mouth care, including cleaning of teeth and gums, should be performed every 4 to 8 hours as a comfort measure and to prevent injury to the gums and loss of teeth resulting from plaque accumulation.

The major complications of ET intubation result from injury to the hypopharynx, larynx, and trachea and are related to the pressure exerted on the upper airway structures by the tube and cuff. Improper tube placement, aspiration, oral and nasal pressure sores, and accidental extubation are also potential problems. Table 61 summarizes the complications seen in patients with ET tubes.

BLOOD TRANSFUSION THERAPY

Description

Traditionally, the term *blood transfusion* meant the administration of whole blood. Blood transfusion now has a broader meaning because of the ability to administer specific components of blood such as platelets, red blood cells (RBCs), or plasma (see Blood Products, p. 708).

Administration Procedure

Blood components can be safely administered through any gauge needle into a free-flowing IV line. Larger gauge needles (e.g., 19 gauge) may be preferred if rapid transfusion is desired; smaller needles are used for platelets, albumin, and cryoprecipitates. The blood administration tubing with a filter should have a stopcock or other means to develop a closed system, with blood open to one port and isotonic saline solution infusing through the other.

- Dextrose solutions or lactated Ringer's should not be used because they induce RBC hemolysis. No other additives (including medications) should be given via the same tubing as the blood unless the tubing is cleared with saline solution.

When the blood or blood components have been obtained from the blood bank, positive identification of the donor blood and recipient must be made.

- Improper product-to-patient identification causes 90% of transfusion reactions, thus placing a great responsibility on nursing personnel to carry out the identification procedure appropriately.

The nurse should follow the policy and procedures at the place of employment.

- The blood should be administered as soon as it is brought to the patient. It should not be refrigerated on the nursing unit. If the blood is not used right away, it should be returned to the blood bank.
- During the first 15 minutes of blood infusion, the nurse should stay with the patient. If there are any unwanted reactions, they are most likely to occur at this time.
- The rate of infusion during this period should be no more than 2 ml/min. Blood should not be infused quickly unless an emergency exists. Rapid infusion of cold blood may cause the patient to become chilled. If rapid replacement of large amounts of blood is necessary, a blood-warming device should be used.
- After the first 15 minutes, the rate of infusion is governed by the clinical condition of the patient and the product being infused. Most patients not in danger of fluid overload can tolerate the infusion of one unit of packed cells over 2 hours.
- The transfusion should not take more than 4 hours to administer. Blood remaining after 4 hours should not be infused because of the length of time it has been removed from refrigeration.

Blood Transfusion Reactions

If a transfusion reaction occurs, the following steps should be taken: (1) stop the transfusion, (2) maintain a patent IV line with saline solution, (3) notify the blood bank and the physician immediately, (4) recheck the identifying tags and numbers, (5) monitor vital signs and urine output, (6) treat the symptoms per physician order, (7) save the blood bag and tubing and send them to the blood bank for examination, (8) complete the transfusion reaction reports, (9) collect the required blood and urine specimens at intervals stipulated by hospital policy to evaluate for hemolysis, and (10) document on the transfusion reaction form and patient chart. The blood bank and laboratory are responsible for identifying the type of reaction.

The complications of transfusion therapy may be significant and necessitate careful evaluation of the patient. Blood transfusion reactions can be classified as acute or delayed (see Tables 29-37 and 29-38, Lewis and others, *Medical-Surgical Nursing,* edition 5, pp. 785-786).

- Acute reactions include hemolysis, febrile reactions, sepsis, allergic reactions, and circulatory overload.
- Delayed reactions include delayed hemolysis, infection (such as hepatitis B and C, HIV, and malaria), iron overload, and graft-versus-host disease.

Autotransfusion

Autotransfusion, or autologous transfusion, consists of removing whole blood from a person and transfusing that blood into the same person. The problems of incompatibility, allergic reactions, and transmission of disease can be avoided. There are various reasons and methods of autotransfusion. These include the following types:

- *Autologous donation* or *elective phlebotomy* (predeposit transfusion). A person donates blood before a planned surgical procedure. The blood can be frozen and stored for up to 3 years. Usually the blood is stored without being frozen and is given to the person within a few weeks of donation.
- *Autotransfusion.* A newer method for replacing blood volume involves safely and aseptically collecting, filtering, and returning the patient's own blood that was lost during a major surgical procedure or from a traumatic injury. This system was originally developed in response to patients' concerns over the safety of blood. However, today it provides an important way to safely replace volume and stabilize bleeding patients. Collection devices can be attached to drains following chest or orthopedic procedures. Sometimes the collection device is a component of the drainage system.

CARDIOPULMONARY RESUSCITATION

Description

Cardiopulmonary resuscitation (CPR) is the process of externally supporting the circulation and respiration of a person who has a cardiac arrest. Resuscitation measures are divided into two components, basic life support (BLS) and advanced cardiac life support (ACLS). The American Heart Association establishes standards for CPR.

Basic Life Support

BLS involves the external support of circulation and ventilation for a patient with cardiac or respiratory arrest through CPR. Artificial respiration (mouth-to-mouth, mouth-to-mask, mouth-to-nose, mouth-to-stoma) and external chest compression substitute for spontaneous breathing and circulation

- The major objective of performing CPR is to provide oxygen (O_2) to the brain, heart, and other vital organs until appropriate care and resuscitation efforts involving advanced life support methods can be initiated, or until resuscitation efforts are ordered to be stopped.

Rapid intervention is the key to success and is critical in preventing biologic death or the death of brain cells. CPR must be initiated within 4 to 6 minutes of cardiac or pulmonary arrest because brain cells begin to die *(brain death)* within 6 minutes of anoxia. National standards for knowledge and technique must be met for personnel to be certified to deliver CPR. Assessment of the victim must be stressed in teaching CPR. Each of the broad areas—**A**irway, **B**reathing, and **C**irculation (the ABCs of CPR)—should be reviewed (see Lewis and others, *Medical-Surgical Nursing,* edition 5, p. 939).

- Rescue breathing and chest compressions are combined for an effective resuscitation effort of the victim of cardiopulmonary arrest. When there is one rescuer, the rate of compression should be 80 to 100 compressions per minute with a compression-ventilation ratio of 15 compressions to 2 ventilations (Table 62). The compression rate for two-rescuer CPR is 80 to 100 per minute with a compression-ventilation ratio of 5:1 (Table 63).
- The victim's condition must be assessed during CPR to determine the effectiveness of compressions and to determine whether the victim has resumed spontaneous circulation and breathing. The pulse should be checked by the ventilating rescuer during compressions to assess the effectiveness of compressions in two-rescuer CPR. Chest compressions are stopped for 5 seconds at the end of the first minute and every few minutes thereafter to determine whether the victim has resumed spontaneous breathing and circulation.
- The goal of CPR is the return of spontaneous breathing and circulation, but it is rarely achieved without more definitive therapy with ACLS.

Advanced Cardiac Life Support

ACLS involves a systematic treatment approach in cardiac emergencies. ACLS includes (1) basic life support (BLS), (2) the use of adjunctive equipment and special techniques for establishing

Table 62 Adult One-Rescuer CPR

Step	Objective	Critical performance
1. Airway	Assessment: determine unresponsiveness.	Tap or gently shake shoulder.
		Shout "Are you okay?"
	Call for help	Call out "Help!"
	Position the victim.	Turn on back as unit, if necessary, supporting head and neck (4-10 sec).
	Open the airway	Use head-tilt/chin-lift maneuver.
2. Breathing	Assessment: determine cessation of breathing.	Maintain open airway.
		With ear over mouth, observe chest: look, listen, feel for breathing (3-5 sec).
	Ventilate twice.	Maintain open airway.
		Seal mouth and nose properly.
		Ventilate two times for 1.5-2 sec/inflation.
		Observe chest rise (adequate ventilation volume).
		Allow deflation between breaths.
3. Circulation	Assessment: determine absence of pulse.	Feel for carotid pulse on near side of victim (5-10 sec).
		Maintain head-tilt with other hand.
	Activate EMS system.	If someone responded to call for help, send person to activate EMS system.

	begin chest compressions.	Kneel by victim's shoulders. Make landmark check before hands are placed. Maintain proper hand position throughout. Keep shoulders over victim's sternum. Maintain equal compression and relaxation. Compress 1.5-2 in. Keep hands on sternum during upstroke. Wait for complete chest relaxation on upstroke. Say any helpful mnemonic (e.g., "one-and-two-and-three-and . . ."). Remember that compression rate is 80-100/min (15/9-11 sec).
4. Compression-ventilation cycles	Do four cycles of 15 compressions and two ventilations.	Maintain proper compression-ventilation ratio of 15 compressions to two ventilations per cycle. Observe chest rise: 1.5-2 sec/inflation; four cycles/52-73 sec.
5. Reassessment	Determine absence of pulse. Ventilate twice.	Feel for carotid pulse (5 sec). If there is no pulse, go to step 6. Ventilate two times. Observe chest rise: 1.5-2 sec/inflation.
6. Continuation of CPR	Resume compression-ventilation cycles.	Feel for carotid pulse every few min.

Source: *Textbook of basic life support for healthcare providers,* 1997, American Heart Association.
CPR, cardiopulmonary resuscitation; *EMS,* emergency medical services.

Table 63   Adult Two-Rescuer CPR

Step	Objective	Critical performance
1. Airway	One rescuer (ventilator): Assessment: determine unresponsiveness. Position the victim. Open the airway.	Tap or gently shake shoulder. Shout "Are you okay?" Turn on back if necessary (4-10 sec). Use a proper technique to open airway.
2. Breathing	Assessment: determine cessation of breathing. Ventilate twice.	Look, listen, and feel for breath (3-5 sec). Observe chest rise: 1.5-2 sec/inflation.
3. Circulation	Assessment: determine absence of pulse. State assessment results. Other rescuer (compressor): get into position for compressions. Locate landmark notch.	Feel for carotid pulse (5-10 sec). Say "No pulse." When another rescuer comes, first rescuer asks if EMS has been activated. Put hands, shoulders in correct position. Check landmark.
4. Compression-ventilation cycles	Compressor: begin chest compressions.	Correct ratio compressions-ventilations is 5:1 Compression rate is 80-100/min (5 compressions/3-4 sec). Say any helpful mnemonic (e.g., "one-and-two-and . . .").

Step		
	Ventilator: ventilate after every fifth compression and check compression effectiveness. (Minimum of 10 cycles)	ventilate once (1.5-2 sec/inflation). Check pulse occasionally to assess compressions. (Time for 10 cycles: 40-53 sec) Give clear signal to change roles. Compressor completes fifth compression. Ventilator completes ventilation after fifth compression.
5. Calling for switch	*Compressor:* call for switch when tired.	
6. Switching	Simultaneously switch: *Ventilator:* move to chest.	Become compressor. Get into position for compressions. Locate landmark notch.
	Compressor: move to head	Become ventilator. Check carotid pulse (5 sec). Say "No pulse." Ventilate once (1.5-2 sec/inflation).
7. Continuation of CPR	Resume compression-ventilation cycles.	Repeat step 4.

Source: *Textbook of basic life support for healthcare providers,* 1997, American Heart Association. *CPR,* Cardiopulmonary resuscitation; *EMS,* emergency medical services.

and maintaining effective ventilation and circulation, (3) ECG monitoring and arrhythmia recognition, (4) the establishment and maintenance of IV access, (5) therapies for emergency treatment of the patient with cardiac or respiratory arrest (including stabilization in the post-arrest phase), and (6) the treatment of the patient with suspected acute myocardial infarction (MI).

- The principle of early defibrillation has been emphasized in national emergency medical care organizations. With the invention of the automated external defibrillator (AED), which is simple to use and available throughout communities, more trained rescuers are available to provide early defibrillation. The importance of early, effective BLS and defibrillation before entrance into the ACLS system cannot be overemphasized.
- Drugs used in ACLS include O_2 therapy, IV fluids, drugs used to control the heart rate (HR) and rhythm, and those used to improve cardiac output (CO) and BP (see Table 34-15, Lewis and others, *Medical-Surgical Nursing,* edition 5, p. 944).

Nursing Role During a Code

- There is a potential for a "code" or cardiopulmonary arrest situation in any clinical setting. The nurse should be well prepared to participate in the resuscitation of a patient. The nurse must be familiar with code protocols, emergency equipment in the crash cart, and keep current with BLS and ACLS skills.
- It is important for the nurse to be familiar with the crash cart's location and contents on the clinical unit. Most crash carts contain all necessary emergency supplies. Ideally, all crash carts in an individual clinic or hospital should be organized in the same fashion.

CASTS

Types of Casts

Immobilization of an acute fracture or soft tissue injury can be accomplished by a variety of casts.

- The *sugar tong splint* is typically used for acute wrist injuries or injuries that may result in significant swelling. Plaster splints are applied to the well-padded forearm. The splinting material is wrapped with either elastic bandage or bias stockingette. The major advantage of this cast is the avoidance of the circumferential effects of a nonelastic cylinder cast, as this splint allows for swelling.

- The *short arm cast* is frequently used for the treatment of stable wrist or metacarpal fractures. An aluminum finger splint can be fabricated into the short arm cast for concurrent treatment of phalangeal injuries. This cast provides wrist immobilization and permits unrestricted elbow motion.
- The *long arm cast* is commonly used for stable forearm or elbow fractures and unstable wrist fractures. It is similar to the short arm cast but extends to the proximal humerus, restricting motion in the wrist and elbow. When a sling is used, the nurse must ensure that the axillary region is well padded to prevent skin maceration associated with direct skin-to-skin contact.
- The *body jacket cast* is frequently used for immobilization and support of stable spine injuries of the thoracic or lumbar spine. This cast is applied around the chest and abdomen and extends from above the nipple line to the pubis.
- The *hip spica* cast is commonly used in treating femoral fractures, especially in children. The purpose of this cast is to immobilize the affected extremity and the trunk securely. It includes two separate casts joined together: (1) the body jacket and (2) the long leg cast. The location of the femoral fracture will determine whether the thigh of the unaffected extremity will have to be immobilized to restrict rotation of the pelvis and possible hip motion on the side of the femur fracture.
- Injuries to the lower extremities are frequently immobilized by either a *long leg* or *short leg cast*. The usual indications for applying a long leg cast are an unstable ankle fracture, soft-tissue injuries, a fractured tibia, or knee injuries. The cast usually extends from the base of the toes to the groin and gluteal crease. The short leg cast can be used for a variety of conditions but is usually used for stable ankle and foot injuries.

Types of Cast Material

Plaster of Paris is wrapped and molded around the affected part after immersion in water. It is anhydrous calcium sulfate embedded in a gauze roll. The strength of the cast is determined by the number of layers of plaster bandage and the technique of application. As the cast dries, it recrystallizes and hardens. Heat is generated during the drying process. Increased edema from increased circulation may occur as a result of heat produced by the drying cast. After the cast is completely dry, it is strong and firm and can withstand stresses.

- The plaster is hard within 15 minutes, so the patient can move around without problems. However, it is not strong enough for weight-bearing until it is dry (after about 24 to 48 hours).

Thermolabile plastic (Orthoplast) and *thermoplastic resins* (Hexcelite) are molded to fit the torso or extremity after being heated in warm water. Polyurethane, which is formed from polyester and cotton fabric impregnated with a chemical, is water activated by immersing it in cool water to start the chemical process.

- Casts made of this fiberglass tape are frequently used because they are lightweight and relatively waterproof and support earlier mobilization. They are appropriate in cases in which severe edema is not present or when multiple cast changes are not anticipated.

Cast Care

Immediately after a plaster cast is applied, there is a short period of exothermic reaction during which heat is released from the plaster. The patient should be alerted to this occurrence, since it can increase edema. A fresh cast should never be covered with a blanket because air cannot circulate and heat builds up in the cast.

- The drying process is usually complete within 24 to 72 hours. During the drying period the cast should not be subjected to any wetness, soiling, or abnormal stresses that can cause weakening or a break in the cast.
- The patient should be turned every 2 hours to reduce continuous pressure and promote even drying of the cast.
- The cast should be carefully handled by the palms of the hands rather than with the fingertips to avoid indentations that will dry and become potential pressure areas.

Regardless of the type of material of which it is made, a cast can interfere with circulation and nerve function from being applied too tightly or because of excessive edema after application. Frequent neurovascular assessments of the immobilized extremity are critical.

- Elevation of the extremity above the level of the heart to promote venous return and applications of ice to control or prevent edema are measures frequently used during the initial phase of immobilization.
- The nurse should instruct the patient to exercise the joints above and below the cast.
- Pulling out cast padding and scratching or placing foreign objects inside the cast is forbidden because it predisposes the patient to skin breakdown and infection within the cast.

A patient teaching guide for cast care is presented in Table 64.

Table 64	Patient Teaching Guide: Cast Care

Do Not
Get cast wet*
Remove any padding
Insert any foreign object inside cast
Bear weight on new cast for 48 hr (Not all casts are made for weight-bearing. Check with health care provider when unsure)
Cover cast with plastic for prolonged periods

Do
Apply ice directly over fracture site for first 24 hr (avoid getting cast wet by keeping ice in plastic bag and protecting cast with cloth)
Check with physician before getting cast wet[†]
Dry cast thoroughly after exposure to water
  Blot dry with towel
  Use hair dryer on low setting until cast is thoroughly dry
Elevate extremity above level of heart for first 48 hr
Move joints above and below cast regularly
Report signs of possible problems to health care provider
- Increasing pain
- Swelling associated with pain and discoloration of toes or fingers
- Pain during movement
- Burning or tingling under cast
- Sores or foul odor under cast
Keep appointment to have fracture and cast checked

*Plaster of Paris cast.
[†]Synthetic cast.

CHEMOTHERAPY

Description

Chemotherapy is a systemic treatment modality for cancer that uses chemicals (drugs). It is primarily used in the treatment of solid tumors, leukemia, and lymphomas. The principle of chemotherapy is to interrupt the cycle of cellular replication and proliferation.

- There are two major types of chemotherapeutic drugs—cell-cycle nonspecific and cell-cycle specific. The aim of a combination approach is to promote a better tumor kill response by using agents that disrupt cellular replication and proliferation by different mechanisms.

Goals of Chemotherapy

The goal of chemotherapy is to reduce the number of cancer cells present in the primary tumor site(s) and also, if present, in the metastatic tumor site(s). Several factors will determine the response of cancer cells to chemotherapy:

1. Mitotic rate of the tissue from which the tumor arises. The more rapid the mitotic rate, the greater the response to chemotherapy.
2. Size of the tumor. The smaller the number of cancer cells, the greater the response to chemotherapy.
3. Age of the tumor. The younger the tumor, the greater the response to chemotherapy. Younger tumors have a greater percentage of proliferating cells.
4. Location of the tumor. Certain anatomic sites provide a protected environment from the effects of chemotherapy. For example, only a few drugs (nitrosoureas and bleomycin [Blenoxane]) cross the blood-brain barrier.
5. Presence of resistant tumor cells. Mutation of cancer cells within the tumor mass can result in variant cells that are resistant to chemotherapy.
6. Physiologic and psychologic status of the host. A state of optimum health and a positive attitude will allow the patient to better withstand aggressive chemotherapy.

One method to prevent the existence of drug-resistant tumor cells is the use of high-dose chemotherapy. The aim of this approach is to maximize drug effects at the cellular level before the problem of resistance occurs.

Types of Chemotherapy

Chemotherapy drugs can be classified according to their mechanism of action (Table 65).

Administration of Chemotherapy

Chemotherapy is most commonly administered by oral or IV routes. A vascular access device allows for chemotherapy to be administered via the large vessels (venous or arterial) and also permits frequent, continuous or intermittent treatment with multiple punctures for vascular access. Types of these devices include silastic right atrial catheters, peripherally inserted central venous catheters, implanted infusion ports, and infusion (external and implanted) pumps.

Table 65 Classification of Chemotherapy Drugs

Mechanisms of action	Examples
Alkylating Agents	
Cell cycle–nonspecific drugs	
Damage DNA by causing breaks in the double-strand helix (similar to the effect of radiation therapy); if repair does not occur, cells will die immediately (cytocidal) or when they attempt to divide (cytostatic)	Mechlorethamine (nitrogen mustard), cyclophosphamide (Cytoxan), chlorambucil (Leukeran), melphalan (Alkeran), thiotepa, busulfan (Myleran), dacarbazine (DTIC), ifosfamide (Ifex), estramustine (Emcyt)
Heavy metal effect on DNA	Cisplatin (Platinol), carboplatin (Paraplatin)
Antimetabolites	
Cell cycle phase–specific drugs	
Interfere with synthesis of DNA by mimicking certain essential cellular metabolites that cell incorporates into synthesis of DNA; cells will die immediately (cytocidal)	Methotrexate (amethopterin), cytarabine (Ara-C, Cytosar), 5-fluorouracil (5-FU), 6-mercaptopurine (6-MP), thioguanine (6-TG), floxuridine (FUDR), vidarabine (Vira-A), 5-azacytidine, hexamethylmelamine, pentostatin (Nipent), fludarabine (Fludara), hydroxyurea (Hydrea)

Continued

DNA, Deoxyribonucleic acid; RNA, ribonucleic acid.

Table 65 — Classification of Chemotherapy Drugs—cont'd

Mechanisms of action	Examples
Antitumor Antibiotics *Cell cycle–nonspecific drugs* Modify function of DNA and interfere with transcription of RNA; cells will die immediately (cytocidal) or when they attempt to divide (cytostatic)	Doxorubicin (Adriamycin), bleomycin (Blenoxane), mitomycin (Mutamycin), daunorubicin (Daunomycin), dactinomycin (actinomycin D), idarubicin (Idamycin), mithramycin (Mithracin)
Plant Alkaloids (Mitotic Inhibitors) *Cell cycle phase–specific drugs* Interrupt cellular replication in mitosis at metaphase; cells will die immediately (cytocidal)	Vinblastine (Velban), vincristine (Oncovin), etoposide (VePesid), paclitaxel (Taxol), vinorelbine (Navelbine), taxotere (Docetaxel), vindesine (Eldisine), teniposide (Vumon)
Nitrosureas *Cell cycle–nonspecific drugs* Has similar effect to alkylating agents and also block specific enzymes needed for the synthesis of purine; cells will die imme-	Carmustine (BCNU), lomustine (CCNU), semustine (Methyl CCNU), streptozocin (STZ), chlorozotozin (DCNU)

Corticosteroids

Cell cycle–nonspecific drugs

Disrupt the cell membrane and inhibit synthesis of protein; decrease circulating lymphocytes; inhibit mitosis; depress immune system; increase feeling of well-being

Cortisone, hydrocortisone, methylprednisone, methylprednisolone, prednisone, dexamethasone (Decadron)

Hormones

Cell cycle–nonspecific drugs

Stimulate the process of cellular differentiation; metastatic lesions are less able to survive in unfavorable environment; decrease the process of cellular proliferation

Androgens (testosterone, fluoxymesterone, [Halotestin]), estrogens (diethylstilbestrol [DES]), progestins (Provera, Delalutin, Megace)

Miscellaneous

Destroys exogenous supply of L-asparagine, which is needed for cellular proliferation; normal cells can synthesize but cannot be synthesized by cancer cells

L-Asparaginase (Elspar)

Antiestrogens used in breast cancer

Tamoxifen (Nolvadex)

Antiadrenal drug blocks adrenal steroid production

Aminoglutethimide (Cytadren)

Produces single- and double-strand breaks in DNA

Amsacrine (m-AMSA)

Suppresses mitosis at interphase; appears to alter preformed DNA, RNA and protein

Procarbazine (Matulane, Natulan)

Suppresses adrenocortical activity; modifies peripheral metabolism of steroids

Mitotane (Lysodren)

Inhibits DNA and RNA synthesis

Mitoxantrone (Novantrone)

- Regional chemotherapy delivers the drug directly to the tumor site. Examples of this type of administration include intraarterial, intraperitoneal, and intrathecal (intraventricular) chemotherapy.

Effects of Chemotherapy

The effects of chemotherapy are caused by (1) the destruction of cells which have a rapid rate of cellular proliferation, (2) the response of the body to products of cellular destruction (cellular waste products in the circulation may cause fatigue, anorexia, and taste alterations), and (3) specific drug toxicities.

The adverse effects of these drugs can be classified as acute, delayed, or chronic. Acute toxicity includes vomiting, allergic reactions, and arrhythmias. Delayed effects include mucositis, alopecia, and bone marrow depression; mucositis can result in mouth sores, gastritis, and diarrhea. Chronic toxicities involve damage to organs such as the heart, liver, kidneys, and lungs. An extensive listing of side effects and problems caused by chemotherapy and radiation therapy is provided in Tables 14-15 and 14-20, Lewis and others, *Medical-Surgical Nursing,* edition 5, p. 291 and p. 303.

Nursing Management

One of the most important responsibilities of the nurse is that of differentiating between the toxic effects of the drug(s) and the progression of the malignant process. The nurse also needs to differentiate between tolerable side effects and acute toxic effects of chemotherapeutic agents. Nausea and vomiting are expected and controllable side effects of many drugs. However, if paresthesia occurs with the use of vincristine (Oncovin) or signs of heart failure appear with the use of doxorubicin (Adriamycin), these serious reactions need to be reported to the physician so that drug dosages can be modified or discontinued.

- Some toxicities associated with chemotherapy may not be reversible. For example, ototoxicity may be an irreversible effect of cisplatin (Platinol) therapy, especially at higher doses. Periodic testing of hearing may be necessary to monitor for this toxicity.
- Results of laboratory studies of the patient who is receiving chemotherapy should be monitored. Particular attention should be given to the white blood cell (WBC), platelet, and red blood cell (RBC) counts.
- If the white blood cell count falls to less than 2000/μL (2 $\times$ 10^9/L), the drug regimen may need to be modified or discontinued. Every measure possible needs to be taken to prevent infections in a patient with leukopenia.
- If the platelet count falls to less than 50,000/μL (50 $\times$ 10^9/L), the patient must be assessed for any signs of bleeding, and measures

should be taken to prevent bleeding. Platelet transfusions may be necessary.

▼ Patient Teaching

Education of the patient is an extremely important part of the nurse's role related to chemotherapy. To decrease the fear and anxiety often associated with chemotherapy, patients must be taught what to expect during a course of treatment.

- The patient's attitude toward treatment should be explored so that any misconceptions or fears can be discussed.
- The patient needs to be told of the possible side effects of chemotherapy that may be experienced during treatment. This may be a discouraging revelation.
- The patient should also be informed that supportive care (e.g., antiemetics and antidiarrheals) will be provided as needed.

Many emotions are experienced and expressed when hair loss occurs, including anger, grief, embarrassment, and fear. For some persons, the loss of hair is one of the most stressful events experienced during the course of the illness.

- Alopecia due to the administration of chemotherapeutic agents is usually reversible. The degree and duration of hair loss depend on the dose of the chemotherapeutic agent, the duration of the treatment, and the nutritional status of the patient.
- Sometimes the hair begins to grow back while the patient is still receiving chemotherapeutic agents, but generally the hair cells do not grow back until the agents are discontinued. Often the new hair has a different color and texture than the hair that was lost.

CHEST TUBES AND PLEURAL DRAINAGE

Description

Chest tubes are inserted into the pleural space to remove air and fluid from the pleural space and to restore normal intrapleural pressure so that the lungs can reexpand.

Chest Tube Insertion

Chest tubes can be inserted in the emergency department (ED), at the patient's bedside, or in the operating room (OR), depending on the situation. In the OR the chest tube is inserted via a thoracotomy incision. In the ED or at the bedside the patient is placed in a sitting position or is lying down with the affected side elevated.

- The area is prepared with antiseptic solution, and the site is infiltrated with a local anesthetic agent. After a small incision is made, one or two chest tubes are inserted into the pleural space.

- One catheter is placed anteriorly through the second intercostal space to remove air (Fig. 6). The other is placed posteriorly through the eighth or ninth intercostal space to drain fluid and blood.
- Tubes are sutured to the chest wall, and the puncture wound is covered with an airtight dressing.
- After the tubes are in place in the pleural space, they are connected to drainage tubing and pleural drainage. Each tube may be connected to a separate drainage system and suction.
- More commonly a Y connector is used to attach both chest tubes to the same drainage system.

Pleural Drainage

Most pleural drainage systems have three basic compartments, each with its own separate function. In early drainage systems, the three compartments were bottles; this was known as the *three-bottle system* (Fig. 7).

- The first compartment, or *collection chamber,* receives fluid and air from the chest cavity. The air in the chamber is vented to the second compartment called the *water-seal chamber,* which acts as a one-way valve. Air enters from the collection chamber via a connector that enters under water in the second compartment. The air bubbles up through the water, and no air can reenter the collection chamber because of the water seal.
- A third compartment, which is used to apply controlled suction to the system, is called the *suction control chamber.*
- Removal of air from the pleural space is facilitated during periods when the patient's intrathoracic pressure is increased, such as during exhalation, coughing, or sneezing. As a result, more air bubbles are noted in the water-seal chamber during these activities.
- A lack of bubbling during exhalation or coughing may indicate a blockage in the chest tube (e.g., kinking, clotting) or expansion of the lung with no further air in the pleural space.

A variety of commercial disposable plastic chest drainage systems are available. Most operate on the same principles as the three-bottle system. One popular system is the Pleur-evac.

Nursing Management

General guidelines for nursing care include the following:

- Keep all tubing as straight as possible and coiled loosely. Do not let the patient lie on it.
- Keep all connections between the chest tubes, drainage tubing, and drainage collector tight. Taping at connections and at the top of the bottle helps prevent air leaks.

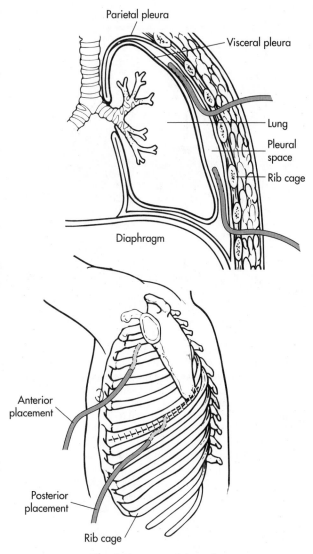

Fig. 6 Placement of chest tubes.

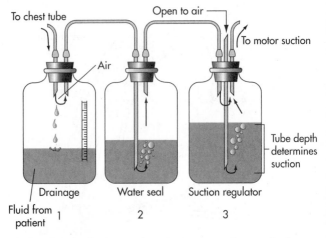

Fig. 7 Three-bottle water-seal suction. *Bottle 1* is drainage bottle. Vertical piece of tape should be applied to outer surface of drainage bottle. Time and fluid level should be marked hourly on tape. *Bottle 2* is water-seal bottle. *Bottle 3* is suction control bottle. Length of glass tube below water surface determines amount of suction.

- Keep the water-seal chamber and suction control chamber at the appropriate water levels by adding sterile water as needed, because water loss by evaporation may occur.
- Mark the time of measurement and the fluid level according to prescribed orders. Any change in the quantity or characteristics of drainage should be reported to the physician.
- Observe for air bubbles in the water-seal chamber and fluctuations in the glass tube or chest tubes. Air should be bubbling out from the glass tube. If no fluctuations are observed (rising with inspiration and falling with expiration in a spontaneously breathing patient; the opposite occurs during positive pressure mechanical ventilation), the drainage system is blocked or the lungs are reexpanded. If bubbling increases there may be an air leak.
- Check for bubbling in the water seal. Normally this is intermittent. When bubbling is continuous and constant, the nurse may determine the source of the air leak by momentarily clamping the tubing at successively distal points away from the patient until the bubbling ceases. Retaping the tubing connections or replacing the drainage apparatus may be necessary to prevent the air leak.

- Monitor the patient's clinical status. Vital signs should be taken frequently, lungs auscultated, and the chest wall observed for any abnormal chest movements.
- Never elevate the drainage system to the level of the patient's chest because this will cause fluid to drain back into the lungs. Drainage bottles should not be emptied unless they are in danger of overflowing.
- Encourage the patient to cough and breathe deeply periodically to facilitate lung expansion.
- If the bottle is overturned and the water seal is disrupted, return it to an upright position and encourage the patient to take a few deep breaths, followed by forced exhalations and cough maneuvers.

Milking and stripping of the chest tubes may briefly increase the amount of negative pressure applied to the pleural space. Increased negative pressure should enhance evacuation of fluid in the chest tubes and prevent the development of clots and obstruction from stagnation of fluids.

- Present practice advocates the use of these procedures when there is bloody drainage or when fluid in the collection bottle tends to clot.
- When chest tubes are used for air collection alone, stripping and milking is not usually performed.
- The nurse should keep in mind that these procedures can cause the patient to experience pain and that dislodgment of the tube may occur if the tube is not stabilized above the area that is being stripped.

Clamping of the chest tubes is no longer advocated as routine clinical practice unless the tubes become disconnected, to momentarily change the drainage apparatus, and to check for air leaks. The danger of a rapid accumulation of air in the pleural space, which causes tension pneumothorax, is greater than that of a small amount of atmospheric air entering the pleural space.

Chest tubes are removed when the lungs are reexpanded and fluid drainage has ceased. The patient with chest tubes may have daily chest x-rays to follow the course of lung reexpansion.

- The tube is removed by cutting the sutures; applying a sterile petroleum jelly gauze dressing; having the patient take a deep breath, exhale, and bear down (Valsalva maneuver); and then removing the tube. Sometimes pain medication is given before chest tube removal.
- The site is covered with an airtight dressing, the pleura seals itself off, and the wound is healed in several days. The wound should be observed for drainage and reinforced if necessary.
- The patient should be observed for any manifestations of respiratory distress, which may signify a recurrent or new pneumothorax.

DIALYSIS

Description

Dialysis is a technique in which substances move from the blood through a semipermeable membrane and into a dialysis solution (dialysate). Dialysis is used to correct fluid and electrolyte imbalances and to remove waste products in renal failure. Dialysis can also be used to treat drug overdoses.

The two methods of dialysis are *peritoneal dialysis* (PD) and *hemodialysis* (HD). Table 66 compares the two methods.

- In PD the peritoneal membrane is used as the semipermeable membrane.
- In HD an artificial membrane (usually made of cellulose-based or synthetic materials) is used as the semipermeable membrane that is in contact with the patient's blood.
- Dialysis is begun when the patient's uremic state can no longer be adequately managed conservatively.
- A general guideline is to start dialysis when the glomerular filtration rate (GFR) (or creatinine clearance) is <5 to 10 ml/min. However, this criterion varies widely in different clinical situations, and the physician determines when to start dialysis on an individual basis. Certain uremic complications, including encephalopathy, uncontrollable hyperkalemia, pericarditis, and accelerated hypertension, indicate a need for immediate dialysis.

Peritoneal Dialysis

In recent years the use of PD to treat chronic renal failure has increased. The large surface area of the peritoneum makes it a good semipermeable membrane for performing clinical dialysis.

Peritoneal Catheters

Peritoneal access is obtained by inserting a catheter through the anterior abdominal wall (Fig. 8). The prototype of the catheter that is used was developed by Tenckhoff in 1968 and is made of silicone rubber tubing. Other types of catheters for chronic PD are variations of the Tenckhoff catheter, including the Toronto-Western, Purdue-Column Disc, and Gore-Tex catheters.

- The tip of the catheter rests in the peritoneal cavity and has many perforations spaced throughout the distal end of the tubing to allow fluid to flow in and out of the catheter.
- Before the start of PD, it is preferable to allow a waiting period of 7 to 14 days for proper sealing of the catheter and for tissue ingrowth. However, some centers start dialysis 5 to 7 days after catheter insertion. About 2 to 4 weeks after catheter

Table 66 Comparison of Peritoneal Dialysis and Hemodialysis

Peritoneal dialysis		Hemodialysis	
Advantages	**Disadvantages**	**Advantages**	**Disadvantages**
Immediate initiation in almost any hospital	Bacterial or chemical peritonitis	Rapid fluid removal	Vascular access problems
Less complicated than hemodialysis	Protein loss into dialysate	Rapid removal of urea and creatinine	Dietary and fluid restrictions
Portable system with CAPD	Exit-site and tunnel infections	Effective K^+ removal	Heparinization may be necessary
Fewer dietary restrictions	Self-image problems with catheter placement	Less protein loss	Extensive equipment necessary
Relatively short training time	Hyperglycemia	Lowering of serum triglycerides	Hypotension during dialysis
Usable in the patient with vascular access problems	Aggravated hyperlipidemia	Home dialysis possible	Added blood loss that contributes to anemia
Less cardiovascular stress	Surgery for catheter placement	Temporary access can be placed at bedside	Specially trained personnel necessary
Home dialysis possible	Contraindication in the patient with multiple abdominal surgeries or trauma		
Preferable for the diabetic patient	Specially trained personnel needed		

CAPD, Continuous ambulatory peritoneal dialysis; K^+, potassium.

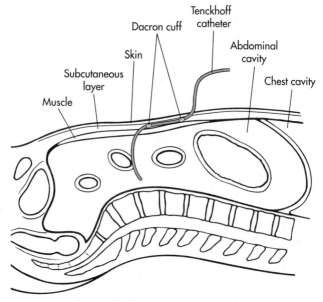

Fig. 8 Tenckhoff catheter in peritoneal dialysis.

implantation, the exit site should be clean, dry, and free of redness and tenderness.

- Once the catheter incision site is healed, the patient may shower and then pat the catheter and exit site dry.
- Daily catheter care includes cleansing with antibacterial soap, application of an antiseptic solution, and a clean dressing, as well as examination of the catheter site for signs of infection.

PD Procedure

The three phases of the PD cycle are *inflow* (fill), *dwell* (equilibration), and *drain* (the three phases together are called an *exchange*).

- During inflow, a prescribed amount of solution, usually 2 L, is infused over about 10 minutes. The flow rate may be decreased if the patient becomes uncomfortable. After the solution has been infused, the inflow clamp is closed before air enters the tubing.
- During the dwell phase, or equilibration, diffusion and osmosis occur between the patient's blood and peritoneal cavity. The duration of dwell time can last 20 to 30 minutes to 8 or more hours, depending on the method of PD.
- Drain time takes 15 to 30 minutes and may be facilitated by gently massaging the abdomen or changing the patient's position.

The cycle starts again with the infusion of another 2 L of solution. For manual PD, a period of about 30 to 50 minutes is required to complete an exchange.

Complications of PD

Complications of PD include exit site infection, peritonitis, abdominal pain, hernias, lower back problems, bleeding, and protein loss. For a discussion of complications, see Lewis and others, *Medical-Surgical Nursing,* edition 5, p. 1324.

Clinically, the patient on PD does at least as well as the patient on HD and sometimes better. There are fewer dietary restrictions and greater mobility is possible than with conventional HD.

- The major disadvantage is the possibility of developing peritonitis. As further improvements in techniques are made (e.g., improved connecting and sterilizing devices, in-line filters, improved catheters), the incidence of peritonitis is decreasing.
- PD is especially indicated for the individual who has vascular access problems and responds poorly to the hemodynamic stresses of HD (e.g., older adult patient with diabetes and cardiovascular disease). The diabetic patient with end-stage renal disease (ESRD) does better on PD than on HD.

Hemodialysis

Vascular Access

In HD, vascular access is needed for the high blood flow required to perform HD (Fig. 9).

An arteriovenous (AV) fistula is created in the forearm or thigh by a side-to-side, end-to-side, or end-to-end anastomosis between an artery (usually radial or ulnar) and a vein (usually cephalic). The fistula provides for arterial blood flow through the vein. The increased pressure of the arterial blood flow through the vein makes the vein dilate and become tough, making it accessible for repeated venipuncture and allowing it to handle the high blood flows required for HD. The vein is accessed using two large gauge needles.

- Grafts used for vascular access are made of synthetic materials (polytetrafluoroethylene [PTFE; Teflon]) and form a "bridge" between the arterial and venous blood supplies. Grafts are surgically anastomosed between an artery (usually brachial) and a vein (usually antecubital). The graft, like the fistula, is under the skin and accessed using two large gauge needles. As grafts are made of manmade materials, they can become infected easily and are thrombogenic.

In some situations when temporary vascular access is required, percutaneous cannulation of the subclavian, internal jugular, or femoral vein is used.

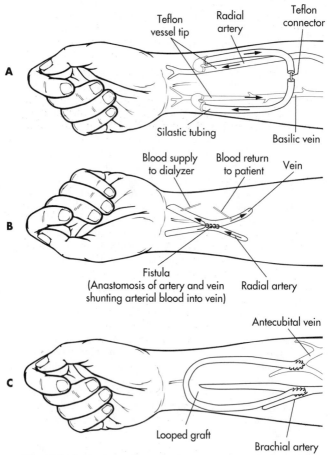

Fig. 9 Methods of vascular access for hemodialysis. **A,** External cannula or shunt. **B,** Internal arteriovenous fistula. **C,** Looped graft in forearm.

Dialyzers

The dialyzer is a long plastic cartridge that contains thousands of parallel hollow tubes or fibers. The fibers are the semipermeable membrane made of cellulose-based or other synthetic materials.

- The blood is pumped through the fibers and dialysis fluid bathes the outside of them, with dialysis and ultrafiltration occurring through the pores of the semipermeable membrane.

Dialysis Procedure

To initiate chronic dialysis two needles are placed in the fistula or graft. The needle closest to the fistula is used to obtain "arterial" blood from the patient and send it to the dialyzer with the assistance of a blood pump. The dialyzer is usually primed with saline solution. The saline solution is infused into the patient as blood fills the dialyzer circuit. Heparin is added to the blood as it flows into the dialyzer to prevent clotting.

- Once the blood enters the extracorporeal circuit, it is propelled through the dialyzer by a blood pump at a flow rate of 200 to 500 ml/min, while the dialysate (warmed to body temperature) circulates in the opposite direction at a rate of 300 to 900 ml/min.
- Blood is returned from the dialyzer to the patient via the "venous" line through the second needle.

In addition to the dialyzer, there is a dialysate delivery and monitoring system. This system pumps the dialysate through the dialyzer countercurrent to the blood flow. Adjustments can be made for ultrafiltration by creating a positive pressure on the blood side, a negative pressure on the dialysate side, or a combination of both. The dialysis system has an alarm system to warn of blood leaking into the dialysate or air leaking into the blood; alterations in dialysate temperature, concentration, or pressure; and extremes in BP readings.

- Dialysis is terminated by flushing the dialyzer with saline solution to return all blood to the patient. The needles are then removed from the patient and firm pressure is applied to the venipuncture sites until the bleeding stops.

Complications of HD

Complications of HD include (1) disequilibrium syndrome with rapid changes in extracellular fluid composition, (2) hypotension due to rapid vascular volume removal, (3) muscle cramps resulting from sodium (Na^+) and water rapid removal, loss of blood from the dialyzer or with a patient who has clotting problems, (4) hepatitis due to blood transfusions, and (5) sepsis at the vascular access site.

HD is still an imperfect technique in treating ESRD. It cannot replace the metabolic and hormonal functions of the kidneys. HD can relieve most of the symptoms of chronic renal failure and, if started early, can prevent certain complications. However, it does not alter the accelerated atherosclerosis.

EMERGENCY PATIENT: PRIMARY AND SECONDARY SURVEY

Recognition of life-threatening illness or injury is one of the most important aspects of emergency care. Before a diagnosis can be made, recognition of the dangerous clinical signs and symptoms with initiation of interventions to reverse or prevent a crisis is essential.

- A triage system identifies and categorizes patients so the most critical are treated first. *Triage* is a French word meaning to "sort".
- The process is based on the premise that patients with a threat to life, vision, or limb should be treated before other patients.

The emergency department (ED) may use a system of words, color coding, numbers for triage acuity, or international codes. See Triage Acuity Systems, p. 738.

The **primary survey** (Table 67) focuses on the airway, breathing, and circulation and serves to identify life-threatening problems so appropriate interventions can be initiated.

The **secondary survey** should not be done until the primary survey is complete. During the primary survey, life-threatening airway, breathing, or circulation problems are corrected as quickly as possible. Once this has been accomplished, a secondary survey is initiated. The secondary survey involves obtaining a history, identifying all injuries, and performing a head-to-toe assessment, including an evaluation of the patient's back (Table 68).

Table 67   Primary Survey of an Emergency Patient

Assessment	Intervention
Airway with Cervical Spine	
Clear and open airway	Suction
Assess for obstructed airway	Jaw thrust
Assess for respiratory distress	Nasal or oral airway, endotracheal tube
Check for loose teeth or foreign objects	Cervical spine immobilization using collar, back board, soft rolls, tape forehead
Assess for bleeding, vomitus, or edema	
Breathing	
Assess ventilation	Ventilate with bag valve mask with 100% oxygen (O_2)
■ Look for chest movements associated with breathing	Prepare to intubate if respiratory arrest
■ Note use of accessory muscles or abdominal muscles	Have suction available
	Give supplemental O_2 via appropriate delivery system
■ Listen for air being expired through nose and mouth	If head trauma, hyperventilate with 100% O_2
■ Feel for air being expelled	If absent breath sounds, perform needle thoracostomy and prepare for chest tube insertion
Observe and count respiratory rate	
Note color of nail beds, mucous membranes, skin	
Auscultate lungs	
Assess for jugular vein distention and position of trachea	

Continued

Table 67   Primary Survey of an Emergency Patient—cont'd

Assessment	Intervention
Circulation	
Check carotid or femoral pulse	If absent pulse, begin chest compressions
Assess color, temperature, and moisture of skin	If shock symptoms or hypotensive, start IVs with at least two large bore
Assess level of consciousness	(14-16 gauge) IV catheters with normal saline or lactated Ringer's solution
Check capillary refill	Administer blood products if ordered
Assess for external bleeding	Consider autotransfusion if isolated chest trauma
	Obtain blood samples for type and cross match
	Control bleeding with direct pressure
Disability	
Assess level of consciousness	Periodically reassess level of consciousness
Assess response to verbal and painful stimuli	
Assess extremity movement (all four)	
Perform Glasgow Coma Scale (pp. 720-721)	
Check pupil response to light	

Table 68   Secondary Survey of an Emergency Patient

Parameter	Assessment
Expose Fahrenheit Get Vital Signs	Remove clothing for adequate examination. Keep patient warm with warm blankets, IV fluids, overhead lights BP Pulse, cardiac rhythm Respiratory rate and effort Temperature Oxygen saturation Urinary catheter if not contraindicated Gastric tube Laboratory studies for presenting condition
History and Head-to-Toe Assessment	*History* Length of time since incident occurred Accident type, location, and patient's position in accident Description of accident, incident, or illness Allergies Medications Past health history, pregnancy Last meal Events leading to accident, incident, or illness

Continued

BP, Blood pressure; *IV,* intravenous; *SC,* subcutaneous.

Table 68   Secondary Survey of an Emergency Patient—cont'd

Parameter	Assessment
History and Head-to-Toe Assessment—cont'd	**Head, Neck, Face** Examine face and scalp for lacerations, bone or soft tissue deformity, tenderness, bleeding, and foreign objects. Examine eyes, ears, nose, and mouth for bleeding, foreign bodies, drainage, pain, deformity, ecchymosis, lacerations Examine head for depressions of cranial or facial bones, contusions, hematomas, areas of softness, bony crepitus Examine neck for stiffness, pain in cervical vertebrae, tracheal deviation, distended neck veins, bleeding, edema, difficulty swallowing, bruising, subcutaneous emphysema, bony crepitus **Chest** Rate, depth, and character of breathing Anterior and posterior chest wall movement Palpate for bony crepitus, SC emphysema Use of accessory muscles External signs of injury: petechiae, bleeding, cyanosis, bruises, abrasions,

Symmetry of external abdominal wall and bony structures
External signs of injury: bruising, abrasions, lacerations, punctures
Assess for masses, guarding, femoral pulses
Type and location of pain
Bowel sounds
Rigidity or distention of abdomen
Assess genitalia for blood at the meatus, priapism, ecchymosis, rectal
    bleeding, and sphincter tone

Extremities
Signs of external injury: deformity, ecchymosis, abrasions, lacerations, swelling
Pain
Movement and strength in arms and legs
Sensation in each limb
Color of skin
Presence and quality of peripheral pulses

Back
Log-roll and inspect and palpate back for deformity, bleeding, lacerations,
    bruising

HEIMLICH MANEUVER

The management of a foreign body obstruction of the airway depends on if the person is conscious or unconscious. Table 69 outlines the actions involved in basic life support and explains how to perform them. Figure 10 illustrates the Heimlich maneuver, which is an emergency procedure for dislodging an obstruction from the trachea to prevent asphyxiation. If repeated attempts to free the airway are unsuccessful, an emergency cricothyrotomy may be done.

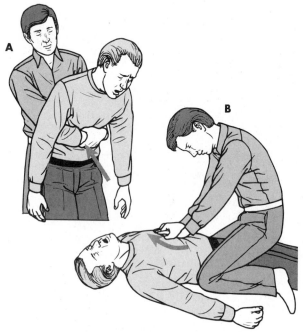

Fig. 10 A, Heimlich maneuver administered to conscious (standing), victim of foreign body airway obstruction. **B,** Heimlich maneuver administered to unconscious (lying) victim of foreign body airway obstruction—astride position.

| Table 69 | Management of Foreign Body Airway Obstruction |

Action	Helpful hints
Conscious Adult	
1. Determine if victim is able to speak or cough.	Rescuer can ask, "Are you choking?" Victim may be using the universal distress signal of choking: clutching the neck between the thumb and index finger
2. Abdominal thrust: perform the Heimlich maneuver until the foreign body is expelled or the victim becomes unconscious (see Fig. 10).	Stand behind victim and wrap arms around victim's waist. Press fist into abdomen with quick inward and upward thrusts.
3. Chest thrust: for victims who are in advanced pregnancy or who are obese.	Chest thrusts: stand behind victim and place arms under victim's armpits to encircle the chest. Press with quick backward thrusts.
Victim Is or Becomes Unconscious	
1. Activate EMS.	Call 911.
2. Check for foreign body obstruction.	Sweep deeply into mouth with hooked finger to remove foreign body.
3. Attempt rescue breathing.	Open airway. Try to give two breaths. If needed, reposition the head and try again.
4. If airway is obstructed, perform Heimlich maneuver.	Kneel astride the victim's thighs. Place the heel of one hand on the victim's abdomen, in the midline slightly above the navel and well below the tip of the xyphoid. Place the second hand on top of the first. Press into the abdomen with quick upward thrusts.
5. Repeat sequence until successful.	Alternate these maneuvers in rapid sequence: finger sweep, rescue breathing attempt, and abdominal thrusts.

EMS, Emergency medical services.
Source: *Textbook of basic life support for healthcare providers*, Dallas, 1997, American Heart Association.

INTESTINAL AND NASOGASTRIC TUBES

Although the physician usually inserts intestinal tubes, the nurse assists with the procedure. Insertion is easier if the patient relaxes, takes deep breaths, and swallows when instructed.

- If insertion of the tube to the small intestine is desired, the patient may be instructed or positioned to lie on the right side to facilitate tube passage through the pylorus.
- In some situations a prokinetic drug such as metoclopramide (Reglan) may be used to facilitate tube movement.
- Once the tube is in place, mouth care is extremely important. Vomiting leaves a terrible taste in the patient's mouth, and fecal odor may be present.

When a nasogastric (NG) tube is in place, the patient breathes through the mouth, drying the mouth and lips.

- The nurse should encourage and assist the patient to brush the teeth frequently. Mouthwash and water for the patient to use in rinsing the mouth and petroleum jelly or a water-soluble lubricant for the lips should be provided at the bedside.
- The patient should be checked for signs of irritation from the NG tube. This area should be cleansed and dried daily with application of a water-soluble lubricant and retaping of the tube.

NG and intestinal tubes should be checked every 4 hours for patency. The patient may be placed on a schedule to clamp the tube every 2 hours for 1 hour, or for 3 out of every 4 hours before removal of the tube.

MECHANICAL VENTILATION

Description

Mechanical ventilation is the process in which air or oxygen (O_2)-enriched air is moved into and out of the lungs mechanically. Mechanical ventilation is not curative. It is a means of supporting patients until they recover the ability to breathe independently. Indicators for mechanical ventilation are listed in Table 63-13, Lewis and others, *Medical-Surgical Nursing,* edition 5, p. 1939.

Types of Mechanical Ventilators

There are two major types of mechanical ventilators: negative-pressure and positive-pressure ventilators.

- *Negative-pressure ventilators* are composed of chambers that encase the chest or body and surround it with intermittent sub-atmospheric or negative pressure. Intermittent negative pressure around the chest wall causes the chest to be pulled outward. This reduces intrathoracic pressure. Air rushes in via the upper airway, which is outside the sealed chamber. Expiration is passive and an artificial airway is not required. Negative-pressure ventilators include the Poncho (Puritan Bennett, Emerson) and Pulmowrap (Lifecare).
- *Positive-pressure ventilation* is the primary method used with acutely ill patients. During inspiration the ventilator forces air into the lungs under positive pressure. Unlike spontaneous ventilation, intrathoracic pressure is raised during lung inflation rather than lowered. Expiration occurs passively as in normal expiration. The three types of positive-pressure ventilators are (1) volume-cycled or volume-limited, (2) time-cycled or time-limited, and (3) pressure-cycled or pressure-limited.

See the detailed information on mechanical ventilation in Lewis and others, *Medical-Surgical Nursing*, edition 5, p. 1939. Nursing management of the patient receiving mechanical ventilation is presented in NCP 63-2, *Medical-Surgical Nursing*, p. 1949.

OSTOMIES

Types of Ostomies

An ostomy is a surgical procedure in which an opening is made to allow the passage of intestinal contents from the bowel to an incision or *stoma*. A stoma is created when the intestine is brought through the abdominal wall and sutured to the skin. It may be permanent or temporary. Fecal matter is diverted from the colon through the stoma to the outside of the abdominal wall.

- An *ileostomy* is an opening from the ileum through the abdominal wall and is also referred to as a *conventional* or *Brooke ileostomy*. It is most commonly used in surgical treatment of ulcerative colitis, Crohn's disease, and familial polyposis.
- A *cecostomy* is an opening between the cecum and the abdominal wall. Both cecostomies and ascending colostomies are uncommon. They are usually temporary and most often are used for fecal diversion before surgery or for palliation.
- A *colostomy* is an opening between the colon and the abdominal wall. The proximal end of the colon is sutured to the skin. Locations for colostomies are shown in Figure 11.

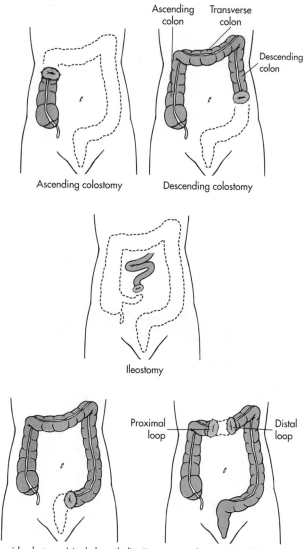

Fig. 11 Types of ostomies.

- A *temporary colostomy* is usually performed to protect an end-to-end anastomosis after a bowel resection or as an emergency measure following bowel obstruction (e.g., malignant tumor), abdominal trauma (e.g., gunshot wound), or a perforated diverticulum. Temporary colostomies are usually located in the transverse colon.
- *Loop colostomy* and *double-barrel colostomy* are most commonly performed as temporary colostomies, but they may be permanent. A comparison of colostomies and ileostomy is shown in Table 70.

The actual procedures to perform ostomy surgeries are discussed in Lewis and others, *Medical-Surgical Nursing,* edition 5, p. 1172.

Nursing Management

In the preoperative period it is important to review the information that the patient has received from the physician. The family and the patient usually have many questions concerning the procedures.

- If available, an enterostomal therapy (ET) nurse or therapist should visit with the patient and the family.
- The nurse or ET nurse must determine the patient's ability to perform self-care, identify support systems, and determine potential adverse factors that could be modified to facilitate learning during rehabilitation.
- The ET nurse marks the stoma site before surgery. An improperly placed stoma complicates rehabilitation by increasing the time and expense of the pouch change routine. It can also contribute to skin irritation and poor adaptation.
- The patient and the family should understand the extent of the surgery as well as the type of stoma and its care.
- If the patient desires a referral and the physician agrees, a trained ostomy visitor from the United Ostomy Association can provide meaningful psychologic support.

Colostomy Care

Postoperative nursing care should focus on assessing the stoma, protecting the skin, selecting the pouch, and assisting the patient to adapt psychologically to a changed body. See NCP 40-4 for the patient with a colostomy or ileostomy, Lewis and others, *Medical-Surgical Nursing,* edition 5. p. 1175.

The stoma should be pink. A dusky-blue stoma indicates ischemia and a brown-black stoma indicates necrosis. The nurse should assess and document stoma color every 8 hours. There is mild to moderate swelling of the stoma the first 2 to 3 weeks after surgery. A skin barrier should be applied to protect the peristomal suture line and skin surrounding the stoma. Solid skin barriers include Stomahesive (Convatec), Coloplast, and Hollister. The skin should be washed with warm water and dried thoroughly before the barrier is applied.

Table 70 Comparison of Colostomies and Ileostomy

	Colostomy			
	Ascending	Transverse	Sigmoid	Ileostomy
Stool consistency	Semiliquid	Semiliquid to semiformed	Formed	Liquid to semiliquid
Fluid requirement	Increased	Possibly increased	No change	Increased
Bowel regulation	No	Uncommon	Yes (if there is a history of a regular bowel pattern)	No
Pouch and skin barriers	Yes	Yes	Dependent on regulation	Yes
Irrigation	No	No	Possible every 24-48 hr (if patient meets criteria)	No
Indications for surgery	Perforating diverticulitis in lower colon; trauma; inoperable tumors of colon, rectum, or pelvis; rectovaginal fistula	Same as for ascending; birth defect	Cancer of the rectum or rectosigmoidal area; perforating diverticulum; trauma	Ulcerative colitis, Crohn's disease, diseased or injured colon, birth defect, familial polyposis, trauma, cancer

- With an open-ended, transparent, plastic, odor-proof pouch it is easy to protect the skin and to observe and collect the drainage. The pouch must fit snugly to prevent leakage around the stoma. The size of the stoma is determined with a stoma measuring card. Although the pouch is applied after surgery, the colostomy functions when peristalsis has been adequately restored.

- The volume, color, and consistency of the drainage are recorded. Each time the pouch is changed, the condition of the skin is observed for irritation. A pouch should never be placed directly on irritated skin without the use of a skin barrier.

- A colostomy in the ascending and transverse colon has semi-liquid stools. The patient needs to be instructed to use a drainable pouch. A colostomy in the sigmoid or descending colon has semiformed or formed stools and can be regulated by the irrigation method. The patient may or may not wear a drainage pouch. A nondrainable pouch should have a gas filter.

- For most patients with colostomies, there are few, if any, dietary restrictions. A well-balanced diet and adequate fluid intake is important. The patient's medical and surgical history needs to be considered when individualizing dietary instructions. For foods and their effects on stomas output, see Table 40-34, *Medical-Surgical Nursing*, p. 1177.

Colostomy irrigations are intended to regulate bowel function, treat constipation, or prepare the bowel for surgery. If control is achieved, there should be little or no spillage between irrigations. The patient who establishes regularity may need to wear only a pad or cover over the stoma. The patient who cannot or chooses not to establish regularity by irrigations must wear a pouch at all times. The procedure for colostomy irrigation is presented in Table 71.

- The procedure should not be rushed; the patient should feel relaxed. The patient or family member must be instructed in the procedure and must be able to demonstrate the ability to irrigate before he or she can be independent. This can be done in the outpatient setting.

▼ **Patient Teaching**

- The patient should be able to perform skin care, control odor, care for the stoma, and identify the signs and symptoms of complications.

- The patient should know the importance of fluids and food in the diet, have names and addresses of the United Ostomy Association, and know when to seek medical care.

- Home care and outpatient follow-up by an ET nurse is highly recommended.

- Patients need to be discharged with written pouch change instructions, teaching literature relevant to the type of stoma they have, a list of equipment they use (including names and phone numbers), a list of equipment retailers, outpatient follow-up appointments with the surgeon and ET nurse, and the phone numbers of the surgeon and nurse.

See Table 40-36 for ostomy teaching guidelines, Lewis and others, *Medical-Surgical Nursing*, edition 5, p. 1178.

Table 71	Patient and Family Home Care Guide: Colostomy Irrigation

Equipment
Lubricant
Irrigation set (1000-2000 ml container, tubing with irrigating cone, clamp)
Irrigating sleeve with adhesive or belt
Toilet tissue to clean around the stoma
Disposal sack for soiled dressing

Procedure
1. Place 500-1000 ml of lukewarm water (not to exceed 105° F) [40.5° C] in container. The volume is titrated for the individual; use enough irrigant to distend the bowel but not enough to cause cramping pain. Most adults use 500-1000 ml of water.
2. Ensure comfortable position. Patient may sit in chair in front of toilet or on the toilet if the perineal wound is healed.
3. Clear tubing of all air by flushing it with fluid.
4. Hang container on hook or IV pole (18-24 in) above stoma (about shoulder height).
5. Apply irrigating sleeve and place bottom end in toilet bowl.
6. Lubricate cone and insert cone tip gently into the stoma and hold tip securely in place.
7. Allow irrigation solution to flow in steadily for 5-10 min.
8. If cramping occurs, stop the flow of solution for a few seconds, leaving the cone in place.
9. Clamp the tubing and remove irrigating cone when the desired amount of irrigant has been delivered or when the patient senses colonic distention.
10. Allow 30-45 minutes for the solution and feces to be expelled. Initial evacuation is usually complete in 10-15 min. Close off the irrigating sleeve at the bottom to allow ambulation.
11. Clean, rinse, and dry peristomal skin well.
12. Replace the colostomy drainage pouch or desired stoma covering.
13. Wash and rinse all equipment and hand dry.

IV, Intravenous.

Ileostomy Care

Care of the ileostomy is presented in the nursing care plan for the patient with a colostomy or ileostomy, Lewis and others, *Medical-Surgical Nursing*, edition 5, p. 1175.

- Immediately after surgery, intake and output must be accurately monitored. The patient should be observed for signs and symptoms of fluid and electrolyte imbalance, particularly potassium (K^+), sodium (Na^+), and fluid deficits.
- In the first 24 to 48 hours after surgery the amount of drainage from the stoma may be negligible. Once peristalsis returns, the patient may experience a period of high volume output of 1000 to 1800 ml per day. Later on, the average amount can be 800 ml daily.

▼ Patient Teaching

The patient should be instructed to drink at least 1 to 2 L of fluid daily; more may be necessary when diarrhea occurs and in the summer, when perspiration is increased. Diarrhea from an ileostomy produces acidosis from the loss of bicarbonate. The physician may instruct the patient to take an electrolyte solution at home (e.g., 1 tsp of salt and 1 tsp of baking soda in 1 qt of water). Fluids rich in electrolytes should be encouraged.

- Usually a low-roughage diet is ordered initially. Fiber-containing foods are reintroduced gradually. Later there are no dietary restrictions except for foods that are troublesome (e.g., high roughage popcorn) for the patient. A return to a normal, presurgical diet is the goal.
- The stoma often bleeds easily when it is touched because it has a high vascular supply. The patient should be told that minimal oozing of blood is normal.

General Nursing Considerations Related to Ostomies

- The patient should not be forced to learn to care for the ostomy. The nurse should watch for clues that the patient is ready. Teaching at the appropriate time is an important part of the care and can contribute to a smooth adjustment process.
- Supportive measures by nursing include helping the patient acquire knowledge, providing or recommending support services, and identifying coping mechanisms that are effective. The nurse provides support by responding to the physiologic needs of stoma care and the psychosocial needs of self-esteem.
- Discussion of sexuality and sexual function needs to be incorporated in the plan of care. The nurse can help the patient understand that sexual function or sexual activity may be affected, but sexuality does not have to be altered.
- The social impact of the stoma is interrelated with the psychologic, physical, and sexual aspects. Concerns of people with

stomas include the ability to resume sexual activity, altering clothing styles, the effect on daily activities, sleeping while wearing a pouch, passing gas, the presence of odor, cleanliness, and deciding when or if to tell others about the ostomy.

OXYGEN THERAPY

Description

The goal of oxygen (O_2) therapy is to supply the patient with adequate O_2 to maximize the O_2-carrying ability of the blood. O_2 is usually administered to treat hypoxemia caused by (1) respiratory disorders such as chronic obstructive pulmonary disease (COPD), cor pulmonale, pneumonia, atelectasis, lung cancer, and pulmonary emboli; (2) cardiovascular disorders such as myocardial infarction (MI), arrhythmias, angina pectoris, and cardiogenic shock; and (3) central nervous system (CNS) disorders such as an overdose of narcotics, head injury, and disordered sleep (sleep apnea).

Methods of Administration

There are various methods of O_2 administration (see Table 27-17, Lewis and others, *Medical-Surgical Nursing,* edition 5, p. 693). The method of administration selected depends on factors such as the fraction of inspired O_2 concentration (FiO_2) and humidification required, patient cooperation, comfort, and cost. Various methods include nasal cannula, face mask, nasal catheter, rebreathing and nonrebreathing masks, transtracheal catheter, and Venturi mask.

- O_2 obtained from cylinders or wall systems is dry. Dry O_2 has an irritating effect on the mucous membranes and dries secretions. Therefore it is important that O_2 be humidified when administered, either by humidification or nebulization.

Complications

O_2 supports combustion and increases the rate of burning. This is why it is important that smoking be prohibited in the area in which O_2 is being used. A "No Smoking" sign should be prominently displayed on the patient's door. The patient should also be cautioned against smoking cigarettes with O_2 prongs or a catheter in place.

- In some cases of respiratory distress such as long-standing COPD, increasing the O_2 flow rate may be quite harmful. When O_2 is administered in high concentrations, the hypoxic stimulus is eliminated and the rate and depth of ventilation decreases. The patient will subsequently develop hypercapnia and eventually *carbon dioxide (CO₂) narcosis*. The patient's mental status and vital signs should be assessed before starting O_2 therapy and frequently thereafter.

Infection can be a major hazard of O_2 administration. Heated nebulizers present the highest risk. Constant use of humidity supports bacterial growth, with the most common infecting organism being *Pseudomonas aeruginosa*. Disposable equipment that operates as a closed system should be used. There should be a hospital policy stating the required frequency of equipment changes based upon the type of equipment. Both equipment and respiratory secretions should be Gram-stained and cultured frequently.

Chronic Oxygen Therapy at Home

An improved prognosis and quality of life has been noted in patients with COPD who receive nocturnal or continuous O_2 to treat hypoxemia. The benefits of long-term continuous O_2 therapy include improved neuropsychologic function, increased exercise tolerance, decreased hematocrit (Hct), and reduced pulmonary hypertension. It also improves sleep and may reduce normal arrhythmias.

- Periodic reevaluations are necessary for the patient who is using chronic supplemental O_2. Generally, the patient should be reevaluated every 6 months during the first year of therapy and annually after that, as long as patient remains stable.

▼ **Patient Teaching**
- Teach the patient and family not to increase the O_2 flow rate unless directed to do so by a physician or nurse to prevent problems related to removing the patient's hypoxic drive.

A home care guide for teaching the patient and family about home O_2 use is in Table 72.

PACEMAKERS

Description

The artificial cardiac pacemaker is an electronic device used in place of the sinoatrial (SA) node, the natural cardiac pacemaker of the heart. The artificial cardiac pacemaker is an electrical circuit in which the battery provides electricity that travels through a conducting wire to the myocardium, and the myocardium stimulates the heart to beat (i.e., it "captures" the heart).

- Recent advances in technology have been applied extensively to pacemakers. This has resulted in sophisticated, noninvasive, programmable single- and dual-chambered pacemakers with

Table 72	Patient and Family Home Care Guide: Home Oxygen Use

Mask/Cannula
- Ensure that the straps are not too tight
- Remove two to three times a day to wash and dry skin where straps are and to stimulate skin
- Pad any pressure points
- Observe tops of ears for skin breakdown from pressure points

Oral and Nasal Mucous Membranes
- Assess oral and nasal mucous membranes two to three times a day
- Use water-based gel on lips and nasal mucosa
- Provide frequent oral hygiene
- Provide humidification via humidifier or nebulizing device

Decreasing Risk for Infection
- Remove mask or collar and cleanse with water two to three times a day
- Cleanse skin carefully at this time and observe for cuts, scratches, and bruises
- Change disposable equipment frequently
- Remove secretions that are coughed out

Decreasing Risk of Fire Injuries
- Post "No Smoking" warning signs in home where they can be seen
- Do not use electric razors, portable radios, open flames, wool blankets, or mineral oils in the area where O_2 is in use
- Do not allow smoking in the home

O_2, Oxygen.
Note: A good resource for patients is *About Oxygen Therapy at Home*, a booklet published by the American Lung Association.

specialized circuits that weigh only 40 to 50 g. Pacemakers have been developed that are more physiologically accurate, pacing both the atrium and ventricle, as well as increasing the heart rate (HR) when appropriate

Types of Pacemakers
Permanent pacemakers are those that are implanted totally within the body and *temporary pacemakers* are those with the power source outside the body.

Table 73	Indications for Permanent Pacemaker Therapy

Sinus node dysfunction
Third-degree AV block
Fibrosis or sclerotic changes of cardiac conduction system
Sick sinus syndrome
Mobitz II second-degree AV block
Hypersensitive carotid sinus syndrome
Chronic atrial fibrillation with slow ventricular response
Tachyarrhythmias
Bifascicular block

AV, Atrioventricular.

- The permanent pacemaker power source is implanted subcutaneously in the chest or abdomen and is attached to pacer electrodes, which are threaded transvenously to the right ventricle (RV) or right atrium (RA). Indications for insertion of a permanent pacemaker are listed in Table 73.
- Temporary pacemakers are used with a lead or wire threaded transvenously to the RV and a wire attached to a power source externally. Indications for temporary pacing are listed in Table 74.

Complications

Pacemaker malfunction is manifested by a failure to sense or a failure to capture. *Failure to sense* occurs when the pacemaker fails to recognize spontaneous atrial or ventricular activity and fires inappropriately. Failure to sense may be caused by pacer lead fracture, battery failure, or electrode displacement. *Failure to capture* occurs when the electrical charge to the myocardium is insufficient to produce atrial or ventricular contraction. Failure to capture may be caused by pacer lead fracture, battery failure, electrode displacement, or fibrosis at the electrode tip.

Complications of invasive temporary or permanent pacemaker insertion include infection and hematoma formation at the site of insertion of the pacemaker power source, pneumothorax, failure to sense or capture with possible bradycardia and significant symptoms, perforation of atrial or ventricular septum by the pacing wire, and the appearance of "end-of-life" battery parameters on testing the pacemaker.

- Measures taken to prevent and assess complications include prophylactic IV antibiotic therapy before and after insertion,

Table 74	Indications for Temporary Pacing

- Maintenance of adequate HR and rhythm during special circumstances such as surgery and postoperative recovery, cardiac catheterization or coronary angioplasty, during drug therapy that may cause bradycardia, and before implantation of a permanent pacemaker
- As prophylaxis after open heart surgery
- Acute anterior MI with second-degree or third-degree AV block or bundle branch block
- Acute inferior MI with symptomatic bradycardia and AV block
- Termination of AV nodal reentry or reciprocating tachycardia associated with WPW syndrome, atrial flutter, or ventricular tachycardia
- Suppression of ectopic atrial or ventricular rhythm
- Electrophysiologic studies to evaluate patient with bradyarrhythmias and tachyarrhythmias

AV, Atrioventricular; *HR,* heart rate; *MI,* myocardial infarction; *WPW,* Wolff-Parkinson-White.

assessment of chest x-ray after insertion to check lead placement and to rule out the presence of pneumothorax, careful observation of the insertion site, and continuous ECG monitoring of patient's rhythm.
- After pacemaker insertion, the patient is kept on bed rest for 12 hours, and minimal arm and shoulder activity is allowed to prevent dislodgment of the newly implanted pacemaker leads.

Nursing Management
Nursing interventions include observation for the signs of infection by assessing the incision for redness, swelling, or discharge. Temperature elevation should also be noted. Careful monitoring of patient's rhythm is used to detect problems with sensing or capturing.
- The patient with a newly implanted pacemaker may frequently have questions about activity restrictions and fears concerning body image and becoming a "cardiac cripple" after the procedure.
- The goal of pacemaker therapy should be to enhance physiologic functioning and the quality of life. This should be emphasized to the patient, and the nurse should give concrete advice on activity restrictions. Patient and family teaching for the patient with a pacemaker is outlined in Table 75.

Table 75	Patient and Family Teaching Guide: Pacemaker

1. Maintain follow-up care with a physician to check the pacemaker site and begin regular pacemaker function checks with magnet and ECG evaluation.
2. Watch for signs of infection at incision site—redness, swelling, drainage.
3. Keep incision dry for 1 week after implantation.
4. Avoid lifting arm on operative side above shoulder level for 1 week.
5. Avoid direct blows to generator site.
6. Avoid close proximity to high-output electrical generators or to large magnets such as an MRI scanner. These devices can reprogram a pacemaker.
7. Microwave ovens are safe to use and do not threaten pacemaker function.
8. Travel without restrictions is allowed. The small metal case of an implanted pacemaker rarely sets off an airport security alarm.
9. The patient should be taught how to take his or her pulse.
10. Carry pacemaker information card at all times.

ECG, Electrocardiogram; *MRI,* magnetic resonance imaging.

RADIATION THERAPY

Description

Radiation therapy is a local treatment modality for cancer. An estimated 60% of all persons with cancer will receive radiation therapy in treating their disease.

- Radiation is the emission and distribution of energy through space or a material medium. The major target of radiation is deoxyribonucleic acid (DNA) damage, resulting in an irreversible loss of proliferative capacity. Cancer cells, which are more likely to be dividing, are at increased risk for permanent damage with cumulative radiation doses. Normal cells usually recover from radiation damage if therapy is kept within certain doses.
- Cellular sensitivity to radiation varies throughout the cell cycle, with cells being most sensitive to lethal damage in the M and G_2 phases, and least sensitive during the S or synthesis phase.
- Table 76 describes the radiosensitivity of various cancerous tumors.

Table 76 Tumor Radiosensitivity

High radiosensitivity	Moderate radiosensitivity	Mild radiosensitivity	Poor radiosensitivity
Ovarian dysgerminoma	Skin carcinoma	Soft tissue sarcomas (e.g., chondrosarcoma)	Osteosarcoma
Testicular seminoma	Oropharyngeal carcinoma	Gastric adenocarcinoma	Malignant melanoma
Hodgkin's disease	Esophageal carcinoma	Renal adenocarcinoma	Malignant gliomas
Non-Hodgkin's lymphoma	Breast adenocarcinoma	Colon adenocarcinoma	Testicular nonseminoma
Wilms' tumor	Uterine and cervical carcinoma		
Neuroblastoma	Prostate carcinoma		
	Bladder carcinoma		

Types of Radiation Therapy

- *External radiation* therapy (telepathy) is given by external beam and is the most common form of treatment.
- *Internal radiation* (brachytherapy) consists of the implantation or insertion of radioactive materials directly into the tumor or in close proximity to the tumor. This method is commonly used for tumors of the head and neck and gynecologic malignancies. Implants, such as prostate implants, may also be permanent, with the insertion of radioactive seeds into tumors.

Side Effects of Therapy

Common side effects from radiation therapy may be divided into phases: *acute effects* occur during treatment and for up to 6 months following the completion of therapy, *subacute effects* occur in the next 6 months following the completion of therapy, and *late effects* occur at 1 year and beyond.

- Actively proliferating tissue, such as GI mucosa, esophageal and oropharyngeal mucosa, and bone marrow, exhibit early, acute responses to radiation therapy. Cartilage, bone, kidney, and central and peripheral nervous tissue manifest subacute or late responses.
- Common therapy side effects are fatigue, anorexia, bone marrow suppression, erythema, mucositis, nausea, vomiting, diarrhea, cough, fever, night sweats, and changes in ovary and testes functioning (see Table 14-15, Lewis and others, *Medical-Surgical Nursing,* edition 5, p. 291).

Nursing Management

Caring for the person with a radioactive implant requires that the nurse be aware that the patient is radioactive. If a patient has a temporary implant, the patient is radioactive during the time the source is in place. If the patient has a permanent implant, radioactive exposure to the outside and others is low, and the patient may be discharged with precautions.

- Helping the patient to cope with the anxiety of receiving radiation is an essential component of the nursing role. The necessity of coming for treatment five times per week forces the individual to confront the cancer on an almost daily basis.
- Demands on the patient and family and the disruption of normal activities created by the treatment schedule are difficult to handle. In conjunction with the social worker, the nurse needs to assist with planning for transportation with available resources such as the American Cancer Society, churches, and community resources.
- The impact of radiation on the quality of life of the patient undergoing therapy may be minimized with information and support.

See Chapter 14, Lewis and others, *Medical-Surgical Nursing,* edition 5, p. 289, for the nursing management of anorexia, skin and oral reactions, GI reactions, pulmonary effects, and reproductive effects.

TOTAL PARENTERAL NUTRITION

Description

Total parenteral nutrition (TPN) is a relatively safe and practical method for delivering total nutritional needs by an IV route. TPN is used when the GI tract cannot be used for the ingestion, digestion, and absorption of essential nutrients.

- The goal of TPN is to meet the patient's nutritional needs and to allow for the growth of new body tissue, which can be drastically depleted by a prolonged inability to eat normally.
- Indications for TPN include patients with severe injury, surgery, or burns and those who are malnourished as a result of medical treatment or disease processes.
- Regular IV glucose solutions contain no protein and have 170 calories/L, whereas TPN contains protein, dextrose (20% to 50% of total calories), electrolytes, trace elements, vitamins, and possibly fat emulsion. All TPN solutions should be prepared by a pharmacist or trained technician using strict aseptic techniques under a laminar flow hood. Nothing should be added to TPN solutions after they are prepared by the pharmacy.
- In general, TPN solutions are good for 24 to 36 hours and must be refrigerated until 30 minutes before use.

Administration of TPN

TPN may be administered via a central line into the superior vena cava (the most common route) or through a single- or double-lumen peripherally inserted central catheter (PICC) usually placed into the basilic or cephalic vein and then advanced into the central circulation.

- Central TPN is indicated when long-term nutritional support is necessary, when the patient has high protein and caloric requirements, and when suitable peripheral veins are not available.
- Peripheral parenteral nutrition (PPN) is administered through a large peripheral vein when (1) nutritional support is needed for only a short time (up to 2 weeks), (2) protein and caloric requirements are not excessively high, (3) the risk of a central catheter is too great, or (4) nutritional support is used to supplement inadequate oral intake.

- Once established for TPN, a single-lumen central catheter should not be used for the administration of blood or antibiotics, the drawing of blood samples, or central venous pressure monitoring.

Nursing Management

Infection is one of the major concerns with TPN solutions. It is essential that proper aseptic techniques be followed.

- Millipore filters should be placed on all parenteral lines. When the filter is used, it should be placed proximal to the catheter hub. Filters are changed every 24 hours.
- The IV tubing is changed with each new bottle of TPN. The tubing and the filter should be clearly labeled with the date and the time they are put into use.

A metabolic complication of TPN is hyperglycemia. At the beginning of TPN therapy, the solution is infused at a gradually increasing rate for 24 to 48 hours. In this way the pancreas can adapt to the increased amount of glucose in the circulation by producing more insulin.

- Blood glucose levels should be checked at the bedside every 4 to 6 hours with a glucose-testing meter. A sliding scale of insulin may be ordered to keep the blood glucose level below 180 to 200 mg/dl.

Nurses must be aware that speeding or slowing the infusion rate is contraindicated. Speeding up the rate results in a large amount of glucose entering the circulation. Conversely, slowing the rate may result in a hypoglycemic state, since it takes time for the pancreatic islet cells to adjust to a reduced glucose level.

- Checking the amount infused and the rate every 30 minutes to 1 hour is recommended. An infusion pump should be used during the administration of TPN so that the infusion rate can be maintained and an alarm will sound if the tubing becomes obstructed.

Vital signs should be monitored every 2 to 4 hours. Daily weights give an indication of the patient's nutritional status as the therapy progresses. Blood levels of glucose, electrolytes, protein, a complete blood count (CBC), and enzyme studies are followed daily until stable and then weekly as the condition warrants.

Dressings covering the catheter site are changed according to institutional protocol, from every other day to once a week. Frequently, specially trained nurses from the IV team or the nutritional support team are responsible for these dressing changes. Some institutions allow the staff nurses to do the dressing changes after special instruction.

- The insertion site is carefully observed for signs of inflammation and infection. Phlebitis can readily occur in the vein as a result of the hypertonic infusion and can become infected. In immunosuppressed patients, signs of inflammation or infection can be subtle, if present at all.

- If an infection is suspected during a dressing change, a culture specimen of the site and drainage should be sent for analysis and the physician should be notified immediately.

The same precautions should be followed in weaning from TPN as when therapy is being initiated, except in the reverse order. The flow rate must be gradually decreased for 4 to 6 hours, while oral intake is increased.

- When the catheter is removed, the dressing should be changed daily until the wound heals. Oral nourishment should be encouraged and a careful record of intake should be maintained.

Additional information related to the nursing management of TPN is presented in NCP 38-2 for the patient receiving total parenteral nutrition, Lewis and others, *Medical-Surgical Nursing,* edition 5, p. 1063.

TRACHEOSTOMY

Description

A *tracheotomy* is a surgical incision into the trachea for the purpose of establishing an airway. A *tracheostomy* is the stoma (opening) that results from a tracheotomy. Correct placement of the tube requires surgical dissection and is therefore not typically an emergency procedure.

Indications for tracheostomy are to bypass an upper airway obstruction, facilitate the removal of secretions, permit long-term mechanical ventilation, and permit oral intake and speech in the patient requiring long-term mechanical ventilation. Patient comfort may be increased because no tube is present in the mouth.

- The patient can eat and speak if the tracheostomy cuff can be deflated or a speaking tube is used. Because the tube is more secure, patient mobility is increased.
- Most clinicians believe a tracheostomy should be performed after 7 to 10 days of mechanical ventilation if extubation is not possible, or earlier if it appears likely that an extended period of mechanical ventilation will be required.
- When the patient can expectorate secretions and maintain adequate gas exchange without mechanical ventilation, the tracheostomy tube can be removed. The stoma is covered with dressing and tape. Epithelial tissue begins to form in 24 to 48 hours, and the opening will close in several days.

Nursing Management

Goals

The patient with a tracheostomy will communicate needs, maintain a patent airway, have a normal white blood cell (WBC) count and temperature, have his or her usual appetite with a normal body weight maintained, and have a normal swallowing function.

See NCP 25-5 for the patient with a tracheostomy, Lewis and others *Medical-Surgical Nursing,* edition 5, p. 598.

Nursing Diagnoses

- Ineffective airway clearance *related to* the presence of a tracheostomy tube and difficulty expectorating sputum
- Altered nutrition: less than body requirements *related to* decreased oral intake, altered taste sensation, and swallowing difficulty
- Impaired verbal communication *related to* the use of an artificial airway and cuff
- Impaired swallowing *related to* the tracheostomy tube
- Ineffective management of therapeutic regimen *related to* a lack of knowledge about the care of a tracheostomy at home
- Risk for infection *related to* the bypass of airway defense mechanisms and impaired skin integrity

Nursing Interventions

Before the tracheotomy, the nurse should explain to the patient and family the purpose of the procedure and inform them that the patient will not be able to speak if an inflated cuff is used. The patient and family should be told that normal speech will be possible as soon as the cuff can be deflated.

Care should be taken to not dislodge the tracheostomy tube during the first few days when the stoma is not mature or healed.

- Retention sutures are often placed in the tracheal cartilage when the tracheotomy is performed. The free ends should be taped to the skin in a place and manner that leaves them accessible if the tube is dislodged.
- Because tube replacement can be difficult, several precautions are required: (1) a replacement tube of equal or smaller size is kept at the bedside, readily available for emergency reinsertion, (2) the first tube change is performed by a physician, usually no sooner than 7 days after the tracheotomy, and (3) tracheostomy tapes are not changed for at least 24 hours after the insertion procedure.
- The cleaning procedure removes mucus that has accumulated on the inside of the tube. If humidification is adequate, this accumulation of mucus should not occur and a tube without an inner cannula can be used. See Table 77 for a detailed listing of tracheostomy care.

▼ Patient Teaching

- Assess the ability of the patient and family to provide care at home, including airway care and the ability to respond

Table 77	Tracheostomy Care

1. Explain procedure to patient.
2. Collect necessary sterile equipment (e.g., suction catheter, gloves, water, basin, drape, tracheostomy ties, tube brush or pipe cleaners, 4 × 4s, hydrogen peroxide (3%), sterile water, and tracheostomy dressing [optional]). Note: clean rather than sterile technique is used at home.
3. Position patient in semi-Fowler's position.
4. Assemble needed materials on bedside table next to patient.
5. Wash hands. Put on goggles and gloves.
6. Auscultate chest sounds. If rhonchi or coarse crackles are present, suction the patient if unable to cough up secretions (Table 25-6, Lewis and others, *Medical-Surgical Nursing*, edition 5, p. 595)
7. Unlock and remove inner cannula, if present. Many tracheostomy tubes do not have inner cannulas. Care for these tubes includes all steps except for inner cannula care.
8. If disposable inner cannula is used, replace with new cannula. If a non-disposable cannula is used:
   a. Immerse inner cannula in 3% hydrogen peroxide and clean inside and outside of cannula using tube brush or pipe cleaners.
   b. Drain hydrogen peroxide from cannula. Immerse cannula in sterile water. Remove the sterile water and shake to dry.
   c. Insert inner cannula into outer cannula with the curved part downward and lock in place.

IV, Intravenous.

appropriately to emergencies, to determine if home care is feasible.

- Teach clean suction technique, good hand washing, home preparation of sterile saline solution, use of one catheter for 24 hours, methods of cleaning and reusing catheters, and clean technique for tracheostomy care.
- Make a referral for a visiting nurse or home health care to provide ongoing assistance and support.
- Provide opportunities for the patient to discuss care and concerns about caring for the tracheostomy at home to alleviate anxiety.

Table 77   Tracheostomy Care—cont'd

9. Remove dried secretions from stoma using 4 × 4 soaked in hydrogen peroxide. Rinse with another 4 × 4 soaked in sterile water. Gently pat area around the stoma dry. Be sure to clean under the tracheostomy face plate, using cotton swabs to reach this area.

10. Maintain position of tracheal retention sutures, if present, by taping above and below the stoma.

11. Change tracheostomy ties. Tie tracheostomy ties securely with room for one finger between ties and skin (Fig. 25-8, *Medical-Surgical Nursing*, p. 597). To prevent accidental tube removal, secure the tracheostomy tube by gently applying pressure to flange of the tube during the tie changes. **Do not change tracheostomy ties for 24 hrs after the tracheotomy procedure.**

12. As an alternative, some patients prefer tracheostomy ties made of velcro, which are easier to adjust. Other patients use plastic IV tubing because it is easily cleaned and dries without the need to replace the ties.

13. Unless excessive amounts of exudate are present, avoid using a tracheostomy dressing since this keeps the site moist and may predispose to infection.

14. If drainage is excessive, place dressing around tube (Fig. 25-8, *Medical-Surgical Nursing*, p. 597). A tracheostomy dressing or unlined gauze should be used. Do not cut the gauze because threads may be inhaled or wrap around the tracheostomy tube. Change the dressing frequently. Wet dressings promote infection and stoma irritation.

15. Repeat care three times a day and as needed.

TUBE FEEDINGS

Indications for tube feedings as a supplemental form of nutrition include:

- The patient who has a functioning GI tract but cannot take oral nourishment
- Persons with anorexia, orofacial fractures, head and neck cancer, neurologic or psychiatric conditions that prevent oral intake, extensive burns, and those who are receiving chemotherapy or radiation therapy.

Tube feedings are easily administered, safer, more physiologically efficient, and less expensive than parenteral nutrition. They are used to provide nutrients by way of the GI tract (alone or as a supplement to oral or parenteral nutrition) or as a treatment for malnutrition.

Types of feeding tubes (Figure 12) include:

- Nastrogastric (NG) tube, which is most commonly used for short-term problems
- Esophagostomy, gastrostomy, or jejunostomy for extended feeding
- Transpyloric tube placement for feeding below the pyloric sphincter

The standard procedure for tube feeding includes (1) having the patient sitting or lying with the head of bed elevated 30 to 45 de-

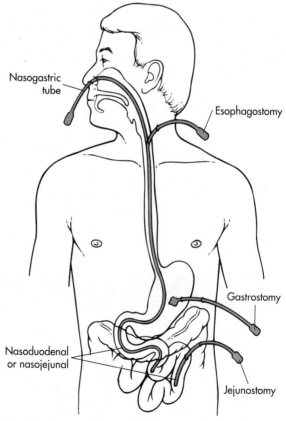

Fig. 12 Common placement locations for enteral feeding tubes.

grees, (2) maintaining tube patency by irrigating before and after each feeding; if feedings are continuous, monitoring the built-in alarm on the feeding pump, and (3) checking proper tube placement before each feeding or every 4 hours with continuous feedings. Feedings should be given at room or body temperature to decrease the likelihood of diarrhea.

Nursing considerations include the following:

- The patient should be weighed daily or several times a week and accurate intake and output records should be maintained.
- The initial blood glucose is checked to assess glucose tolerance.
- Feedings that have been opened and not refrigerated or feedings that have been infusing longer than 8 hours should be discarded to minimize bacterial growth.
- Feedings should be labeled with the date and time they are initially used.
- If a pump is being used, the tubing should be changed every 24 hours.

The type of problems encountered in patients receiving tube feedings and corrective measures are presented in Table 38-18, Lewis and others, *Medical-Surgical Nursing,* edition 5, p. 1058.

URINARY CATHETERIZATION

The process of inserting a catheter into a body cavity or passage is termed *catheterization.* Indwelling catheters often have self-retaining balloons to keep the catheter in place. Nursing responsibilities include understanding the reason for catheterization, the scientific principles involved, aseptic technique, and the appropriate care of the patient after catheterization.

Indications for urinary catheterization are listed in Table 78. Two reasons that are *not* indications for catheterization are (1) the routine acquisition of a sterile specimen for laboratory analysis and (2) the convenience for the nursing staff or the patient's family. Catheterization for sterile urine specimens may occasionally be indicated when patients have complicated urinary infection histories. A catheter should be the final means of providing the patient with a dry environment for the prevention of skin breakdown and protection of dressings or skin lesions.

While the patient has a catheter in place, nursing actions should include maintaining catheter patency, managing fluid intake, providing for the comfort and safety of the patient, and preventing infection. Attention should be given to the psychologic implications of urinary drainage. Concerns of the patient can include embarrassment related

| **Table 78** | **Indications for Urinary Catheterization** |

1. Relief of urinary retention caused by lower urinary tract obstruction, paralysis, or inability to void
2. Bladder decompression preoperatively and operatively for lower abdominal or pelvic surgery
3. Facilitation of surgical repair of urethra and surrounding structures
4. Splinting of ureters or urethra to facilitate healing after surgery or other trauma in area
5. Instillation of medications into bladder
6. Accurate measurement of urinary output in critically ill patient
7. Measurement of residual urine after urination
8. Study of anatomic structures of urinary system
9. Urodynamic testing
10. Collection of sterile urine sample in selected situations

to exposure of the body, an altered body image, and fear concerning the care of the catheter that results in increased dependency.

- Catheters vary in construction materials, tip shape, and the size of the lumen. Catheters are sized according to the French scale. Each French unit equals 0.33 mm of diameter. The diameter measured is the internal diameter of the catheter. The size used varies with the size of the individual and the purpose for catheterization.
- The most common route of urethral catheterization is insertion of the catheter through the external meatus into the urethra, past the internal sphincter, and into the bladder.

Suprapubic catheterization is the simplest and oldest method of urinary diversion. The two methods of insertion of a suprapubic catheter into the bladder are (1) through a small incision in the abdominal wall and (2) by the use of a trocar. A suprapubic catheter is placed while the patient is under general anesthesia for another surgical procedure or at the bedside with a local anesthetic. The catheter may be sutured into place, but a Foley catheter is usually used.

- The suprapubic catheter is used in temporary situations such as bladder, vesical neck, prostate, and urethral surgery. The suprapubic catheter is also used long-term in selected patients.
- Nursing care includes taping the catheter to prevent dislodgment. The care of the tube and catheter is similar to that of the urethral catheter. A pectin-base skin barrier (e.g., Stomahesive) is effective around the insertion site in protecting the skin from breakdown.

The suprapubic catheter is prone to poor drainage because of mechanical obstruction of the catheter tip by the bladder wall, sediment, and clots. Nursing interventions to ensure the patency of the tube include (1) preventing tube kinking by coiling the excess tubing and maintaining gravity drainage, (2) having the patient turn from side to side, and (3) milking the tube. If these measures are not effective, the catheter is irrigated with sterile technique after a physician's order has been obtained.

- If the patient experiences bladder spasms that are difficult to control, urinary leakage may result. Oxybutinin (Ditropan) or other oral antispasmodics or belladonna and opium (B + O) suppositories may be prescribed to decrease bladder spasms.

An alternative approach to a long-term indwelling catheter is *intermittent catheterization*. It is being used with increasing frequency in conditions characterized by neurogenic bladder (e.g., spinal cord injuries, chronic neurologic diseases). This type of catheterization may also be used in the oliguric and anuric phases of acute renal failure to reduce the possibility of infection from an indwelling catheter. Intermittent catheterization is also used postoperatively, often after a surgical procedure for female incontinence or radioactive seed implantation into the prostate for cancer.

- The main goal of intermittent catheterization is to prevent urinary retention, stasis, and compromised blood supply to the bladder due to prolonged pressure.
- The technique consists of inserting a urethral catheter into the bladder every 3 to 5 hours. Some patients do intermittent catheterization only once or twice a day to measure residual urine and to assure an empty bladder.
- Patients should be instructed to wash and rinse the catheter and their hands with soap and water before and after catheterization. Lubricant is necessary for men and may make catheterization more comfortable for women.
- The catheter may be inserted by the patient or the care provider. The bladder is emptied and the catheter is removed.
- The same catheter can be used for weeks at a time. In general, patients should change the catheter every 2 to 4 weeks. In the hospital, a sterile technique is used. For home care, a clean technique that includes good hand washing with soap and water is used.
- The patient is taught to observe for signs of urinary tract infection (UTI) so that treatment can be instituted early. If indicated, some patients are placed on a regimen of prophylactic antibiotics.

PART THREE

REFERENCE APPENDIX

ABBREVIATIONS

°C	degrees Centigrade
°F	degrees Fahrenheit
μg	microgram
μm	micrometer
@	at
ABG	arterial blood gas
ac	before meals
ad lib	freely as desired
ADL	activity of daily living
AIDS	acquired immunodeficiency syndrome
ALS	amyotrophic lateral sclerosis
AM	morning
a.m.a.	against medical advice
AMI	acute myocardial infarction
amp	ampule
BE	barium enema
bid	two times a day
BM, bm	bowel movement
BMR	basal metabolic rate
BP	blood pressure
BPH	benign prostatic hyperplasia
BRP	bathroom privileges
BUN	blood urea nitrogen
c̄	with
c/o	complains of
Ca	calcium, cancer, carcinoma
CAD	coronary artery disease
cap	capsule
cath.	catheter, catheterize
CBC	complete blood count
CBR	complete bed rest
CC	chief complaint
cc	cubic centimeter
CCU	coronary care unit, critical care unit
CDC	Centers for Disease Control and Prevention
CEA	carcinoembryonic antigen
CHF	congestive heart failure
CHO	carbohydrate
Cl	chlorine
cm	centimeter
cm^3	cubic centimeter
CNS	central nervous system
CO	carbon monoxide
CO_2	carbon dioxide
COPD	chronic obstructive pulmonary disease

CPR	cardiopulmonary resuscitation
CSF	cerebrospinal fluid
CT	computed tomography
CVA	cerebrovascular accident, costovertebral angle
CVP	central venous pressure
D&C	dilation and curettage
D5W	5% dextrose in water
db, dB	decibels
dc	discontinue
DIC	disseminated intravascular coagulation
diff	differential blood count
DJD	degenerative joint disease
dl	deciliter
DNR	do not resuscitate
DOE	dyspnea on exertion
dx, DX	diagnosis
EBV	Epstein-Barr virus
ECF	extracellular fluid
ECG	electrocardiogram
ECT	electroconvulsive therapy
EEG	electroencephalogram
elix	elixir
EMG	electromyogram
ER	emergency room
ERG	electroretinogram
ESR	erythrocyte sedimentation rate
ESRD	end-stage renal disease
EST	electroshock therapy
f℥	fluid ounce
FANA	fluorescent antinuclear antibody test
Fe	iron
FEV	forced expiratory volume
FRC	functional residual capacity
FUO	fever of unknown origin
Fx, fx	fracture, fractional urine test
g, gm, Gm	gram
Gc, GC	gonococcus
GI	gastrointestinal
gr	grain
gtt, gt	drop, drops
GTT	glucose tolerance test
GU	genitourinary
GYN, Gyn	gynecological
H_2O	water
h	hour
H^+	hydrogen ion

h/o	history of
H&P	history and physical examination
HAV	hepatitis A virus
Hb	hemoglobin
HBAg	hepatitis B antigen
HBV	hepatitis B virus
Hct, HCT	hematocrit
Hg	mercury
Hgb	hemoglobin
HIV	human immunodeficiency virus
HLA	human leukocyte antigen
hs	at bedtime
HSV	herpes simplex virus
I&O	intake and output
ICP	intracranial pressure
ICU	intensive care unit
Ig	immunoglobulin
IM	intramuscular
IOP	intraocular pressure
IPPB	intermittent positive pressure breathing
IV	intravenous
IVP	intravenous push, intravenous pyelogram
JRA	juvenile rheumatoid arthritis
K	potassium
kg	kilogram
KUB	kidney, ureters, and bladder (radiograph)
KVO	keep vein open
L	liter
L&A	light and accommodation
LBBB	left bundle branch block
LE	lupus erythematosus
LLL	left lower lobe
LLQ	left lower quadrant
LMP	last menstrual period
LNMP	last normal menstrual period
LP	lumbar puncture
LUL	left upper lobe
LUQ	left upper quadrant
LVH	left ventricular hypertrophy
m	meter
m, min, ɱ	minim, minute
MAP	mean arterial pressure
mcg	microgram
MCH	mean corpuscular hemoglobin
MCHC	mean corpuscular hemoglobin concentration
MCV	mean cell volume, mean corpuscular volume

mg	milligram
Mg	magnesium
MG	myasthenia gravis
MI	myocardial infarction
MICU	medical intensive care unit
ml	milliliter
mm	millimeter
mm^3	cubic millimeter
mm Hg	millimeters of mercury
MRI	magnetic resonance imaging
MS	multiple sclerosis
MW	molecular weight
N	nitrogen
Na	sodium
NIH	National Institutes of Health
nm	nanometer
NMR	nuclear magnetic resonance
NPO	nothing by mouth
NS	normal saline
O_2	oxygen
OD	right eye, optical density, overdose
OL	left eye
OOB	out of bed
ORIF	open reduction and internal fixation
OT	occupational therapy
OTC	over-the-counter
oz	ounce
$PaCO_2$	partial pressure of carbon dioxide in arterial blood
PaO_2	partial pressure of oxygen in arterial blood
PAT	paroxysmal atrial tachycardia
PAWP	pulmonary artery wedge pressure
pc	after meals
PCO_2	partial pressure of carbon dioxide
PCP	pulmonary capillary pressure, phencyclidine
PCV	packed cell volume
PE	pulmonary embolism, physical examination
PEEP	positive end expiratory pressure
per	through, by way of
PERRLA	pupils equal, round, and reactive to light and accommodation
PET	positron emission tomography
PG	prostaglandin
pH	hydrogen ion concentration (acidity and alkalinity)
PID	pelvic inflammatory disease
PKU	phenylketonuria
PM	evening

PMS	premenstrual syndrome
PND	paroxysmal nocturnal dyspnea, postnasal drip
PO_2	partial pressure of oxygen
PO, po	orally
PPD	purified protein derivative
ppm	parts per million
prn	when required, as often as necessary
PT	physical therapy; prothrombin time
PTT	partial thromboplastin time
PVC	premature ventricular contraction
q	every
q2hr	every 2 hours
q3hr	every 3 hours
q4hr	every 4 hours
qd	every day
qhr	every hour
qid	four times a day
qn	every night
qod	every other day
R/O	rule out
RA	rheumatoid arthritis
RBBB	right bundle branch block
RDA	recommended daily (dietary) allowance
RDS	respiratory distress syndrome
Rh+	positive Rh factor
Rh−	negative Rh factor
RHD	rheumatic heart disease
RLL	right lower lobe
RLQ	right lower quadrant
RML	right middle lobe
ROM	range of motion
ROS	review of systems
RS	Reiter's syndrome
RUL	right upper lobe
RUQ	right upper quadrant
Rx	take; treatment
s̄	without
SC	subcutaneous
sib	sibling
SICU	surgical intensive care unit
Sig	write on label
SLE	systemic lupus erythematosus
sol	solution, dissolved
sos	if necessary
sp gr, SG, sg	specific gravity
SQ, subq	subcutaneous

ss	half
STAT	immediately
STD	sexually transmitted disease
STS	serologic test for syphilis
susp	suspension
T&A	tonsillectomy and adenoidectomy
TAH	total abdominal hysterectomy
TAT	tetanus antitoxin; thematic apperception test
TB, TBC	tuberculosis
TBG	thyroxin-binding globulin
TIA	transient ischemic attack
TIBC	total iron-binding capacity
tid	three times a day
TKO	to keep open
TLC	total lung capacity; thin layer chromatography
TPN	total parenteral nutrition
TPR	temperature, pulse, and respirations
tr, tinct	tincture
URI	upper respiratory infection
UTI	urinary tract infection
VC	vital capacity
VD	venereal disease
VDH	valvular disease of the heart
VDRL	Venereal Disease Research Laboratory (test for syphilis)
VS	vital signs
VSD	ventricular septal defect
V_T	tidal volume
WBC	white blood cell, white blood count
WNL	within normal limits

Note: abbreviations in common use can vary widely from place to place. Each institution's list of acceptable abbreviations is the best authority for its records.

Source: Potter PA, Perry AG: *Fundamentals of nursing,* ed 4, St Louis, 1997, Mosby.

CHARACTERISTICS OF COMMON ARRHYTHMIAS

Pattern	Rate and rhythm	P wave	PR interval	QRS complex
NSR	60-100 bpm and regular	Normal	Normal	Normal
Sinus bradycardia	<60 bpm and regular	Normal	Normal	Normal
Sinus tachycardia	>100 bpm and regular	Normal	Normal	Normal
PAC	Usually 60-100 bpm and irregular	Abnormal shape	Normal or variable	Normal (usually)
PSVT	100-300 bpm and regular	Abnormal shape, may be hidden	Variable	Normal (usually)
Atrial flutter	Atrial: 250-350 bpm and regular Ventricular: >100 bpm and irregular	Sawtooth	Variable	Normal (usually)
Atrial fibrillation	Atrial: 350-600 bpm and irregular Ventricular: >100 bpm and irregular or possibly any rate	Chaotic	Not measurable	Normal (usually)
Junctional rhythms	40-140 bpm and regular	Abnormal (may be hidden)	Variable	Normal (usually)

bpm, Beats per minute; *NSR,* normal sinus rhythm; *PAC,* premature atrial contraction; *PSVT,* paroxysmal supraventricular tachycardia; *PVC,* premature ventricular contraction.

Continued

CHARACTERISTICS OF COMMON ARRHYTHMIAS—cont'd

Pattern	Rate and rhythm	P wave	PR interval	QRS complex
First-degree heart block	Normal and regular	Normal	0.20 sec	Normal
Second-degree heart block				
Type I (Mobitz I, Wenckebach)	*Atrial:* normal and regular *Ventricular:* slower and irregular	Normal	Progressively lengthened	Normal QRS width, with pattern of one nonconducted QRS
Type II (Mobitz II)	*Atrial:* usually normal and regular or irregular *Ventricular:* slower and regular or irregular	P wave occurs in multiples	Normal or prolonged	Widened QRS, preceded by two or more P waves
Third-degree heart block	Ventricular rate 20-40 bpm and regular	Normal, but no connection with QRS complex	Variable	Normal or widened; no connection with P waves
PVC	60-100 bpm and irregular	Not usually present	Not measurable	Wide and distorted
Ventricular tachycardia	100-250 bpm and regular or irregular	Not usually present	Not measurable	Wide and distorted
Ventricular fibrillation	Not measurable and irregular	Absent	Not measurable	Not measurable

BLOOD GASES
Normal Values

	Arterial (sea level)	**Venous**
pH	7.35-7.45	7.34-7.37
pO_2*	80-100 mm Hg	30-40 mm Hg
pCO_2	35-45 mm Hg	41-51 mm Hg
HCO_3	22-26 mEq/L	24-30 mEq/L
O_2 sat	95%-99%	60%-80%
Base excess	-2 to $+2$	0 to $+4$

*In a patient >60 years old, PaO_2 is equal to 80 mm Hg minus 1 mm Hg for every year over 60. Expected $PaO_2 = FiO_2 \times 5$.

Interpreting ABGs
1. Check pH   ↑ = Alkalosis; ↓ = acidosis
2. Check pCO_2 ↑ = CO_2 retention (hypoventilation); respiratory acidosis or compensating for metabolic alkalosis
   ↓ = CO_2 blown off (hyperventilation); respiratory alkalosis or compensating for metabolic acidosis
3. Check HCO_3 ↑ = Nonvolatile acid is lost; HCO_3 gained (metabolic alkalosis or compensating for respiratory acidosis)
   ↓ = Nonvolatile acid is added; HCO_3 is lost (metabolic acidosis or compensating for respiratory alkalosis)
4. Determine imbalance
5. Determine if compensation exists

Determining the Imbalance in ABGs

If: pH ↑ and pCO_2 ↓
or
pH ↓ and pCO_2 ↑   }   **Then** respiratory disorder

If: pH ↑ and HCO_3 ↑
or
pH ↓ and HCO_3 ↓   }   **Then** metabolic disorder

If: pCO_2 ↑ and HCO_3 ↑
or
pCO_2 ↓ and HCO_3 ↓   }   **Then** compensation is occurring

If: pCO_2 ↑ and HCO_3 ↓
or
pCO_2 ↓ and HCO_3 ↑   }   **Then** mixed imbalance

BLOOD LABORATORY VALUES

Test	Conventional units	SI units
Complete Blood Count		
RBC	$4.5\text{-}6.0 \times 10^6/\mu L$ (males)	$4.5\text{-}6.0 \times 10^{12}/L$
	$4.0\text{-}5.0 \times 10^6/\mu L$ (females)	$4.0\text{-}5.0 \times 10^{12}/L$
WBC	$4.0\text{-}11.0 \times 10^3/\mu l$	$4.0\text{-}11.0 \times 10^9/L$
Hb	13.5-18 g/dl (males)	135-180 g/L
	12-16 g/dl (females)	120-160 g/L
Hct	40%-51% (males)	0.40-0.51
	38%-44% (females)	0.38-0.44
Chemistry		
Albumin	3.5-5 g/dl	507-725 μmol/L
Alkaline phosphatase	30-120 U/L	0.5-2.0 μkat/L
Alanine amino-transferase (ALT)	5-36 U/L	0.08-0.6 μkat/L
Ammonia	30-70 μg/dl	17.6-41.1 μmol/L
Amylase	0-130 U/L	0-2.17 μkat/L
Aspartate amino-transferase (AST)	7-40 U/L	0.12-0.67 μkat/L
Bilirubin		
Total	0.2-1.3 mg/dl	3.4-22.0 μmol/L
Direct	0.1-0.3 mg/dl	1.7-5.1 μmol/L
Indirect	0.1-1.0 mg/dl	1.7-17 μmol/L
BUN	10-30 mg/dl	1.8-7.1 mmol/L
BUN:Cr ratio	10:1-15:1	
Calcium	9-11 mg/dl	2.25-2.74 mmol/L
Cholesterol	140-200 mg/dl (age dependent)	3.6-5.2 mmol/L
HDL	>45 mg/dl (males)	>1.2 mmol/L
	>55 mg/dl (females)	>1.4 mmol/L
LDL	<130 mg/dl	<3.4 mmol/L

HDL, High density lipoprotein; *LDL,* low density lipoprotein.

Test	Conventional units	SI units
Chloride	95-105 mEq/L	95-105 mmol/L
CO_2	20-30 mEq/L	20-30 mmol/L
Creatinine	0.5-1.5 mg/dl	44-133 μmol/L
Glucose	70-120 mg/dl	3.89-6.66 mmol/L
Iron	50-150 μg/dl	9.0-26.9 μmol/L
Lactic dehydro-genase (LDH)	50-150 U/L	0.83-2.5 μkat/L
Lipase	0-160 U/L	0-2.66 μkat/L
Magnesium	1.5-2.5 mEq/L	0.75-1.25 mmol/L
Osmolality	285-295 mOsm/kg	285-295 mmol/kg
Phosphorus	2.8-4.5 mg/dl	0.90-1.45 mmol/L
Potassium	3.5-5.5 mEq/L	3.5-5.5 mmol/L
Protein	6-8 g/dl	60-80 g/L
Sedimentation rate	<15 mm/hr (males)	
	<20 mm/hr (females)	
Sodium	135-145 mEq/L	135-145 mmol/L
T_3	110-230 ng/dl	1.7-3.5 nmol/L
T_4	5-12 μg/dl	64-154 nmol/L
Triglyceride	40-150 mg/dl	0.45-1.69 mmol/L
Uric acid	2.5-6.5 mg/dl	149-387 μmol/L
Coagulation		
Platelets	150-400 $\times$ 10^3/μL	150-400 $\times$ 10^9/L
PT	10-14 sec	Same as conventional unit
APTT	30-45 sec	Same as conventional unit
FSP	<10 mg/L	Same as conventional unit

APTT, Activated partial thromboblastin time; FSP, fibrin split products; PT, prothrombin time.

BLOOD PRODUCTS*

Description	Special considerations	Indications for use
Packed RBCs Packed RBCs are prepared from whole blood by sedimentation or centrifugation. One unit contains 250-350 ml.	Use of RBCs for treatment allows remaining components of blood (e.g., platelets, albumin, plasma) to be used for other purposes. There is less danger of fluid overload. Packed RBCs are preferred RBC source because they are more component specific.	Severe or symptomatic anemia, acute blood loss.
Frozen RBCs Frozen RBCs are prepared from RBCs using glycerol for protection and frozen. They can be stored for 3 yr at $-188.6°$ F ($-87°$ C).	They must be used within 24 hr of thawing. Successive washings with saline solution remove majority of WBCs and plasma proteins.	Autotransfusion, patient with previous febrile reactions to transfusions. Infrequently used because filters remove most WBCs.
Platelets Platelets are prepared from fresh whole blood within 4 hr after collection. One unit contains 30-60 ml of platelet concentrate.	Multiple units of platelets can be obtained from one donor by plateletpheresis. They can be kept at room temperature for 1-5 days, depending on type of collection and storage bag used. Expected	Bleeding caused by thrombocytopenia, platelet levels <10,000-20,000/μL (10-20 × 10^9/L).

Fresh Frozen Plasma

Liquid portion of whole blood is separated from cells and frozen. One unit contains 200-250 ml. Plasma is rich in clotting factors but contains no platelets. It may be stored for 1 yr. It must be used within 2 hr after thawing.

Use of plasma in treating hypovolemic shock is being replaced by pure preparations such as albumin plasma expanders.

Bleeding caused by deficiency in clotting factors (e.g., DIC, hemorrhage, massive transfusion).

Albumin

Albumin is prepared from plasma. It can be stored for 5 yr. It is available in 5% or 25% solution.

Albumin 25 g/100 ml is osmotically equal to 500 ml of plasma. Hyperosmolar solution acts by moving water from extravascular to intravascular space.

Hypovolemic shock, hypoalbuminemia.

Cryoprecipitates and Commercial Concentrates

Cryoprecipitate is prepared from fresh frozen plasma, with 10-20 ml/bag. It can be stored for 1 yr. Once thawed, must be used.

See Table 29-19 in Lewis and others, *Medical-Surgical Nursing*, edition 5, p. 761.

Replacement of clotting factors, especially factor VIII and fibrinogen.

*Component therapy has replaced use of whole blood, which accounts for <10% of all transfusions.

DIC, Disseminated intravascular coagulation; *Hct,* hematocrit; *RBC,* red blood cell; *WBC,* white blood cell.

BREATH SOUNDS
Normal Sounds

Type	Normal site	Duration	Characteristics
Vesicular	Peripheral lung	I > E	Soft and swishing sounds; abnormal when heard over the large airways
Bronchial	Trachea and bronchi	E > I	Louder, coarser, and of longer duration than vesicular; abnormal if heard over peripheral lung
Bronchovesicular	Sternal border of the major bronchi	E = I	Moderate in pitch and intensity; abnormal if heard over peripheral lung

E, Expiration; *I*, inspiration.

Adventitious Sounds

Type	Waveform	Characteristics	Possible clinical condition
Coarse crackle		Discontinuous, explosive, interrupted; loud; low in pitch	Pulmonary edema; pneumonia in resolution stage
Fine crackle		Discontinuous, explosive, interrupted; less loud than coarse crackles, lower in pitch, and of shorter duration	Interstitial lung disease; heart failure; atelectasis
Wheeze		Continuous, of long duration, high-pitched, musical, hissing	Narrowing of airway; bronchial asthma; chronic obstructive pulmonary disease
Rhonchus		Continuous, of long duration, low-pitched, snoring	Production of sputum (usually cleared or lessened by coughing)
Pleural friction rub		Grating, rasping noise	Rubbing together of inflamed parietal linings; loss of normal pleural lubrication

CANCER SCREENING GUIDELINES: SPECIFIC CANCER SITES

High-risk profile	Screening	Medium- and low-risk profile	Screening
Lung Cancer			
History of 20 pack-years of smoking (1 pack a day for 20 years); exposure to airborne carcinogens, especially asbestos, uranium, hydrocarbons; age range 40 to 80 years; chronic lung disease	Early detection method not available; chest x-rays (advised by some physicians); observation by patient for change in respiratory status; increased frequency of infections and change in cough, sputum, breathing, voice	History of less than 20 pack-years of smoking; non-smokers exposed to passive cigarette smoke from smokers; nonsmokers; former smokers after 10 years	Early detection method not available
Colon and Rectal Cancer			
History of familial polyposis, ulcerative colitis, Crohn's disease; personal or family history of colon or rectal cancer; diet high in fat and low in fiber; age range 40 to 75 years	Guaiac test on stools and digital rectal examination annually after age 40; sigmoidoscopic examination every 3 to 5 years with beginning age based on advice of physician; observation by patient for changes in bowel pattern: diarrhea, constipation, pain, flatus, black tarry stools,	Persons with no known risk factors	Guaiac test on stools and digital rectal examination annually after age 40; sigmoidoscopy, preferably flexible, as a baseline at age 50; after two normal examinations, repeated proctosigmoidoscopic examination every 3 to 5 years

		Presence of one risk factor, excluding age	Digital rectal examination and PSA blood test annually age 50 and over
Prostate Cancer			
Presence of prostatic hyperplasia or presence of prostatic infection; African-American; increased risk with age	Digital rectal examination and PSA blood test annually age 50 and over; observation by patient for dysuria, blood in urine, difficulty in producing stream of urine		
Cervical Cancer		No known risk factors	Pap test and pelvic examination every year after age 18; after three or more normal examinations in a row, at least every 3 years. Pap test may be performed less frequently at the discretion of the physician.
Early intercourse (before age 18) with multiple partners or with partners who have had multiple partners; poor personal hygiene, infected with the HIV virus; genital warts, chlamydia, gonorrhea, cervical dysplasia; smoking	Pap test and pelvic examination every year for women who are or have been sexually active or who have reached age 18; colposcopy if suspicious area is noted; observation by patient for abnormal vaginal bleeding or discharge, pain, or bleeding with sexual intercourse		

Continued

BSE, Breast self-examination; PSA, prostate specific antigen.
Based on the American Cancer Society 1996 Recommendations.

CANCER SCREENING GUIDELINES: SPECIFIC CANCER SITES—cont'd

High-risk profile	Screening	Medium- and low-risk profile	Screening
Endometrial Cancer			
Infertility; never having children; early menarche; late menopause, ovarian dysfunction, obesity, uterine bleeding; estrogen replacement therapy and tamoxifen over long period of time; diabetes, hypertension, gall bladder disease; exposure to pelvic radiation; over age 50	Pap test every year; pelvic examination every year; endometrial biopsy for women at menopause and at high risk; observation by patient for abnormal uterine bleeding, pain, change in menstrual pattern	Presence of one risk factor, excluding estrogen therapy, over long period of time	Pap test and pelvic examination, observation by patient for abnormal uterine bleeding, pain, change in menstrual pattern
Skin Cancer			
Prolonged exposure to sun; three or more blistering sunburns during adolescence; previous radiation exposure; fair, thin skin; positive family history of dysplastic nevus syndrome	Self-examination monthly; physical examination every year; observation by patient for sore that does not heal or change in size, shape, or color of wart or mole	Presence of one risk factor, excluding prolonged exposure to sun	Self-examination, physical examination each year; observation by patient for sore that does not heal or change in size, shape, or color of wart or mole

Breast Cancer

Risk Factors	Recommendation	Risk Factors	Recommendation
Caucasian; early menarche, late menopause, fibrocystic breast disease, infertility; over age 30 for first pregnancy; personal history of breast cancer; mother or sister with history of breast cancer; obesity; age range 35 to 65	Monthly BSE; breast examination every 3 years for women age 20 to 40 and every year after age 40; baseline mammogram at age 40, every 1 to 2 years between ages 40 and 49, and every year after age 49; observation by patient for lump or thickening discharge from nipple, pain in breast	Excluding family history of breast cancer, fewer than two risk factors	Monthly BSE; breast examination by health professional every 3 years for women age 20 to 40 and every year after age 40; baseline mammogram at age 40, every 1 to 2 years between ages 40 and 49, and every year after age 49; observation by patient for lump or thickening discharge from nipple, pain in breast

BSE, Breast self-examination.

COMMONLY USED FORMULAS

Parameter	Formula	Normal range
Alveolar-arterial oxygen gradient ($AaDO_2$)	$PaO_2 - PaO_2$	<15 mm Hg
Alveolar partial pressure of oxygen (PAO_2)	$FiO_2 (713) - PaCO_2/0.8$	
Anion gap	$Na - (HCO_3 + Cl)$	8-16 mEq/L
Cardiac index (CI)	CO/Body surface area (BSA)	2.2-4.0 L/min/m^2
Cardiac output (CO)	$HR \times SV$	4-8 L/min
Cerebral perfusion pressure (CPP)	$MAP - ICP$	80-100 mm Hg
Ejection fraction (EF)	$\dfrac{SV}{\text{End diastolic volume}} \times 100$	60% or greater
Mean arterial pressure (MAP)	$\dfrac{2\,(DPB) + SBP}{2}$	70-105 mm Hg

Pulmonary vascular resistance (PVR)	$\dfrac{PAM - PAWP}{CO} \times 80$	<200 dyne sec/cm
Pulmonary vascular resistance index (PVRI)	$\dfrac{PAM - PAWP}{CI} \times 80$	160-380 dyne sec m^2/cm^5
Stroke volume (SV)	$\dfrac{CO \times 1000}{HR}$	60-180 ml/beat
Stroke volume index (SVI)	$\dfrac{SV}{BSA}$ or $\dfrac{CI}{HR} \times 1000$	30-65 ml/m^2/beat
Systemic vascular resistance (SVR)	$\dfrac{MAP - CVP}{CO} \times 80$	800-1200 dyne sec/cm^5
Systemic vascular resistance index (SVRI)	$\dfrac{MAP - CVP}{CI} \times 80$	1970-2390 dyne sec m^2/cm^5

DBP, Diastolic blood pressure; *FiO$_2$,* fraction of inspired oxygen; *ICP,* intracranial pressure; *PAM,* mean pulmonary artery pressure; *PAWP,* pulmonary artery wedge pressure; *SBP,* systolic blood pressure.

CONVERSION FACTORS

1 kg	= 1 L fluid	1/150 gr	= 0.4 mg
1 mg	= 1000 μg	1 tsp	= 5 ml
1 kg	= 2.2 lb	1 tbsp	= 15 ml
1 gr	= 60 or 65 mg	1 oz	= 30 ml
1/100 gr	= 0.6 mg	1 mm Hg	= 1.36 cm H_2O

ELECTROCARDIOGRAM (ECG) MONITORING: WAVEFORM

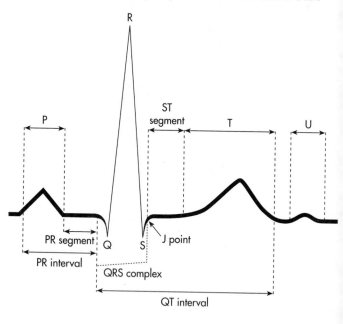

P wave	Represents atrial depolarization.
PR segment	Represents time required for impulse to travel through atrioventricular (AV) node, where it is delayed, and through bundle of His, bundle branches, and Purkinje fiber network, just before ventricular depolarization.
PR interval	Represents time required for atrial depolarization and impulse to travel through conduction system and Purkinje fiber network, inclusive of P wave and PR segment. It is measured from beginning of P wave to end of PR segment. Normally measures 0.12 to 0.20 sec in duration.
QRS complex	Represents depolarization of both ventricles and is measured from beginning of Q (or R) wave to end of S wave. Also measured from end of PR interval to J point. Normally measures from 0.04 to 0.12 sec.
J point	Represents junction where QRS complex ends and ST segment begins.
ST segment	Represents early ventricular repolarization. Measured from J point to beginning of T wave.
T wave	Represents ventricular repolarization.
U wave	Represents late ventricular repolarization. Not normally seen in all leads.
QT interval	Represents total time required for ventricular depolarization and repolarization and is measured from beginning of QRS complex to end of T wave.

GLASGOW COMA SCALE

Category of response	Appropriate stimulus
■ Eyes open	Approach to bedside Verbal command Pain
■ Best verbal response	Verbal questioning with maximum arousal
■ Best motor response	Verbal command (e.g., "raise your arm, hold up two fingers") Pain (pressure on proximal nail bed)

Response	Score
Spontaneous response	4
Opening of eyes to name or command	3
Lack of opening of eyes to previous stimuli but opening to pain	2
Lack of opening of eyes to any stimulus	1
Untestable	U
Appropriate orientation, conversant, correct identification of self, place, year, and month	5
Confusion, conversant, but disorientation in one or more spheres	4
Inappropriate or disorganized use of words (e.g., cursing), lack of sustained conversation	3
Incomprehensible words, sounds (e.g., moaning)	2
Lack of sound, even with painful stimuli	1
Untestable	U
Obedience of command	6
Localization of pain, lack of obedience but presence of attempts to remove offending stimulus	5
Flexion withdrawal,* flexion of arm in response to pain without abnormal flexion posture	4
Abnormal flexion, flexing of arm at elbow and pronation, making a fist	3
Abnormal extension, extension of arm at elbow usually with adduction and internal rotation of arm at shoulder	2
Lack of response	1
Untestable	U

*Added to the original scale by many centers.

HEART SOUNDS
Normal Sounds

Sound	Auscultation site	Timing	Pitch
S_1 (M_1 T_1)	Apex	Beginning of systole	High
S_1 split	Apex	Beginning of systole	High
S_2 (A_2 P_2)	A_2 at 2nd ICS, RSB; P_2 at 2nd ICS, LSB	End of systole	High
S_2 physiologic split	2nd ICS, LSB	End of systole	High
S_2 persistent (wide) split	2nd ICS, LSB	End of systole	High
S_2 paradoxic (reversed) split (P_2 A_2)	2nd ICS, LSB	End of systole	High
S_2 fixed split	2nd ICS, LSB	End of systole	High
S_3 (ventricular gallop)	Apex	Early in diastole just after S_2	Dull, low
S_4 (atrial gallop)	Apex	Late in diastole just before S_1	Low

CAD, Coronary artery disease; *CHF,* congestive heart failure; *ICS,* intercostal

Clinical occurrence	End-piece/ pt. position
Closing of mitral and tricuspid valves; normal sound	Diaphragm/ pt. supine
Ventricles contracting at different times due to electrical or mechanical problems (e.g., longer time span between M_1 T_1 caused by right bundle-branch heart block, or reversal [T_1 M_1] caused by mitral stenosis)	
Closing of aortic and pulmonic valves; normal sound	Diaphragm/ pt. supine
Accentuated by inspiration; disappears on expiration; sound that corresponds with respiratory cycle due to normal delay in closure of pulmonic valve during inspiration; accentuated during exercise or in individuals with thin chest walls; heard most often in children and young adults	Same as S_2
Heard throughout respiratory cycle; caused by late closure of pulmonic valve or early closure of aortic valve; occurs in atrial septal defect, right ventricular failure, pulmonic stenosis, hypertension, or right bundle-branch heart block	Same as S_2
Because of delayed left ventricular systole, aortic valve closes after pulmonic valve rather than before it (normally during expiration the two sounds merge); causes may include left bundle-branch heart block, aortic stenosis, severe left ventricular failure, MI, and severe hypertension	Same as S_2
Heard with equal intensity during inspiration and expiration due to split of pulmonic and aortic components, which are unaffected by blood volume or respiratory changes; may be heard in pulmonary stenosis or atrial septal defect	Same as S_2
Early and rapid filling of ventricle, as in early ventricular failure, CHF; common in children, during last trimester of pregnancy, and possibly in healthy adults over age 50 yr	Bell/patient in left lateral or supine position
Atrium filling against increased resistance of stiff ventricle, as in CHF, CAD, cardiomyopathy, pulmonary artery hypertension, ventricular failure; may be normal in infants, children, and athletes	Same as S_3

space; *LSB,* left sternal border; *MI,* myocardial infarction; *RSB,* right sternal border.

Murmurs

Type	Timing	Pitch	Quality	Auscultation site	Radiation
Pulmonic stenosis	Systolic ejection	Medium-high	Harsh	2nd ICS, LSB	Toward left shoulder, back
Aortic stenosis	Mid-systolic	Medium-high	Harsh	2nd ICS, RSB	Toward carotid arteries
Ventricular septal defect	Late systolic	High	Blowing	4th ICS, LSB	Toward right sternal border
Mitral insufficiency	Holosystolic	High	Blowing	5th-6th ICS, left MCL	Toward left axilla
Tricuspid insufficiency	Holosystolic	High	Blowing	4th ICS, LSB	Toward apex
Aortic insufficiency	Early diastolic	High	Blowing	2nd ICS, RSB	Toward sternum
Pulmonary insufficiency	Early diastolic	High	Blowing	2nd ICS, LSB	Toward sternum
Mitral stenosis	Mid-late diastolic	Low	Rumbling	5th ICS, left MCL	Toward axilla
Tricuspid stenosis	Mid-late diastolic	Low	Rumbling	4th ICS, LSB	Usually none

ICS, Intercostal space; LSB, left sternal border; MCL, midclavicular line; RSB, right sternal border.

MEDICATION ADMINISTRATION
Equivalent Weights and Measures

Metric	Apothecary	Household
Weight		
1 kg	2.2 pounds	
1000 mg = 1 gram	gr xv	
60 or 65 mg	gr i	
30 mg	gr ss (one half)	
1 µg (mcg) = 0.0001 mg		
Volume		
	4 quarts	1 gallon
1000ml = 1 liter = 1000 cc	Approx. 1 quart	1 quart
500 ml	Approx. 1 pint (½ qt)	16 ounces
240 or 250 ml	ʒ viii (8 fluid ounces)	1 cup or 1 glass
30 ml = approx. 30 cc	ʒ i (1 fluid ounce)	2 tbsp
16 ml = approx. 16 cc	ʒ iv (4 fluidrams)	1 tbsp
8 ml	ʒ (2 fluidrams)	2 tsp
4 to 5 ml	ʒ (1 fluidram)	1 tsp
1 ml = approx. 1 cc	Minims xv or xvi	

Drug Calculations

Ratio and proportion:

1. To set up a ratio and proportion, put on the right-hand side what you already have or what you already know (e.g., 1000 mg:1 ml).
2. On the left-hand side put X, or what you want to know (e.g., 750 mg:X).
3. The equation should look like this:
   750 mg:X = 1000 mg:1 ml
4. Multiply the two inside numbers. Multiply the two outside numbers.
   1000X = 750
5. Solve for X:
   $$X = \frac{750}{1000} = 0.75 \text{ ml}$$

IV Drip Rate

$$\frac{\text{Total number of milliliters to be infused}}{\text{Total number of minutes infusion is to run}} \times \text{Drop factor}$$

$$= \text{Rate (drops per minute)}$$

Abbreviations for Medication Administration

Abbrev.	Unabbrev. form	Meaning
a	ante	before
ac	ante cibum	before meals
ad lib	ad libitum	freely
AM	ante meridiem	morning
bid	bis in die	twice each day
c̄	cum	with
cap	capsule	capsule
cc, cm³	cubic centimeter	cubic centimeter (ml)
D/C or DC	discontinue	terminate
elix	elixir	elixir
g, gm	gram	1000 milligrams
gr	grain	60 milligrams
gtt	gutta	drop
h, hr	hora	hour
hs	hora somni	at bedtime
IM	intramuscular	into a muscle
IV	intravenous	into a vein
IVPB	IV piggyback	secondary IV line
kg	kilogram	2.2 lb (1000 g)
KVO	keep vein open	very slow infusion rate
Ⓛ	left	left
L	liter	liter
μg, mcg	microgram	one millionth of a gram
mg	milligram	one thousandth of a gram
mEq	milliequivalent	the number of grams of solute dissolved in 1 milliliter of a normal solution
min or m	minim	minim ($\frac{1}{15}$ or $\frac{1}{16}$ ml)
ml, mL	milliliter	one thousandth of a liter
ng	nanogram	one billionth of a gram
ō	no or none	no or none
OD	oculus dexter	right eye
OS	oculus sinister	left eye
os	os	mouth
OTC	over-the-counter	nonprescription drug
OU	oculus uterque	each eye

Abbrev.	Unabbrev. form	Meaning
pc	post cibum	after meals
PM	post meridiem	after noon
PO	per os	by mouth, orally
prn	pro re nata	according to necessity
pt	patient	patient
q	quaque	every
qd	quaque die	every day
qh	quaque hora	every hour
q4hr, q4°	every 4 hours	every 4 hours around the clock
qid	quater in die	four times each day
qod	quaque aliem die	every other day
qs	quantum satis	sufficient quantity
®	right	right
℞	receipt	take
s̄	sine	without
SL	sub linguam	under the tongue
SOS	si opus sit	if necessary
ss	semis	a half
stat	statim	at once
SC, SQ	subcutaneous	into subcutaneous tissue
tbsp	tablespoon	tablespoon (15 ml)
tid	ter in die	three times a day
TO	telephone order	order received over the telephone
tsp	teaspoon	teaspoon (4 or 5 ml)
U	unit	a dosage measure for insulin, penicillin, heparin
VO	verbal order	order received verbally
t, tt	one, two	one, two (as in "gr t," "gr tt")
ℨ	dram	4 or 5 ml
℥	ounce or fluid-ounce	ounce (30 milliliters)
×	times	as in two times a week
>	greater than	greater than
<	less than	less than
=	equal to	equal to

Techniques of Administration
Angles of Injection

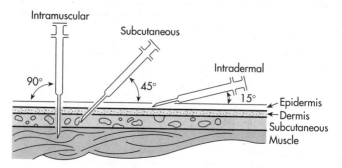

Injection Sites
Subcutaneous

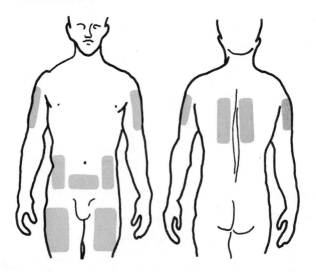

Intramuscular: deltoid muscle

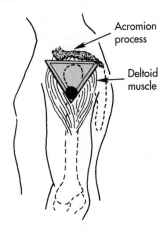

Intramuscular: dorsogluteal muscle

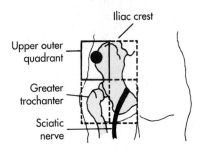

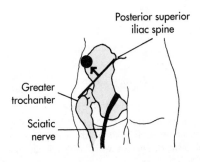

Intramuscular: vastus lateralis muscle

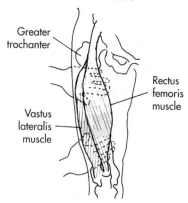

Intramuscular: ventrogluteal muscle

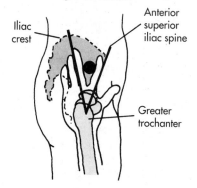

Z-Track Technique

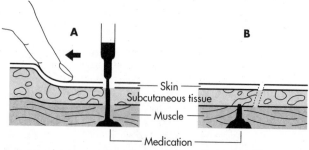

A, In Z-track intramuscular injection, skin is pulled laterally, then injection is administered. **B,** After needle is withdrawn, skin is released. This technique helps prevent medication from leaking.

Intermittent IV

Peripheral vein intermittent infusion device

1. Irrigate device with 1 ml of normal saline.
2. Administer prescribed medication.
3. Irrigate device with 1 ml of normal saline after medication administration is completed.
4. If policy, perform a final irrigation with 1 ml of heparin solution (100 units of heparin per ml of normal saline).

Central vein intermittent infusion device

1. Irrigate device with 2 to 5 ml of normal saline (volume depends on type of infusion catheter and agency policy).
2. Administer prescribed medication.
3. Irrigate device with 2 to 5 ml of normal saline when medication administration is completed.
4. Irrigate device with 2 to 5 ml of heparin solution (100 units of heparin per ml of normal saline).

Heparin Flush

Peripheral vein intermittent infusion device

1. Irrigate device with 1 ml of normal saline.
2. Administer prescribed medication.
3. Irrigate device with 1 ml of normal saline after medication administration is completed.
4. If policy, perform a final irrigation with 1 ml of heparin solution (100 units of heparin per ml of normal saline).

Central vein intermittent infusion device

1. Irrigate device with 2 to 5 ml of normal saline (volume depends on type of infusion catheter and agency policy).
2. Administer prescribed medication.
3. Irrigate device with 2 to 5 ml of normal saline when medication administration is completed.
4. Irrigate device with 2 to 5 ml of heparin solution (100 units of heparin per ml of normal saline).

Intravenous Needle Site Complications

	Infiltration	Phlebitis
Assessment		
Color	Pale	Red
Temperature	Cool to cold	Warm to hot
Swelling	Rounded	Cordlike vein path
Pain	Yes, usually	Yes
Flow	Slowed or stopped	No change or may be slowed
Nursing Actions	Tourniquet proximally (flow continues—infiltration)	Discontinue IV; usually call IV team
	Lower bottle (blood in tubing—no infiltration)	Note irritating solution (Valium, Keflin, KCl running too fast)
	Discontinue IV	Warm compresses; elevate and immobilize part
	Call IV team	
	Get order for warm compresses and elevate part	

NURSING DIAGNOSES
GROUPED BY FUNCTIONAL HEALTH PATTERNS
Health Perception–Health Management Pattern
Development, Altered: Risk for
Energy Field Disturbance
Growth, Altered: Risk for
Health Maintenance, Altered
Health-Seeking Behaviors
Infection, Risk for
Injury, Risk for
Management of Therapeutic Regimen, Ineffective (Community)
Management of Therapeutic Regimen, Ineffective (Family)
Management of Therapeutic Regimen, Ineffective
Noncompliance
Poisoning, Risk for
Protection, Altered
Suffocation, Risk for
Surgical Recovery, Delayed
Trauma, Risk for

Nutritional-Metabolic Pattern
Aspiration, Risk for
Breastfeeding, Effective
Breastfeeding, Ineffective
Breastfeeding, Interrupted
Dentition, Altered
Fluid Volume Deficit
Fluid Volume Deficit, Risk for
Fluid Volume Excess
Fluid Volume Imbalance, Risk for
Hyperthermia
Hypothermia
Infant Feeding Pattern, Ineffective
Latex Allergy Response
Latex Allergy Response, Risk for
Nausea
Nutrition, Altered: Less than Body Requirements
Nutrition, Altered: More than Body Requirements
Nutrition, Altered: Risk for More than Body Requirements
Oral Mucous Membrane, Altered
Skin Integrity, Impaired
Skin Integrity, Impaired: Risk for
Swallowing, Impaired
Temperature, Risk for Altered Body
Thermoregulation, Ineffective
Tissue Integrity, Impaired

Elimination Pattern
Constipation
Constipation, Colonic
Constipation, Perceived
Constipation, Risk for
Diarrhea
Incontinence, Bowel
Incontinence, Functional Urinary
Incontinence, Reflex Urinary
Incontinence, Stress
Incontinence, Total
Incontinence, Urge
Urinary Elimination, Altered
Urinary Retention

Activity-Exercise Pattern
Activity Intolerance
Activity Intolerance, Risk for
Airway Clearance, Ineffective
Breathing Pattern, Ineffective
Cardiac Output, Decreased
Disuse Syndrome, Risk for
Diversional Activity Deficit
Dysreflexia
Dysreflexia, Risk for Autonomic
Energy Field Disturbance
Failure to Thrive
Fatigue
Gas Exchange, Impaired
Growth and Development, Altered
Home Maintenance Management, Impaired
Infant Behavior, Disorganized
Infant Behavior, Potential for Enhanced Organized
Infant Behavior, Risk for Disorganized
Mobility, Impaired: Bed, Physical, Wheelchair
Perioperative Positioning Injury, Risk for
Peripheral Neurovascular Dysfunction, Risk for
Self-Care Deficit, Bathing/Hygiene
Self-Care Deficit, Dressing/Grooming
Self-Care Deficit, Feeding
Self-Care Deficit, Toileting
Surgical Recovery, Delayed
Tissue Perfusion, Altered
Transfer Ability, Impaired
Ventilation, Inability to Sustain

Ventilatory Weaning Response, Dysfunctional
Walking, Impaired

Sleep-Rest Pattern
Sleep Deprivation
Sleep Pattern Disturbance

Cognitive-Perceptual Pattern
Adaptive Capacity, Decreased, Intracranial
Confusion, Acute
Confusion, Chronic
Decisional Conflict
Environmental Interpretation Syndrome, Impaired
Knowledge Deficit
Memory, Impaired
Nausea
Pain
Pain, Chronic
Sensory-Perceptual Alterations
Thought Processes, Altered
Unilateral Neglect

Self-Perception–Self-Concept Pattern
Anxiety
Body Image Disturbance
Death Anxiety
Fear
Hopelessness
Personal Identity Disturbance
Powerlessness
Self-Esteem, Chronic Low
Self-Esteem Disturbance
Self-Esteem, Situational Low
Self-Mutilation, Risk for

Role-Relationship Pattern
Caregiver Role Strain
Caregiver Role Strain, Risk for
Communication, Impaired Verbal
Family Processes, Altered
Grieving, Anticipatory
Grieving, Dysfunctional
Parental Role Conflict
Parenting, Altered
Parenting, Altered: Risk for
Relocation Stress Syndrome

Role Performance, Altered
Social Interaction, Impaired
Social Isolation
Violence, Risk for: Directed at Others
Violence, Risk for: Self-Directed

Sexuality-Reproductive Pattern
Rape Trauma Syndrome
Rape Trauma Syndrome: Compound Reaction
Rape Trauma Syndrome: Silent Reaction
Sexual Dysfunction
Sexuality Patterns, Altered

Coping–Stress-Tolerance Pattern
Adjustment, Impaired
Coping, Defensive
Coping, Ineffective Community
Coping, Ineffective Individual
Coping, Potential for Enhanced Community
Denial, Ineffective
Failure to Thrive, Adult
Family Coping, Ineffective: Compromised
Family Coping, Ineffective: Disabling
Family Coping: Potential for Growth
Post-Trauma Syndrome
Post-Trauma Syndrome, Risk for
Sorrow, Chronic

Value-Belief Pattern
Spiritual Distress (Distress of Human Spirit)
Spiritual Well-Being, Potential for Enhanced

Modified from *NANDA nursing diagnoses: definitions and classification 1999-2000,* North America Nursing Diagnosis Association; and Gordon M: *Manual of nursing diagnoses,* St Louis, 1997, Mosby.

TEMPERATURE CONVERSION FACTORS

°C	°F	°C	°F	°C	°F	°C	°F
34.0	93.2	36.4	97.5	38.8	101.8	41.2	106.1
34.2	93.6	36.6	97.9	39.0	102.2	41.4	106.5
34.4	93.9	36.8	98.2	39.2	102.6	41.6	106.8
34.6	94.3	37.0	98.6	39.4	102.9	41.8	107.2
34.8	94.6	37.2	99.0	39.6	103.3	42.0	107.6
35.0	95.0	37.4	99.3	39.8	103.6	42.2	108.0
35.2	95.4	37.6	99.7	40.0	104.0	42.4	108.3
35.4	95.7	37.8	100.0	40.2	104.4	42.6	108.7
35.6	96.1	38.0	100.4	40.4	104.7	42.8	109.0
35.8	96.4	38.2	100.8	40.6	105.2	43.0	109.4
36.0	96.8	38.4	101.1	40.8	105.4		
36.2	97.2	38.6	101.5	41.0	105.9		

°C = Temperature in Celsius (centigrade) degrees. $(°C \times 9/5) + 32 = °F$.
°F = Temperature in Fahrenheit degrees. $(°F - 32) \times 5/9 = °C$.

TRIAGE ACUITY SYSTEMS

	Emergent	Urgent	Nonurgent	Expectant
Color	Red	Yellow	Green	Black
Numbers	Priority I	Priority II	Priority III	Priority 0
Urgency	Life-threatening; needs immediate attention	Needs treatment in 20 minutes to 2 hours	Can wait hours or days	Dying or dead
Example	Trauma, chest pain, respiratory distress, chemicals in the eyes, arm or leg amputation, shock	Fever >104° F (>40° C), diastolic blood pressure >130 mm Hg, kidney stone, simple fracture	Sprain, minor laceration, flulike symptoms, rash, chronic headache	Massive head trauma, cardiopulmonary arrest

URINE LABORATORY VALUES

Test	Normal	Abnormal finding and significance
▪ Color	Amber yellow	Dark, smoky color suggests hematuria. Yellow brown to olive green indicates excessive bilirubin. Orange red or orange brown is caused by phenazopyridine (Pyridium) or urobilin in excess. Cloudiness of freshly voided urine indicates infection. Colorless urine indicates excessive fluid intake, renal disease, or diabetes insipidus.
▪ Smell	Aromatic	On standing, urine becomes more ammonia-like in smell. In urinary tract infections, urine smells unpleasant.
▪ Protein	0-150 mg/24 hr 0-18 mg/dl	Persistent proteinuria is characteristic of acute and chronic renal disease, especially involving glomeruli. In absence of disease, positive finding may be caused by high-protein diet, strenuous exercise, dehydration, fever, or emotional stress. Vaginal secretions may contaminate urine specimen and give positive finding.
▪ Glucose	None	Glycosuria indicates diabetes mellitus or low renal threshold for glucose reabsorption (if blood glucose level is normal). Small amounts may be found after glucose loading (e.g., glucose tolerance test).
▪ Ketones	None	Altered carbohydrate and fat metabolisms indicate diabetes mellitus and starvation. Findings can also be seen in dehydration, vomiting, and severe diarrhea.
▪ Bilirubin	None	Presence of bilirubinuria is as significant as jaundice in detection of liver disorders. Bilirubin may appear in urine before jaundice becomes visible or may be present in persons with hepatic disorders who do not have recognizable jaundice.

Continued

URINE LABORATORY VALUES—cont'd

Test	Normal	Abnormal finding and significance
▪ Specific gravity	1.003-1.030	Specific gravity of morning urine specimen reflects maximum concentrating ability of kidney and is 1.025 to 1.030. Low specific gravity indicates dilute urine and possibly excessive diuresis. High specific gravity indicates dehydration. If it becomes fixed at about 1.010, this indicates renal inability to concentrate urine, suggesting that kidney is progressing to end-stage renal disease.
▪ Osmolality	300-1300 mOsm/kg	Measurement is a more accurate method than specific gravity for determining diluting and concentrating ability of kidneys. Deviations from normal indicate tubular dysfunction. Findings indicate if kidney has lost ability to concentrate or dilute urine. (Not part of routine urinalysis.)
▪ pH	4.0-8.0 (average 6.0)	If more than 8.0, finding may be the result of standing of urine or urinary tract infections because bacteria decompose urea to form ammonia. If less than 4.0, may indicate respiratory and metabolic acidosis.
▪ RBC	0-4/hpf	Bleeding in urinary tract is caused by calculi, cystitis, neoplasm, glomerulonephritis, tuberculosis, kidney biopsy, or trauma.
▪ WBC	0-5/hpf	Increased number of WBCs in urine (pyuria) indicates urinary tract infection or inflammation.
▪ Casts	None—occasional hyaline	Casts are molds of the renal tubules and may contain protein, WBCs, RBCs, or bacteria. Noncellular casts are hyaline in appearance, and a few may be found in normal urine. Casts indicate renal dysfunction or urinary tract infections.
▪ Culture for organisms	No organisms in bladder, <10^4 organisms/ml result of normal urethral flora	Bacteria counts >10^5/ml indicate urinary tract infection. Organisms most commonly found in urinary tract infections are *Escherichia coli,* enterococci, *Klebsiella, Proteus,* and streptococci.

hpf, High-powered field; *RBC,* red blood cell; *WBC,* white blood cell.